KU-227-425

Handbook of Dissociation

Theoretical, Empirical, and Clinical Perspectives

Handbook of Dissociation

Theoretical, Empirical, and Clinical Perspectives

Edited by

Larry K. Michelson and **William J. Ray**

The Pennsylvania State University
University Park, Pennsylvania

PLENUM PRESS • NEW YORK AND LONDON

Library of Congress Cataloging-in-Publication Data

On file

ISBN 0-306-45150-6

A Division of Plenum Publishing Corporation
233 Spring Street, New York, N. Y. 10013

10 9 8 7 6 5 4 3 2 1

Printed in the United States of America

To my wife Sandra, for her love, light, and laughter

—LKM

To my parents, my spouse, and my children,
who have shown me the varieties of loving relationships

—WJR

Contributors

Pamela C. Alexander, Department of Psychology, University of Maryland, College Park, Maryland 20742

Catherine L. Anderson, Northwest Center for Community Mental Health, Reston, Virginia 22091

Peter M. Barach, Horizons Counseling Services, Inc., Cleveland, Ohio 44130

Alexandre Bennett, Department of Psychiatry, Yale University School of Medicine, and National Center for PTSD, Department of Veterans Affairs Medical Center, West Haven, Connecticut 06516

J. Douglas Bremner, Department of Psychiatry, Yale University School of Medicine, and National Center for PTSD, Department of Veterans Affairs Medical Center, West Haven, Connecticut 06516

Etzel Cardeña, Department of Psychiatry, Uniformed Services University of the Health Sciences, Bethesda, Maryland 20814

Dennis S. Charney, Department of Psychiatry, Yale University School of Medicine, and National Center for PTSD, Department of Veterans Affairs Medical Center, West Haven, Connecticut 06516

James A. Chu, Dissociative Disorders Program, McLean Hospital, Belmont, Massachusetts 02178; and Department of Psychiatry, Harvard Medical School, Boston, Massachusetts 02115

Catherine Classen, Department of Psychiatry and Behavioral Sciences, Stanford University School of Medicine, Stanford, California 94305

Barry M. Cohen, P.O. Box 9853, Alexandria, Virginia 22304

Pamela M. Cole, Department of Psychology, Pennsylvania State University, University Park, Pennsylvania 16802

Christine M. Comstock, Horizons Counseling Services, Inc., Cleveland, Ohio 44130

Philip M. Coons, Department of Psychiatry, Indiana University School of Medicine, Indianapolis, Indiana 46202

George H. Faust, 2515 Kemper Place, Shaker Heights, Ohio 44120

Catherine G. Fine, Dissociative Disorders Unit, Institute of Pennsylvania Hospital, Philadelphia, Pennsylvania 19139

Edna B. Foa, Center for the Treatment and Study of Anxiety, Medical College of Pennsylvania, Eastern Pennsylvania Psychiatric Institute, Philadelphia, Pennsylvania 19129

Jean M. Goodwin, Department of Psychiatry, University of Texas Medical Branch, Galveston, Texas 77555-0428

George B. Greaves, 1175 LaVista Road, Apartment #205, Atlanta, Georgia 30324

Diana Hearst-Ikeda, National Center for Posttraumatic Stress Disorder, Women's Health and Sciences Division, Boston Department of Veterans Affairs Medical Center, Boston, Massachusetts 02130

Nancy L. Hornstein, Department of Psychiatry, Child Division, University of Illinois at Chicago and Institute for Juvenile Research, Chicago, Illinois 61612

Richard P. Kluft, Dissociative Disorders Program, The Institute of Pennsylvania Hospital, Philadelphia, Pennsylvania 19139

Cheryl Koopman, Department of Psychiatry and Behavioral Sciences, Stanford University School of Medicine, Stanford, California 94305

John H. Krystal, Department of Psychiatry, Yale University School of Medicine, and National Center for PTSD, Department of Veterans Affairs Medical Center, West Haven, Connecticut 06516

Richard J. Loewenstein, Dissociative Disorders Service Line, Sheppard Pratt Health Systems, Baltimore, Maryland 21285; and Department of Psychiatry and Behavioral Sciences, University of Maryland School of Medicine, Baltimore, Maryland 21201

Mary Main, Department of Psychology, University of California at Berkeley, Berkeley, California 94720

Richard Moraga, Department of Psychology, Pennsylvania State University, University Park, Pennsylvania 16802

Hillary Morgan, Department of Psychology, University of California at Davis, Davis, California 95616

Michael R. Nash, Department of Psychology, University of Tennessee at Knoxville, Knoxville, Tennessee 37996

Judith A. Peterson, Phoenix Counseling, Consulting, and Forensic Services, 3303 Chimney Brook Lane, Houston, Texas 77068

William J. Ray, Department of Psychology, Pennsylvania State University, University Park, Pennsylvania 16802

Colin A. Ross, Dissociative Disorders Unit, Charter Behavioral Health System of Dallas, Plano, Texas 75024

Roberta G. Sachs, Highland Park Psychological Resources, 660 LaSalle Place, Highland Park, Illinois 60035

David K. Sakheim, 1610 Ellington Road, South Windsor, Connecticut 06074

Steven M. Southwick, Department of Psychiatry, Yale University School of Medicine, and National Center for PTSD, Department of Veterans Affairs Medical Center, West Haven, Connecticut 06516

David Spiegel, Department of Psychiatry and Behavioral Sciences, Stanford University School of Medicine, Stanford, California 94305

Marlene Steinberg, Department of Psychiatry, Yale University School of Medicine, New Haven, Connecticut 06510

Moshe S. Torem, Department of Psychiatry and Behavioral Sciences, Akron General Medical Center, Akron, Ohio 44307; and Department of Psychiatry, Northeastern Ohio Universities College of Medicine, Akron, Ohio 44272

Onno Van der Hart, Department of Clinical and Health Psychology, Utrecht University, and the Regional Institute for Ambulatory Mental Care, Amsterdam South/New West, The Netherlands

Johan Vanderlinden, Department of Behavior Therapy, University Center St. Jozef, B-3070 Kortenberg, Belgium

Katalin Varga, Department of Experimental Psychology, Eötvös Lorand University, Budapest, Hungary

Helen H. Watkins, Department of Psychology, University of Montana, Missoula, Montana 59801

John G. Watkins, Department of Psychology, University of Montana, Missoula, Montana 59801

Jonathan E. Whalen, Department of Psychology, University of Tennessee at Knoxville, Knoxville, Tennessee 37996

Linda J. Young, National Treatment Center for Traumatic and Dissociative Disorders, Del Amo Hospital, Torrance, California 90505

Walter C. Young, National Treatment Center for Traumatic and Dissociative Disorders, Del Amo Hospital, Torrance, California 90505

Theodore P. Zahn, Laboratory of Psychology and Psychopathology, National Institute of Mental Health, Bethesda, Maryland 20892

Preface

Within the last decade there has been a tremendous explosion in the clinical, theoretical, and empirical literature related to the study of dissociation. Not since the work done at the turn of the century by Pierre Janet, Morton Prince, William James, and others have the psychological and medical communities shown this great an interest in describing and understanding dissociative phenomena. This volume is the result of this significant expansion. Presently, interest in the scientific and clinical progress in the field of dissociation is indicated by the following:

1. The explosion of conferences, workshops, and seminars devoted to dissociative disorders treatment and research.
2. The emergence of NIMH-supported investigations that focus on dissociation.
3. The burgeoning literature on dissociation. According to a 1992 bibliographic analysis of the field by Goettman et al. (1992), 72% of all writings on the topic have appeared in the past decade, with about 1000 published papers scattered across diverse disciplines and journals.
4. Current interest in dissociation as reflected in the appearance of major articles and special issues in respected psychology and psychiatry journals.
5. The initiation of a journal entitled *Dissociation* (Richard Kluft, MD, Editor) devoted to the area.
6. The development of scientific organizations such as the International Society for the Study of Dissociation, as well as dissociation presentations within such organizations as the Society for Experimental and Clinical Hypnosis, the American Society of Clinical and Experimental Hypnosis, and special interest groups within both the American Psychological Association and the American Psychiatric Association.
7. The growing awareness of the prevalence of childhood sexual abuse and its sequelae in relation to dissociative phenomena.
8. The rapidly expanding database from psychology, psychiatry, medicine, and epidemiology on the comorbidity of dissociation and affective, anxiety, and posttraumatic stress disorders, in addition to eating, somatoform, and personality disorders.
9. Growing international interest in dissociation as manifested by significant

increases in research, papers, and conferences from outside of North America.

10. Recent studies revealing the relatively high prevalence of dissociative phenomena and disorders among inpatient, outpatient, and "normal" populations, indicating it will likely remain a permanent and significant area for conceptual, scientific, and clinical inquiry.
11. An increasing number of individuals presenting for treatment with dissociative disorder.
12. The publication of three volumes, two on dissociative identity disorder (multiple personality disorder) by Frank Putnam and Colin Ross and an edited volume on theoretical and clinical perspectives of dissociation by Steven Lynn and Judith Rhue.

However, from the outset it should be noted that with this renewed interest also has come great controversy. Articles and letters have been written to scientific journals suggesting that not only are dissociative disorders overestimated but that certain disorders such as dissociative identity disorder may not exist at all. Since early trauma and sexual abuse have been associated with the presence of dissociative disorders, there has been a growing concern as to valid methods for establishing past trauma or sexual abuse. As part of this approach, authors have debated the ability of a given individual to recover lost memories of trauma or sexual abuse. Those of us who have tried to follow these debates quickly learn that the search for objectivity and truth remains a complex process in the midst of highly rhetorical presentations. Clearly, untrained therapists, in spite of their best motivations, seek signs of abuse or dissociative disorders where they may not exist, and thus do not act in the best interests of either their patients or the field of dissociation. However, there are also individuals who move through the mental health system with unrecognized dissociative processes and remain untreated.

Presently there are few published volumes that provide a comprehensive, state-of-the-art text that simultaneously addresses theoretical, conceptual, diagnostic, assessment, treatment, ethical, and legal dimensions of the field of dissociation. The luminary status of the volume's contributors, whose expertise spans the entire spectrum of dissociative phenomena, has resulted in a stimulating, comprehensive, and in-depth volume. The text's potential significance includes, but is certainly not limited to, the following: (1) Highly respected theorists, scientists, clinical-researchers, and psychotherapists share their expertise, resulting in an integrated volume that reflects the cutting edge of the field; (2) the presence of a "critical mass" of theory, research, and practice in the field of dissociation, which was awaiting compilation into a substantive, cohesive, multidisciplinary volume; and (3) likely audiences for the text include psychologists, psychiatrists, social workers, and other mental health professionals, graduate students, interns, residents, university libraries, and institutions of higher learning.

We believe the volume has much potential for stimulating dialogue in the dissociation field, which is rapidly expanding and making fertile interconnections with other disciplines and sciences. Further, we hope the text will serve as a primary source for elucidation of both current and emerging theory, research, and treatment of dissociative phenomena.

The volume is divided into seven parts. Part I, Foundations, entails historical, epidemiological, phenomenological, etiological, normative, and cross-cultural dimensions of dissociative phenomena, providing an empirical foundation for the remaining chapters. Part II, Developmental Perspectives, represents a newly emerging area that focuses on developmental aspects of dissociative processes, including the potential role of incest and attachment in the development of dissociative processes, as well as a description of dissociative disorders in childhood and adolescence. Part III, Theoretical Models, encompasses contemporary conceptual and research dimensions from a variety of perspectives. These contributions include psychobiological, information-processing models of dissociation, and the relation of dissociation to hypnotic phenomena, moving beyond earlier theoretical frameworks for elucidating the etiopathogenesis of dissociation. Part IV, entitled Assessment, comprises three interrelated chapters devoted to the diagnosis, psychological, and psychophysiological assessment of clients with dissociative disorders.

Part V, Diagnostic Classifications, offers clinicians and researchers an overview of current nosology, differential diagnoses, as well as conceptual and clinical implications of the varied dissociative disorders. In Part VI, Therapeutic Interventions, eight chapters are presented that provide a wealth of information for clinicians treating clients with dissociative disorders, posttraumatic stress disorders, and survivors of sexual abuse and/or assault. These chapters reflect leading clinical perspectives in the amelioration of dissociative disorders and related sequelae of abuse. In Part VII, the final section, Special Topics, two chapters address ritual abuse and ethical-legal issues in dissociative disorders that should be considered as important readings for clinicians working with dissociative disorder clients.

In our clinical and research endeavors with clients with myriad dissociative disorders, we have been sensitized to both the advances in theory, research, and treatment, as well as, unfortunately, the many "black holes" of knowledge that await further scientific study. We were struck by the need for a comprehensive volume on dissociation that would be useful to the professional as well as for graduate-level courses and seminars, providing a timely, balanced, and cogent review of the controversial tributaries in the field. Hence, we endeavored to have the contributors address both fundamental domains as well as issues that have generated much debate in scientific and clinical spheres.

We hope the reader finds the volume as intellectually and clinically rewarding as we have in helping it come to fruition. We would like to extend our sincere appreciation to the outstanding contributors who so generously offered their cumulative wisdom and expertise. To the clients who so courageously shared their experiences and whose quest for healing has enlightened us all, we want to express our deepest gratitude and respect.

Larry K. Michelson
William J. Ray

REFERENCES

Gotteman, C., Greaves, G., & Coons, P. (1992). *Multiple personality and dissociation, 1791-1990: A complete bibliography*. Atlanta: Greaves.

Contents

I. FOUNDATIONS

II. DEVELOPMENTAL PERSPECTIVES

VII. SPECIAL TOPICS

I

FOUNDATIONS

This section begins with the unique history of dissociation and the dissociative disorders within the fields of psychology and psychiatry. In Chapter 1, Ross suggests that dissociative processes have been recorded since the earliest times and treated throughout history by shamans and priests in a tradition that continues throughout the world up to the present time. Scientifically, dissociation represents an important topic area that had its initial flowering in the 1800s and brought forth explanations and descriptions by some of the great creative thinkers of the time, including William James, Pierre Janet, Carl Jung, and Morton Price. During the twentieth century, this tradition was largely ignored and forgotten until about 10 years ago. A number of factors are described in the chapters of this section related to the disappearance of scientific and clinical discussions of dissociative processes. These include the rise of behaviorism in academic circles, the strength of psychoanalysis with its emphasis on repression rather than dissociation, as well as the term "schizophrenia" initially being used to describe dissociative symptoms.

An important theme found in the three chapters of this section is consistency of the phenomenology of dissociative processes across a variety of cultures and levels of pathology. The overall picture is that samples from the United States, Canada, the Netherlands, Central Europe, and Japan show similarities even in the more psychopathological forms of dissociation (e.g., dissociative identity disorder). In fact, it is pointed out in this section that no clinical report from anywhere in the world shows marked deviancy in its description of dissociative identity disorder.

Another important theme addressed in this section is the epidemiology of dissociative processes. This is a new area but results are appearing that help to determine the relative occurrence of each dissociative disorder, which Ross discusses in Chapter 1. Throughout the three chapters of this section, dissociative experiences in the general population are discussed. Interestingly enough, both Ross, using an adult nonclinical population in Winnipeg, Canada, and Ray (Chapter 3), using a college student population at a Big Ten university, found similar factor structures using the best-studied dissociation scale. Ray further determined the relationships between scores on this dissociation scale and other measures such as absorption, absentmindedness, and hypnotic susceptibility, as well as health, stress, and abuse. One intriguing finding from these data is that an orthogonal relationship exists between dissociative tendencies and hypnotic susceptibility. This lack of relationship has been seen consistently in a number of samples collected involving over 2000 college students.

In Chapter 2, Johan Vanderlinden and his colleagues describe the progress in studying dissociative processes in Western and Central Europe. They first describe the modification and development of dissociation questionnaires targeted at the European population. These researchers further compare the report of dissociative experiences in the Netherlands and Belgium with those reported in Hungary as it moved from a communist to a more democratic form of government.

1

History, Phenomenology, and Epidemiology of Dissociation

Colin A. Ross

The dissociative disorders have a unique history within psychology and psychiatry. Our understanding of this history, particularly the contributions of Pierre Janet in the nineteenth century (Ellenberger, 1970; Nemiah, 1989; Putnam, 1989; Ross, 1989; van der Hart & Friedman, 1989), has shifted radically since 1980. Intertwined with this development, a detailed, replicated description of the phenomenology of dissociation has been built up, based primarily on research in North America (North, Ryall, Ricci, & Wetzel, 1993), with significant contributions from the Netherlands and Belgium (Boon & Draijer, 1993; Vanderlinden, 1993). A considerable amount of work has been done on the epidemiology of dissociation within clinical populations and a lesser amount among college students (Frischholtz et al., 1990; Ross, Ryan, Anderson, Ross, & Hardy, 1989e; Ross, Ryan, Voigt, & Eide, 1990c; Sanders, McRoberts, & Tollefson, 1989). One general population survey of dissociation has been completed in North America (Ross, 1991; Ross, Joshi, & Currie, 1990a, 1991b).

In this chapter, I will review the history, phenomenology, and epidemiology of dissociation and the dissociative disorders, using the *Diagnostic and Statistical Manual of Mental Disorders*, 4th Edition (DSM-IV) nomenclature (American Psychiatric Association, 1994). The five DSM-IV dissociative disorders are dissociative amnesia disorder, dissociative fugue disorder, depersonalization disorder, dissociative identity disorder (multiple personality disorder), and dissociative disorder not otherwise specified. For an exhaustive list of references on dissociation, the reader

Colin A. Ross • Dissociative Disorders Unit, Charter Behavioral Health System of Dallas, Plano, Texas 75024.

Handbook of Dissociation: Theoretical, Empirical, and Clinical Perspectives, edited by Larry K. Michelson and William J. Ray. Plenum Press, New York, 1996.

is referred to the bibliography by Goettman, Greaves, and Coons (1994), entitled *Multiple Personality and Dissociation, 1791-1990: A Complete Bibliography* (available from Dr. George Greaves at 529 Pharr Road, Smyrna, Georgia 30305).

Because the study of dissociative identity disorder (DID)/multiple personality disorder (MPD) has been the major focus of the dissociative disorders field, it is not possible to discuss dissociation without giving significant attention to DID. Therefore, I will discuss the extreme form of dissociation, DID, and its complexity, chronicity, and morbidity, to illustrate principles that apply to dissociation in general and to the close relationship between trauma and dissociation.

HISTORY

The history of dissociation begins in prehistory, with the ecstatic experiences of the shamans (Eliade, 1964). Dissociation appears to be a fundamental and universal component of human psychology. The psychological foundations of DID and other complex dissociative disorders are illustrated by the trance and possession states found in most cultures throughout history. In Western civilization, demonic possession is the historical precursor of DID (Crabtree, 1985; Oesterreich, 1974; Ross, 1989), and surprisingly a substantial number of contemporary MPD patients have been treated unsuccessfully with exorcism (Bowman, 1993).

The structural components of MPD and other complex dissociative disorders are switches of executive control from one identity to another and amnesia. In *somnambulistic possession*, there is amnesia for the period during which the possessing entity is in executive control, while in *lucid possession* there is no amnesia, but the person does not experience himself as the agent of his body's actions, and there is a direct, palpable experience of the presence of the possessing entity. At the structural level, DID is based on universal human psychological phenomena that have been harnessed to cope with overwhelming childhood trauma. In our culture, the traumatized girl creates a tough secular adolescent male protector personality, while in another culture the protector would be a deity, spirit guide, or mythological figure. There is variation at the level of content, but the structure is probably universal. In many cultures, extreme forms of dissociation are normal and even prized and sought after through study, fasting, self-immolation, peyote, solitude in the wilderness, or other techniques.

The Psychopathology of Dissociation in the Nineteenth Century

The dominant model of dissociation in nineteenth-century psychology and psychiatry was a psychopathological one, in which dissociation occurred because of a defect or deficit in ego strength (Janet, 1965/1907, 1977/1901). The relationship between trauma and dissociation was well understood (Breuer & Freud, 1986/1895), and there was a body of clinical, experimental, and theoretical literature on DID, trauma, dissociation, hypnosis, and the paranormal. Some leading figures such as Janet and Freud were not interested in the paranormal, while others like Myers (1920) had no interest in trauma. Jung (1977/1902), in comparison, was interested in all four components.

The late nineteenth-century dissociative models of psychopathology were not narrowly focused on the disorders classified as dissociative in DSM-IV. They were broad-based and included conversion disorder, somatization disorder, somnambulism, some forms of obsessive-compulsive disorder, and everything encompassed under the term hysteria. Splitting of consciousness, and the sequestering of traumatic memories and unacceptable impulses and ideas in dissociated packets of psyche, was thought by scientists like Breuer, Myers, Janet, Prince, and Binet to be the mechanism underlying paranormal phenomena, mediumship, possession states, and a wide range of psychopathologies.

In their *Studies on Hysteria*, Breuer and Freud (1986/1891) presented cases that meet DSM-IV criteria for DID and dissociative disorder not otherwise specified, and childhood sexual trauma is reported in many of the case histories. Breuer and Freud's treatments were based on a trauma-dissociation model of psychopathology, and the sexual trauma was a key focus of treatment. Their thinking was consistent with the clinical understanding of other psychologists and psychiatrists on both sides of the Atlantic who both preceded and followed them, including Binet (1977a/1896, 1977b/1890), James (1983/1890), Prince (1978/1905), and Janet (1965/1907, 1977/1901). In the two decades from 1890 to 1910, trauma and dissociation were major, mainstream themes on the center stage of psychology and psychiatry on both sides of the Atlantic.

The Decline in Interest in Dissociation in the Early Twentieth Century

The curve of interest in dissociation from 1890 to 1994 is unique within psychology and psychiatry. From a peak in the last two decades of the nineteenth century, the curve drops off exponentially in the first two decades of the twentieth century, to virtually zero (Goettman et al., 1991). This occurred so quickly and the magnitude of the change was so great that the process cannot be explained by passive forgetting, a gradual shift of interest to other priorities, or similar mechanisms. There had to have been an active dissociation of dissociation from mainstream psychiatry and psychology.

What were the factors that led to dissociation virtually disappearing from mainstream academia early in the twentieth century? The first was Freud's repudiation of the seduction theory, which was accompanied by his denigration of hypnosis and his shift from a dissociation to a repression model of psychopathology. If the women with dissociative disorders who were coming to Freud for treatment for the long-term sequelae of childhood sexual trauma were never actually abused, then how should they be understood and treated? By invalidating the childhood sexual abuse, Freud disallowed the possibility of treatment of dissociative symptoms within a trauma model, and dissociative diagnoses became irrelevant to mainstream clinical practice. The fundamental issue was not DID or dissociation but the endemic nature of childhood sexual abuse and society's need to disavow the reality of both the abuse itself and its long-term consequences.

The second factor was the creation of the term *schizophrenia* by Bleuler, who wrote in 1924 that, "it is not alone in hysteria that one finds an arrangement of different personalities one *succeeding* the other: through similar mechanisms schizophrenia produces different personalities existing *side by side*" (quoted in Boon & Draijer, 1993, p. 119). To the contemporary student of schizophrenia, it is not obvious why Bleuler decided that *dementia praecox* should be called *split mind disorder*, which is the meaning of the Greek term schizophrenia, since splitting of mental functions is not a topic addressed in the contemporary schizophrenia literature. The explanation for Bleuler's choosing the term schizophrenia is that his clinical descriptions of schizophrenia are often descriptions of DSM-IV dissociative identity disorder.

Subsequent to the coining of the term schizophrenia, many DID patients were transferred into a biomedical organic brain model, which is the model of schizophrenia that dominates contemporary psychiatry. Patients who several decades earlier would have received a dissociative diagnosis and treatment focused on their childhood sexual trauma were now triaged in one of two directions within the mental health field: they were defined as hysterics and prescribed psychoanalysis for their sexual fantasies, or they received a diagnosis of schizophrenia and were assigned to a biomedical pathway.

The third factor was the rise of behaviorism. The intellectual gestalt of strict behaviorism does not allow consideration of internal states of consciousness, divided consciousness, or symptoms that evolve from causes 20 or 30 years in the patient's past. As behaviorism acquired more academic territory, the time and energy available for study of dissociation decreased (Hilgard, 1987).

Within a few decades, it was no longer possible to have a serious clinical, theoretical, or phenomenological interest in the paranormal, dissociation, hypnosis, or childhood sexual abuse, despite the fact that all four subjects had been on center stage in the recent past. These interrelated topics were banished beyond the fringes of psychology and psychiatry by active exclusion.

During the years 1920 to 1950, academic interest in DID dwindled to a handful of publications per year in the entire world literature. If one searches the *Index Medicus* even in the 1970s and 1980s, one will find hundreds of topics with more citations than DID. No other disorder has been subject to this kind of exclusion from mainstream psychological and medical study.

Resurgence of Interest in Dissociation in the 1970s and 1980s

During the 1980s, the curve of interest in dissociation turned upward and the field began to undergo exponential growth. The number of annual publications on DID and the number of cases reported increased by thousands of percents from 1979 to 1993. To use personal measures of the epidemiological shift, about 200 cases had been reported in the world literature in 1980, whereas my Dissociative Disorders Unit admits more patients than this per year, and I have published or presented independent series of 236 (Ross, Norton, & Wozney, 1989d), 102 (Ross, et al., 1990b), and 107 cases of MPD (C. A. Ross, J. Ellason, & D. Fuchs, unpublished data).

The upturn in the curve has occurred against resistance from mainstream psychology and psychiatry, which is the inverse of the process that occurred 80 years ago. What factors resulted in this exponential upward growth at this point in history? The overwhelmingly important factor is childhood physical and sexual abuse being brought out of the closet by the women's movement. In the three-volume 1980 edition of the *Comprehensive Textbook of Psychiatry* (Kaplan, Freedman, & Sadock, 1980), which is the main textbook of North American psychiatry, there is a tiny section on incest that includes a reference to a 1955 study that found a prevalence of incest of one family out of a million in North America. This estimate was out by a factor of at least 10,000, because incest actually occurs in more than one family out of 100 in our culture (Bagley & King, 1990).

When Chris Sizemore, who is Eve of *The Three Faces of Eve* (Thigpen & Cleckley, 1957), was diagnosed, she was told that she was probably the only person on the planet with DID. If less than 100 families in North America at any given time have experienced incest, and if severe, chronic childhood trauma is the foundation of dissociative psychopathology, then Eve being the only person alive with DID is a reasonable estimate. If at least 5% of boys and 15% of girls experience unwanted, sexually abusive treatment before age 18 in our culture, however, as Bagley and King (1990) conclude from their review of the literature, then dissociative psychopathology might be common and of mainstream clinical interest.

Although academic psychiatry and psychology can no longer maintain that severe, chronic childhood trauma is rare, for the most part it is still considered clinically peripheral. For instance, in the August 1993 special issue of the *Canadian Journal of Psychiatry* on child and adolescent psychiatry, there are 12 articles and 2 editorials with a total of 467 references. Childhood sexual abuse is mentioned once and referenced once in the entire issue, in an article entitled, "Public Health Nurse Home Visitation for the Tertiary Prevention of Child Maltreatment: Results of a Pilot Study" (MacMillan & Thomas, 1993). In this study, a history of sexual abuse was used as an exclusion criterion for enrolling families, a fact that generated the single reference on sexual abuse.

In the other 11 articles with a total of 428 references, there is not a single reference to childhood physical or sexual abuse. In one article there are two references to studies on child maltreatment, but they are discussed only in terms of the psychometrics of the instruments used in the studies. The articles in the issue deal with topics such as family factors in adolescent unipolar depression, psychiatric follow-up of adoptees, attachment and conduct disorder, disruptive behavior problems, and child survivors of the Holocaust. These are all topics in which childhood sexual trauma is of central interest.

It is not possible to understand the dissociative disorders or professional resistance to them without a prior understanding of childhood sexual abuse. Any attempt to debate the validity of DID is premature if there is no agreement that chronic childhood trauma is a major etiologic theme in psychopathology.

The second factor helping to bring the dissociative disorders back into the mainstream was the Vietnam War. For sociological reasons originating outside psychology and psychiatry, the Vietnam War and the posttraumatic stress disorder (PTSD) that arose from it were not forgotten when the veterans returned home, as had been the case in the two world wars and the Korean War. The realization that real, severe trauma could have serious long-term psychopathological consequences was forced on society as a whole by Vietnam. Once this principle was accepted, it was a short leap to the conclusion that severe childhood trauma might have serious sequelae lasting into adulthood.

The third factor was publication of the books *The Three Faces of Eve* (Thigpen & Cleckley, 1957) and *Sybil* (Schreiber, 1973), both of which were made into successful Hollywood movies. These two cases brought dissociation into mainstream consciousness.

The fourth factor was the appearance of DSM-III in 1980 (American Psychiatric Association, 1980). In DSM-III, the dissociative disorders were for the first time given a separate section of their own, and operationalized diagnostic criteria for multiple personality disorder were included for the first time. This development in the DSM process provided a major impetus to the phenomenological research on DID that was conducted in the 1980s.

Current Scientific State of the Art

In 1980, the dissociative disorders' field was in a prescientific state of development. Since then, dissociation has become an established field of scientific study, a fact that made this handbook possible. The transition to scientific status was achieved remarkably quickly, given the small number of serious investigators in the field and the small amount of grant money devoted to dissociation in the 1980s compared to other aspects of psychopathology such as anxiety, depression, psychosis, and substance abuse.

The majority of the clinical and research effort on dissociation since 1980 has been devoted to DID for a number of reasons: it is the most interesting dissociative disorder; it carries the most morbidity; undiagnosed DID patients often fare poorly in the mental health system and receive numerous different diagnoses and ineffective treatments; specific psychotherapy can result in dramatic improvement in function and reduction in symptoms (see Chapter 16, this volume); and the disorder has the most to teach us of any dissociative disorder. Most of my brief review will therefore focus on DID.

Several self-report measures of dissociation have been developed (Boon & Draijer, 1993), of which the Dissociative Experiences Scale (DES) (Bernstein & Putnam, 1986) is by far the most studied. The DES may become established as the equivalent for dissociation of the Beck Depression Inventory (North et al., 1993). The DES is a highly robust measure of dissociation with three factors that are stable across a number of large series in the general population and in clinical populations (Carlson et al., 1993; Frischholtz et al., 1990, 1991; Ross et al., 1991b). The factors are absorption, amnesia, and depersonalization-derealization.

There are two structured interviews for diagnosing dissociative disorders: the Dissociative Disorders Interview Schedule (DDIS) (Ross et al., 1989c), and the Structured Clinical Interview for DSM-III-R Dissociative Disorders (SCID-D) (Boon & Draijer, 1993; Bremner, Steinberg, Southwick, Johnson, & Charney, 1993; Steinberg, Rounsaville, & Cicchetti, 1990). Both the DDIS and the SCID-D require further research on their validity and reliability, but both make a diagnosis of DID with an interrater kappa of .95-.96, which is higher than the kappa for any diagnosis made by the Structured Clinical Interview for DSM-III-R (Spitzer, Williams, & Gibbon, 1987).

The sensitivity of the DDIS for DID in 396 subjects with that clinical diagnosis was 95%, and in over 500 administrations of the structured interview to subjects without clinical diagnoses of DID, the false-positive rate for the diagnosis of DID has been 1% (C. A. Ross, unpublished data, 1993). Structured interviews for nondissociative diagnoses do not approach this level of diagnostic precision. Thus, although further research is required, it appears that DID can be diagnosed with higher reliability, greater sensitivity, and fewer false positives than any other disorder in DSM-IV.

The validity of DID in terms of treatment outcome is profound at the clinical anecdote level and in preliminary financial cost-benefit analyses (Fraser & Raine, 1992; Ross & Dua, 1993). The treatment outcome data are nowhere near well-enough developed to convince skeptics of the validity of the disorder, however. Anyone who has treated a severely impaired individual with DID to stable integration cannot help but have been deeply impressed by the power of the DID treatment model, as outlined in this handbook and in texts by Putnam (1989) and Ross (1989).

The scientific study of dissociation in childhood is in very early stages, as are transcultural studies. In the Netherlands, DID has the same clinical profile as in North America (Boon & Draijer, 1993), and this is also true in Japan according to studies done there with translated versions of the DES and DDIS (Berger et al., 1992). It appears that DID can be readily diagnosed in Scotland (Macilwain, 1992), Puerto Rico (Martinez-Taboas, 1989), and New Zealand (Altrocchi, 1992) by clinicians who inquire systematically for its features. DID personality systems I have treated in native North Americans have the same features as those described in the research literature. DID has also been reported sporadically from Switzerland (Modestin, 1992) and a variety of other countries (Coons, Bowman, Kluft, & Milstein, 1991).

The major foci for systematic research on DID in the 1990s will be further demonstrating the reliability and validity of the disorder, exploring comorbidity, tracking treatment outcome, and better defining childhood DID. For dissociation in general, the focus of research will be on establishing its prevalence in various clinical populations and the general population and demonstrating its correlations with childhood trauma and other forms of psychopathology. An important book by North et al. (1993) demonstrated that DID has begun to be taken seriously as a subject of legitimate scientific study by investigators well grounded in research methodology, who are not members of the small group of writers and researchers that dealt with dissociative disorders in the 1980s.

A Paradigm Shift in Progress in Psychiatry and Psychology

Classical paradigm shifts as defined by Thomas Kuhn (1962) do not occur very frequently. Psychiatry, I believe, is currently in the process of a paradigm shift from endogenous-reductionist models of psychopathology, which effectively ignore environmental variables, to a trauma model of psychopathology, one driven by research on DID and childhood trauma (Ross, 1992). Through most of the twentieth century, DID has been an anomaly from the point of view of normal science psychiatry and has been ignored as such. In the last 5 years it has becoming increasingly evident that the DID is a paradigm-threatening anomaly.

Unlike the paradigm shift in physics from Newtonian to relativistic and quantum-mechanical models, however, the shift to a trauma model in psychiatry will to a large extent represent a return to a prior paradigm dominant from 1880 to 1900. I mention this paradigm shift briefly, without making any argument for its validity, to alert those interested in the philosophy of science to an opportunity to study a paradigm shift in progress. The content of this handbook provides the substance of the argument.

PHENOMENOLOGY

The phenomenology of dissociation in clinical populations, college students, and the general population has been studied in the last half decade, as mentioned above. Dissociation consists of three factors: absorption-imaginative involvement, amnesia, and depersonalization-derealization. Absorption is by far the most common subcomponent of dissociation in all populations studied, while the other two factors tend to be clearly psychopathological in nature when elevated item scores occur.

As Frankel (1990) warned, assessment of the severity of dissociative symptoms has a lower interrater reliability when milder degrees of dissociation are being assessed and high reliability when severe symptoms in DID patients are being assessed (Boon & Draijer, 1993). The significance of statistically significant but numerically small differences in DES scores within the general population is unknown, but unlikely to be of any marked clinical significance.

In this section I will describe the dissociative continuum, the relationship between borderline personality disorder and this continuum, and the phenomenology of dissociative identity disorder, because it illustrates dissociation in the extreme. I will briefly describe the other dissociative diso.ders by presenting the DSM-IV criteria.

The DSM-IV Dissociative Disorders

The following are the DSM-IV criteria for the five dissociative disorders (American Psychiatric Association, 1993):

300.12 Dissociative Amnesia

A. The predominant disturbance is one or more episodes of inability to recall important personal information, usually of a traumatic or stressful nature, that is too extensive to be explained by ordinary forgetfulness.
B. The disturbance does not occur exclusively during the course of Dissociative Identity Disorder and is not due to the direct effects of a substance (e.g., drugs of abuse, medication) or a general medical condition (e.g., Amnestic Disorder due to head trauma).

300.13 Dissociative Fugue

A. The predominant disturbance is sudden, unexpected travel away from home or one's customary place of work, with inability to recall one's past.
B. Confusion about personal identity or assumption of a new identity (partial or complete).
C. The disturbance does not occur exclusively during the course of Dissociative Identity Disorder and is not due to the direct effects of a substance (e.g., drugs of abuse, medication) or a general medical condition (e.g., temporal lobe epilepsy).

300.14 Dissociative Identity Disorder (Multiple Personality Disorder)

A. The presence of two or more distinct identities or personality states (each with its own relatively enduring pattern of perceiving, relating to, and thinking about the environment and self).
B. At least two of these identities or personality states recurrently take control of the person's behavior.
C. Inability to recall important personal information that is too extensive to be explained by ordinary forgetfulness.
D. Not due to the direct effects of a substance (e.g., blackouts or chaotic behavior during Alcohol Intoxication) or a general medical condition (e.g., complex partial seizures). Note: In children, the symptoms are not attributable to imaginary playmates or other fantasy play.

300.6 Depersonalization Disorder

A. Persistent or recurrent experiences of feeling detached from, and as if one is an outside observer of, one's mental processes or body (e.g., feeling like one is in a dream).
B. During the depersonalization experience, reality testing remains intact.
C. The depersonalization causes clinically significant distress or impairment in social, occupational, or other important areas of function.
D. The depersonalization experience is not better accounted for by another disorder, such as Schizophrenia, Dissociative Identity Disorder, or Panic Disorder, and is not due to the direct effects of a substance (e.g., drugs of abuse, medication) or a general medical condition (e.g., temporal lobe epilepsy).

300.15 Dissociative Disorder Not Otherwise Specified

This category is reserved for disorders in which the predominant feature is a dissociative symptom (i.e., a disturbance or alteration in the normal integrative functions of identity, memory, or consciousness) but the criteria are not met for any specific Dissociative Disorder. Examples include:

1. Clinical presentations similar to Dissociative Identity Disorder that fail to meet full criteria for this disorder. Examples include presentations in which: (a) there are not two or more distinct personality states, or (b) amnesia for important personal information does not occur.
2. Derealization unaccompanied by depersonalization in adults.
3. States of dissociation that occur in individuals who have been subjected to periods of prolonged and intensive coercive persuasion (e.g., brainwashing, thought reform, or indoctrination while the captive of terrorists or cultists).
4. Dissociative trance disorder: single or episodic alterations in the state of consciousness that are indigenous to particular locations and cultures. Dissociative trance involves narrowing of awareness of immediate surroundings or stereotyped behaviors or movements that are experienced as being beyond one's control. Possession trance involves replacement of the customary sense of personal identity by a new identity, attributed to the influence of a spirit, power, deity, or other person, and associated with stereotyped "involuntary" movements or amnesia. Examples include *amok* (Indonesia), *bebainan* (Indonesia), *latah* (Malaysia), *pibloktoq* (Artic), *phil bob* (Thailand), *vimbuza* (Nigeria), *ataque de nervios* (Latin America), and

possession (India). The dissociative or trance disorder is not a normal part of a broadly accepted collective cultural or religious practice.
5. Loss of consciousness, stupor, or coma not attributable to a general medical condition.
6. Ganser's syndrome: the giving of "approximate answers" to questions, commonly associated with dissociative amnesia or fugue.*

The Dissociative Continuum

The idea that the dissociative disorders lie on a continuum of increasing complexity, chronicity, and severity related to more extreme trauma was initially proposed by Ross (1985) and Braun (1986); but this conceptualization is general to the field and was likely arrived at independently by a large number of clinicians working with the dissociative disorders. At the left-hand of the continuum is normal dissociation, as represented by daydreaming, trancing out for a few blocks while driving a car, absorption in a book or movie, and normal childhood imaginative play. Next come more pathological forms of dissociative and trance-state phenomena such as highway hypnosis, which are not freestanding psychiatric disorders. Further to the right are simple dissociative disorders such as dissociative amnesia disorder. These are followed by more complex and chronic forms of dissociative disorder not otherwise specified (DDNOS), with DID at the far right-hand end of the continuum.

It is widely accepted clinically in the dissociative disorders field, and in DSM-IV, that many individuals with DDNOS have partial, not fully crystallized forms of DID, and require a similar treatment involving memory retrieval and processing, integration of dissociated ego states, and resolution of conflicts between the ego states. But what empirical evidence is there to support the concept of a dissociative spectrum?

So far, only three published studies address this issue (Boon & Draijer, 1993; Coons, 1992; Ross et al., 1992b), and all support the continuum hypothesis. Boon and Draijer's study is the most comprehensive and is based on Dutch versions of the DES and Structured Clinical Interview for DSM-III-R Dissociative Disorders (SCID-D). The DES, SCID-D, and DDIS can differentiate clinically diagnosed DID from DDNOS at high levels of statistical significance on many different symptom clusters. The continuum concept is widely accepted among clinicians in the dissociative disorders field, and the only studies investigating it have supported the model; therefore, it appears that future research is likely to confirm this conceptualization. We can anticipate the appearance of more complex versions of the model as our data base increases.

Borderline Personality Disorder and the Dissociative Disorders

The relationship between borderline personality disorder and the dissociative disorders has been complicated rather than clarified in DSM-IV, because a ninth criterion for borderline personality disorder has been added: "transient, stress-related paranoid ideation or severe dissociative symptoms" (American Psychiatric

*Reprinted by permission from *Diagnostic and Statistical Manual of Mental Disorders*, Fourth Edition. Copyright 1994 American Psychiatric Association.

Association, 1993). One now has to meet five of nine rather than five of eight criteria, as was the case in DSM-III and DSM-III-R, in order to receive a borderline diagnosis.

There are no exclusion criteria in the borderline diagnostic set, so there are no specific rules for determining when severe dissociative symptoms should result in an Axis I dissociative diagnosis and when there should be no Axis I diagnosis but a positive dissociative criterion on Axis II. Nor is it specified whether one can have a positive dissociative borderline criterion on Axis II and a concurrent Axis I dissociative disorder.

While there is no systematic data set concerning dissociative symptoms and disorders in a sample of borderlines, the inverse is not true. Beginning with a study of Horevitz and Braun (1984), there have been several replications of the finding that 38 to 70% of patients with DID meet criteria for borderline personality disorder (Boon & Draijer, 1993; Fink & Golinkoff, 1990; Ross, Ellason, & Fuchs, 1992c; Ross, Heber, Norton, & Anderson, 1989a; Ross et al., 1990b). In a sample of 102 clinically diagnosed DID subjects, the average subject was positive for 5.2 (SD 2.3) borderline criteria on the DDIS. The number of positive borderline criteria differentiates DID from panic disorder, eating disorders, and schizophrenia (Ross et al., 1989a), and from temporal lobe epilepsy (Ross et al., 1989b).

It is well-established that borderline personality disorder patients have high rates of childhood trauma (Gunderson & Sabo, 1993), although Axis I dissociative comorbidity was not examined in any of the supporting studies. To my way of thinking, borderline personality disorder is a simple form of DID in which the personality states are less crystallized, less personified, fewer in number, and not separated by the same degree of amnesia. Inversely, DID is a complex variant of borderline personality disorder.

Data to support this conceptualization come from Boon and Draijer (1993), who showed that borderline personality disorder exists on a continuum of increasing severity, with DDNOS having a greater degree of complexity than pure borderline personality and DID the greatest degree of elaboration and crystallization. They demonstrated this with SCID-D data and compelling clinical observation.

The relationship between trauma, dissociation, and DSM-IV borderline criteria is a rich topic for future research. Large numbers of subjects should be compared on the DES, SCID-D, and DDIS, as well as other measures, in future studies, and the subject groups should include pure borderline personality disorder without an Axis I dissociative disorder and DDNOS and DID groups with and without concurrent borderline personality. Correlational analyses will likely demonstrate powerful relationships between the degree of childhood trauma, the complexity of dissociation, and the number of positive borderline criteria.

At the present time, the existing data unequivocally refute the commonly advanced proposition that DID patients are "really just borderlines." Fink (1991) has provided the most comprehensive clinical discussion of the interaction between DID and Axis II psychopathology.

The Phenomenology of Dissociative Identity Disorder

The phenomenology of DID is consistent in samples from Canada, the United States, the Netherlands, and Japan studied with the DES, SCID-D, and DDIS, as stated above. There are no clinical reports from anywhere in the world of a markedly different form of DID, and there are no studies that have not confirmed the symptom profile. DID can be diagnosed by the DDIS or SCID-D with an interrater reliability unsurpassed by any other DSM-IV diagnosis. The kappa value for the interrater reliability of DID on structured interview is .95-.96, compared with an overall average for Axis I of .68 using the Structured Clinical Interview for DSM-III-R, which does not make dissociative diagnoses (Spitzer et al., 1987).

The core phenomenology of the disorder is the existence of distinct personality states that take turns being in executive control of the body and are separated by varying degrees of amnesia. This phenomenon does not occur in any other disorder, and is described in detail in texts by Putnam (1989) and Ross (1989). From the core phenomenology, one can predict most of the secondary features of the disorder: the frequency of the secondary features in a sample of 102 DID cases is readily available (Ross et al., 1990b).

The secondary features include such items as blank spells or periods of missing time; coming out of blank spells in unfamiliar surroundings, unsure of how one got there; being told of disremembered events; finding objects present or missing in the environment that cannot be accounted for; distinct changes of handwriting; referring to onself as "we" or "us"; and auditory hallucinations, which may include voices commenting, voices conversing with one another, command hallucinations, and other variations of internal voices and conversations.

The secondary features each exist on a spectrum from normal to severe forms increasingly specific for DID. For instance, internal dialogues and monologues are part of common experience, but to have a fully ego-alien voice shouting commands for suicide inside one's head intermittently for decades is outside the range of normal experience.

The subtle phenomenology of DID is mostly due to intrusions, influences, and interactions of alter personalities not involving full switches of executive control. For instance, laceration of the wrist may occur in a depersonalized state during which the person experiences herself as not being the agent of the cutting. In full DID, there will, in addition, often be command hallucinations to cut and episodes of cutting for which the host personality is amnesic. In DID, a specific alter personality that does the cutting can be contacted directly and engaged in conversation; this degree of elaboration does not occur in DDNOS or pure borderline personality, although depersonalized self-mutilation can occur at any point on the spectrum. The general differential diagnostic principle is that patients with full DID exhibit all the phenomenology of DDNOS, but in addition have crystallized symptoms due to fully personified and differentiated personality states that do not occur in DDNOS.

DID patients have an extreme degree of Axis I and II comorbidity. In a sample of 107 DID patients treated at Charter Behavioral Health System of Dallas, we found, using the SCID-I and SCID-II, that the average patient met DSM-III-R criteria for 3.6 different personality disorders and 7.3 different Axis I disorders, in addition to the DID, which is not diagnosed by the SCID (C. A. Ross et al., unpublished data). The most common comorbid diagnoses include depression, panic disorder, PTSD, substance abuse, and eating disorders.

On Axis II, borderline, paranoid, avoidant, and self-defeating personality disorders each occurred in 43.7-56.3% of the 107 cases. The most common Axis II diagnoses are in Cluster C, and a pure Cluster B profile (histrionic, narcissistic, borderline, or antisocial) occurs in only 4.9% of cases. Histrionic personality disorder is one of the least common Axis II diagnoses with a frequency of 8.7% in the sample of 107 patients.

Why so much comorbidity? This can be understood by considering the case of a 24-year-old, highly hypnotizable woman with no preexisting psychopathology who is raped by a stranger. She copes with the assault by blocking out all memory of it, and therefore has dissociative amnesia. This Axis I disorder might not require treatment if it were not for the comorbidity that develops as part of the normal human reaction to extreme psychological trauma. The rape victim develops either subthreshold or a diagnostic level of many different DSM-IV disorders.

She begins to phobically avoid the area of the rape and experiences intense anxiety if she does not do so (panic disorder with agoraphobia). She feels dirty and showers four times a day (obsessive-compulsive disorder). Her relationship with her lover becomes strained, and she develops inhibited sexual arousal and anorgasmia, although she was previously normally adjusted sexually. Her relationship with her somewhat chauvinistic boss at work becomes stormy, stressful, and conflicted; if this pattern had been present since adolescence, we would call it a personality disorder.

Because of postraumatic numbing, intrusions, hypervigilance, nightmares, and avoidance, she meets full criteria for PTSD and has trouble sleeping because of nightmares. The feelings of dirtiness, self-blame for poor performance as a sexual partner, and fatigue and interpersonal difficulties at work are demoralizing and may result in her reaching threshold for a clinical depression. To sleep better, she begins to drink excessively before bedtime. Within 6 weeks, this young woman, who was well until raped, now meets or nearly meets criteria for mood, anxiety, dissociative, sleep, psychosexual, and substance abuse disorders and has more than one diagnosis in some categories.

If the onset of the trauma had been in childhood, if the perpetrators had been close relatives, and if the duration had been a decade or more, it is not difficult to see why there would be the kind of comorbidity that is the norm in DID. The comorbidity results in the average DID patient in two large series spending 6.8 years in the mental health system prior to diagnosis of the dissociative disorder (Putnam, 1989; Ross, 1989), receiving numerous other diagnoses, and undergoing trials of many different treatments.

Undiagnosed DID patients received incorrect diagnoses of schizophrenia in 25% and 40% of cases in two large series (Putnam, 1989; Ross, 1989), while in one series 12% and in the other 16% had received electroconvulsive therapy. Over half of 102 DID patients in a third large series had been treated with neuroleptics (Ross et al., 1990b). All available data unequivocally support the contention that undiagnosed DID patients are perceived as suffering from severe mental illnesses by treating clinicians.

DID can usually be diagnosed in a single standard psychiatric assessment once a decision tree for the diagnosis is incorporated into the interview. The mental status assessment of DID has been described by Loewenstein (1991). The major screening items for DID are a history of childhood physical and/or sexual abuse, recurrent blank spells, auditory hallucinations, presence of positive borderline criteria, and absence of a thought disorder. Subjects with this constellation are highly likely to have either DDNOS or DID. When the blank spells are sharply demarcated, recurrent, and chronic, and the voices fully ego-alien, out loud, and internal, DID is the most likely diagnosis, even in the absence of any further clinical information. Although direct observation of switching of personality states is desirable for final confirmation of the diagnosis, DSM-IV rules do not state that this is necessary and direct observation of the active phase of the disorder is not required for any other Axis I disorder; therefore, to require it for DID would be uniquely stringent.

Clinicians in the dissociative disorder field, by consensus, regard DID as the paradigmatic example of the psychological response to severe, chronic childhood trauma, and therefore view it as exhibiting the relationship between trauma and all types of symptomatology through its primary and secondary features and comorbidity. DID patients are the extreme cases illustrating general principles of the trauma response.

The Other Dissociative Disorders

The other dissociative disorders have not been studied as thoroughly as DID. The best recent reviews are by Putnam (1993), Kluft (1993), Loewenstein (1993), Steinberg (1993), Nemiah (1993), and Spiegel (1993). These chapters were originally published in the American Psychiatric Press' annual *Review of Psychiatry* (Vol. 10). As described above, partial forms of DID currently classified as DDNOS clearly fall into the dissociative spectrum and are related to substantial but less severe histories of childhood trauma than those in DID.

Boon and Draijer (1993) found that 19 of 20 subjects in their study with an initial diagnosis of DDNOS proved to have full DID on 1-year followup. The function of the DDNOS category is in part to provide a preliminary dissociative diagnosis for patients in whom DID is possible or suspected, but cannot be confirmed.

Dissociative amnesia commonly occurs in survivors of severe childhood trauma who do not have a more complex dissociative disorder. It takes a number of different forms. There can be complete amnesia for all life events from age 12 or 14 back, with a sudden onset of normal memory at a specific age. At other times, there can be complete amnesia for a period of several years, with intact memory before and afterward. Differentiating traumatic amnesia for childhood from normal forgetting can be difficult in marginal cases. One clinical clue is the ability of younger siblings to recall details of vacations and other nontraumatic events that the index sibling has dissociated.

Some survivors block out only the traumatic memories, leaving intact their memories of the rest of childhood, while others block out everything. Although definitive epidemiological studies have not been done, amnesia for childhood trauma is probably the most common form of dissociative amnesia disorder. Amnesias for part or all of single-episode, adult-onset trauma has been recognized in combat and other conditions for many years, however (Loewenstein, 1993).

There is no consensus in the field yet as to how often depersonalization disorder exists as an independent disorder (Steinberg, 1993). Depersonalization commonly occurs as a predominant symptom in mood, substance abuse, organic, and psychotic disorders. In sexual abuse survivors, reports of floating up to the ceiling or into the wall, or escaping into internal fantasy during abuse are the most common form of depersonalization. Depersonalization can be pervasive and nonspecific or can involve a detailed, time-limited, out-of-body experience. An interesting largely unexamined question is whether the body image distortions occurring in anorexia nervosa and body dysmorphic disorder are often dissociative in nature.

Most clinicians in the dissociative disorders field have seen only a few cases of pure dissociative fugue, although fugue episodes are common in DID. A diagnosis of fugue should always prompt the clinician to carefully rule out DID by longitudinal assessment.

A common pattern is for a patient to meet criteria for both dissociative amnesia and depersonalization disorder by DSM-IV rules. Although we lack any research data on the problem, clinical experience tells me that most of these patients have either full or partial forms of DID, and therefore should be classified as DDNOS. The problem is that DDNOS can be diagnosed only in the absence of any other dissociative disorder. This common problem in differential diagnosis within the dissociative disorders will require attention in DSM-V and DSM-VI. I favor the creation of a category for partial forms of DID, the presence of which would be an exclusion criterion for diagnosis of dissociative amnesia or depersonalization disorder.

The phenomenology of the dissociative disorders is rich, complex, and described in detail in the referenced literature, as well as elsewhere in this volume.

EPIDEMIOLOGY

At the time of publication of the texts by Putnam (1989) and Ross (1989), there was no information on the epidemiology of dissociation in the general population and very little in clinical populations. Since then, an increasing body of research has begun to fill this gap in the literature. However, we still lack an adequate data base of multicenter replicated findings. Therefore, everything said about epidemiology is necessarily tentative.

Epidemiology of Dissociation in the General Population

Studies of the prevalence of dissociative experiences were not possible before the development of reliable measures, of which the first was the DES (Bernstein & Putnam, 1986). General population surveys have been completed in Canada using the DES (Ross, 1991) and in the Netherlands and Belgium using the Dissociation Questionnaire (DIS-Q) (Vanderlinden, 1993), in addition to surveys of college student populations. All studies have yielded the same finding of a highly left-skewed distribution of scores, with the mean DES score in Canada being 10.8 (SD 10.1) and the median score 7.0. In the Netherlands, the mean DIS-Q score is 1.61 (SD 0.40). DES and DIS-Q scores correlate with each other at very high levels in both the Netherlands (Vanderlinden, 1993) and the United States (Sainton, Ellason, Mayran, & Ross, 1993).

The DES yields three factors in the general population ($N = 1055$) (Ross et al.,

1991b): absorption-imaginative involvement; activities of dissociated states (an amnesia factor); and depersonalization-derealization. The DIS-Q has four subscales similar to those of the SCID-D, called identity confusion, loss of control, amnesia, and absorption. It is evident that dissociation is not a unitary phenomenon and that there are at least three aspects to the overall phenomenology.

In all surveys completed to date, the items in the absorption-imaginative involvement factor are by far the most frequently endorsed. For instance, in the sample of 1055 respondents in Winnipeg, Canada who completed the DES (Ross et al., 1990a), the mean score for DES Item 2 from the absorption factor was 24.3 (SD 22.1); 83% of subjects endorsed the item and 28.9% of subjects reported that they had this experience more than 30% of the time. In comparison, DES Item 4 from the amnesia factor had a mean score of 1.9 (SD 8.5), was endorsed by only 13.6% of subjects, and was experienced more than 30% of the time by only 1.5% of subjects.

The frequency distributions of scores for these two items are shown in Table 1. The DES is scored such that individual items can have scores only at intervals of 5: the 28 items are summed and divided by 28 to yield an overall score ranging from 0 to 100, with overall scores usually expressed to one decimal point.

It is likely that high scores on the amnesia factor of the DES predict the presence of a dissociative disorder, but no studies testing this prediction have been reported to date. Dissociation in normal populations is discussed in greater detail in Chapter 3, this volume.

The distribution of DES scores in Canada led Ross, Joshi, and Currie (1991b) to predict that the lifetime prevalence of dissociative disorders in the general population might be in the range of 5 to 10%, while DIS-Q scores in the Netherlands and Belgium led Vanderlinden (1993) to predict a prevalence of 1-3% in those countries. Epidemiological studies with the DDIS and/or SCID-D will be required to determine the prevalence of DSM-IV dissociative disorders in different countries.

Table 1. Frequency Distribution of Two DES Items in the General Population

	Number of subjects[a]			Number of subjects[a]	
Score	Item 2	Item 4	Score	Item 2	Item 4
0	179	912	55	26	0
5	95	81	60	15	2
10	119	27	65	18	2
15	102	9	70	19	0
20	99	3	75	18	1
25	90	6	80	9	2
30	65	2	85	9	1
35	54	2	90	6	0
40	42	0	95	4	2
45	42	3	100	1	0
50	43	1			

[a]N = 1055.

Epidemiology of Dissociative Disorders in the General Population

Only one study of the prevalence of dissociative disorders in the general population has been conducted (Ross, 1991). This survey, a stratified cluster sample (N = 454), was conducted in Winnipeg, Canada: the 454 subjects completing the DDIS were a subset of 1055 subjects who completed the DES in the same project (Ross et al., 1990a).

The study has a number of limitations. A much larger, multicenter sample is required, the validity of the DDIS in the general population has not been established, and validating interviews by "blind" clinicians were not undertaken. The results of this survey must be considered a first approximation only. Until further research is conducted, however, the results are consistent with DES data from the larger sample and with the large number of undiagnosed cases detected in screening studies in clinical populations.

Subsequent to publication of the sample of 454 subjects, further interviews were completed for a final sample of 502 subjects completing the DDIS. The lifetime prevalence of the dissociative disorders in Winnipeg, Canada from this expanded sample of 502 subjects is shown in Table 2. According to the DSM-III-R diagnostic criteria for multiple personality disorder embedded in the DDIS, 3.0% of subjects were positive for the disorder. However, inspection of the DDIS profiles revealed that only six of these subjects reported trauma histories and endorsed the symptom profile for multiple personality disorder; therefore, the corrected estimate for the prevalence of DID in the general population is 1%. Whether the other nine subjects had another dissociative disorder or not is unknown; therefore, the corrected estimate for the lifetime prevalence of dissociative disorders is in the range of 10 to 12%. If this is accurate, dissociation is a major form of psychopathology comparable in prevalence to anxiety, depression, and substance abuse.

Epidemiology of Dissociation in Clinical Populations

Studies in clinical populations using the DES, DDIS, SCID-D, and DIS-Q have consistently found high rates of dissociative symptoms (Boon & Draijer, 1993; Chu & Dill, 1990; Demitrack, Putnam, Brewerton, Brandt, & Gold, 1990; Kolodner & Frances, 1993; North et al., 1993; Quimby & Putnam 1991; Ross, Anderson, Fleisher,

Table 2. Prevalence of DSM-III-R Dissociative Disorders in the General Population[a]

Diagnosis	Percentage of respondents positive
Psychogenic amnesia	6.0
Psychogenic fugue	0.2
Depersonalization disorder	2.8
Multiple personality disorder	3.0
Dissociative disorder not otherwise specified	0.2
A dissociative disorder of some kind	12.2

[a]N = 502.

& Norton, 1991a; Ross et al., 1992d; Vanderlinden, 1993). Dissociation is much more common in clinical populations than in the general population across a wide spectrum of settings and diagnostic categories, just as anxiety and mood symptoms are encountered at elevated levels throughout the mental health field.

Future research into the treatment implications of dissociative comorbidity will likely yield powerful predictors of differential treatment responses by highly dissociative subjects (Ross, 1989, 1992). This may be the case in eating disorders (Demitrack et al., 1990; Vanderlinden, 1993), substance abuse (Kolodner & Frances, 1993; Ross et al., 1992d), and a wide range of different diagnostic categories.

The factor structure of the DES in clinical populations appears to be similar to that in the general population, with the item scores and overall scores being elevated and the distribution of scores therefore shifted right compared with nonclinical samples.

Epidemiology of Dissociative Disorders in Clinical Populations

In two studies published to date surveying general adult psychiatric inpatients with the DES and DDIS, previously undiagnosed DID was found in 5% of subjects in Winnipeg (Ross et al., 1991a) and 4% of subjects in Boston (Saxe et al., 1993). The frequency of the dissociative disorders overall in the two studies was 20.7% in Winnipeg and 15% in Boston.

In a sample of 100 chemical dependency subjects in Winnipeg, 43 reported a history of childhood physical and/or sexual abuse, while 39 met DDIS criteria for a dissociative disorder, including 14 with DID (Ross et al., 1992d). Kolodner and Frances (1993) found 13 cases of DID and 13 cases of DDNOS in a chemical dependency population in the Washington, DC area. Other studies reporting clinical detection of DID and other dissociative disorders have not used standardized measures (Bliss & Jeppsen, 1985; Putnam, Loewenstein, Silberman, & Post, 1984)

Based on screening studies to date, it appears that the minimum rate of undiagnosed DID in severely disturbed clinical populations such as general psychiatric inpatients is 5% (Ross et al., 1991a; Saxe et al., 1993). Given the likelihood that other subjects with DDNOS or other dissociative disorders are likely to have undiagnosed DID as well (Boon & Draijer, 1993), the actual rate may be in the range of 15 to 20% in chemical dependency inpatients, general adult psychiatric inpatients, and similar groups. The prevalence of all of the dissociative disorders combined in these populations appears to be at least 20%.

If these findings are replicated and accepted, the differential diagnosis and management of dissociative disorders will become part of daily mainstream clinical practice.

CONCLUSIONS

The history of the dissociative disorders, with a peak of interest in the late nineteenth century, then almost complete suppression of serious study for most of the twentieth century prior to an exponential upsurge in interest in the 1980s, is unique in the mental health field. The field shifted from a prescientific to a scientific state in the second half of the 1980s, and it should be a mainstream component of psychiatry and psychology by the end of the century. The resurgence in interest occurred against political and ideological resistance.

Studies in North America, Japan, and Europe with a variety of standardized measures and structured interviews have confirmed a stable, core set of symptoms for the most complex dissociative disorder: DID. The ability of structured interviews to differentiate DID from DDNOS and borderline personality disorder has been demonstrated, and preliminary evidence of the prevalence of dissociative symptoms and disorders in clinical populations and the general population is available.

The dissociative disorders as a group appear to have a lifetime prevalence of about 10% in the general population in North America, including a prevalence of about 1% for DID. These figures are expected to vary from country to country based on differential rates of chronic childhood trauma and cultural factors. Dissociative comorbidity may prove to be a powerful predictor of differential treatment response in a variety of clinical populations.

REFERENCES

Altrocchi, J. (1992). "We don't have that problem here": MPD in New Zealand. *Dissociation, 5*, 109-110.

American Psychiatric Association (1980). *Diagnostic and statistical manual of mental disorders* (3rd ed.). Washington, DC: Author.

American Psychiatric Association (1993). *DSM-IV draft criteria*. Washington, DC: Author.

Bagley, C., & King, K. (1990). *Child sexual abuse*. New York: Tavistock/Routledge.

Berger, D., Saito, S., Ono, Y., Tezuka, I., Shirahase, J., Kuboki, T., & Suematsu, H. (1992). Dissociative symptomatology in an eating disorder cohort in Japan. Paper presented at the Japanese Stress Science Conference, Tokyo.

Bernstein, E. M., & Putnam, F. W. (1986). Development, reliability, and validity of a dissociation scale. *Journal of Nervous and Mental Disease, 174*, 727-735.

Binet, A. (1977a). *Alterations of personality*. Washington, DC: University Publications of America. (Original work published in 1896)

Binet, A. (1977b). *On double consciousness*. Washington, DC: University Publications of America. (Original work published in 1890)

Bliss, E. L., & Jeppsen, E. A. (1985). Prevalence of multiple personality among inpatients and outpatients. *American Journal of Psychiatry, 142*, 250-251.

Boon, S., & Draijer, N. (1993). *Multiple personality disorder in the Netherlands*. Amsterdam: Swets & Zeitlinger.

Bowman, E. (1993). Clinical and spiritual effects of exorcism in 15 patients with MPD. In B. G. Braun & J. Parks (Eds.), *Proceedings of the 10th international conference on multiple personality/dissociative states*, (p. 79). Chicago: Rush.

Braun, B. G. (1986). Issues in the psychotherapy of multiple personality disorder. In B. G. Braun (Ed.), *Treatment of multiple personality disorder* (pp. 1-28). Washington, DC: American Psychiatric Press.

Bremner, J. D., Steinberg, M., Southwick, S. M., Johnson, D. R., & Charney, D. S. (1993). Use of the structured clinical interview for DSM-IV dissociative disorders for systematic assessment of dissociative symptoms in posttraumatic stress disorder. *American Journal of Psychiatry, 150*, 1011-1014.

Breuer, J., & Freud, S. (1986). *Studies on hysteria*. New York: Pelican Books. (Original work published in 1895.)

Carlson, E. B., Putnam, F. W., Ross, C. A., Torem, M., Coons, P., Dill, D. L., Loewenstein, R. J., & Braun, B. G. (1993). Validity of the dissociative experiences scale in screening for multiple personality disorder: A multicenter study. *American Journal of Psychiatry, 150*, 1030-1036.

Chu, J. A., & Dill, D. L. (1990). Dissociative symptoms in relation to childhood physical and sexual abuse. *American Journal of Psychiatry, 147*, 887-892.

Coons, P. M. (1992). Dissociative disorder not otherwise specified: A clinical investigation of 50 cases with suggestions for typology and treatment. *Dissociation, 5*, 187-195.

Coons, P. M., Bowman, E. S., Kluft, R. P., & Milstein, V. (1991). The cross-cultural occurence of MPD: Additional cases from a recent survey. *Dissociation, 4*, 124-128.

Crabtree, A. (1985). *Multiple man: Explorations in possession and multiple personality*. Toronto: Collins.

Demitrack, M. A., Putnam, F. W., Brewerton, T. D., Brandt, H. A., & Gold, P. W. (1990). Relation of clinical variables to dissociative phenomena in treating disorders. *American Journal of Psychiatry, 147*, 1184-1188.

Eliade, M. (1964). *Shamanism*. Princeton: Princeton University Press.

Ellenberger, H. (1970). *The discovery of the unconscious*. New York: Basic Books.

Fink, D. (1991). The comorbidity of multiple personality disorder and DSM-III-R Axis I disorders. *Psychiatric Clinics of North America, 14*, 547-566.

Fink, D., & Golinkoff, M. (1990). Multiple personality disorder, borderline personality disorder, and schizophrenia. *Dissociation, 3*, 127-134.

Frankel, F. H. (1990). Hypnotizability and dissociation. *American Journal of Psychiatry, 147*, 823-829.

Fraser, G. A., & Raine, D. A. (1992). Cost analysis of the treatment of multiple personality disorders. In B. G. Braun (Ed.), *Proceedings of the ninth international conference on multiple personality/dissociative states*. Chicago: Rush.

Frischholtz, E. J., Braun, B. G., Sachs, G. R., Hopkins, L., Shaeffer, D. M., Lewis, J., Leavitt, F., Pasquotto, J. N., & Schwartz, D. R. (1990). The dissociative experiences scale: Further replication and validation. *Dissociation, 3*, 151-153.

Frischholtz, E. J., Braun, B. G., Sachs, R. G., Schwartz, D. R., Lewis, J., Schaeffer, D., Westergaard, C., & Pasquotto, J. (1991). Construct validity of the dissociative experiences scale (DES): 1. The relationship between the DES and other self report instruments. *Dissociation, 4*, 185-188.

Goettman, C., Greaves, G. B., & Coons, P. (1994). *Multiple personality and dissociation 1791-1992: A complete bibliography*. Atlanta, GA: Greaves.

Gunderson, J. G., & Sabo, A. N. (1993). The phenomenological and conceptual interface between borderline personality disorder and PTSD. *American Journal of Psychiatry, 150*, 19-27.

Hilgard, E. R. (1987). Multiple personality and dissociation. In *Psychology in America: A historical survey* (pp. 303-315). San Diego: Harcourt Brace Jovanovich.

Horevitz, R. P., & Braun, B. G. (1984). Are multiple personalities borderline? *Psychiatric Clinics of North America, 7*, 69-87.

James, W. (1983). *The principles of psychology*. Cambridge: Harvard University Press. (Original work published in 1890)

Janet, P. (1965). *The major symptoms of hysteria*. New York: Hafner. (Original work published in 1907)

Janet, P. (1977). *The mental state of hystericals*. Washington, DC: University Publications of America. (Original work published in 1901)

Jung, C. G. (1977). On the psychology and pathology of so-called occult phenomena. In *Psychology and the occult* (pp. 6-91). Princeton: Princeton University Press. (Original work published in 1902)

Kaplan, H. I., Freedman, A. M., & Sadock, B. J. (1980). *Comprehensive textbook of psychiatry/III*. Baltimore: Williams & Wilkins.

Kluft, R. P. (1993). Multiple personality disorders. In D. Spiegel (Ed.), *Dissociative disorders: A clinical review* (pp. 17-44). Lutherville, MD: Sidran Press.

Kolodner, G., & Frances, R. (1993). Recognizing dissociative disorders in patients with chemical dependency. *Hospital and Community Psychiatry, 44*, 1041-1043.

Kuhn, T. (1962). *The structure of scientific revolutions*. Chicago: University of Chicago.

Loewenstein, R. J. (1993). Psychogenic amnesia and psychogenic fugue. In D. Spiegel (Ed.), *Dissociative disorders: A clinical review* (pp. 45-78). Lutherville, MD: Sidran Press.

Macilwain, I. F. (1992). Multiple personality disorder (letter). *British Journal of Psychiatry, 161*, 863.

MacMillan, H., & Thomas, B. H. (1993). Public health home nurse visitation for the tertiary prevention of child maltreatment: Results of a pilot study. *Canadian Journal of Psychiatry, 38*, 436-442.

Martinez-Taboas, A. (1989). Preliminary observations on MPD in Puerto Rico. *Dissociation, 2*, 128-134.

Modestin, J. (1992). Multiple personality disorder in Switzerland. *American Journal of Psychiatry, 149*, 88-92.

Myers, F. W. H. (1920). *Human personality and its survival of bodily death*. London: Longman's, Green and Company.

Nemiah, J. C. (1989). Janet redivivus: The centenary of *L'automatisme psychologique*. *American Journal of Psychiatry, 146*, 1527-1529.

Nemiah, J. C. (1993). Dissociation, conversion, and somatization. In D. Spiegel (Ed.), *Dissociative disorders: A clinical review* (pp. 104-116). Lutherville, MD: Sidran Press.

North, C. S., Ryal, J. E., Ricci, D. A., & Wetzel, R. D. (1993). *Multiple personalities, multiple disorders*. New York: Oxford University Press.

Oesterreich, T. K. (1974). *Possession demoniacal and other*. Secaucus, NJ: Citadel Press. (Original work published 1921)

Prince, M. (1978). *The dissociation of a personality*. New York: Oxford University Press. (Original work published in 1905)

Putnam, F. W. (1989). *Diagnosis and treatment of multiple personality disorder*. New York: Guilford Publications.

Putnam, F. W. (1993). Dissociative phenomena. In D. Spiegel (Ed.), *Dissociative disorders: A clinical review* (pp. 1-16). Lutherville, MD: Sidran Press.

Putnam, F. W., Loewenstein, R. J., Silberman, E. K., & Post, R. M. (1984). Multiple personality disorder in a hospital setting. *Journal of Clinical Psychiatry, 45*, 172-175.

Quimby, L. G., & Putnam, F. W. (1991). Dissociative symptoms and aggression in a state mental hospital. *Dissociation, 4*, 21-24.

Ross, C. A. (1985). DSM-III: Problems in diagnosing partial forms of multiple personality disorder. *Journal of the Royal Society of Medicine, 75*, 933-936.

Ross, C. A. (1989). *Multiple personality disorder. Diagnosis, clinical features, and treatment*. New York: John Wiley & Sons.

Ross, C. A. (1991). Epidemiology of multiple personality disorder and dissociation. *Psychiatric Clinics of North America, 14*, 503-518.

Ross, C. A. (1992). Childhood sexual abuse and psychobiology. *Journal of Child Sexual Abuse, 1*, 95-102.

Ross, C. A., & Dua, V. (1993). Psychiatric health care costs of multiple personality disorder. *American Journal of Psychotherapy, 47*, 103-112.

Ross, C. A., Heber, S., Norton, G. R., & Anderson, G. (1989a). Differences between multiple personality disorder and other diagnostic groups on structured interview. *Journal of Nervous and Mental Disease, 177*, 487-491.

Ross, C. A., Anderson, G., Heber, S., Norton, G. R., Anderson, B., del Campo, M., & Pillay, N. (1989b). Differentiating multiple personality disorder and complex partial seizures. *General Hospital Psychiatry, 11*, 54-58.

Ross, C. A., Heber, S., Norton, G. R., Anderson, G., Anderson, D., & Barchet, P. (1989c). The dissociative disorders interview schedule: A structured interview. *Dissociation, 2*, 169-189.

Ross, C. A., Norton, G. R., & Wozney, K. (1989d). Multiple personality disorder: An analysis of 236 cases. *Canadian Journal of Psychiatry, 34*, 413-418.

Ross, C. A., Ryan, L., Anderson, G., Ross, D., & Hardy, L. (1989e). Dissociative experiences in adolescents and college students. *Dissociation, 2*, 239-242.

Ross, C. A., Joshi, S., & Currie, R. (1990a). Dissociative experiences in the general population. *American Journal of Psychiatry, 147*, 1547-1552.

Ross, C. A., Miller, S. D., Reagor, P., Bjornson, L., Fraser, G. A., & Anderson, G. (1990b). Structured interview data on 102 cases of multiple personality disorder from four centers. *American Journal of Psychiatry, 147*, 596-601.

Ross, C. A., Ryan, L., Voigt, H., & Eide, L. (1990c). High and low dissociators in a college student population. *Dissociation, 3*, 147-151.

Ross, C. A., Anderson, G., Fleisher, W. P., & Norton, G. R. (1991a). The frequency of multiple personality disorder among psychiatric inpatients. *American Journal of Psychiatry, 148*, 1717-1720.

Ross, C. A., Joshi, S., & Currie, R. (1991b). Dissociative experiences in the general population: A factor analysis. *Hospital and Community Psychiatry, 42*, 297-301.

Ross, C. A., Anderson, G., Fleisher, W. P., & Norton, G. R. (1992a). Dissociative experiences among psychiatric inpatients. *General Hospital Psychiatry, 14*, 350-354.

Ross, C. A., Anderson, G., Fraser, G. A., Reagor, P., Bjornson, L., & Miller, S. D. (1992b). Differentiating multiple personality disorder and dissociative disorder not otherwise specified. *Dissociation, 5*, 88-91.

Ross, C. A., Ellason, J., & Fuchs, D. (1992c). Axis I and II comorbidity of MPD. In B. G. Braun & E. B. Carlson (Eds.), *Proceedings of the 9th international conference on multiple personality/dissociative states* (pp. 000). Chicago: Rush.

Ross, C. A., Kronson, J., Koensgen, S., Barkman, K., Clark, P., & Rockman, G. (1992d). Dissociative comorbidity in 100 chemically dependent patients. *Hospital and Community Psychiatry, 43*, 840-842.

Sainton, K., Ellason, J., Mayran, L., & Ross, C. A. (1993). Reliability of the new form of the Dissociative Experiences Scale (DES) and the Dissociation Questionnaire (DIS-Q). In B. G. Braun & J. Parks (Eds.), *Proceedings of the 10th international conference on multiple personality/dissociative states* (pp. 125). Chicago: Rush.

Sanders, B., McRoberts, G., & Tollefson, C. (1989). Childhood stress and dissociation in a college population. *Dissociation, 2*, 17-23.

Saxe, G. N., van der Kolk, B. A., Berkowitz, R., Chinman, G., Hall, K., Lieberg, G., & Schwartz, J. (1993). Dissociative disorders in psychiatric inpatients. *American Journal of Psychiatry, 150*, 1037-1042.

Schreiber, F. R. (1973). *Sybil*. Chicago: Henry Regnery.

Spiegel, D. (1993). Dissociation and trauma. In D. Spiegel (Ed.), *Dissociative disorders: A clinical review* (pp. 117-131). Lutherville, MD: Sidran Press.

Spitzer, R. L., Williams, J. B. W., & Gibbon, M. (1987). *Structured clinical interview for DSM-III-R (SCID)*. New York: New York State Psychiatric Institute, Biometrics Research.

Steinberg, M. (1993). The spectrum of depersonalization: Assessment and treatment. In D. Spiegel (Ed.), *Dissociative disorders: A clinical review* (pp. 79-103). Lutherville, MD: Sidran Press.

Steinberg, M., Rounsaville, B., & Cicchetti, D. V. (1990). The structured clinical interview for DSM-III-R dissociative disorders: Preliminary report on a new diagnostic instrument. *American Journal of Psychiatry, 147*, 76-82.

Thigpen, C. H., & Cleckley, H. M. (1957). *The three faces of Eve*. New York: McGraw-Hill.

van der Hart, O., & Friedman, B. (1989). A reader's guide to Pierre Janet on dissociation: A neglected intellectual heritage. *Dissociation, 2*, 3-16.

Vanderlinden, J. (1993). *Dissociative experiences, trauma and hypnosis*. Delft: Eburon Delft.

2

European Studies of Dissociation

Johan Vanderlinden, Onno Van der Hart, and Katalin Varga

INTRODUCTION

Apart from the Netherlands and Belgium, clinical interest and research in Europe in the field of dissociation and the dissociative disorders are lagging far behind North American developments. In most European countries, strong professional ignorance and skepticism still exist. After a brief description of the clinical field in Europe, in particular in the Netherlands and Belgium, the main focus of this chapter is on European studies on dissociation and dissociative disorders. Special attention is given to studies on the development of a scale for the assessment of dissociative experiences and symptoms and on the prevalence of these phenomena in both general populations and psychiatric patient samples.

DISSOCIATIVE DISORDERS IN EUROPE

While rapid developments are taking place in the field of the dissociative disorders in the Netherlands and Belgium, most other European countries are

Johan Vanderlinden • Department of Behavior Therapy, University Center St. Jozef, B-3070 Kortenberg, Belgium. **Onno Van der Hart** • Department of Clinical and Health Psychology, Utrecht University, and the Regional Institute for Ambulatory Mental Care, Amsterdam South/New West, The Netherlands. **Katalin Varga** • Department of Experimental Psychology, Eötvös Lorand University, Budapest, Hungary.

Handbook of Dissociation: Theoretical, Empirical, and Clinical Perspectives, edited by Larry K. Michelson and William J. Ray. Plenum Press, New York, 1996.

lagging far behind (cf. Van der Hart, 1993). Most clinicians are still ignorant of the phenomenology and treatment of dissociative disorders, and research is nonexistent. While in Britain official psychiatry exhibits a negative attitude, as is shown in some publications in the *British Journal of Psychiatry* (e.g., Fahy, 1988), there is nevertheless a growing number of therapists who are treating adult or child patients with dissociative identity disorder (DID) (e.g., Karle, 1992; Macilwain, 1992) and who are organizing themselves into an informal network. At the University of Warwick, Coventry, Dr. John S. Davis is carrying out a prevalence study using the Dissociative Experiences Scale (DES) and the Dissociative Disorders Interview Schedule (DDIS) on reported dissociative disorders. At the University College in London, Waller and colleagues are studying the prevalence of dissociative symptoms in eating disordered patients compared to non-eating disordered women (see Everill, Waller, & Macdonald, 1995). In Germany, until recently, DID was an almost completely unknown diagnostic category, although the general public was informed by the publication of a few translated biographies of DID patients. Since then, a few workshops on diagnosis and treatment of DID, given by Dutch clinicians, have had a snowball effect. A number of serious publications in women's magazines have attracted the attention of both the general public and psychotherapists. In 1995, Huber published the first German handbook on the treatment of DID (Huber, 1995). In Scandinavian countries, there are a few clinicians treating dissociative disorder patients, but professional ignorance is still strong. An important exception is the Rogaland Psychiatric Hospital in Stavanger, Norway, which is very active in the diagnosis and treatment of dissociative disorders. Currently, a prevalence study using the DES and the SCID-D is being carried out in this hospital.

In Switzerland, a study has been carried out about how frequently DID is diagnosed. Modestin (1992) sent all qualified Swiss psychiatrists a questionnaire on DID along with the *Diagnostic and Statistical Manual of Mental Disorders*, 3rd edition (DSM-III) description of MPD and three classical nineteenth-century case examples. Thirty-nine percent of the 770 respondents reported they had not known the concept of DID before the present study. Three percent reported that they were treating or examining one or more patients meeting DSM-III criteria for DID. Ten percent indicated that they had seen DID at least once during their professional career. Modestin concluded that MPD is relatively rare. However, with more refined and updated information on DID phenomenology, he would probably have found a higher prevalence. His study falls very short of the serious prevalence studies in North America, Belgium, the Netherlands, and Norway, where validated diagnostic instruments such as the Structured Clinical Interview for DSM-III-R Dissociative Disorders (SCID-D) and the DDIS are used.

In Italy, Dalle Grave and colleagues are doing promising work studying the prevalence of dissociative symptoms using the Dissociation Questionnaire (DIS-Q) in a large sample of eating-disordered people and college students (Dalle Grave, Rigamonti, & Todisco, in press) at the hospital Casajdi Cura in Garda. Meanwhile, at the University of Padua Institute of Clinical Psychiatry, Favaro and Santonastaso are studying the prevalence of dissociative symptoms in a student population sample (Favaro & Santonastaso, 1995). At the University of Madrid in Spain, Iconan and Orengo-Garcia are planning a validation study of the DES.

In most other European countries, much less can be reported. However, there is an increase of information exchange between clinicians and researchers in different countries, resulting, at least in Hungary, in a prevalence study on dissociative experiences having been carried out.

THE NETHERLANDS

In the Netherlands, interest in the dissociative disorders developed in the early 1980s and was fostered and furthered by workshops on diagnosis and treatment presented by North American specialists in the field, notably Drs. Bennett G. Braun, Richard P. Kluft, and Roberta Sachs. Van der Hart (1991) reported on 60 DID patients being treated in the Netherlands. Since then, Boon and Draijer (1993a,b) have been able to get collaboration for their study of 71 Dutch DID patients treated by 60 clinicians. Van der Hart (1993) subsequently estimated that roughly 400 DID patients were treated by 250 clinicians in the Netherlands.

The prominence of the Netherlands in the dissociative disorders field in Europe was exemplified by the fact that the International Conference on Multiple Personality Disorder and Dissociative States, with 465 participants, was held in Amsterdam, May 21-23, 1992 and again May 11-13, 1995, with more than 500 participants. Currently, there is a lot of media interest in DID. An increasing number of mental health institutions are providing treatment for DID patients. A few outpatient institutions have their own dissociative disorders teams, and the first inpatient DID unit has recently been opened.

Clinical Studies

In the Netherlands and the Flemish part of Belgium, a number of clinical studies on diagnosis and treatment have been published (e.g., Boon & Van der Hart, 1988a,b), 1989; Nijenhuis, 1994, 1995; Van der Hart, 1991). In 1991, Van der Hart edited a book on trauma, dissociation, and hypnosis, which was widely read by a professional audience and, due to his success, reprinted in 1995. Noteworthy in these works is the return of the eminent French philosopher and psychiatrist Pierre Janet (1859-1947) to the pioneering clinical and theoretical studies on trauma and dissociation (cf. Van der Hart, 1986, 1988; Van der Hart & Horst, 1989). Around the turn of the century, Janet (1889, 1898, 1907, 1919) was probably the first author to systematically study the relationship between traumatic experiences and dissociation in the etiology of a wide range of psychiatric problems, including the DSM-III-R dissociative disorders and eating disorders. Janet's old definition of hysteria (i.e., the dissociative disorders) seems to be as important today as it was a century ago:

> A form of mental depression characterized by the retraction of the field of personal consciousness and a tendency to the dissociation and emancipation of the systems of ideas and functions that constitute personality. (Janet, 1907, p. 332)

Janet's descriptions and analyses of traumatic experiences, traumatic memories, and the transformation of traumatic memories into narrative memories serve as important guidelines for modern treatment approaches of severely traumatized patients. International cooperation has produced a number of English-language publications showing the importance of Janet's pioneering observations and notions to an international professional audience (cf. Van der Hart & Friedman, 1989; Van der Hart, Brown, & Van der Kolk, 1989; Van der Hart, Brown, & Turco, 1990; Van der Hart & Horst, 1989; Van der Hart, Steele, Boon, & Brown, 1993a; Van der Hart, Witztum, & Friedman, 1993b; Van der Kolk & Van der Hart, 1989, 1991).

Empirical Studies

In a survey of sexual abuse of girls by relatives, Draijer (1988, 1990) found in a representative sample of 1054 women that 15.6% reported childhood sexual abuse by relatives. She concluded that such abuse is much more common than is usually believed. Draijer found indications that those women who were probably most severely abused were the least able to provide information about it. These women presented symptoms indicating the existence of a dissociative disorder.

Ensink and Van Otterloo (1989) validated a Dutch version of the DES (Bernstein & Putnam, 1986). In a study of 100 women having been sexually abused in childhood, Ensink (1992), using among other scales the DES (Bernstein & Putnam, 1986), found that more than one third (36%) gained scores as high as patients with DID. A cutoff score on the DES of 30 was used (F. W. Putnam, personal communication, 1990). Ensink found that a high level of dissociation (>30 on the DES) tended to be reported by: (1) women having a childhood history of sexual abuse during which they feared they would be killed; (2) women who as children were subjected to group rapes in which unknown perpetrators were involved; (3) women who were sexually abused as children at the hands of multiple perpetrators; (4) women who were physically assaulted as children by the perpetrator before the sexual abuse started; (5) women who as children experienced physical aggression associated with sexual abuse for a considerable amount of time; and (6) women whose mothers were involved in the sexual abuse. A multiple regression analysis showed four characteristics significantly contributing to the level of dissociation: (1) cumulation of childhood trauma; (2) age at onset of sexual abuse; (3) physical aggression preceding sexual abuse; and (4) being forced to have sexual contact with unknown perpetrators.

In a prevalence study on 160 psychiatric inpatients, Draijer and Langeland (1993) found that at least 5% of this group suffered from DID, a finding that is remarkably similar to North American findings (Ross, Anderson, Fleisher, & Norton, 1991b; Saxe et al., 1993). These and other findings indicate that, contrary to some opinions voiced in Europe (e.g., Aldridge-Morris, 1989), DID is *not* a North American culture-bound phenomenon, but probably occurs as often in Europe as in North America. Findings of Boon and Draijer (1993b) on the characteristics of DID patients in the Netherlands indicate also that the phenomenology of European and North American DID patients is similar. In harmony with North American findings on DID patients (Ross, 1989), Cohen, Wallage, and Van der Hart (1992) found in 80 successive referrals to a Regional Institute for Ambulatory Mental Health Care that their DES scores correlated highly with reports on somatic complaints for which no physical cause could be found, which the authors regarded as mainly dissociative in nature. This result seems to support the fact that in the *ICD-10 Classification of Mental and Behavioural Disorders* (World Health Organization, 1992) conversion disorders are classified as dissociative disorders of movement and sensation.

In 1993, Boon and Draijer published their findings on a large study of the reliability and validity of the SCID-D (Steinberg, Rounsaville, & Cichetti, 1990), a diagnostic instrument for the assessment of dissociative disorders (Boon & Draijer, 1993a,b). Several parts of this study were published before (Boon & Draijer, 1991). Besides the SCID-D, two other instruments were employed: the DES (Bernstein & Putnam, 1986) and the Structured Trauma Interview (STI) (Draijer, 1990). First, a pilot study carried out in 44 patients showed an interrater reliability of 97.7% for the SCID-D. Ninety patients (45 with a dissociative disorder and 45 with another psychiatric diagnosis) participated in the main study designed to validate the SCID-D. All diagnoses of dissociative disorders by clinicians were confirmed by the SCID-D. In the control condition, the diagnosis of a dissociative disorder was excluded in 43 cases. In two cases (both diagnosed as borderline personality disorder only), the diagnosis of a dissociative disorder was detected with the SCID-D. The validity of the SCID-D was assessed for total score and severity of specific dissociative symptoms. Overall ANOVA results showed a significant difference among the two groups ($p < .0001$) at all levels of assessment. Patients with a dissociative disorder reported a cluster of severe and chronic dissociative symptoms, while patients without a dissociative disorder reported only minor dissociative symptoms, mainly associated with episodes of stress or depression, psychosis or mania. These findings caused Boon and Draijer (1993b) to remark that it is no longer acceptable to conceptualize dissociation on a continuum: dissociative symptoms in patients with dissociative disorders are qualitatively different and much more severe compared to dissociative symptoms in patients without a dissociative disorder.

Besides the SCID-D scores, Boon and Draijer (1993b) also compared the DES scores between the two groups. Patients with a dissociative disorder gained a significantly higher score on the DES: their mean DES score was 47.6 (SD = 16.3; range, 11.6–81.3). Patients without a dissociative disorder had a mean DES score of 12.0 (SD = 11.4; range, 0.0–38.6). A high Pearson correlation of .78 was found between the DES and total SCID-D score, a finding further supporting the congruent validity of the SCID-D. Boon and Draijer (1993b) also studied the utility of the Dutch version of the DES as a screening instrument to discriminate between patients with and without dissociative disorder. They found that a cutoff score of 25 yielded a good-to-excellent sensitivity and specificity. In spite of these optimistic results, Boon and Draijer (1993b) remarked that a clinical assessment or the use of a standardized interview such as the SCID-D is required in order to diagnose the presence or absence of a dissociative disorder.

Their study of the clinical phenomenomogy of the DID patients showed that 94.4% of these patients reported a history of childhood physical and/or sexual abuse, and 80% met criteria for posttraumatic stress disorder. Investigating the relationship between traumatic experiences and dissociative symptoms and disorders, Boon and Draijer (1993b) found that the childhood traumatic experiences were significantly more prevalent and severe in dissociative disorder patients than in patients without a dissociative disorder. These findings confirmed research data from other researchers in the Netherlands (Ensink, 1992): The severity of the dissociative symptoms was closely related to the severity of childhood trauma, especially sexual abuse, together with the age at which the trauma started. The younger the age of the patient at which the abuse started, the more severe the dissociative symptoms.

Boon and Draijer (1993b) concluded that the SCID-D is a reliable and valid diagnostic instrument to make an assessment of dissociative symptoms and dissociative disorders. They remarked:

> Although the clinical awareness of MPD is growing rapidly in the Netherlands, this diagnostic category deserves more systematic attention to prevent MPD patients from spending years in the mental health system, without appropriate treatment. Screening for dissociative pathology should become an integral part of routine diagnostic assessment. (Boon & Draijer, 1993b, pp. 269–270)

Recently, Nijenhuis, Spinhoven, Van Dyck, Van der Hart and Vanderlinden (1995), starting from clinically observed (dissociative) state-dependent somatoform phenomena, have developed the 20-item Somatoform Dissociation Questionnaire (SDQ-20). Statistical analyses revealed that the items were strongly scalable on a unidimensional scale and that the reliability was high. Further analyses derived five items (SDQ-5) that yielded optimal sensitivity (94%; capacity of a test to select true positives; here dissociative disorder cases) and specificity (96%; capacity to select true negatives; here cases with other DSM-IV diagnoses). Trying to explain some of these somatoform dissociative phenomena and the widely divergent psychophysiological reactions that are displayed in various dissociative states, Nijenhuis and Vanderlinden (1996) drew an analogy between animal defensive states and human dissociative states. Animal defense is of radical different topography, depending on the stage of imminence. For example, while in the postencounter (with a predator) stage tone, freezing behavior is functional; in the circa-strike stage development of analgesia and the recuperative post-strike stage return of pain perception are adaptive responses. Interestingly, the SDQ-items for a substantial part relate to inability to move, analgesia, anesthesia, and pain. According to Nijenhuis (1994, 1995), exposure to severe threat constitutes a classical conditioning procedure, in which various stages of imminence (unconditioned stimuli) automatically evoke particular evolutionary prepared defensive states (unconditioned responses), which will be associated with salient stimuli that signal or refer to threat. These conditioned stimuli ("triggers") will posttraumatically re-elicit representations of the traumatic event and, by consequence, the defensive states of relevance. Nijenhuis (1994, 1995) further argues that posttraumatic confrontations between states that are "loaded" with trauma and states that are not, also constitute classical conditioning procedures. These internal exposures to threat are aversive, and may cause a *phobia for traumatic memories*, and a *phobia for dissociative states* that encompass these representations and associated defensive reactions. Both phobias maintain dissociative responding; functional defenses thus may turn into pathology.

THE DISSOCIATION QUESTIONNAIRE STUDIES IN BELGIUM

Development of the Dissocation Questionnaire

Encouraged by the interesting pioneering work of Bernstein and Putnam (1986) and because a European dissociation questionnaire was lacking (sociocultural factors may play an important role in the experience of dissociative phenomena), Vanderlinden and colleagues decided to construct their own dissociation questionnaire (DIS-Q) (Vanderlinden, Van Dyck, Vertommen, & Vandereycken, 1992b; Vanderlinden, Van Dyck, Vandereycken, Vertommen, & Verkes, 1993a) (see Appendix).

Method

The item pool has been based (1) on statements by patients with dissociative disorders and (2) on a selection of items of the three existing dissociation questionnaires [DES, Perceptual Alteration Scale (PAS), and Questionnaire of Experiences of Dissociation (QED)]. After translation into Dutch, the latter items were reformulated and modified to make them more suitable to the sociocultural situation in Belgium and the Netherlands. In this way a pool of 95 items was composed. These items were submitted to five clinicians (both psychologists and psychiatrists) who had experience in dealing with dissociative disorder, with the request to evaluate to which extent each item reflected something about a dissociative experience. Based on their responses, 26 items were eliminated and 69 items were retained.

Five different answer categories were chosen: the subjects had to circle one of the five numbers, indicating to what extent that item or statement is applicable to that particular subject (1 = not at all; 2 = a little bit; 3 = moderately; 4 = quite a bit; 5 = extremely). While using the DES questionnaire, it was learned that some patients found it difficult to answer the items of the DES by making a slash on a 100-mm line to indicate the percentage of time they experienced this particular experience. Therefore, it was decided to use another way of answering the items in the DIS-Q. All DIS-Q scores are average scores and can vary between 1 and 5. The DIS-Q also gathers data on the age, sex, educational level, and demographic status of the subject involved and contains a small trauma list. Subjects are asked "if they remember having experienced severely damaging or life-threatening experiences." When this question is positively answered, subjects are asked to describe the kind of trauma of which several possibilities are given: severe bodily injury, state of war, sexual abuse by family and nonfamily members, serious emotional maltreatment by parents, and so forth.

Factor Analysis of the DIS-Q

The DIS-Q was first administered to a representative sample of the population (n = 374) (Vanderlinden, Van Dyck, Vandereycken & Vertommen, 1991). A factor analysis was performed on the scores of the total sample and four subscales were detected, which together accounted for 77% of the common variance: (1) *identity confusion-fragmentation* (referring to experiences of derealization and depersonalization); (2) *loss of control* over behavior, thoughts, and emotions (referring to experiences of losing control over behavior, thoughts, and emotions); (3) *amnesia* (referring to experiences of memory lacunas); and (4) *absorption* (referring to experiences of enhanced concentration, which are supposed to play an important role in hypnosis). Since then, several other factor analytic studies have been carried out on different subject samples: on a second representative subject sample from the Dutch population (N = 378) and on a group of psychiatric patients with mixed diagnoses ($N = 261$) (Vanderlinden, 1993; Vanderlinden et al., 1993a). After rotation, again the four-factor solution turned out to most adequately represent the underlying latent structure in the DIS-Q data of both samples. An iterative Gulliksen item analysis was performed on the items with a Pearson r of more than .30, and not a single item has been eliminated.

Reliability and Validity Studies of the DIS-Q

The Cronbach's alpha coefficients showed that the DIS-Q has a good internal consistency: .96 for the total scale and .94, .93, .88, and .67 for the four subscales. Test-retest reliability was measured by giving the DIS-Q to a group of 50 subjects randomly selected from the general population (25 adolescents and 25 adults) on two occasions with an interval of 3 to 4 weeks. The DIS-Q total score test-retest reliability coefficient is .94 ($p < .0001$) and, respectively, .92, .92, .93, and .75 for the four subscales. These results show that the DIS-Q scores are stable over time. Next, the DIS-Q was administered to different psychiatric patient samples (diagnosed following DSM-III-R criteria): dissociative disorders [DID ($n = 30$) and dissociative disorder not otherwise specified (DDNOS) ($n = 23$)]; posttraumatic stress disorder ($n = 13$); schizophrenics ($n = 31$); eating disorders ($n = 98$); obsessive-compulsive disorders ($n = 29$); and borderline personality disorder ($n = 17$) (see Table 1).

A one-way analysis of variance (ANOVA) on the scores of the different groups showed highly significant differences between the groups for the total DIS-Q scores ($DF = 7, 618$; $F = 133{,}50$; $p < .0001$) and subscale scores ($p < .0001$). To compare the DIS-Q scores of the different psychiatric categories, the Bonferroni procedure for multiple comparisons was done (alpha was set at $p < .05$): the results showed that the DID subgroup gained a significantly higher score than all other psychiatric categories. Pearson r correlations have been assessed between the DES and DIS-Q in a sample of 100 psychiatric patients and the results strongly supported the con-

Table 1. Mean and SD of DIS-Q Scores among Normal Subjects and Several Patient Groups

		DIS-Q total		DIS-Q1[a]		DIS-Q2		DIS-Q3		DIS-Q4	
	N	Mean	SD	Mean	SD	Mean	SD	Mean	SD	Mean	SD
Normals	378	1.5	0.4	1.4	0.4	1.7	0.5	1.4	0.4	1.9	0.6
Obsessive-compulsive	29	2.0	0.5	2.0	0.8	2.1	0.5	1.5	0.4	2.4	0.7
Schizophrenics	31	2.0	0.6	2.0	0.7	2.1	0.6	1.9	0.6	2.5	0.8
Eating disorders	98	2.2	0.5	2.4	0.6	2.4	0.6	1.6	0.5	2.7	0.7
PTSD[b]	13	2.7	0.6	2.8	0.9	3.0	0.7	2.3	0.4	2.4	0.4
BPD	32	2.8	0.6	2.8	0.8	3.1	0.6	2.3	0.7	2.8	0.6
DDNOS	23	2.9	0.6	3.0	0.8	3.1	0.7	2.5	0.8	2.7	0.9
DID	30	3.5	0.4	3.8	0.5	3.2	0.5	3.3	0.6	3.1	0.5

[a]DIS-Q1, identity confusion; DIS-Q2, loss of control; DIS-Q3, amnesia; DIS-Q4, absorption.
[b]PTSD, posttraumatic stress disorder; DDNOS, dissociative disorder not otherwise specified; BPD, borderline personality disorder; DID, Dissociative Identity Disorder.

struct validity of both the DES and DIS-Q ($r = .85$ between the total DES and DIS-Q scores).

Recently the reliability and validity of the DIS-Q have also been studied in a North American setting (Sainton, Ellason, Mayran, and Ross, 1993). The DIS-Q and DES were administered to subjects with a clinical diagnosis of DID (n = 87), inpatients with a primary chemical dependency diagnosis (n = 26), and undergraduate students (n = 83). Cronbach's alpha of the DIS-Q was above .90 in all three subject groups. The Pearson correlation between DES and DIS-Q was .87 ($p <$ .0001). Even more important was the fact that the average DIS-Q scores of American undergraduate students and DID patients closely resembled the average scores of European students and DID patients: respectively, 1.79 (SD = 0.58) versus 1.70 (SD = 0.50) for the students and 3.63 (SD = 0.58) versus 3.5 (SD = 0.4) for the DID patients (see also Table 1). Sainton et al. (1993) concluded that no other area of psychiatry has produced self-report measures with greater reliability and validity than the DES and the DIS-Q.

The present findings show that the DIS-Q has (1) a clear factorial structure; (2) a good-to-excellent internal consistency and test-retest reliablity; (3) differentiates clearly between patients with dissociative disorder and other subjects; and (4) has good construct validity. Moreover, recent data (Sainton et al., 1993) show that the DIS-Q can be assumed to be a valid measure of dissociation also in North America.

Dissociative Experiences in the General Population

First Study in Belgium and the Netherlands

Subjects. In a first study, the DIS-Q was sent to 500 subjects in the Netherlands and to 300 Flemish subjects in Belgium (see also Vanderlinden et al., 1991). In all, 374 questionnaires were collected (235 Dutch and 139 Flemish subjects), showing an almost perfect male-female ratio: 119 (50.6%) men versus 116 (49.6%) women in the Dutch sample and 69 (49.6%) men versus 70 (50.4%) women in the Flemish sample. The sample was representative in terms of sex and educational level, but not fully representative for the variables of marital status and age distribution.

Results. First, the specific effect of several variables on the DIS-Q scores, such as age, sex, demographic status, marital status, and nationality, was studied by means of ANOVA. Whenever the ANOVA was significant, two-tailed t-tests of Scheffe's were done. The average item result (mean ± SD) for the total scale was 1.61 ± 0.40. With regard to the total DIS-Q score, it was found that age is the only variable having a significant effect on the scores (DF = 1, $F = 30.89, p < .0001$). These results confirmed Ross' findings (Ross & Ryan 1989; Ross, Joshi, & Currie, 1990, 1991a), indicating that dissociative experiences decline with age. Significant differences ($p < .05$) were found between subjects aged 10-20 years and subjects aged 40-50 and > 60 years. With regard to the DIS-Q subscale scores, it was found that only the subscale loss of control significantly ($p < .05$) declined with age. The decline of dissociative experiences with age in the general population seemed to be mainly related to the scores on the subscale loss of control.

No differences were found between men and women for the total DIS-Q score (1.66 ± 0.45 for men versus 1.60 ± 0.37 for women). Educational level, nationality, and marital status had no significant effect on the DIS-Q scores.

Prevalence of Dissociative Symptoms. To study the prevalence of dissociative experiences in the general population, first a cutoff score for the total DIS-Q score was assessed: The scores of the normal sample (*N* = 374) were compared with the scores of a patient group with dissociative disorders (*N* = 53). When a cutoff score of 2.5 was used, an excellent sensitivity (the ability to correctly identify true positive cases or subjects with dissociative disorder) and specificity (ability to correctly identify true negative cases or subjects without dissociative disorder) was detected: sensitivity was 91% and specificity 97%. These data indicated that 11 subjects or 2.94% of the total sample reported serious dissociative experiences. In this group, four subjects (1.06% of the total sample) had DIS-Q scores as high as the scores of patients with DID, suggesting that they, too, had a severe dissociative disorder. Next, several characteristics of this group with scores above 2.5 on the DIS-Q were analyzed (*N* = 11). With regard to the sex of these subjects, a surprising finding was that the majority were men (7 men vs. 4 women) in both groups (Flemish and Dutch sample). This finding is in contrast with some earlier data from the literature on the prevalence of DID, indicating a male–female ratio of 1:9 (cf. Ross, Norton, & Wozney, 1989). Six subjects were Flemish, five Dutch, seven subjects were married, three single, and one divorced; the mean age was 34. The subjects had very different educational levels.

Second Study in the Netherlands

Method. Within the framework of further standardization and validation, the DIS-Q was sent to a second representative sample (*N* = 1000) of the Dutch population (Vanderlinden, Van Dyck, Vandereycken & Vertommen, 1993c). Besides studying the prevalence of dissociative experiences, this study was also aimed at exploring the relationship between self-reported trauma experiences (reported on the small trauma list of the DIS-Q) and dissociative symptoms of the subjects involved. It was assumed that subjects reporting a history of sexual abuse [such as rape or unwanted sexual experiences by nonfamily members and/or by relatives (incest)], would indicate a higher prevalence of dissociative symptoms, as compared with all other subjects. Hence, it was decided to compare three groups: subjects reporting no history of abuse (nontrauma group), subjects reporting sexual abuse (major trauma group), and all other trauma categories (minor trauma group).

Data analysis consisted of deriving descriptive statistics and mean plus standard deviation values for the several subscale scores of the DIS-Q. First, an ANOVA was done to study the effect of the different variables on the DIS-Q scores. Next *t*-tests were performed to compare the trauma versus the nontrauma group. To evaluate the effects of the traumatic experience (minor vs. major trauma) on the different variables of the four questionnaires, a general linear model (GLM) procedure was carried out. When the GLM procedure turned out to be significant, the Bonferroni procedure for multiple comparisons was done (alpha was set at $p < .05$).

Subjects. This second group (*N* = 1000), obtained through random sampling from the central register of population of a Dutch city, was representative of the Dutch population in terms of age, sex, demographic status, and educational level. Three hundred seventy-eight subjects returned the questionnaire fully completed. The proportion of men to women was 141 (37.3%) versus 237 (62.7%). The data showed that this sample was representative of the Dutch population in terms of age distribution and educational level. However, with regard to sex and demographic status, both women and married subjects were overpresented.

Average Scores and Frequency Distribution of the DIS-Q. The average item result for the total group was 1.50 ± 0.35 (range, 1 to 3.6); this result does not differ significantly from the average result of the previous Dutch sample (1.55 ± 0.40; range, 1-3.73). The average subscale results and standard deviations were as follows: (1) identity confusion-fragmentation: 1.35 ± 0.38 (range, 1-4.04); (2) loss of control: 1.69 ± 0.47 (range, 1-3.83); (3) amnesia: 1.36 ± 0.31 (range, 1-2.92); and (4) absorption: 1.85 ± 0.62 (range, 1-4.33). These results confirmed the findings from the first study: Dissociative experiences are relatively common experiences in the general population. The subscales loss of control and absorption had the highest variation (standard deviation) in the population, while the subscales identity disorder and amnesia had the lowest frequency, suggesting that these scales probably measure the most pathological dissociative experiences. When studying the effects of the different variables on the DIS-Q scores, the results roughly confirmed the findings from the first study. Again, the ANOVA indicated that age significantly influences the total DIS-Q result (DF = 5, $F = 2.43$, $p < .035$). Younger respondents (10-20 and 21-30 years) show much higher scores on loss of control than the older age groups (51-60 and > 60 years). Men and women showed no significantly different scores on the total DIS-Q. However, there was a clear difference for the subscale loss of control: Women showed significantly higher scores than men ($p < .008$), but these differences are chiefly encountered in the age group 20-30 years. In harmony with the findings of the first study, training level had no influence at all on the DIS-Q results. The demographic status, on the other hand, appeared to exert a minor influence on the results.

Prevalence of Dissociative Experiences. In order to get an indication of the possible prevalence of dissociative experiences in the general population, the same cutoff score as used in the first study was employed. If a cutoff score of 2.5 (total result on the DIS-Q) was used, eight subjects (2.1%) gained a DIS-Q score higher than 2.5. Two subjects (0.52%) gained scores comparable to the scores of a patient group with DID. These percentages were lower than the findings from the first study, where 11 subjects (2.94%) obtained a result above the cutoff score and 4 subjects (1.06%) a score comparable to the group of patients with DID. Unlike the first study, the majority of the high scores were females (7 women vs. 1 man). Reckoning with the number of men and women in this sample, there was a proportion of 2.9% women versus 0.7% men (a proportion of 4 to 1) with a DIS-Q result above the 2.5 cutoff. As for the other characteristics of this subgroup, four respondents were married, two divorced and two single. The average age was 33.75 years (SD = 12.26, range, 19-56 years). By means of the trauma list of the DIS-Q, six subjects of this group reported having experienced serious trauma in their life: loss of a child ($n = 1$), loss of a father ($n = 1$), incest ($n = 1$), sexual abuse by a nonfamily member ($n = 1$), divorce ($n = 1$), war and emotional maltreatment ($n = 1$). Two subjects mentioned no trauma at all.

Self-Reported Trauma in the General Population. About 25% of the subjects ($n = 93$) reported on the trauma list of the DIS-Q of having experienced at least one of eight different traumatic situations: (1) physical or bodily injury;

(2) state of war; (3) sexual abuse; (4) serious emotional neglect by parents; (5) death of a family member; (6) specific strain on the family (such as alcohol abuse by a family member, serious fights between the parents, psychiatric problem of a family member); (7) divorce or separation of the subject involved; and (8) psychiatric problem of the subject involved. About 20% of the subjects reported more than one traumatic situation. A remarkable finding was the fact that men reported mostly two trauma categories: severe bodily injury (9.9%) and state of war (9.2%), while women reported various traumatic experiences: loss of a family member (often the loss of a child) (6.7%), state of war (4.6%), incest and sexual abuse by nonfamily members (together, 5%), strain on the family (4.6%), and severe bodily injury (4.6%). By using χ^2 tests, only one significant difference between men and women for the trauma category sexual abuse was found ($p < .004$). The results of the total group showed that state of war (7.1%), severe bodily injury (6.6%), and loss of a family member (5.6%) were most frequently reported. Remarkably enough, not one subject of the sample reported physical abuse.

The Relationship between Trauma and Dissociative Experiences. By using χ^2 tests, no significant differences were found between the trauma group (n = 93) and the nontrauma group (n = 285) with regard to the following characteristics: sex, demographic status, and educational level. An ANOVA showed no difference for age between the two groups. A comparison was made between the subscale scores of the trauma group compared with the nontrauma group. Next, the three groups (major trauma, minor trauma, and no trauma) were compared, using a GLM procedure. The results clearly indicated that the trauma group gained significantly higher DIS-Q scores for both total result ($p < .0001$) and the four subscales, especially identity confusion ($p < .0001$) and absorption ($p < .0002$). Hence, subjects who mentioned a trauma reported significantly more dissociative symptoms than subjects who mentioned no trauma.

When comparing the sexually abused group (n = 11) with the two other groups [no trauma (n = 279) and minor trauma (n = 84)], the results strongly suggested that sexual abuse provoked significantly more dissociative experiences than all other trauma categories (see Table 2). Another remarkable finding was that the sexually

Table 2. Comparison of Subscale Scores of Nontrauma versus Minor/Major Trauma

	Nontrauma (N = 279)		Minor trauma (N = 84)		Major trauma (N = 11)			
variable	Mean	SD	Mean	SD	Mean	SD	F (df = 2)	p^b
DIS-Q1[a]	1.30	.32	1.48	.48	1.83	.51	17.12	.0001*
DIS-Q2	1.64	.44	1.77	.50	2.31	.57	12.73	.0001*
DIS-Q3	1.34	.28	1.39	.35	1.73	.39	9.16	.0001*
DIS-Q4	1.77	.58	2.08	.72	2.04	.66	8.84	.0001
DIS-Q total	1.45	.31	1.60	.43	1.96	.39	16.66	.0001*

[a]DIS-Q1, identity confusion-fragmentation; DIS-Q2, loss of control; DIS-Q3, amnesia; DIS-Q4, absorption.

[b]*, Significant after application of Bonferroni correction for multiple comparisons ($p < .05$).

abused subjects reported significantly ($p < .0001$) more amnesia experiences (DIS-Q3) as compared to all other groups.

Dissociative Experiences in Eating Disorders. After Janet's pioneering studies of dissociation and eating disorders, interest in this subject disappeared for more than half a century but has reemerged in recent decades (Torem, 1986; Vanderlinden & Vandereycken, 1988, 1990). The presence of minor dissociative "hysterical" mechanisms in bulimic patients was already reported by Russell in 1979. Demitrack, Putnam, Brewerton, Brandt, and Gold (1990) studied dissociative experiences in 30 female eating-disorder patients, compared with 30 age-matched normal female subjects, and found that the patients demonstrated significantly higher levels of dissociative psychopathology than the control subjects.

The goal of the following studies was to explore the presence of trauma and dissociative experiences in eating disorders. A first pilot study in a sample of 50 eating-disorder patients (Vanderlinden, Vandereycken, Van Dyck, & Delacroix, 1992a) showed a self-reported trauma rate of 16%, much lower than the rates reported in the literature. Compared with a group of normal control subjects ($n = 378$), the eating-disorder patients had significantly higher scores on the DIS-Q. In an analysis of several subgroups of eating-disorder patients, those with bulimic and atypical eating disorders appeared to report significantly higher scores on the DIS-Q and these higher scores were partly related to the presence of traumatic experiences.

These interesting findings stimulated a more refined study of the relationship between trauma and dissociation in a larger sample of eating-disorder patients. In this second study (Vanderlinden, Vandereycken, Van Dyck, & Vertommen, 1993b), the different subgroups of eating disorders were better matched for age, sex, duration of illness, demographic status, and educational level. The relationship between specific traumatic experiences and particular dissociative phenomena were studied in detail.

Method. To assess the presence of dissociative experiences, the DIS-Q was administered. Past traumatic experiences (incest, sexual and/or physical abuse, serious parental rejection) were explored by means of a self-reporting questionnaire about past sexual experiences (Lange, 1990) and a clinical interview.

Subjects. The sample consisted of 98 patients (2 males, 96 females) who were consecutively admitted to the inpatient Eating Disorders Unit of the University Center in Kortenberg. In case of DSM-III-R anorexia nervosa, a distinction was made between the restricting type, i.e., pure fasters or abstainers ($n = 34$; 34.7%), and the mixed type, i.e., combined with bingeing and/or purging ($n = 24$; 24.5%). Normal-weight bulimia nervosa was diagnosed in 28.6% ($n = 28$), while 12.2% ($n = 12$) showed an atypical eating disorder (lacking one or more criteria of the previous diagnoses). The mean age of this patient sample was 24.3 (SD = 6.68; range, 14–42 years). The duration of illness averaged 6.38 (SD = 5.25; range, 0.5–11 years) with an average age at onset of 17.7 (SD = 4.3; range, 11–33 years). The four eating disorder subgroups did not differ, except for the typical eating pathology.

Dissociative Experiences in Eating Disorders Compared to Normals. An ANOVA and Scheffe's *t*-test were used to compare the DIS-Q scores of eating-disorder patients and age-matched female controls ($n = 66$). The results of this study confirmed the findings of a former study (Vanderlinden et al., 1992a) that showed that eating-disorder patients (especially bulimics and atypical eating disorders) report significantly higher levels of dissociative experiences than normal control subjects. About 12% of the patient sample reported DIS-Q scores as high as the scores of patients with dissociative disorders. The results supported the assumed relationship between overwhelming trauma and a dissociative reaction, i.e., the more serious the trauma, the higher the DIS-Q scores. Most interesting are the high scores on the amnesia subscale in the case of incest and sexual abuse (see Table 3). This finding seems to endorse Janet's conceptualization of dissociation, which postulates that amnesia (the escape from conscious awareness of the idée fixe relating to the trauma) is the most specific clinical characteristic in trauma-induced dissociation (see also Chu & Dill, 1990; Van der Kolk & Van der Hart, 1991).

An important subgroup of the eating-disorder patients, about 12%, reported pathological dissociative experiences. The great majority of these patients had experienced a serious trauma during their life. Thus it may be concluded that in a considerable subgroup of eating disorders (especially bulimia nervosa and atypical eating disorder), trauma-induced dissociative experiences may play an important role in the development of the eating disorder. Hence, those patients with both a history of trauma and high scores on the DIS-Q should also be screened for the diagnosis of dissociative disorder.

A Follow-up Study on Dissociative Symptoms in Eating Disorders. Recently, a follow-up study has been carried out, studying the presence of dissociative symptoms in 62 eating disordered patients upon admission to a specialized unit, six months after admission, and one year after admission (Vanderlinden, Vandereyken, and Probst, 1995). Scores in the DIS-Q decreased in restricting anorectics and bulimics, but remained virtually unchanged for binging and purging anorectics. Patients with a history of abuse had a worse outcome (compared to the non-abused group), suggesting that abuse definitely must be considered as a risk factor for the outcome in eating disorders.

Table 3. DIS-Q Scores According to Different Forms of Trauma in Eating Disorders

		Total		DIS-Q1[a]		DIS-Q2		DIS-Q3		DIS-Q4	
	N	Mean	SD	Mean	SD	Mean	SD	Mean	SD	Mean	SD
Nontrauma	71	2.2	0.5	2.3	0.7	2.3	0.6	1.5	0.4	2.6	0.7
Total trauma group	27	2.4*	0.6	2.5	0.7	2.6	0.6	1.9**	0.6	2.8	0.8
Incest	8	2.5*	0.6	2.6	0.8	2.7	0.5	2.1***	0.9	2.9	0.9
Sexual abuse[b]	12	2.5*	0.6	2.7	0.8	2.7*	0.6	1.9**	0.5	2.8	0.8
Physical abuse	3	2.1	0.3	2.0	0.4	2.5	0.4	1.7	0.3	2.2	0.5
Neglect	8	2.1	0.5	2.2	0.7	2.3	0.6	1.8	0.5	2.4	0.6
Loss of family member	5	2.3	0.4	2.3	0.6	2.5	0.2	1.9*	0.6	2.4	0.6

[a]DIS-Q1, identity confusion; DIS-Q2, loss of control; DIS-Q3, amnesia; DIS-Q4, absorption. * $p < .05$; ** $p < .005$; *** $p < .002$.
[b]By other than family members.

Recently, the DIS-Q has been translated into the Hungarian language by Katalin Varga and Eva Banyai, two psychologists and researchers at the Eötvös Lorand University in Budapest. (This research was made possible due to the financial support of the grant OTKA [no. 284 0313, Eva Banyai and Katalin Varga]). The goal was to replicate the DIS-Q studies carried out in the general population of Belgium and the Netherlands in a Hungarian population sample. The results could give more insight into possible sociocultural factors that might influence the DIS-Q scores. Hungary is a former Communist country, currently struggling with a major economic crisis and searching for a new identity. The end of the Communist regime first resulted in a euphoric atmosphere ("finally we are free"), but very soon changed to general frustration, confusion, and an important identity crisis for the population. Taking into account these considerations, it was assumed that higher DIS-Q scores would be obtained in the Hungarian population, compared to Belgium and the Netherlands.

Method

The DIS-Q was administered to 311 subjects of the general population in Hungary. Psychology students were asked to get data of the DIS-Q of about 300 subjects from the general population, according to the Hungarian age and sex distribution. The students could give the DIS-Q questionnaire to anyone who wanted to participate in the study. The only restriction was that the subject "was not under hospital care currently or in the past 5 years." Hence, most subjects came from the psychology students' families and friends. No money or other reward was given to the subjects. Some preliminary data of this study are reported below.

Results

Subjects. In all, 456 DIS-Q questionnaires were collected. Since the distribution of age of this sample was not fully representative for the Hungarian population, a representative sample was chosen. This way, 311 subjects were selected: The sample was representative for the Hungarian population for the variables of age, sex (166 females and 145 males), and education.

Mean Scores and Frequency Distribution. Compared to the DIS-Q scores of the second study in the Netherlands, the Hungarian sample gained significantly higher DIS-Q scores on the DIS-Q total score ($p < .0001$) and all subscales (see Table 4). Several findings of the Dutch and Belgium DIS-Q studies were confirmed: The subscales loss of control and absorption had the highest variation (standard deviation) in the Hungarian population, while the subscales identity confusion and amnesia had the lowest frequency.

Although the differences may not seem to be impressive (1.5 vs. 1.7 for the total DIS-Q score), they become much more important with regard to the frequency distribution of the DIS-Q scores. In Flemish and Dutch studies, 3% and 2% of the subjects, respectively, gained DIS-Q scores above the 2.5 cutoff score. In Hungary,

Table 4. Mean and SD DIS-Q Scores of Netherlands versus Hungary

		DIS-Q[a] total		DIS-Q1		DIS-Q2		DIS-Q3		DIS-Q4	
	N	Mean	SD	Mean	SD	Mean	SD	Mean	SD	Mean	SD
Netherlands	378	1.5*	0.5	1.5**	0.5	1.7*	0.5	1.4*	0.4	1.9*	0.6
Hungary	311	1.7	0.5	1.6	0.5	1.9	0.7	1.6	0.5	2.3	0.8

[a]DIS-Q1, identity confusion; DIS-Q2, loss of control; DIS-Q3, amnesia; DIS-Q, absorption. * $p < .0001$; ** $p < .004$.

the frequency distribution shows that 10.6% of this sample scores above the cutoff score and reports severe dissociative symptoms; 2.6% scored as high as DID patients. This result is much higher compared to the previous studies, where 1% and 0.5%, respectively, gained scores as high as DID patients. These data support the assumption of higher levels of dissociative symptoms in the Hungarian population.

Effect of the Different Variables on the DIS-Q Scores. By means of ANOVA, the effects of the variables of sex and age on the DIS-Q scores were studied. Whenever the ANOVA was significant, the Bonferroni procedure for multiple comparisons was done (alpha was set at $p < .05$). Again, the results showed that age was the only variable significantly influencing the DIS-Q total score (DF = 5, 310; $F = 26.22$; $p < .0001$). Younger respondents (age 10–20 years) scored significantly higher on the DIS-Q total scores (mean = 2.1; $p < .05$) and on subscales identity confusion (mean = 2.0; $p < .05$) and loss of control (mean = 2.5; $p < .05$) compared to all the other age categories. These findings correspond with the data of all previous population studies on the prevalence of dissociative experiences: These experiences are more frequently present in adolescents and young adults, and they decline with age (Ross, 1991).

When comparing the scores of the male and female subjects, no significant differences were found. These results confirm the data from our previous studies (Vanderlinden et al., 1991, 1993c).

CONCLUDING REMARKS

The state of the art in Europe with regard to diagnosis, treatment, and study of the dissociative disorders still leaves much to be desired. Important developments are nevertheless taking place, in particular, in the Netherlands and Belgium. There also are signs that in countries such as Germany, the United Kingdom, Norway, Italy, Hungary, and Spain, promising developments in the clinical field are underway. There is an increasing number of studies on the prevalence of dissociative experiences being done, both in the general population and in psychiatric patient samples using the DES or the DIS-Q. Apart from the Dutch validation study of the SCID-D, there are currently studies being carried out on the prevalence of dissociative disorders in different populations using the SCID-D and the DDIS. A number of related studies are planned, such as the research being done by Nijenhuis and collegues in the Netherlands and Belgium on the development of a new self-reporting questionnaire to assess somatic and somatoform aspects of dissociation:

the Somatoform Dissociation Questionnaire. As exemplified by the DIS-Q study in Hungary, there is a growing tendency for researchers from different European countries to collaborate on common projects. Perhaps the time has come for North American and European researchers to join ranks in conducting intercontinental studies on dissociation and the dissociative disorders.

Appendix I: DISSOCIATION QUESTIONNAIRE (DIS-Q)

This questionnaire consists of two parts. The first part contains a few general questions about your background. In the second part you are asked to indicate to what extent the following experiences apply to you. The experiences mentioned in the questionnaire may occur when people are under the influence of alcohol, drugs or medicines. It is intended to answer this questionnaire regarding your condition without the use of any such means. You are asked to react to the statements by circling the figure that applies to you. Any answer is good, so long as it reflects your own view. Please react to all (of the) statements.

Example: To what extent does the following statement apply to you?

I find it hard to make up my mind. 1 2 3 4 5

By circling one of the figures, you can indicate whether that statement is more or less applicable to you. If the statement "Moderately," as in the above-mentioned example, is applicable to you, you will circle number 3. Against each statement, you will put a figure that is most applicable to you.

1 = This is not at all applicable.
2 = This a little bit applicable.
3 = This is moderately applicable.
4 = This is quite a bit applicable.
5 = This is extremely applicable.

Part 1

Name: ______________________

Date: ______________________

Will you please fill in and cross where appropriate?

Your age: ________ years
Your sex: □ Male
□ Female

Your marital status: □ Single
□ Married
□ Living together

☐ Divorced
☐ Widower/Widow

Your training:

☐ Elementary education

☐ First-grade secondary: ☐ General educational ☐ Technical ☐ Vocational

☐ Second-grade secondary: ☐ General educational ☐ Technical ☐ Vocational

☐ Higher nonuniversity
☐ University training

Please cross the training that corresponds most to your own training.

Do you remember having experienced severely damaging, life-threatening or traumatic events?

☐ No

☐ Yes, i.e. (several answers being possible):

- ☐ Severe bodily injury
- ☐ Physical abuse
- ☐ State of war
- ☐ Sexual abuse by family members
- ☐ Sexual abuse by others (non-family members)
- ☐ Emotional maltreatment
- ☐ Otherwise: namely:

Part 2

1 = Not at all 2 = A little bit 3 = Moderately 4 = Quite a bit 5 = Extremely

1.	At times I have the feeling that I am dreaming.	1	2	3	4	5
2.	I regularly have the feeling that everything is unreal.	1	2	3	4	5
3.	At times it appears that I have lost contact with my body.	1	2	3	4	5
4.	I gorge myself with food without thinking about it.	1	2	3	4	5
5.	While driving and/or bicycling, I suddenly realize that I cannot remember what happened on the way.	1	2	3	4	5
6.	I can, without reason, without wanting to, burst out laughing or crying.	1	2	3	4	5
7.	It happens that I have the feeling that I am somebody else.	1	2	3	4	5

8. It happens that I am listening to someone and suddenly realize that I have not heard part or the whole of the story.	1	2	3	4	5
9. When I am tired, it seems as if a strange power from outside takes possession of me and decides for me what to do.	1	2	3	4	5
10. I get into situations in which I do not want to be.	1	2	3	4	5
11. At times I feel a great distance between myself and the things I think and do.	1	2	3	4	5
12. At times I wonder who I am exactly.	1	2	3	4	5
13. It happens that I find new articles among my things without being able to remember having ever purchased these.	1	2	3	4	5
14. I regularly feel an urge to eat something, even when I am not hungry.	1	2	3	4	5
15. It happens that I get angry without wanting to be at all.	1	2	3	4	5
16. It happens that I am determined to do something, but my body acts quite differently against my own will.	1	2	3	4	5
17. It happens that I feel confused.	1	2	3	4	5
18. At moments I cannot remember where I was the day (or days) before.	1	2	3	4	5
19. It happens that I am told that I act as if friends or family members were strangers to me.	1	2	3	4	5
20. In particular situations I experience myself as a split personality.	1	2	3	4	5
21. It happens that I cannot remember anything about certain important events in my life, such as my final examinations or wedding day.	1	2	3	4	5
22. It happens that I am about to say something, but then something quite different crosses my lips.	1	2	3	4	5
23. There can be a sudden, complete change in my mood.	1	2	3	4	5
24. It happens that I do something without thinking about it.	1	2	3	4	5
25. I immediately forget what other people tell me.	1	2	3	4	5
26. It happens that I am doing something and that I am suddenly struck by a blackout.	1	2	3	4	5
27. It occurs that I look at myself in the mirror without recognizing myself.	1	2	3	4	5
28. It happens that I get the feeling that my body undergoes an alteration.	1	2	3	4	5
29. It happens that I have the feeling that other people, other things and the world surrounding me, are not real.	1	2	3	4	5
30. I have the feeling that my body is not (really) mine.	1	2	3	4	5
31. When I watch television, I do not notice anything about what goes on around me.	1	2	3	4	5

32. It happens that entire blocks of time drop out and that I cannot remember what I did then.	1	2	3	4	5
33. I can remember so vividly something that happened formerly, that I have the feeling that I am reliving it.	1	2	3	4	5
34. It happens that it seems as if someone else inside me decides what I do.	1	2	3	4	5
35. Some imes I discover that I have done something without remembering anything about it.	1	2	3	4	5
36. I wonder how I can prevent myself from doing certain things.	1	2	3	4	5
37. Sometimes I suddenly notice that I find myself in a place that is unknown to me, without knowing how I got there.	1	2	3	4	5
38. It happens that I am not sure whether certain memories have really taken place, or if I merely dreamed about them.	1	2	3	4	5
39. Sometimes I find myself in a well-known place that appears strange and unknown to me.	1	2	3	4	5
40. I have the feeling that I do certain things without knowing why.	1	2	3	4	5
41. Sometimes I think or do something against my liking in a way that does not suit me at all.	1	2	3	4	5
42. I notice that I watch myself closely in everything I do.	1	2	3	4	5
43. I can enclose myself in fantasies or daydreaming so much that it seems to be really happening.	1	2	3	4	5
44. It happens that I am staring aimlessly, without thinking about anything.	1	2	3	4	5
45. I often think about nothing.	1	2	3	4	5
46. I find it very hard to resist bad habits.	1	2	3	4	5
47. I sometimes forget where I have put something.	1	2	3	4	5
48. When eating, I do so without thinking about it.	1	2	3	4	5
49. It happens that I catch myself day-dreaming.	1	2	3	4	5
50. I wish I had more control of myself.	1	2	3	4	5
51. When I walk, I am aware of each step I make.	1	2	3	4	5
52. In particular situations, I notice that I am able to do certain things with the greatest ease, that I find very hard to do in others (e.g. sports, work, social contacts).	1	2	3	4	5
53. When eating, I am aware of every bite I take.	1	2	3	4	5
54. I lose every notion of time.	1	2	3	4	5
55. It happens that I cannot remember whether I have really done something or if I merely planned it.	1	2	3	4	5
56. It happens that I want to do two things at the same time and that I notice that I am arguing with myself the pros. and cons.	1	2	3	4	5
57. It happens that I have the feeling that my mind is split up.	1	2	3	4	5

58. It happens that I find notes, drawings or annotations of my own, without remembering having ever made these. 1 2 3 4 5
59. I have the feeling that I am made up of two (or more) persons. 1 2 3 4 5
60. I often do something without thinking about it. 1 2 3 4 5
61. It happens that I hear voices in my head telling me what I am to do or making comment on what I am doing. 1 2 3 4 5
62. I see myself differently from the way other people see me. 1 2 3 4 5
63. It happens that I feel I am looking at the world through a haze, so that the people and things surrounding me appear remote or vague. 1 2 3 4 5

Appendix II: DIS-Q Scoring Form

Name: ______________________

Born: ______________________

Date: ______________________

DIS-Q1 Identity-confusion fragmentation		DIS-Q2 Loss of control		DIS-Q3 Amnesia		DIS-Q4 Absorption	
Nr	Score	Nr	Score	Nr	Score	Nr	Score
2		1		13		33	
3		4		18		42	
7		5		19		51	
9		6		21		52	
10		8		25		53	
11		14		26		56	
12		15		31			
16		17		32			
20		23		35			
22		24		37			
27		38		45			
28		43		47			
29		44		55			
30		46		58			
34		48					
36		49					
39		54					
40		60					

(*continued*)

Appendix II: DIS-Q Scoring Form (*Continued*)

DIS-Q1 Identity-confusion fragmentation		DIS-Q2 Loss of control		DIS-Q3 Amnesia		DIS-Q4 Absorption	
Nr	Score	Nr	Score	Nr	Score	Nr	Score
41							
50							
57							
59							
61							
62							
63							
Sum =		Sum =		Sum =		Sum =	
Sum: 25 =		Sum: 18 =		Sum: 14 =		Sum: 6 =	

TOTAL DIS-Q score =
TOTAL SUM: 63 =

REFERENCES

Aldridge-Morris, R. (1989). *Multiple personality: An exercise in deception*. Hillsdale, NJ: L. Erlbaum Associates.

American Psychiatric Association. (1980). *Diagnostic and statistical manual of mental disorders* (3rd ed.). Washington, DC: Author.

American Psychiatric Association, (1987). *Diagnostic and statistical manual of mental disorders* (3rd ed., rev.). Washington, DC: Author.

Bernstein, E. M., & Putnam, F. W. (1986). Development, reliability, and validity of a dissociation scale. *Journal of Nervous and Mental Disease, 174*, 727-735.

Boon, S., & Draijer, N. (1991). Diagnosing dissociative disorders in the Netherlands: A pilot study with the structured clinical interview for DSM-III-R dissociative disorders. *American Journal of Psychiatry, 148*, 458-462.

Boon, S., & Draijer, N. (1993a). Multiple personality disorder in the Netherlands: A clinical investigation of 71 patients. *American Journal of Psychiatry, 150*, 489-494.

Boon, S., & Draijer, N. (1993b). *Multiple personality disorders in the Netherlands. A study on reliability and validity of the diagnosis*. Amsterdam/Lisse: Swetz & Zeitlinger.

Boon, S., & Van der Hart, O. (1988a). Dissocieren als overlevingsstrategie bij fysiek en seksueel geweld [Dissociation as survival strategy for physical and sexual abuse]. *Maandblad Geestelijke Volksgezondheid, 43*, 1197-1207.

Boon, S., & Van der Hart, O. (1988b). Het herkennen van dissociatieve stoornissen, in het bijzonder de multiple persoonlijkheidsstoornis [Recognition of dissociative disorders, in particular multiple personality disorder]. *Maandblad Geestelijke Volksgezondheid, 43*, 1208-1225.

Boon, S., & Van der Hart, O. (1989). De behandeling van de multiple persoonlijkheidsstoornis [Treatment of multiple personality disorder]. *Maandblad Geestelijke Volksgezondheid, 44*, 1283-1299.

Carlson, E. B., Putnam, F. W., Ross, C. A., (1990) A discriminant analysis on the D.E.S.: A multicenter study. In B. G. Braun & E. B. Carlson (Eds.), *Dissociative disorders 1990. Proceedings of the 7th international conference on multiple personality/dissociative states* (p. 141). Chicago: Rush.

Chu, J. A., & Dill, D. L. (1990). Dissociative symptoms in relation to childhood physical and sexual abuse. *American Journal of Psychiatry, 147*, 887-892.

Cohen, M., Wallage, P., & Van der Hart, O. (1992). *De prevalentie van dissociatieve verschijnselen en traumatische jeugdervaringen bij een RIAGG populatie* [The prevalence of dissociative phenomena and traumatic experiences in childhood in population of a Regional Institute for Ambulatory Mental Health Care]. Amsterdam: Riagg Zuid/Nieuw West.

Dalle Grave, R., Rigamanti, R., & Todisco, P. (in press). Trauma and dissociative experiences in eating disorders. *European Eating Disorders Review.*

Demitrack, M. A., Putnam, F. W., Brewerton, T. D., Brandt, H. A., & Gold, P. W. (1990). Relation of clinical variables to dissociative phenomena in eating disorders. *American Journal of Psychiatry, 147,* 1184-1188.

Draijer, N. (1988). *Seksueel misbruik van meisjes door verwanten* [Sexual abuse of girls by relatives]. The Hague: Ministerie van Sociale Zaken en Werkgelegenheid.

Draijer, N. (1990). *Seksuele traumatisering in de jeugd: Gevolgen op lange termijn van seksueel misbruik van meisjes door verwanten* [Sexual traumatization in childhood: Long-term consequences of sexual abuse of girls by relatives]. Amsterdam: SUA.

Draijer, N., & Langeland, W. (1993). Dissociatieve symptomen bij opgenomen psychiatrische patienten: Prevalentie en de relatie met trauma [Dissociative symptoms in psychiatric inpatients: Prevalence and the relationship with trauma]. *Maandblad Geestelijke Volksgezondheid.*

Ensink, B. J. (1992). *Confusing realities: A study on child sexual abuse and psychiatric symptoms.* Amsterdam: VU University Press.

Ensink, B. J., & Van Otterloo, D. (1989). A validation of the DES in the Netherlands. *Dissociation, 2,* 221-223.

Everill, J., Waller, G., & MacDonald, W. (1995). Dissociation in bulimic and non-eating-disordered women. *International Journal of Eating Disorders, 17,* 127-134.

Fahy, T. A. (1988). The diagnosis of multiple personality disorder: A symptom of psychiatric disorder. *British Journal of Psychiatry, 154,* 99-101.

Favaro, A., & Santonastaso P. (1995). Dissociative experiences, trauma and eating disorders in a female college sample. *Euopean Eating Disorders Review, 3,* 136-200.

Huber, M. (1995). *Multiple persönlichkeiten: Überlebenden extremer gewalt. Ein handbuch.* [*Multiple personality disorder: Survivors of extreme abuse,* A handbook.] Frankfurt: Fischer.

Janet, P. (1889). *L' Automatisme psychologique.* Paris: Félix Alcan.

Janet, P. (1898). *Névroses et idées fixes* (Vol. 1). Paris: Félix Alcan.

Janet, P. (1907). *The major symptoms of hysteria.* London & New York: Macmillan. (Second edition with new matter: 1920. Facsimile of 1920 edition: Hafner, New York, 1965)

Janet, P. (1919). *Les médications psychologiques.* Paris: Félix Alcan. (*Psychological Healing.* New York: MacMillan, 1925)

Karle, H. (1992). *The filthy lie.* London: Hamish Hamilton.

Lange, A. (1990). Vragenlijst sexuele ervaringen uit het verleden [Questionnaire of sexual experiences in the past]. University of Amsterdam: Unpublished report.

Macilwain, I. F. (1992). Multiple personality disorder (Letter). *British Journal of Psychiatry, 161,* 863.

Modestin, J. (1992). Multiple personality disorder in Switzerland. *American Journal of Psychiatry, 149,* 88-92.

Nijenhuis, E. R. S. (1994). *Dissociatieve stoornissen en psychotrauma* [*Dissociative disorders and psychotrauma*]. Pratijkreeks Gedragstherapie. Houten, Bohn Stafleu Van Loghum.

Nijenhuis, E. R. S. (1995). Dissociatie en leertheorie: Trauma geinduceerde dissociatie als klassiek geconditioneerde defensie [Dissociation and learning theory: trauma induced dissociation as classiclally conditioned defense]. In K. Jonker, J. J. Derksen, & F. J. S. Donker (Eds.), *Dissociatie: Een fenomeen opnieuw belicht* [*Dissociation: A phenomenon illuminated afresh*]. Houten: Bohn Stafleu Van Loghum.

Nijenhuis, E. R. S., & Vanderlinden, J. (in press). Dierlijke defensieve reacties als model voor dissociatieve reacties op psychotrauma [Animal defensive reactions as a model for trauma-induced dissociative reactions]. *Tijdschript voor Psychiatrie.*

Nijenhuis, E. R. S., Spinhoven, Ph. Van Dyck, R., Van der Hart, O., & Vanderlinden, J. (1995, May 10-13). *The development of the Somatoform Dissociation Questionnaire as screener for dissociative disorders.* Paper presented at the Fifth Annual Spring Conference of the International Society for the Study of Dissociation, Amsterdam, The Netherlands.

Ross, C. A. (1989). *Multiple personality disorder: Diagnosis, clinical features and treatment.* New York: John Wiley.

Ross, C. A. (1991). Epidemiology of multiple personality disorder and dissociation. *Psychiatric Clinics of North America, 14*(3), 503-517.

Ross, C. A., & Ryan, L. (1989). Dissociative experiences in adolescents and college students. *Dissociation, 2*, 239-242.

Ross, C. A., Norton, G. R., & Wozney, K. (1989). Multiple personality disorder: An analysis of 236 cases. *Canadian Journal of Psychiatry, 34*, 413-418.

Ross, C. A., Joshi, S., & Currie, R. (1990). Dissociative experiences in the general population. *American Journal of Psychiatry, 147*, 1547-1552.

Ross, C. A., Joshi, S., & Currie, R. (1991a). Dissociative experiences in the general population: A factor analysis. *Hospital and Community Psychiatry, 42*, 297-301.

Ross, C. A., Anderson, G. A., Fleisher, W. P., & Norton, G. R. (1991b). The frequency of multiple personality disorder among psychiatric inpatients. *American Journal of Psychiatry, 148*, 1717-1720.

Russell, G. (1979). Bulimia nervosa: An ominous variant of anorexia nervosa. *Psychological Medicine, 9*, 429-449.

Sainton, K., Ellason, J., Mayran, L., & Ross, C. (1993). Reliability of the new form of the Dissociative Experiences Scale (DES) and the Dissociation Questionnaire (DIS-Q). In B. G. Braun & J. Parks (Eds.), *Dissociative disorders 1993: Proceedings of 10th international conference on multiple personality/dissociative states* (p. 125). Chicago: Rush.

Saxe, G. N., Van der Kolk, B. A., Berkowitz, R., Chinman, G., Hall, K., Lieberg, G., & Schwartz, J. (1993). Dissociative disorders in psychiatric inpatients. *American Journal of Psychiatry, 150*, 1037-1042.

Steinberg, M., Rounsaville, B., & Cicchetti, D. V. (1990). The structured clinical interview for DSM-III-R dissociative disorders: Preliminary report on a new diagnostic instrument. *American Journal of Psychiatry, 147*, 76-82.

Torem, M. (1986). Dissociative states presenting as an eating disorder. *American Journal of Clinical Hypnosis, 23*, 137-142.

Van der Hart, O. (1986). Pierre Janet over hysterie en hypnose [Pierre Janet on hysteria and hypnosis]. *Directieve Therapie, 5*, 223-246.

Van der Hart, O. (1988). Een overzicht van Janets werk over hysterie en hypnose [An overview of Janet's works on hysteria and hypnosis]. *Directieve Therapie, 8*, 336-365.

Van der Hart, O. (Ed.) (1991). *Trauma, dissociatie en hypnose*. [Trauma, dissociation and hypnosis]. Amsterdam: Swets & Zeitlinger (reprinted 1995).

Van der Hart, O. (1993). The state of diagnosis and treatment of multiple personality disorder in Europe: Impressions. *Dissociation, 6*(2/3), 102-118.

Van der Hart, O., & Friedman, B. (1989). A reader's guide to Pierre Janet on dissociation: A neglected intellectual heritage. *Dissociation, 2*(1), 3-16.

Van der Hart, O., & Horst, R. (1989). The dissociation theory of Pierre Janet. *Journal of Traumatic Stress, 2*, 397-412.

Van der Hart, O., Brown, P., & Van der Kolk, B. A. (1989). Pierre Janet's treatment of posttraumatic stress. *Journal of Traumatic Stress, 2*, 379-396.

Van der Hart, O., Brown, P., & Turco, R. (1990). Hypnotherapy for traumatic grief: Janetian and modern approaches integrated. *American Journal of Clinical Hypnosis, 32*(4), 263-271.

Van der Hart, O., Steele, K., Boon, S., & Brown, P. (1993a). The treatment of traumatic memories: Synthesis, realization and integration. *Dissociation, 6*(2/3), 162-180.

Van der Hart, O., Witztum, E., & Friedman, B. (1993b). From hysterical psychosis to reactive dissociative psychosis. *Journal of Traumatic Stress, 6*, 43-64.

Van der Kolk, B. A., & Van der Hart, O. (1989). Pierre Janet and the breakdown of adaptation in psychological trauma. *American Journal of Psychiatry, 146*, 1530-1540.

Van der Kolk, B. A., & van der Hart, O. (1991). The intrusive past: The flexibility of memory and the engraving of trauma. *American Imago, 48*, 425-454.

Vanderlinden, J. (1993). *Dissociative experiences, trauma and hypnosis. Research findings and clinical applications in eating disorders*. Delft: Eburon.

Vanderlinden, J., & Vandereycken, W. (1988). The use of hypnotherapy in the treatment of eating disorders. *International Journal of Eating Disorders, 7*, 673-679.

Vanderlinden, J., & Vandereycken, W. (1990). The use of hypnosis in the treatment of bulimia nervosa. *International Journal of Clinical and Experimental Hypnosis, 38*, 101-111.

Vanderlinden, J., Van Dyck, R., Vandereycken, W., & Vertommen, H. (1991). Dissociative experiences in the general population of Belgium and the Netherlands. *Dissociation*, *4*, 180-184.

Vanderlinden, J., Vandereycken, W., Van Dyck, R., & Delacroix, O. (1992a). Hypnotizabilty and dissociation in a group of fifty eating disorder patients. Preliminary findings. In W. Bongartz (Ed.), *Hypnosis, 175 years after Mesmer* (pp. 291-296). Konstanz: Universitäts-Verlag

Vanderlinden J., Van Dyck, R., Vertommen, H., & Vandereycken, W. (1992b). De Dissociation Questionnaire (DIS-Q). Ontwikkeling en karakteristieken van een dissociatievragenlijst [Development and characteristics of a dissociation questionnaire]. *Nederlands Tijdschrift voor de Psychologie*, *47*, 134-147.

Vanderlinden, J., Van Dyck, R., Vandereycken, W., Vertommen, H., & Verkes, R. J. (1993a). The Dissociation Questionnaire (DIS-Q). Development and characteristics of a new self-report questionnaire. *Clinical Psychology and Psychotherapy*, *1*, 21-27.

Vanderlinden, J., Vandereycken, W., Van Dyck, R., & Vertommen, H. (1993b). Dissociative experiences and trauma in eating disorders. *International Journal of Eating Disorders*, *13*, 187-194.

Vanderlinden, J., Van Dyck, R., Vandereycken, W., & Vertommen, H. (1993c). Trauma and psychological (dys)functioning in the general population of the Netherlands. *Hospital and Community Psychiatry*, *44*, 786-788.

Vanderlinden, J., Vandereycken, W., & Probst, M. (1995). Dissociative symptoms in eating disorders: A follow-up study. *European Eating Disorder Review*, *3*, 174-184.

World Health Organization (1992). ICD-10: The ICD-10 classification of mental and behavioural disorders. Geneva: Author.

3

Dissociation in Normal Populations

William J. Ray

INTRODUCTION

Historically, dissociation was an important clinical and theoretical topic at the beginning of the 1900s. The term psychological dissociation (*désagrégations psychologiques*) was developed by Pierre Janet (Janet, 1889), and his work has been discussed by a number of sources (see Ellenberger, 1970; Haule, 1986; Quen, 1986; Sjövall, 1967, for historical overviews). Dissociation for Janet was the resultant of stress, with some individuals being seen as more susceptible to dissociation than others. Janet and other nineteenth-century investigators studied unusual cases of psychogenic memory disorder, dramatic changes in personality, discontinuities in consciousness and awareness, and sensorimotor disturbances that were attributed to the basic mechanism of dissociation (Nemiah, 1985, 1991). However, interest increasingly waned throughout subsequent decades. Historically, this decline can be attributed to both a rise of behaviorism in academic circles and the strength of psychoanalysis in clinical practice. Theoretically, the works of Janet, Jung, and others concerning dissociation were largely ignored in favor of Freud's rival hypothesis of repression (Ellenberger, 1970; Frey-Rohn, 1974; Nemiah, 1985, 1991). However, we have recently seen a shift in perspective. With renewed interest in multiple personality disorder (MPD) (Putnam, 1989; Ross, 1989) and posttraumatic stress disorder (PTSD) in the 1980s, dissociation again has become an important theoretical and clinical consideration.

William J. Ray • Department of Psychology, Pennsylvania State University, University Park, Pennsylvania 16802.

Handbook of Dissociation: Theoretical, Empirical, and Clinical Perspectives, edited by Larry K. Michelson and William J. Ray. Plenum Press, New York, 1996.

Likewise, the scientific study of dissociation is also regaining a place of importance, both for the role played by dissociation processes in psychopathology, as well as its potential value in understanding normal states of cognitive-emotional-motoric processing and the relationship with underlying brain states. In terms of recent conceptualizations of the construct itself, dissociation has been seen clinically and theoretically to involve alternations in consciousness that appear to involve a variety of individual memory processes (cf. Kihlstrom et al., 1994). These processes or the lack thereof in turn manifest themselves in a variety of ways. Some of these include: (1) depersonalization and derealization in the sense of not experiencing aspects of one's self or environment as real; (2) amnesia of either a short- or long-term nature; (3) absorption such as the ability to be lost in the task at hand whether watching a movie, reading a book, or driving down the highway; (4) the existence of subpersonalities that may be experienced as separate; and (5) various forms of both trance experiences and nonnormal processing and experience within everyday life. Many of these states can occur in everyone's daily life as manifested by forgetfulness, absentmindedness, or absorption into books or films. Other dissociative processes may be more rare and found only in psychopathological states. Such extreme dissociative processes as seen in fugue states, extreme depersonalization, or dissociative identity disorders clearly represent an important area of study as illustrated by the majority of chapters within this volume. However, a number of theoretical questions remain to be answered in terms of the relationship between normal and pathological states of dissociation as well as the manner in which each is developed (see Chapter 4 for a discussion of dissociation considered within normal developmental processes and Chapter 6 for a discussion of children who develop disorganized modes of relating).

INDIVIDUAL DIFFERENCES

Conceptually, individual differences in dissociation have been discussed as lying on a continuum, although this idea has not been thoroughly tested. Bernstein and Putnam (1986) discuss the concept of such a continuum which they date to at least the turn of the century with the work of Janet, Prince, and James. The standard continuum is conceptualized as ranging from the normal dissociative processes of everyday life to the inclusion of major psychopathological processes (e.g., multiple personality disorder and fugue states). From this perspective, one would assume that dissociative tendencies (e.g., absentmindedness, "spacing out," etc.) seen in the normal population lie at the basis of the more pathological forms seen in patient populations. However, until recently there was little empirical research to help us understand dissociative experiences as seen in normal populations.

An important research aspect of the study of dissociation has been the development of objective instruments for the identification of dissociative processes. Four self-report scales have been developed independently to identify the prevalence of dissociative processes. These are the Dissociative Experiences Scale (DES), the Perceptual Alteration Scale (PAS), the Questionnaire of Experiences of Dissociation (QED), and the Dissociation Questionnaire (DIS-Q) (Bernstein & Putnam, 1986; Sanders, 1986; Riley, 1988; Vanderlinden, Van Dyke, Vandereycken, & Vertommen,

1991, respectively). The DIS-Q was developed originally for use in Europe and is discussed in Chapter 2. The DES, with 28 items, has been most extensively developed with abnormal populations (Bernstein & Putnam, 1986; Ross, Heber, Norton, & Anderson, 1989). The PAS, with 60 items, was developed as a scale of altered perceptual experiences, especially as related to dissociation and binge eating (Sanders, 1986). The QED, with 26 items, was developed based on the responses of over 1700 subjects (mainly undergraduates) with a true-false response format (Riley, 1988). In terms of brief assessment devices with psychometric properties based on large-scale samples, the DES and QED offer the best available scales of dissociation at this time. These two scales describe experiences ranging from normal dissociation (e.g., absorption while watching a movie or loss of awareness while driving) to those of a more psychopathological nature (e.g., amnesia for significant aspects of one's life).

Although a number of theoretical factors have been assumed to be comprehended within the domain of dissociation, there have been limited attempts to describe these empirically. For example, the BASK model of dissociation (Braun, 1988) posits discontinuity of behavior, affect, sensation, and knowledge, one or more of which may be temporally disconnected from the main stream of consciousness, whereas the American Psychiatric Association (1987, 1994) identifies identity, memory, and consciousness as the domains of disunity. The inclusion by Sanders (1986) of somatic and behavioral control aspects of dissociative process is more consistent with the theory and clinical observations of the early 1900s than with current diagnostic distinctions. Our current taxonomy may or may not reflect natural structural divisions of dissociated experience. If little is understood about the structure of pathological dissociation, less is known about the structure of normal dissociative processes and the extent to which structural elements covary in different populations. It is unknown whether dissociative processes differ in structure, extent, or both, between the disordered and the normal population and whether both are reflected on an identical association–dissociation continuum (Spiegel, 1963). It is the purpose of the present chapter to focus on dissociative processes as found within normal populations from a variety of perspectives.

BROAD-BASED NORMAL SAMPLES

One of the first studies of dissociative experiences within the general population was conducted by Ross, Joshi, and Currie (1990) in the city of Winnipeg, Canada. From an initial population of 650,000 people, these authors used a three-part stratified random sampling technique to select 1055 individuals over the age of 18. The final sample included 41.7% males and 58.3% females with a mean age of early 40s for both males and females. During the interview demographic information was collected and the DES was administered. The DES requests the person to rate on a 0% ("this never happens to me") to 100% ("this always happens to me") scale the amount of time that a particular experience has occurred. Traditional scoring requires that the items be summed and divided by 28. Thus, a score of 30 would suggest that a particular person acknowledges that the average of these 28 experiences happens to them 30% of the time. Previous research has suggested scores in the 20 to 30 range as a cutoff for psychopathological responding (Ross et al., 1989, 1990; Carlson & Putnam, 1993). Using the DES, Ross and co-workers found a mean score of 10.8 (±10.2) for the Winnipeg sample. Further analysis showed 5% of the Winnipeg sample scored above 30, 8.4% above 25, and 12.8% above 20 on the DES, suggesting that dissociative experiences are very common with at least 25% of this population. Overall, Ross and co-workers concluded that dissociative experiences are: (1) common in the general population; (2) do not differ in terms of gender of respondent; and (3) are reported less by older respondents.

Whether the dissociative experiences reported by the Winnipeg sample are indicative of psychopathology is of course a very different question; but these results do suggest future directions for research. For example, in the Winnipeg study a negative correlation (−0.23) was found between DES score and age. Other research by Ryan and Ross reported that responding to dissociation items declines between early adolescence and college (Ryan, 1988; Ryan & Ross, 1988; described in Ross, 1989), which brings forth the possibility that dissociative experiences are in some manner a life span developmental process in that their occurrence in normal populations decreases with age. However, there exists little research examining the aging process in more psychopathological populations. A related area of future research involves the potential differential pattern of responding between normal and psychopathological groups. That is to say, even with similar scores, psychopathological groups may respond to very different items on the DES than the normal population. For example, 29% of the Winnipeg subjects reported that they "... find that sometimes they are listening to someone talk and they suddenly realize that they did not hear part or all of what was said," whereas less than 2% of the subjects reported that they "... have the experience of looking in a mirror and not recognizing themselves." We begin such exploration in Table 1, which we will discuss in more detail later in the chapter. One approach is to examine the factor structure of the DES which we now turn to for the Winnipeg population.

Ross, Joshi, and Currie (1991a), using principal components analysis, identified three dimensions based on the data from the Winnipeg study. The first factor was an absorption-imaginative involvement factor that accounted for 47.1% of the variance. This factor included such items as "missing part of a conservation" and "absorption in television." The second factor reflected activities of dissociated states such as "finding oneself in a place but unaware how one got there" or "finding oneself dressed in clothes one can't remember putting on." The third factor was a depersonalization-derealization factor that included items such as "other people and objects do not seem real" and "feeling as though one's body is not one's own."

In two studies limited to college-age populations Ray and his colleagues (Ray, June, Turaj, & Lundy, 1992; Ray & Faith, 1995) examined the frequency of dissociative experiences using both the DES and QED. In the initial study with 264 subjects, a seven-factor solution was produced for the DES and a six-factor solution for the QED. The follow-up study with 1090 subjects produced a four-factor solution for the DES that basically matched the first original four factors in the earlier study. The first five factors on the QED were the same in both samples with slight variations involving individual items. Overall, the DES produced four factors that, in order of variance explained, were: (1) absorption-derealization; (2) depersonalization;

(3) segment amnesia; and (4) in situ amnesia. The QED produced five factors that were: (1) depersonalization; (2) process amnesia; (3) fantasy-daydream; (4) dissociated body behavior; and (5) trance. The factor structure of the two scales are shown in Tables 1 and 2.

Sanders and Green (1994) gave the DES to 566 female and 294 male college students. These authors found three basic factors that they referred to as: (1) imaginative involvement; (2) depersonalization-derealization; and (3) amnesia. These factors are similar to both those found on the DES by both Ross's and Ray's laboratories and not unlike those found in psychiatric populations (cited in Sanders & Green, 1994; compare Carlson & Putnam, 1993).

With factor analytic techniques it is possible to specify the number of factors. Since Ross and co-workers had reported a three-factor solution, the Ray and Faith data were reanalyzed to fit such a solution. Table 3 shows the factor solutions for the DES found in this reanalysis and compares them with those of Ross et al.

Table 1. DES Factors Based on Data from Ray and Faith (1995)

Item number	Item
Factor 1	Absorption-derealization
17	Absorbed in TV/movie
23	Amazing ease in certain situations
20	Stare into space
18	Absorbed in fantasy
14	Remember events as if real
15	Not remember if something really happened
22	Act differently as if two different people
19	Able to ignore pain
21	Talk out loud when alone
24	Not know if actually did event
16	Familiar place seems strange
Factor 2	Depersonalization
12	Other people not real
13	One's body does not belong
11	Not recognize self in mirror
28	Look at world through fog
7	Standing next to themself
27	Hear voices in head
Factor 3	Segment amnesia
5	Finding things did not buy
26	Find writing/drawing did not do
6	Approached by people do not know
10	Accused of lying
25	Do things do not remember doing
8	Do not recognize friends
9	No memory for important events
Factor 4	In situ amnesia
1	Space out driving
3	Find self in place don't remember
4	Dressed in clothes don't remember
2	Space out while listening

Table 2. QED Factors Based on Data from Ray and Faith (1995)

Item numbers	Item
Factor 1	Depersonalization
2	Feel like someone else
4	Wonder who I really am
1	Things are not real
5	Stranger in mirror
6	Removed from thoughts and actions
7	Confused and in a daze
Factor 2	Process amnesia
18	Mind goes blank
8	Couldn't remember where I had been
3	Mind blocks and goes empty
9	Words don't come out right
17	Forget where I put things
Factor 3	Fantasy-daydream
21	I daydream
15	Daydreamed in school as child
19	Rich fantasy life
11	Off in world of my own
20	Stare off into space
Factor 4	Dissociated body behavior
13	Someone inside directing actions
12	Body undergoing transformation
14	Limbs move on their own
10	Come to without knowing how I got there
16	Problems understanding speech
Factor 5	Trance
25	Gone into trance
23	Able to hypnotize myself
22	Soul leaves my body
24	Had imaginary companions
26	Periods of déjà vu

(1991a). An examination of this table portrays a number of interesting relationships in the two samples. First, the initial absorption-derealization factor matches almost item for item for the DES in both samples. Likewise, a similar depersonalization factor is found in both samples. Whereas Ross and co-workers found a single amnesia factor, Ray and Faith reported that these items differentiated into two factors in this college-age population. The first amnesia factor (Factor III) reflects particular past events (e.g., buying particular items) for which the person is not aware that the events have occurred, whereas the second amnesia factor (Factor IV) reflects a coming to awareness that the person has not been conscious of the current situation (e.g., realizing that one has been spaced out while driving). As expected, when a three-factor solution is required, a single amnesia factor comes forth that includes all of the items found by Ross and co-workers to compose this factor. Thus, the factors found in both the Winnipeg and the college-age study on the DES show a high degree of similarity. It should also be noted that there were

Table 3. Means of Each DES Item and Percent of Subjects Scoring above Either 3 (Ray data) or 30 (Ross data)[a]

Item numbers	Item	Ray 0-9 > 3		Ross 0-100 >30	
		Mean	Percent	Mean	Percent
Factor 1	Absorption-derealization				
17	Absorbed in TV/movie	4.37	59.4	20.2	24.2[1]
23	Amazing ease in certain situations	3.99	56.6	22.8	22.4[1]
20	Stare into space	4.12	65.8	15.3	25.7[1]
18	Absorbed in fantasy	3.49	44.8	10.0	10.9[1]
14	Remember events as if real	3.65	49.3	17.4	19.2[1]
15	Not remember if something really happened	4.14	56.1	12.6	12.5[1]
22	Act differently as if two different people	3.17	40.5	11.5	11.8[1]
19	Able to ignore pain	3.48	46.4	25.6	33.4[1]
21	Talk out loud when alone	3.54	45.2	15.2	17.7[1]
24	Not know if actually did event	3.67	49.2	21.2	24.7[1]
16	Familiar place seems strange	2.52	30.2	(8.6	8.2)[0]
2	Space out while listening	5.08	77.4	24.9	29.0[1]
Factor 2	Amnesia				
5	Finding things did not buy	1.03	8.3	4.5	4.1[2]
26	Find writing/drawing did not do	1.59	17.0	(6.7	6.3)[0]
25	Do things do not remember doing	2.37	27.2	(13.5	14.3)[1]
4	Dressed in clothes don't remember	0.53	1.5	1.9	1.4[2]
3	Find self in place don't remember	1.18	10.8	2.8	2.0[2]
6	Approached by people do not know	2.03	23.4	(12.4	4.1)[0]
8	Do not recognize friends	0.66	4.3	5.1	4.6[2]
10	Accused of lying	2.12	23.9	(7.3	6.0)[0]
9	No memory for important events	1.03	9.6	(8.8	9.5)[0]
Factor 3	Depersonalization				
12	Other people not real	1.7	19.3	4.9	4.1[3]
13	One's body does not belong	1.2	10.9	3.9	3.6[3]
11	Not recognize self in mirror	0.72	5.8	1.8	1.2[3]
28	Look at world through fog	1.2	11.6	4.7	4.0[3]
7	Standing next to themself	1.27	14.0	(5.3	4.3)[0]
27	Hear voices in head	1.59	17.9	5.3	7.3[3]

[a]Three factors DES solution based on Ray data. Note similarity with Ross factor analytic solution. Ross factors shown as superscripts. See text for more detail.

differences in frequency of dissociative experiences between the results found in the Winnipeg and college-age population. Consistent with developmental theory as well as other findings, college-age subjects report a higher incidence of absorption and depersonalization experiences than the older populations of Ross et al. Overall, these data suggest that as one matures, one experiences a decrease in both experiences of depersonalization and of absorption-derealization. On the other hand, there exist a few items such as finding oneself dressed in clothes one doesn't remember putting on or an inability to recognize friends that are experiences with equal and low frequencies across the lifespan.

What the relationship is between high scores on such sound psychometric measures as the DES and day-to-day experiences of individuals who achieve these scores is an important question. That is to say, are there unique descriptive properties of a given individual's experience not adequately reflected in the DES and would these experiences in a normal population be consistent with psychopathological diagnoses? To help answer this question, both Ross, Ryan, Voigt, & Eide (1991b) and Ray and Lukens (1995) interviewed college students who scored high on the DES.

From an original sample of 345, Ross et al. (1991b) interviewed 22 college students who scored above 22.6 and 20 who scored below 5 on the DES. These subjects were asked to complete a widely used measure of general psychopathology, the Symptom Checklist (SCL-90), and a personality measure [Millon Multiaxial Clinical Inventory (MMCI)] as well as being interviewed with the Dissociative Disorders Interview Schedule (DDIS) (Ross, 1989; Ross et al., 1989). Although the high- and low-DES subjects did not differ in terms of demographics, the high-DES subjects did show higher overall and subscales on the SCL-90 and a higher score on the borderline subscale of the MMCI than the low-DES subjects. In terms of the diagnostic interview, 70% (14) of the high-DES subjects met criteria for one or more dissociative disorders. As expected, none in the low-DES group met any of the criteria.

Another measure of psychopathological dissociation is the Structured Clinical Interview for the DSM-IV Dissociative Disorders (SCID-D) (Steinberg, 1993). Although the DSM-IV categories of dissociative disorders and this instrument are discussed in greater detail in Chapter 12, it can be noted that this is a semistructured interview that assesses five dissociative symptom clusters. These clusters are amnesia, depersonalization, derealization, identity confusion, and dissociative identity disorder (the DSM-IV designation of MPD). Ray and Lukens (1995) used the SCID-D with a sample of 17 college students who had scored high on the DES. All of the high-DES subjects scored above the equivalent 20–30 score range that has been seen as suggestive of psychopathology. However, in terms of the SCID-D, only 3 of the 17 high-DES subjects met all criteria for a dissociative disorder. An additional 3 subjects met all criteria except the requirement for distress. DSM-IV states this requirement as follows: "The symptoms cause clinically significant distress or impairment in social, occupational, or other important areas of functioning." The requirement for distress is an interesting one since all of the high-DES subjects we interviewed denied ever seeking services for dissociative symptoms as well as not being currently in therapy. Thus, although dissociative experiences are reported in this normal population, these experiences do not seem to be an extremely disruptive aspect of these subjects' life. Without considering distress as a requirement, approximately one third of the high-DES subjects described dissociative experiences consistent with a DSM-IV dissociative disorder. The other two thirds of high-DES subjects also reported dissociative experiences, but these did not meet criteria for a DSM-IV dissociative disorder.

One aspect the Ray and Lukens study sought to understand was the undiagnosed presence of dissociative experiences. The dissociative experiences reported in the interview ranged from mild symptoms to severe difficulties. For example, in response to the questions concerning amnesia, subjects reported gaps in memory lasting from a few hours to an entire day. One person reported an amnesia experience as recently as one day before the interview was conducted. Another person reported that she would walk through town and the next moment she would "wake up" standing in line at a store's cash register with unfamiliar store items in her hands. She also reported feeling embarrassed at having no explanation for her actions. With regard to the depersonalization items, one individual reported, "While I was sitting in my room, I zoned out and then as a third person or camera, I watched myself, my body, leave the room to visit a friend. I then returned to my room whereupon I snapped out of it. An hour had passed." She continued to say that the experience was very different from that of dreaming or daydreaming. In fact, it made such an impact on her that she felt the need to call her friend to see if she had actually visited, which she had not. Another subject described in some details her experiences of derealization, part of which is described: "I have episodes where I see everything differently, everything starts blending ... things look more fluid. I snap out of it on purpose because it is a disturbing experience. I can't tell what is real and what is not." Other subjects report derealization experiences in which "things were moving in slow motion," "voices echoed," and the surroundings became "cartoonlike." Finally, some subjects described situations in which they rose above or to the side of their body. From this perspective, they would watch their own actions. These results seem consistent with more anecdotal reports in that the experience of being outside of one's body are not uncommon experiences for individuals with dissociative tendencies.

Overall, the studies from the Ross and Ray laboratories suggest that dissociative experiences are common within the normal population. Further, these experiences or tendencies do not seem to carry with them high levels of distress, which raises questions in terms of referring to these dissociative experiences in a psychopathological manner.

RELATIONSHIP TO OTHER INDIVIDUAL DIFFERENCE FACTORS

In order to understand how dissociative tendencies are related to and separate from other individual difference factors, we have examined the relationship between two major dissociative scales and a variety of individual difference measures. At this point, we have collected data from more than 2000 college students over a 5-year period, although not all subjects received every individual difference measure. In the following section we will discuss some of these measures.

Absentmindedness

One important question asks if dissociative tendencies share a common root with other types of lapses of awareness such as absentmindedness or other types of simple forgetfulness. Absentmindedness and other types of lapses of awareness have been topics of great interest in the human factors literature (cf. Reason, 1984). In this literature, distinctions have been make between "slips" and "mistakes." Slips would be considered actions not in accord with the overall goal in the case where one had a good plan but it was poorly execution. Mistakes, on the other hand, would be considered planning failures and the resultant of errors of judgement, inference, and so forth. With a mistake one accurately follows the plan, but the plan is faulty. Thus, in this section, to use the terminology of human factors, we are interested in slips, lapses, and accidents but not mistakes.

We all know that accidents happen to people and that they are unpredictable and random, as opposed to something someone plans to do. However, we can ask if people who make one type of slip or error (e.g., attention) also make other types of errors (e.g., memory). To help answer this question, at least two questionnaires have been developed to assess error proneness. The first was developed by Broadbent and referred to as the Cognitive Failures Questionnaire (Broadbent, Cooper, FitzGerald, & Parks, 1982). The second was developed by Reason and Mycielska (1982) and referred to as the absentmindedness questionnaire. In our own work we have found that these two questionnaires correlate highly with each other ($r = .68$). Other research in the human factors area has reported that: (1) there exists a general factor found in all questionnaires of absentmindedness or cognitive failures; (2) it is difficult in general to find cognitive laboratory measures that discriminate between high and low scorers on these questionnaires; (3) distributed attention tasks appear to differentiate high and low scores especially when more than one task is attempted simultaneously; and (4) subjects scoring high in absentminded or cognitive failure cope by using more mental effort to deal with or suppress emotions, whereas low subjects use more action-oriented techniques such as seeking support from others. Such data have led Reason to suggest that high-scoring subjects have a less adaptive coping style. Other research suggests that although stress may increase the likelihood of cognitive failure, it is not a necessary condition for its occurrence. However, Broadbent et al. (1982) suggest high cognitive failures scores are related to increased vulnerability to externally imposed stress. In terms of data collected with our college student population, we found that Broadbent's Cognitive Failures Questionnaire correlates .47 (n = 541) with the DES and Reason's Absent-Mindedness Questionnaire correlates .56 (n = 249). Given these correlations, it is possible to speculate that there may exist similar processes that underlie both normal absent-mindedness and more severe dissociative tendencies.

Absorption

Tellegen and Atkinson (1974) developed the Tellegen Absorption Scale (TAS), which is a scale of openness to absorption. In a number of studies the TAS has been shown to have low positive correlation with hypnotic susceptibility (.21 and .11 in our samples of 243 and 278 subjects, respectively). Tellegen (1992) has described absorption as a "marked restructuring of the phenomenal self and world." In terms of dissociative tendencies, Tellegen suggests that "these more or less transient states may have a dissociated or an integrative and peak-experience-like quality." The finding in our samples of a moderately high correlation (.55 and .59 in samples of 243 and 278 subjects, respectively) supports this speculation.

Hypnotic Susceptibility

The phenomena of dissociation and hypnosis have been closely associated in both the scientific and popular literature since at least the 1880s. The investigation of clinical dissociative phenomena and the use of hypnosis in their study and treatment was practiced by Janet and many of his contemporaries, including Charcot and Freud (Ellenberger, 1970). Since many of these dissociative phenomena could be produced under hypnosis and were studied and treated within the context of hypnosis, there was a natural association of the two phenomena. Historically, the association between hypnosis and dissociation is based on empirical, theoretical, and clinical grounds such as the similarity of hypnotic and dissociative states (Hilgard, 1965; Spiegel & Cardeña, 1991) and the reported high hypnotizability of dissociative clinical groups (Bliss, 1986; Frischholz, Lipman, Braun, & Sachs, 1992; Putnam, 1989). In terms of the dimensions of hypnotizability and dissociative experiences in normal populations, little research exists that is available to answer the question of whether the same individuals who are hypnotically susceptible are also individuals who report experiencing dissociative processes. This was the question we sought to answer (Faith and Ray, 1994). To study the relationship between hypnotizability and dissociation in a nonclinical population, we report the results of a large-scale correlational study, conducted over 3 years, using two separate measures of dissociation (the DES and QED) and a highly regarded scale of hypnotizability, that of the Harvard Grove Scale of Hypnotic Susceptibility (HGSHS).

Across four administrations (866 subjects), correlation coefficients were computed between the two dissociation scales and the hypnotizability scale. Correlations between the DES and the QED for the entire sample was .81, which is consistent with the findings of other studies (Angiulo & Kihlstrom, 1991; Ray et al., 1992; Ray & Faith, 1995; Riley, 1988). For all subjects combined, correlations between the dissociation scales (DES and QED) and the hypnotic susceptibility scale (HGSHS:A) were .09 and .10, respectively. Therefore, for the sample as a whole, the variance in hypnotizability scores explained by dissociation scales is approximately 1%. It can also be noted that similar correlations between the dissociation scales and the hypnotic susceptibility scales were found with each administration.

Although there was little correlation between dissociation and hypnotizability, there still existed a possibility of a nonlinear relationship. That is, the relationship could exist only for selected aspects of the distribution such as high hypnotizability subjects. This possibility was investigated using scatterplots of the data. QED and DES scores were plotted independently against the HGSHS:A scores. Figure 1 shows these results for the DES. The QED showed similar results, which are not reproduced in this chapter. Inspection of the plot does not support a nonlinear relationship. Dissociation scores were scattered uniformly across the range of hypnotizability scores.

Another possibility is that separate factors on the HGSHS:A would correlate differentially with dissociative experiences. Several distinct content dimensions have repeatedly emerged in factor analytic studies of hypnotic susceptibility (Hilgard, 1965). In summary of Hilgard's presentation, these factors are: (1) a general hypnotizability or direct suggestion factor; (2) a motor inhibition factor; (3) a cognitive and sensory inhibition factor; and (4) a positive hallucination factor. The cognitive-sensory inhibition factor includes amnesia and negative hallucinations. However, some of the factors represent more difficult items than others.

To investigate whether difficulty level of hypnotic challenges, as reflected in

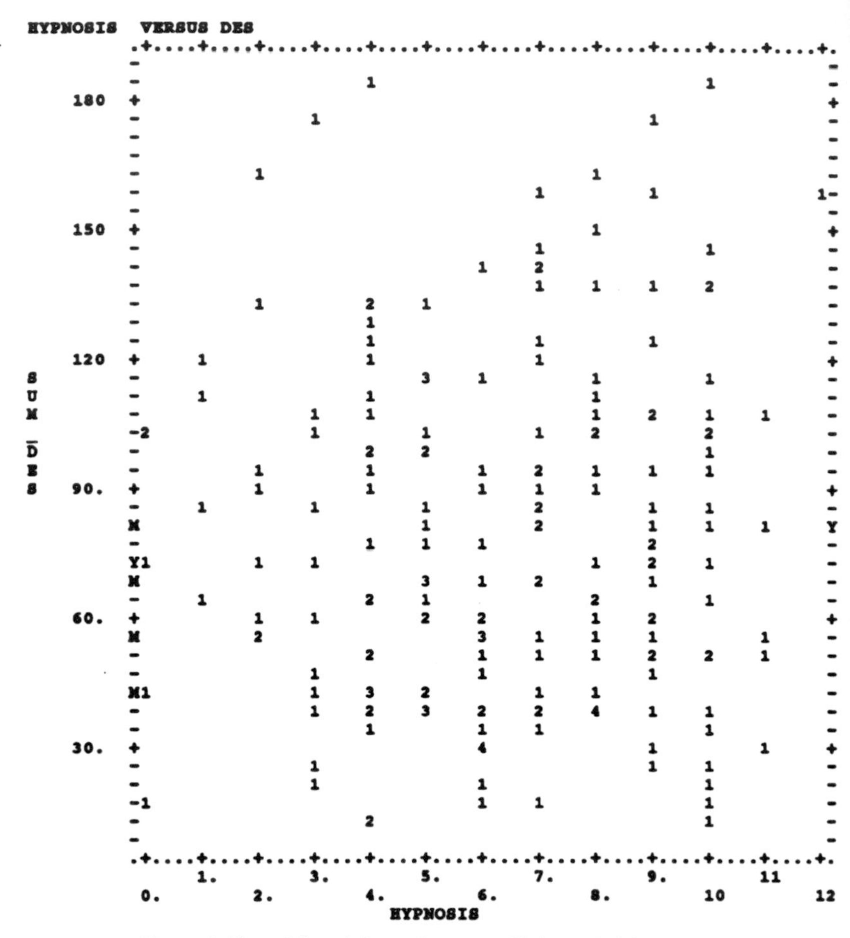

Figure 1. Plots of dissociation scale scores with hypnotizability scores.

factorial structure, was related to dissociative experiences, we performed a factor analysis (BMDP 4M with varimax rotation) on the HGSHS:A items with the present subject sample. The factors that were found quite closely approximated those reported in the literature (Hilgard, 1965; Peters, Dhanens, Lundy, & Landy, 1974). Factor scores on the hypnotic susceptibility scale were computed for 858 subjects and then correlated with DES and QED scores. All correlations ranged from −.06 to .12 and were nonsignificant. The data suggest no relationship between response difficulty and dissociation score, since the factors with items of greater difficulty (posthypnotic suggestion, posthypnotic amnesia) were not associated with a report of more dissociative experiences (DES or QED scores).

Further, psychophysiological data suggest a differential of responding in individuals selected as high in hypnotic susceptibility and dissociative tendencies. That is, although previous EEG baseline data demonstrate a differentiation of EEG activity, especially in the theta band, in hypnotically susceptible subjects (Graffin, Ray, & Lundy, 1995), no differentiation of baseline EEG characteristics was found in college-age subjects scoring high on the DES (Ray & Faith, 1993). Thus, in terms of both psychometric and psychophysiological studies, an orthogonal relationship between hypnotizability and dissociation exists, at least in normal populations.

Health, Stress, and Abuse

It is widely accepted that psychopathological forms of dissociation have at their basis previous experiences of trauma, especially in childhood. In 100 MPD cases surveyed by the National Institutes of Mental Health, 97% reported significant childhood trauma, incest being the most commonly reported (Putnam, Guroff, Silberman, Barban, & Post, 1986). Similar incidence rates of trauma in MPD are reported by other researchers (Braun & Sachs, 1985; Coons & Milstein, 1984; Ross, 1989). Individuals with dissociative disorders other than MPD also frequently report early abuse histories (Coons, Bowman, & Pellows, 1989). Likewise, among individuals with nondissociative disorders, reported childhood abuse predicts dissociative symptoms (Spiegel & Cardeña, 1991). However, there is as yet little empirical substantiation of the relationship between dissociative tendencies and abuse in nonclinical populations. Thus, our first task was to examine the relationship between self-reported abuse and dissociative tendencies. In a sample of 737 college students, we found an overall positive relationship (r = .38) between all forms of childhood abuse (sexual abuse, punishment, and neglect) and dissociative tendencies. Looking at specific types of abuse, the strongest relationship was found between experiences of neglect and dissociative tendencies (r = .34). That is, subjects who reported being neglected, as in the case of inaccessible parents (e.g., alcoholic or frequently fighting parents), reported higher experiences of dissociative tendencies than those who reported sexual abuse (r = .19) or physical punishment (r = .28).

In terms of the relationship between reporting dissociative experiences and health and stress, a moderate relationship was found. There was a positive correlation (r = .25, n = 492) between reporting dissociative experiences on the DES and the amount of time an individual felt to be under stress or felt to be upset/angry/sad (r = .26, n = 739). Likewise, scores on the DES correlated with both scores on the Beck Depression Inventory (r = .30, n = 415) and the State Trait Anxiety Inventory (r = .31, n = 414). In terms of specific health symptoms, there was a positive correlation between scores on the DES and the follow specific complaints: joint pains/sore muscles (r = .41, n = 739); sweaty palms or underarms/nervous stomach/flushed (r = .30, n = 739); bowel problems/indigestion (r = .25, n = 739); aware of heart rate/short of breath/feeling dizzy (r = .36, n = 739); headaches (r = .26, n = 739); colds/flu/being sick (r = .34, n = 739); and using alcohol/drugs (r = .33, n = 739).

Given the previous correlations relating abuse, stress, health, and dissociative experiences, the time is ripe to return to the original questions of Janet as to constitutional predispositions of certain individuals to stress and dissociative tendencies. It is also time to examine the developmental time line or order of events that function as mediating or moderating factors in term of dissociatve processes and their function in psychopathology. Empirical and theoretical implications of such developmental processes are discussed in other chapters.

DEVELOPMENT OF DISSOCIATION IN NORMAL POPULATIONS

Given that the research reported in this chapter with normal subjects reported few subjects that did not endorse some type of dissociative experience, it is difficult to view dissociation as other than a normal cognitive process. Our current way of viewing dissociation is to suggest that all individuals come into this world in a dissociative state. This may result from either an immature nervous system that is yet to form or even from a break of a physiological entrainment process between the mother and her infant in the womb. That is to suggest that previous to birth the physiological organizing principle of the developing nervous system is that of the mother. With birth, this entrainment process is broken and the various aspects of the child's nervous systems function in a less than totally integrative manner. If indeed the development of physiological, emotional, cognitive, and motoric integration continues throughout a child's development until a unifying principle, generally referred to as "self," develops, then dissociation can be seen as the resultant of an interruption of that normal process. As has been pointed out by others, such disorders as multiple personality disorder are not actually a number of personalities but the lack of any strong personality or coherent system. At this point trauma of various forms appears to be the more likely candidate for producing an interruption in normal development that would lead to such psychopathological dissociative states. However, Janet's original suggestion of constitutional weakness must also be considered.

Although few physiological data exist at this point, it is important to consider recent work in relation to the functioning of perceptual binding mechanisms, although this mechanism takes place on a more micro level. Recent research suggests that an approximately 40- to 70-Hz EEG signal appears in a variety of areas across the brain when responding to a similar stimulus and that this serves to combine our awareness into a coherent whole (cf. Gray & Singer, 1989). Crick and Koch (1990) go further to suggest that such synchronous firing is not only a means of combining perceptions but also of establishing consciousness. Although a conceptual leap, it could be possible that with certain dissociative disorders (e.g., dissociative identity disorder), different binding mechanisms could be connected with different "personalities." Of more interest to cognitive scientists is the further suggestion that this binding process is the mechanism for placing cognitions into working memory. If this same or a similar mechanism is not only involved in bringing the various aspects of stimulus perception into a coherent whole externally but is also involved with internal experiences, then it would lie at the heart of such dissociative experiences as amnesia and depersonalization-derealization.

American Psychiatric Association, (1987). *Diagnostic and statistical manual of mental disorders* (3rd ed., rev.). Washington, DC: Author.

American Psychiatric Association. (1994). *Diagnostic and statistical manual of mental disorders*. (4th ed.). Washington, DC: Author.

Angiulo, M., & Kihlstrom, J. (1991). Dissociative experiences in a college population. Unpublished Manuscript, University of Arizona.

Bernstein, E., & Putnam, F. (1986). Development, reliability, and validity of a dissociation scale. *Journal of Nervous and Mental Disease, 174*, 727-735.

Bliss, E. L. (1986). *Multiple personality, allied disorders, and hypnosis*. New York: Oxford University Press.

Braun, B. G. (1988). The BASK model of dissociation. *Dissociation, 1*, 4-23.

Braun, B. G., & Sachs, R. G. (1985). The development of multiple personality disorder: Predisposing, precipitating, and perpetuating factors. In R. P. Kluft (Ed.), *Childhood antecedents of multiple personality disorder* (pp. •). Washington, DC: American Psychiatric Press.

Broadbent, D., Cooper, P., FitzGerald, P., & Parks, K. (1982). Cognitive Failures Questionnaire (CFQ) and its correlates. *British Journal of Clinical Psychology, 21*, 1-16.

Carlson, E., & Putnam, F. (1993). An update on the Dissociative Experiences Scale. *Dissociation, 6*, 16-27.

Coons, P. M., & Milstein, V. (1984). Rape and post-traumatic stress in multiple personality. *Psychological Reports, 55*, 839-845.

Coons, P. M., Bowman, E. S., & Pellows, T. A. (1989). Post-traumatic aspects of the treatment of victims of sexual abuse and incest. *Psychiatric Clinics of North America, 12*, 325-337.

Crick, F., & Koch, C. (1990). Toward a neurobiological theory of consciousness. *Seminars in the Neurosciences, 2*, 263-275.

Ellenberger, H. F. (1970). *The discovery of the unconscious*. New York: Basic Books.

Faith, M., & Ray, W. J. (1994). Hypnotizability and dissociation in a college age population: Orthogonal individual differences. *Personality and Individual Differences, 17*, 211-216.

Frey-Rohn, L. (1974). *From Freud to Jung*. Boston: Shambhala.

Frischholz, E., Lipman, L., Braun, B., & Sachs, R. (1992). Psychopathology, hypnotizability, and dissociation. *American Journal of Psychiatry, 149*, 1521-1525.

Graffin, N., Ray, W., & Lundy, R. (1995). EEG concomitants of hypnosis and hypnotic susceptibility. *Journal of Abnormal Psychology, 104*, 123-131.

Singer, W., & Grey, C. (1989). Stimulus-specific neuronal oscillations in orientation columns of cat visual cortex. *Proceedings of the National Academy of Sciences USA, 86*, 1698-1702.

Haule, J. R. (1986). Pierre Janet and dissociation: The first transference theory and its origins in hypnosis. *American Journal of Clinical Hypnosis, 29*, 86-94.

Hilgard, E. R. (1965). *Hypnotic suggestibility*. New York: Harcourt, Brace & World.

Janet, P. (1889). *L'automatisme psychologique*. Paris: Félix Alcan.

Kihlstrom, J. F., Glisky, M., & Angiulo, M. J. (1994). Dissociative tendencies and dissociative disorders. *Journal of Abnormal Psychology, 103*, 117-124.

Nemiah, J. C. (1985). Dissociative disorders. In H. Kaplan & B. Sadock (Eds.), *Comprehensive textbook of psychiatry* (4th ed., pp. 942-957. Baltimore: Williams & Wilkins.

Nemiah, J. C. (1991). Dissociation, conversion, and somatization. In D. Spiegel (Ed.), Dissociative disorders. *American Psychiatric Press Review of Psychiatry, 10*, 248-275.

Peters, J., Dhanens, T., Lundy, R., & Landy, F. (1974). A factor analytic investigation of the Harvard Group Scale of Hypnotic Susceptibility, Form A. *International Journal of Clinical and Experimental Hypnosis, 22*, 377-387.

Putnam, F. W. (1989). *Diagnosis and treatment of multiple personality disorders*. New York: Guilford.

Putnam, F. W., Guroff, J. J., Silberman, E. K., Barban, L., & Post, R. M. (1986). The clinical phenomenology of multiple personality disorder: A review of 100 recent cases. *Journal of Clinical Psychiatry, 47*, 285-293.

Quen, J. (1986). *Split minds/split brains*. New York: New York University Press.

Ray, W. J., & Faith, M. (1993). EEG processing of emotional material in high and low dissociative individuals. *Psychophysiology, 30*, S52.

Ray, W., & Faith, M. (1995). Dissociative experiences in a college age population: Follow-up with 1190 subjects. *Personality and Individual Differences, 18*, 223-230.

Ray, W. J., June, K., Turaj, K., & Lundy, R. (1992). Dissociative experiences in a college age population: A factor analytic study of two dissociation scales. *Personality and Individual Differences, 13*, 417-424.

Ray, W., & Lukens, S. (1995). Dissociative experiences and their relation to psychopathology in a college-age population. Paper presented at the Society for Psychopathology Research annual meeting, Iowa City, IA.

Reason, J. (1984). Lapses of attention in everyday life. In R. Parasuraman & D. Davies (Eds.), *Varieties of attention* (pp. 515-549). London: Academic Press.

Reason, J., & Mycielska, K. (1982). *Absent-minded? The psychology of mental lapses and everyday errors*. Englewood Cliffs, New Jersey: Prentice-Hall.

Riley, K. (1988). Measures of dissociation. *Journal of Nervous and Mental Disease, 176*, 449-450.

Ross, C. (1989). *Multiple personality disorder*. New York: John Wiley.

Ross, C., Heber, S., Norton, G., & Anderson, G. (1989). Differences between multiple personality disorder and other diagnostic groups on structured interview. *Journal of Nervous and Mental Disease, 177*, 487-491.

Ross, C., Joshi, S., & Currie, R. (1990). Dissociative experiences in the general population. *American Journal of Psychiatry, 147*, 1547-1552.

Ross, C., Ryan, L., Voigt, H., & Eide, L. (1991b). High and low dissociators in a college student population. *Dissociation, 4*, 147-151.

Ryan, L. (1988). *Prevalence of dissociative disorders and symptoms in a university population*. Unpublished doctoral dissertation, California Institute of Integral Studies, San Francisco.

Ryan, L., & Ross, C. (1988). Dissociation in adolescents and college students. In B. G. Braun (Ed.), *Proceedings of the fifth international conference on multiple personality/dissociative states* (p. 19). Chicago: Rush Presbyterian St. Luke's Medical Center.

Sanders, B., & Green, J. (1994). The factor structure of the dissociative experiences scale in college students. *Dissociation, 7*, 23-27.

Sanders, S. (1986). The perceptual alteration scale: A scale measuring dissociation. *American Journal of Clinical Hypnosis, 2*, 95-102.

Sjövall, B. (1967). *Psychology of tension: An analysis of Pierre Janet's concept of "tension psychologique" together with an historical aspect*. Stockholm: Svenska Bokföflaget.

Spiegel, D., & Cardeña, E. (1991). Disintegrated experience: The dissociative disorders revisited. *Journal of Abnormal Psychology, 100*, 366-378.

Spiegel, H. (1963). The dissociation-association continuum. *Journal of Nervous and Mental Disease, 136*, 374-378.

Steinberg, M. (1993). *Structured Clinical Interview for DSM-IV Dissociative Disorders (SCID-D)*. Washington, DC: American Psychiatric Press.

Tellegen, A. (1992). *Note of structure and naming of the MPQ Absorption Scale*. Unpublished manuscript, University of Minnesota, Minneapolis.

Tellegen, A., & Atkinson, G. (1974). Complexity and measurement of hypnotic susceptibility: A comment on Coe and Sarbin's alternative interpretation. *Journal of Personality and Social Psychology, 33*, 142-148.

Vanderlinden, J., Van Dyck, R., Vandereycken, W., & Vertommen, H. (1991). Dissociative experiences in the general population in the Netherlands and Belgium: A study with the Dissociative Questionnaire (DIS-Q). *Dissociative, 4*, 180-184.

II
DEVELOPMENTAL PERSPECTIVES

This section begins with the important relationship between dissociative disorders and childhood trauma. Although there is ample evidence to suggest an association between dissociative disorders and previous trauma, there has been little theory and research to understand these processes within a developmental perspective. Part II begins to approach this important theme and to place dissociative processes within a developmental perspective. In Chapter 4, Pamela Cole and her colleagues ask how dissociation can be understood from the standpoint of normative development and emotional regulation. These researchers begin with the assumption that early childhood trauma affects developing patterns of emotional regulation and they examine the conditions under which trauma might promote dissociative disorders. For example, they suggest that ages 3 to 5 represent a critical period in which sexual abuse can lead to more severe dissociative disorders such as dissociative identity disorder. However, the story may not be quite so simple as these authors demonstrate. They point out the importance of not only understanding a trauma situation but also examining the developmental characteristics of the victim prior to the trauma, during the trauma, and after the trauma is over. To help clarify this relationship, the focus of Chapter 4 is on father-daughter incest. The important question to ask is what are the co-occurring developmental processes that are present with the onset of incest in particular and any trauma in general.

In Chapter 5, Goodwin and Sachs begin by describing stories of abuse from the popular press and continue with survey data from professionals treating dissociative disorders. From their review, they suggest a strong relationship between dissociative disorders and previous trauma. Throughout their discussion they raise a number of intriguing questions as to the etiology of dissociative processes. First, these authors note the similarity between patients with severe dissociative disorders and shell-shocked combat veterans. Second, they ask if there exists a similarity in mechanism between those processes, found in both animals and humans, that place the organism in a deep trance during conditions of stress and those underlying dissociative processing. Third, the question is raised as to why not all individuals who experience severe child abuse develop dissociative disorders. And fourth, the question of abuse and dissociation running in families is raised. Overall, this chapter helps us to understand some of the questions that need to be asked in future research as well as the difficulty of finding simple answers.

All children proceed through certain developmental stages that include shifts in perceptual, motor, and emotional development. Bowlby emphasized the emotional attachment seen in infants with their caregivers, generally their mothers. Developmental researchers have been interested in early attachment relationships and later social competence. As will be described in great detail in the chapters, the nature of these attachments can be classified into distinct patterns. In Chapter 6, Main and Morgan ask if one of the these distinct patterns—the disorganized-disoriented pattern—has a phenotypic resemblance to dissociative states. Not unlike the trance states of animals described by Goodwin and Sachs, Main and Morgan describe certain infants as "freezing all movement." Interestingly enough, there also appears to be a characteristic response of the parents of such infants, again raising the question of intergenerational transition of traumatic behaviors and responses. Main and Morgan describe one possible mechanism for such transmission in a case report in which an infant learns to respond in a psychopathological manner to the parents' responses to their own traumatic memories. The chapters in this section also raise the important question as to why some individuals who experience severe trauma never manifest dissociative experiences. Perhaps a better understanding of attachment events and development sequences will hold the key to this important question.

The final chapter in the section, by Hornstein, focuses on formal descriptions of dissociative disorders in children and adolescents. As can be seen from the chapter, dissociative experiences of children do not exist in isolation, but co-occur with a variety of affective, attentional, and behavioral problems, making exact differentiation difficult. As with adults, children who are diagnosed with dissociative disorders also have received a variety of previous psychiatric diagnoses, the most common of which are depression, depressive psychosis, posttraumatic stress disorder, oppositional defiant disorder, conduct disorder, and attention deficit hyperactivity disorder.

4

Dissociation in Typical and Atypical Development

Examples from Father–Daughter Incest Survivors

Pamela M. Cole, Pamela C. Alexander, and Catherine L. Anderson

Dissociation has been characterized as the lack of normal integration of thoughts, feelings, and experiences into the stream of consciousness and memory (Nemiah, 1981; Putnam, 1984). The term is used to describe clinical conditions in which individuals lose awareness or memory of events and their attendant internal states. In addition, the term is sometimes used to describe normative regulatory processes by which an individual modulates internal state (e.g., intense emotion) and external input (e.g., aversive stimulation). For example, denial and dissociation have been described as primary defense mechanisms for children prior to school age (Cramer, 1991). Dissociation also appears to be a universal response to trauma at all ages (Putnam, 1985). The disconnection of affective content from conscious awareness at the time of trauma helps the individual both to mobilize for action without being flooded by emotion and to tolerate trauma until it is ended and physical and psychological help is available. Therefore, it may be that dissociation can be understood from the standpoint of normative development and emotion regulation.

It is not known whether more common dissociative processes should be regarded as being on a continuum of functionality with dissociative disorders, or

Pamela M. Cole • Department of Psychology, Pennsylvania State University, University Park, Pennsylvania 16802. **Pamela C. Alexander** • Department of Psychology, University of Maryland, College Park, Maryland 20742. **Catherine L. Anderson** • Northwest Center for Community Mental Health, Reston, Virginia 22091.

Handbook of Dissociation: Theoretical, Empirical, and Clinical Perspectives, edited by Larry K. Michelson and William J. Ray. Plenum Press, New York, 1996.

whether dissociative disorders represent a discrete and distinct set of processes. One possibility is that a normative regulatory process, under conditions of severe and/or sustained stress, may develop a dysfunctional quality. For example, if an individual experiences intense emotional distress in childhood, she may become primarily reliant on dissociative coping throughout development. Such an outcome would interfere with her ability to function in an attuned and flexible manner in adult relationships and to conduct the responsibilities of adult life. The prevailing wisdom is that severe dissociation, including conditions like multiple personality disorder (MPD), is particularly likely to occur in conjunction with early childhood trauma. Retrospective research indicates that the development of a condition like MPD is associated with sexual abuse that begins between the ages of 3 to 5 when dissociation may be a primary normative emotion regulatory strategy (see Cole & Putnam, 1992, for a developmental discussion).

Emotion regulation, a term that conveys that emotions are subject to regulation and that they are regulatory of other functions (e.g., attention), can be used to provide an integrative perspective on typical and atypical development related to dissociation. Although emotion regulation is a moment-to-moment process, several theorists contend that stable patterns of emotion regulation form a core of personality (e.g., Izard, 1979; Malatesta, 1990; Rothbart & Ahadi, 1994; Watson & Clark, 1984). From this perspective, a habitual reliance on a particular method of regulating emotion can come to characterize an individual's style of coping. If that style is dissociative, the likelihood is that there will be serious impairment in the individual's ability to act responsively and responsibly in life. Potential for serious impairment exists as experiences, particularly emotion-laden experiences, become temporally disconnected and episodes of time are thus lost from consciousness and memory. In the most extreme forms of dissociative disorder, this style of emotional functioning interferes with the integration of personality and promotes the development of the experience of multiplicity of separate selves.

This chapter on developmental perspectives on dissociation is organized around the assumption that early childhood trauma affects developing patterns of emotion regulation and that under certain conditions that trauma can promote dissociative disorders. The basis of our clinical perspective is our experience with clients and research participants with a history of childhood sexual abuse. Dissociative disorder has been noted to occur among many, but by no means all, survivors of childhood sexual abuse (Gelinas, 1983). Dissociation serves as both an initial protective response to emotional trauma and, for some, as a subsequent style of functioning and a form of psychopathology (Sexton, Harralson, Hulsey, & Nash, 1988). As a result of exposure to repeated, severe, inescapable, and unpredictable sexual victimization by a previously trusted individual, a child's ability to regulate distress is quickly overtaxed (Braun, 1989; Putnam, 1989; Sanders, McRoberts, & Tollefson, 1989; Spiegel, 1986). In the case of incest, abuse may occur without adequately soothing, restorative relationships that help the victim regulate emotional distress (Kluft, 1984). As a result, many abused children appear to spontaneously enter trance states in their self-regulatory attempts to find relief and to maintain emotional equilibrium in the presence of continuing, inescapable, and unpredictable trauma (Bliss, 1988).

In this chapter, we offer a developmental perspective on dissociation in both its typical and atypical presentations. Unfortunately, the empirical evidence is sparse and more questions are raised than answered. By using a *developmental psychopathology* perspective, we hope to suggest that dissociation can be explored as a normative phenomenon and that particular conditions may promote the development of atypical dissociative patterns. Such a perspective requires a description of dissociation in relation to normal child, adult, and family development (Rutter & Garmezy, 1983; Sroufe & Rutter, 1984). To focus our discussion, we rely on our clinical and research experiences with girls and women who have been victims of father-daughter incest. Psychological vulnerabilities in reaction to a disturbed parent-child relationship are conceptualized in terms of developmental factors that influence the child's capacity to regulate the emotional trauma, specific developmental tasks that are compromised by the trauma, and familial conditions that promote and sustain dissociative functioning as a primary means of regulating emotion. We depict how incest can arise in families that cope through denial and dissociation, how dissociation helps the child victim survive the incest, and how the incest experience in its familial context can promote the consolidation of a dissociative disorder.

THE RELATIONSHIP BETWEEN INCEST AND DISSOCIATION

Dissociation often occurs as a response to trauma, such as incest. Unlike many other forms of trauma, however, incestuous behavior by a father is rarely a discrete event. More typically, the incest is a disturbance in an existing primary relationship that has as its focal point numerous episodes of unwanted sexual contact. In our view, incest involves an extreme form of trauma in which psychological and often physical injury occur regularly and chronically to the child. Although unwanted sexual contacts provide a defining core of this particular form of abuse, incest may be most debilitating in terms of the emotional injury to the relationship between the child and her family. Therefore, the level of the child's emotional distress may be determined more by the meaning of the sexual incidents and disturbed relationship than by the incidents themselves. Her psychological interpretation of the events determines the quality of her posttraumatic adaptation at any given point (van der Kolk, 1987).

Most incest victims must cope with multiple aspects of the experience: (1) physical and psychological trauma in the form of the actual sexual experiences, including violation of one's body; (2) extended periods of apprehension, guilt, and fear between sexual contacts; and (3) the damage to and potential loss of a relationship with one or more emotionally significant family members. The intense and sustained nature of incest places excessive demands on the child's developing ability to regulate emotional states and compromises her ability to acquire alternative coping strategies as she matures. The incest violates whatever basic sense of trust she has formed, deprives her of reliance on family members for comfort and problem-solving, and interferes with her ability to seek and form emotionally satisfying and soothing relationships with others. Therefore, the incest victim experiences sustained, pervasive trauma that she cannot diminish or control in reality. As a result, it is thought that dissociation affords the young victim the most reasonable recourse in the face of an abusive parental relationship.

Emotion regulation is often discussed in terms of the intrapsychic processes involved in managing emotion. It is equally important to emphasize that incest emerges within a context of broader family dysfunction. Incestuous families are not a homogeneous group, and a specific preexisting familial dysfunction has not been isolated. Nonetheless, incest does not emerge at random. Instead, it reflects intergenerational vulnerabilities that lead two adults to form a marriage and a family in which a father perpetrates sexual abuse on his daughter. The incestuous family environment promotes the child's dissociative processes by serving as (1) a *predisposing* climate in which dissociative processes are the primary means of the family's emotional functioning, (2) a *precipitating* factor by virtue of the trauma of the abuse, and (3) a *perpetuating* force in the maintenance of dissociation as a means for the family to tolerate the trauma (Braun, 1984). For these reasons, we focus not on the specific nature of the abuse but rather on the development of the family and the incest victim at three different stages—before the incest begins, during the incest, and after the sexual acts have ended.

THE DEVELOPMENTAL PERSPECTIVE

Child Development and Family Functioning in the Preincestuous Period

In describing child development and family functioning in the incestuous family, we assume that (1) family relationships are one of the most important units of analysis, (2) family relationships have continuity and coherence over time such that they are predictable across individuals and generations, (3) individuals internalize family relationships, and (4) these internalized relationships are carried forward into the next generation (Sroufe & Fleeson, 1988). We begin our review by discussing the nature of emotional development in the first years of childhood and the nature of the family context out of which father-daughter incest eventually emerges.

Child Development. The ability to regulate one's own emotional state begins in infancy and appears to be influenced by biologically governed dispositional factors (temperament, certain cognitive capabilities) and socially governed experiences (parent-child relationships, exposure to stress). For example, infants use gaze aversion to reduce and seek stimulation from external sources and self-sucking to reduce the level of internal autonomic activity (Rothbart, Ziaie, & O'Boyle, 1992; Stifter & Moyer, 1991). These early behaviors indicate that the human is equipped at the earliest stage to begin to regulate emotional experience by refocusing attention (Wolff, 1987). It has been suggested that the capacity of infants and toddlers to enter rapidly into deep trance states is indicative of a capacity to dissociate from external events (Gardner & Olness, 1981).

Infants must rely, however, primarily on adult caregivers to regulate their emotional states through responsive parenting. Parental regulatory behavior may contribute to the rudiments of a normative dissociative capacity in young children by stimulating state shifts through stroking, rocking, and singing (Gardner & Olness, 1981). Furthermore, young children appear to adopt these strategies to sooth themselves. For example, the young son of a colleague became terrified at a fireworks display. His mother took him to the car and caressed him until he fell asleep. He did not recall having been upset when they discussed it the next day. The next time the family went to a fireworks display, the boy began stroking his hair and spontaneously fell asleep.

Prior to age 8–10 months, infants do not appear to appreciate the continuity of objects in space and time. For example, it is only during the end of the first year that they begin to search for hidden objects (see Harris, 1983). Therefore, an accomplishment of infancy is the discovery that things exist beyond one's immediate, concrete experience of them. This accomplishment, often called *object permanence* or *constancy*, includes the capacity to temporarily hold onto the sense of maternal emotional comfort during mother's absence and to delay distress until she has returned (Ainsworth, Blehar, Waters, & Wall, 1978).

Developmental psychologists use the construct of *attachment* (Bowlby, 1969) to conceptualize the manner in which emotion regulatory interactions take place in the larger context of the infant–caregiver relationship. The quality of the attachment relationship has been shown to predict later social competence (Waters, Wippman, & Sroufe, 1979), formation of self-identity and self-understanding (Cicchetti & Beeghly, 1990), and even the quality of adult relationships with partners and children (Main & Goldwyn, 1984).

Infants' attachment-related behaviors have been used to characterize the attachment as secure or insecure (Ainsworth et al., 1978). Secure attachment involves the infant's ability to tolerate negative affect for short periods of time with the confidence that the parent will be available presently and to experience solace from the caregiver as needed. Insecure attachment involves deviations from this pattern. The two most commonly described forms of insecure attachment are avoidant attachment in which the infant blunts negative emotions and remains detached from the parent, and resistant attachment in which the infant actively attempts to engage the parent but often without solace.

A third and more rare form of insecure attachment has been noted to occur among children with a history of abuse. Disorganized attachment is defined by simultaneous approach–avoidance, freezing, apprehension, and dazed expressions when the child is reunited with the parent (Carlson, Cicchetti, Barnett, & Braunwald, 1989; Main & Solomon, 1986, 1990). For example, a child might rock on hands and knees after unsuccessfully approaching the parent, may move away from the parent while simultaneously displaying fearfulness about approaching anyone else, or may freeze in posture for several seconds en route to approaching the parent. It is thought that these stultifying behaviors reflect a confusion about approach and avoidance that results in their mutual inhibition (Main & Hesse, 1990; Main & Solomon, 1986). The apparent similarity of these behaviors to dissociation is noteworthy.

This approach–avoidance tends to occur specifically in the presence of a parent who exhibits what Main and Hesse (1990) refer to as "frightened and/or frightening" behavior and who frequently has a history of traumatic loss or sexual abuse. The parent, for example, may suddenly invade the infant's personal space, such as looming into the infant's face or sliding his or her hands across the infant's throat (Main & Hesse, 1990, 1992). Alternatively, the parent may appear to be frightened as the infant reaches toward the parent's face. Thus, the parent appears to flee from the child (through expressions of fear, dissociation, or actually leaving, precisely at as time when the child is most in need of reassurance and nurturance from the parent (Liotti, 1992). Liotti (1992) speculates that the parent's own unresolved attachment history, memories of which may be triggered or amplified by the presence of the child, appear to cause the parent to unconsciously look to the child for soothing and comfort. This role reversal has been observed in the relationship between parents and disorganized children (Main & Cassidy, 1988). When the child fails to adequately nurture the parent, the parent is likely to become angry and aggressive (i.e., frightening) toward the child (Bowlby, 1985). Thus the child finds herself in the untenable position of relating to a parent who is simultaneously the source of the solution and the source of the problem (Main & Solomon, 1986). The breakdown of the child's strategies for experiencing the security of the attachment during times of stress are thwarted and this situation is thought to result in dissociated states.

Much of emotional development during toddlerhood is characterized by the child's learning about her own and others' emotions and instrumental behaviors for dealing with distress (Dunn, 1988; Kagan, 1981; Kopp, 1982; Stipek, Gralinski, & Kopp, 1990; Zahn-Waxler, Radke-Yarrow, & King, 1979). These newly acquired skills are limited, and toddlers are easily overwhelmed by life's emotional challenges. Parents attempt to support the child's developing emotional autonomy, often using techniques such as distraction to manage toddler distress rather than the physical caregiving that they provided in infancy. For example, when toddlers are upset by minor problems, adults often redirect children's attention to interesting toys or activities. This attentional shift separates the first event (the distress) from the subsequent event (the toy). This normative use of distraction may promote or extend the child's capacity to dissociate.

During these same years, language is rapidly developing and children are learning labels for their internal states, e.g., emotions (Bretherton, Fritz, Zahn-Waxler, & Ridgeway, 1986). Young children gain experience communicating about emotion with their parents and siblings, and emotion words develop at approximately the same time as self-referent terms like *me* and *I* (Bloom, 1991). Fischer (1980) has theorized that development is characterized by the acquisition of individual, specific skills and subsequent organization of sets of skills into units. For example, toddlers acquire words for naming emotions, but they cannot use those emotion terms in all the ways that an adult can. Also, a child may use and understand positively and negatively valenced affective terms (e.g., nice and mean) but be unable to integrate these two separate understandings. The acquisition of component skills prior to their reorganization into more sophisticated skill units is the basis for *affective splitting*, the inability to coordinate or integrate negative valences about events that leads to them being treated as separate, unrelated events (see also Harter, 1983).

The preschool years (ages 2 through 5 or 6) mark the transition from infancy to childhood. During this period, children face the task of integrating their experience of being an agentic self with the restrictions and sanctions of the social world. Their developing cognitive skills and broadening social experience are associated with a rapidly expanding ability to control their own actions and emotions (Kopp, 1982; Dunn, 1988). Cognitive advances also allow the child to imagine possibilities beyond the concrete realities of her experience. The preschool child can engage in symbolic play to explore the nature of experience (Garvey, 1977). Through interactions and through play, preschoolers learn the limits of and differences between what is real and what is not real and can experiment with imaginary characters and scenarios for problem resolution (Wolf, 1990). That is, through the cognitive and social activities of early childhood, children have experiences that help them explore imagination and reality and promote the development of reality-based coping with emotional distress.

In situations where preschoolers lack cognitively articulated scripts for coping, denial (behaving as if a problematic situation did not happen or is not true) appears to be a common coping mechanism (Cramer, 1991; Fraiberg, 1959; Freud, 1966; Trad, 1989). Anna Freud argued that denial and dissociation are normative in young children in part because they are promoted by techniques parents use to help young children cope (e.g., when preparing a child for an immunization injection, saying "Now, this won't hurt"). Empirical research has supported this description of preschoolers' coping (Cramer, 1991; Dunn, 1988; Schibuk, Bond, & Bouffard, 1989).

It is during the preschool years that children first appear to be able to integrate positive and negative qualities of a person or an event. For example, with play objects, older preschoolers can represent a single doll as a character who is nice and then mean. But she is likely to be unable to conceptually represent the possibility that two people interacting can be simultaneously nice and mean (see Fischer & Pipp, 1984, for an extended discussion). Analyses of young children's play and conversations indicate that they develop the capacity during the preschool years to play out events by assigning roles to characters. They are able to assume roles and to switch them fluidly during pretend play, to generate imaginary friends, and to blame their own misdeeds on someone else or use a "pretend identity" (Dunn, 1988; Wolf, 1990).

Dissociative capacity is reported to increase during the preschool years. In addition, denial, visual hallucinations, spontaneous trance states, amnesias, rapid shifts in demeanor, imaginary playmates, and sleepwalking may be more common in the preschool years (Cramer, 1991; Gardner & Olness, 1981; Putnam, 1991). Although these behaviors may cause concern if seen in older children, they may allow younger children to isolate and tolerate confusing and complex aspects of their emotional worlds. Until they are able to coordinate and integrate multiple, diverging aspects of experience intellectually, young children simply ignore one part of an experience in order to dwell on the other. This dissociative pattern has been called "fractionation" (Fischer & Pipp, 1984).

In sum, the data suggest that there is a period between infancy and elementary school age during which young children may be capable of and tend to engage in mental strategies that allow them to disconnect events in time, to play with manipulating reality, and to organize experiences into different characters and roles. At the same time, they are having many experiences that promote and assist them with coping in a reality-based way (e.g., parents use of reviewing events and reasoning about them).

In a family where there is clearly something wrong, and the parents continually reassure the child that everything is all right and fail to provide opportunities for labeling the distress, it seems logical that a child could develop a reliance on dissociative coping—failing to cognize about distressful states and events, resorting to manipulations of reality in fantasy, and subjugating the experience of distress to the parental "worldview" that everything is well. Recent data indicate that maltreated toddlers are less likely to use internal state language than nonmaltreated toddlers and that these differences are not attributable to differences in expressive language skill (Beeghly & Cicchetti, 1994). In addition, Fischer and Ayoub (1994) have shown in case studies and research samples of young children the powerful influences of maltreatment on the development of the abilities to isolate and integrate affective and cognitive information. Therefore, it is clear that family violence and maltreatment interfere with the development of important skills that allow the child to understand and integrate multiple aspects of their worlds.

The relation between the normative fluidity of young children's thinking and feeling and instances of pathological dissociation is not understood, and the question of whether pathological dissociation can take place in preschool age children is unresolved. There are reports in the psychiatric literature of cases of child multiple personality disorder (Kluft, 1985; Peterson, 1991), but the developmental status of young children makes it particularly challenging to discriminate normative from atypical patterns. Examination of the child's history may show evidence of extreme or unremitting dissociative qualities that exceed that noted in typical development.

For example, a 4-year-old boy who had been an incest victim for most of his life was seen for evaluation to determine whether he was "psychotic." The presenting problem was that he was completely unresponsive when he was being scolded for his misdeeds. Some of his wrongdoing was very serious, including trapping the pet cat in the oven and turning on the oven, breaking all the mirrors in the house, putting objects in an infant sibling's anus, and setting sheets on fire. When scolded, he would enter a trancelike state during which he would not flinch if a loud sound was made behind him. He appeared to have no recollection of the misdeeds or reprimands. This phenomenon of dissociating himself this completely from what these types of events is not typical of children this age. The casework history revealed that he had been subjected to sexual abuse by his mother since infancy.

Studies designed from a developmental psychopathology framework are needed to assess the various capacities of nonrisk young children and at-risk children and to follow children's progress over time. Additionally, individual development must be considered in the context of the family. We now turn to a developmental discussion of the formation of incestuous families.

Family Functioning. Abusive family relationships are so imbedded in generations of family dysfunction that it is hard to define a beginning point. We begin with the formation of the family in which incest is first identified. As stated previously, even in the typical and adaptively functioning family, parents engage in processes that promote the dissociative capacity of the young child. In the context of a supportive, responsive family system that allows the flexibility to cope in diverse ways, parents' and children's dissociation are but one of a variety of emotion regulatory devices, including those that provide a context for the child to advance to more sophisticated strategies. However, other families appear to function predominantly in terms of denial of interpersonal distress and via dissociation in the recognition and interpretation of emotionally significant events.

We believe that one way that this pattern emerges is when dissociative style characterizes the psychological functioning of one, and usually both, parents. In fact, we would argue that there is a tendency for young adults with dissociative styles to select each other as marital partners due to a shared history of child abuse. We argue that these parents become active participants in the intergenerational transmission of psychological patterns that promote the continuation of abuse across generations.

Attachment theory, which hypothesizes four distinct patterns of attachment, provides a useful model for understanding the intergenerational transmission of patterns of emotional functioning. In particular, Main and Goldwyn (1984) suggest that adult attachment provides a means of conceptualizing how functional or dysfunctional relationships in one's family of origin are internalized and replicated in the family of procreation. Secure attachment in adulthood is reflected in the ability to recall emotionally positive and negative childhood experiences with ease and integration. Insecure attachment in adults is associated with difficulty and inconsistency in memories of childhood. Adults with a dismissing pattern of attachment idealize childhood. They fail to access negative memories and devalue the importance of their attachment relationships; this pattern exists even when they provide evidence of events that would suggest that childhood was far from ideal and highly aversive. Adults with a preoccupied pattern of attachment are characterized by heightened affect, excessive dependency on intimate relationships, and an inability to move beyond the relationships with the caregivers.

A final category—unresolved-fearful adult attachment—may be particularly important in the understanding of the development of incestuous relationships and of dissociative disorders as a consequence of those relationships. Main and Hesse (1990) used this category to describe the behavior of parents whose children were classified as disorganized in their attachment. These parents appeared frightened and/or frightening to their children and frequently had a history of their own traumatic loss or sexual abuse. This same pattern of adult attachment has been found to be prevalent among incest survivors (Alexander et al., 1995) and to be significantly correlated with the degree of dissociation and borderline personality disorder in incest survivors (Alexander et al., 1995; Anderson & Alexander, 1995). That is, the unresolved, conflictual attachment history of the parent is likely to co-occur with dissociative symptoms and negatively impinge on the child's ability to use the parent as a secure base.

Secure attachment provides an individual with the ability to be effective in his or her own emotional regulation and to be attuned to the emotional needs of others. These qualities protect against the emergence of incest by guiding the secure adult both in selecting a well-adjusted marital partner and in organizing the parent's emotional responses to the challenges presented by children. Therefore, secure attachment is less likely to be seen in abusive parents and their partners.

Preexisting insecure attachment, on the other hand, can set the stage for abusive behavior (Alexander, 1992). In this regard, the unresolved-fearful pattern may be the most predictive of incestuous abuse. Because of the lack of resolution about their own trauma or loss in childhood, adults characterized by an unresolved-fearful attachment are inextricably connected to their families of origin by the competing fears of intimacy and abandonment. They are enmeshed with their own parents in patterns that are similar to those described by Main and Cassidy (1988) for the disorganized child. That is, their relations with their own parents are conflictual and reflect the approach-avoidance conflict that paralyzes the young child. For example, Alexander and Schwartz (1995) found that dissociation is significantly correlated with both fusion and triangulation with one's family of origin. This intense emotional involvement with the parents and an inability to resolve these ambivalent relationships interfere with the adult's ability to form loyalties and intimacy with a marital partner and increases the likelihood that he or she will act out the same approach-avoidance conflicts with the partner.

Research evidence indicates that the marital relationship of an adult who is unresolved is compromised both by her difficulty in separating from her family of origin as well as her social discomfort with and avoidance of intimacy (Alexander et al., 1995). Many such adults never marry but for those who do, the result is frequently a couple which, as a consequence of their own difficulties in emotion regulation, is susceptible to patterns of rapid escalation of negative emotion during conflicts (Kobak & Hazan, 1991). The threatening quality of the emotional escalation activates the attachment system and the pattern of vacillation between intense enmeshment and emotional distancing between the partners. They cannot satisfactorily resolve conflict or derive support and nurturance from one another. Fear of abandonment, however, may preclude the dissolution of this unhappy, ultimately destructive marriage.

When a child is born into this dysfunctional family system, the stage is set for the stabilization of the family pattern and for the intergenerational repetition of the incestuous pattern. Adults who have failed to resolve the fear and dependency of their early attachment relationships and who have been abused at an early age are likely to abuse younger children. In fact, perpetrators who abuse preschool-age children have been distinguished from those who abuse older children; the former appear to be motivated by unresolved conflicts related to nurturance, abandonment, and separation, whereas those who abuse older children are more motivated by power and dominance (Waterman, 1986).

The psychological functioning of adults who are unresolved with regard to attachment, and who may exhibit the related dissociative and borderline personality disorders, is characterized by splitting and projective identification (Alexander et al., 1995; Everett, Halperin, Volgy, & Wissler, 1989). These defenses permeate all relationships in the dissociative family (Sachs, Frischolz, & Wood, 1988) and interfere with the parent's ability to distinguish the child's needs from the adult's needs and to help the child integrate experience (Everett et al., 1989; Kluft, Braun, & Sachs, 1984). Finally, the emotional demands that the child places on the parent challenge the parent's sense of adequacy (Cole, Woolger, Power, & Smith, 1992), which further activates dissociative functioning (Main, Kaplan, & Cassidy, 1985).

The young child enters this system with presumably normal emotional responses that organize her affiliative behavior. However, if the child's very presence triggers a dissociative response from the parent or if the parent appears inexplicably frightened or dissociates when interacting with the child, the impact on the child is distressing. In such distress, the child is likely to feel an increased need to access her attachment figure (the parent). This may in turn increase the parent's withdrawal, fear, and dissociation. This emotional cycle is thought to lead to the dissociative-disorganized attachment pattern observed in children (type D). The child's resulting multiple and incompatible experiences of self may include the self as vulnerable, as threatening, as rescuer of the frightened, vulnerable parent, and as abandoned and unlovable (Liotti, 1992). Thus, the child is susceptible to the development of a dissociative disorder even before the experience of abuse has occurred.

We have taken considerable time to discuss the role of dissociation in early childhood and parental risk factors that jeopardize family functioning and child development *prior* to the onset of incest. It is important to recognize that the trauma of incest may not cause dissociative disorder directly, but may be a product of a larger intergenerational phenomenon in which a dissociative style creates a climate in which sexual abuse can occur and be tolerated. In such a predisposing atmosphere, it becomes difficult for the child to advance beyond a reliance on dissociation as a primary means of emotion regulation. In this case, the onset of sexual abuse in early childhood may create risk for the development of a severe dissociative disorder. We now turn to the qualities of the child and family during the incestuous period that could serve to support and sustain a reliance on dissociative processes.

Child Development and Family Functioning during the Incest

The Child. In the years that precede the onset of puberty, there is a reported decrease in the reliance on denial and dissociation as a method of emotion regulation (Cramer, 1991). The socioemotional tasks of the childhood years include the development of an increasing sense of one's own cognitive and social competence and sense of control (Connell, 1990; Harter, 1983), and coming to understand oneself in terms of intangible, psychological characteristics (thoughts, feelings, motivations) and in relation to others (Harter, 1983; Ruble, Boggiano, Feldman, & Loebl, 1980; Selman, 1980). Around age 8 or 9, conscious self-criticism and awareness of feelings like shame and pride are more evident (Ferguson, Stegge, & Damhuis, 1991; Harter, 1982; Selman, 1980).

The child is faced with understanding her social and private selves as having both positive and negative qualities. A major developmental task of this period is the integration of multiple aspects of self, including the integration of positive and negative qualities; in younger children, "opposite" qualities (good and bad, happy and sad, mean and nice) are cognitively incomprehensible, and they deny one or the other quality (Fischer, Shaver, & Carnochan, 1990; Harter, 1983). The integration of these multiple aspects is facilitated by the development of operational thought and metacognitive processes that permit reflection upon the self as an object of thought.

School-age children are also embarking on forming and maintaining relationships of choice (Damon, 1983), which further aid them in their developing understanding and evaluation of themselves and others. They understand that friends share enjoyable activities and are cooperative with one another, are sensitive to peer evaluation, and begin to incorporate others' perspectives into their interpersonal transactions (Selman, 1980). As they approach adolescence, they achieve more cognitively sophisticated experiences of loyalty and trust in their friendships

(Berndt, 1981; Selman, 1980). They also come to inhibit impulsive or selfish acts for the sake of social relations, to reconceptualize wrongdoing and experience guilt in terms of how they view themselves rather than on the concrete consequences of wrongful actions (e.g., punishment), and to internalize a sense of how others see them. Inference, reflection, and reasoning provide more latitude in problem-solving. The cognitive and social advances of the childhood years may promote the use of blaming (actual) others and rationalizing wrongdoing and a decrease in denying or forgetting misdeeds (Cramer, 1991; Douglas, 1965; Freud, 1966; Schibuk et al., 1989).

The timing of the onset of incest in most cases co-occurs with the timing of these developmental tasks. The average age at which the first sexualized contact between father and child occurs is between 7 and 9 years (Kendall-Tackett & Simon, 1988). Abuse prior to or at this time compromises the child's successful acquisition of all of the developmental tasks of childhood. Unable to relate realistically to emotionally intense experiences and lacking adequate models for flexible self-control, the child's behavior may vacillate between diminished and rigid control. Intense guilt, shame, and confusion diminish the likelihood of feeling secure enough to build friendships and to receive social support outside the home. Data show that physically abused school-age children are less liked by their peers (Dodge, Pettit, & Bates, 1994) and that they develop an internal sense of themselves as unlovable and others as unloving (McCrone, Egeland, Kalkoske, & Carlson, 1994). However, it is not simply a case of the development of a negative view of the self and the world; instead, dissociative processes interfere with an *integrated* view. Moreover, many perpetrators actively confuse the victim about the meaning and content of events through the use of both denial and confusion techniques. For example, one of our clients said that her father would ask her what had happened between them after each sexual incident and then shout at her that she was wrong and crazy and that he would kill her if she ever said such untruths. Thus, while denial and dissociation typically decrease during this period, they appear to remain elevated in sexually abused children (Adams-Tucker, 1985; Trickett, MacBride-Chang, & Putnam, 1994). These family dynamics interfere with the integration of positive and negative aspects of self and realistic self-appraisal.

The Adolescent. Father–daughter incest is believed to have the longest duration of all forms of childhood sexual abuse (Wyatt & Newcomb, 1990). Therefore, the experience of incest usually compromises the child's resolution of the tasks of adolescent development. The most salient of these tasks is adjustment to the onset of puberty and emerging sexuality. In typical development, adolescence is marked by cognitive advances that permit the adolescent to conceptualize psychological intimacy and to experience the intimacy of self-revelation and intense closeness in friendships. This is also the period during which the developing articulated sense of self begins to consolidate as a stable, whole experience (Damon & Hart, 1982) and as a self-contained secure base for exploring the world that no longer requires extensive regulation by parents. During this stage of development toward a consolidated sense of self, youths also experience normative multiplicity of self as they try on personae and attempt to discover and define who they "really" are (Harter & Monsour, 1992). Transient experiences of depersonalization and derealization are not atypical (Putnam, 1985).

At a point when the typical adolescent girl has the developmental base from which to absorb her changing sexual identity and to incorporate this into her peer relationships, the incest victim has had precocious exposure to sexuality, experiences herself as different from any and all of her peers, and has a distorted sense of her self as a partner in relationships. Moreover, the continuing developmental task of integrating the multiple and changing aspects of self into a coalesced, coherent whole is probably significantly jeopardized. The nature of the adult outcomes uniquely linked to incest suggest that this integration is profoundly compromised by early-onset incest (Cole & Putnam, 1992). If it is the case that the emotional demands of being an incest victim promote a reliance on dissociation of experience, then the alternatives of reflecting upon, reasoning about and planning in relation to problems may be preempted. In fact, many adolescent victims act impulsively or recklessly, engage in substance abuse, sexual acting out, and running away, and self-destructive behavior.

Family Functioning. Several characteristics of the incestuous family, and particularly the dissociation-generating incestuous family, serve to maintain the abusive relationship and subsequent dissociation. The first characteristic of the incestuous family that maintains the child's dissociative processes for coping with the abuse is the dynamic of *secrecy and isolation* (Braun, 1984). While any form of childhood sexual abuse is associated with a victim's shame and a strong motivation for secrecy, children who have grown up in adaptively functioning families can often overcome these feelings and utilize someone in their support system in the interest of terminating the abuse. Families with parents characterized by unresolved attachment are more likely to depend solely on each other and to avoid social contacts that might provide opportunities for disclosure (Alexander et al., 1995). In any primary relationships, their fear of abandonment will preclude their revelation of the incest. The abuse is therefore less likely to be detected and more likely to continue into adolescence. Consequently, the child victims are isolated from more mature adults who might provide a context for social support and affirmation of reality. The fear of abandonment that permeates such a family further reinforces avoidance of conflict in coping with the incest and the fear that disclosure will dissolve the family.

The second characteristic of the family that generates and maintains dissociation is *intense dysregulated affect*. A cluster analysis of data from incestuous families showed that individuals with clinical levels of dissociative symptoms described their families as significantly more conflictual than individuals with lower levels of dissociation (Alexander & Schaeffer, 1994). Both the fathers and the mothers from these families were significantly more physically abusive to their children and to each other than were the parents of incest survivors with lesser dissociative tendencies. These conflicts, characterized by intense emotion and poor impulse control, convey a very real sense of danger to the child and fosters the dissociation of her own aggressive feelings as a necessary defense against the overwhelming conflict she feels between fear of and dependence on the parents.

Finally, the *nature of the abuse* can help to maintain both the abusive relationship and the dissociative response as a primary means of tolerating it. As stated previously, incest associated with an outcome of dissociative disorder typically has an onset at an early age. This early onset interferes with the fundamental aspects of the development of self (Cole & Putnam, 1992), unlike the temporal dissociation more common among victims who are older at the age of onset (Speigel, 1986). In addition, the perpetrating father is often a primary attachment figure for the child; he alternates the abuse with active expressions of nurturance and affection (Braun & Sachs, 1987). In the course of experiencing some form of emotional sustenance from the father, the victim may perceive and be told by others that she was unwilling or unable to resist her perpetrator, framing her dependence on him as active collusion in the abuse. These discontinuities between abusive and loving behavior and between the victim's own fear and dependence are so confusing and overwhelming to the young child that dissociation is perhaps the only recourse for functioning. Young children, who are not able to integrate opposite qualities into their understandings (Harter, 1983), must select one side of the paradox. This aspect of the child's development then supports the unspoken parental dictum that the paradox not be addressed or acknowledged, contributes to the family's secretiveness, and can be translated into a lack of co-consciousness as in the case of MPD (Spiegel, 1986).

Dissociation as a primary means of coping with incest is also promoted by severe and bizarre abusive behaviors. Sometimes highly unusual and disturbing behaviors are perpetrated by fathers who are otherwise perceived as successful, prominent, admirable members of the community (Kluft et al., 1984). For example, one of our clients was forced to drink her father's urine after he sexually abused her; in his public life, he was a CEO and highly respected member of the church and community. This discrepancy increases the child's sense of dissonance and unreality and diminishes the likelihood that her disclosure would be believed and the abuse would be ended. Moreover, the dramatic and sudden shifts between the perpetrator's public persona and his abusive behavior actually model for the child discontinuity in mental states (Kluft et al., 1984).

The final characteristic of the incestuous family that sustains dissociative processes is the *absence of a restorative, nurturant relationship* that disrupts the abuse and helps the child deal with the trauma. Many incest victims, despite the abusive behavior of their fathers, also experienced some convincing love and affection from him. The resulting ambivalence was heightened by the contrasting perception of their mothers as emotionally unavailable and punitive. Victims who later develop MPD often describe their relationships with their abusive fathers as preferable to the abusive and/or neglectful relationships with their mothers (Anderson & Alexander, 1995). Thus, the victim may feel motivated to sustain the one supportive relationship she perceives, resulting in the omission of many facts and perceptions from her consciousness and memory.

Although not all incestuous families are alike, we believe that these are a number of dimensions that serve to promote and support coping through the reliance on dissociative processes. Unfortunately, many of these qualities persist even if the sexual activity ceases. We now turn to a discussion of developmental issues in the period after the sexual activity has ended.

Adult Development and Family Functioning after the Incest

The Adult Child. The family processes that support and sustain the dissociative process continue into adulthood unless intervening events, such as treatment, reshape them. We therefore focus this section solely on the victim's adult development. Adulthood from a developmental perspective is marked by a set of events and transitions that are more self-directed than are the transitions of childhood (Cowan, 1991). These include marriage, birth of the first and last child, and an "expansion" phase that follows the birth of the last child and marks a period of relative stability (Elder, 1991). Although the order of these events may be variable, most American adults have identified themselves in terms of one or more of these developmental tasks by their late 20s and early 30s. The changes are reflected in self and social development as one becomes identified in terms of a number of roles—worker, wife, mother—and integrates one's own identity with those of others (Fischer, 1980). The individual has responsibilities to other individuals that must be fulfilled and that require yet another level of ability to regulate self in such a way as to accomplish these things maturely. Child-rearing, for example, demands that the adult regulate his or her own time, activity, and affective state as well as the state of young children, a particularly emotionally demanding experience (Dix, 1991).

By the mid-30s, typical adults have established an adult lifestyle and enter the expansion phase characterized by the accumulation of experiences over time that affords an opportunity for reflection upon these life circumstances and choices. In terms of self-development, the youthful question, "What will I be when I grow up?" has been transformed to the reflective question, "Who have I become?" The years between 28 to 38 seem to be characterized by the awareness of the limitations and imperfections of one's chosen paths and a sense of the narrowing of one's horizons (Back & Gergen, 1968; Levenson, 1978).

By the time the incest survivor reaches adulthood, the cumulative impairments to her self and social functioning may preclude a normal transition into adulthood and the roles of adult women (Cole & Putnam, 1992; Downs, 1993). These impairments may be reflected in the timing and sequence of major adult decisions, such as when to marry or bear children. We have had clients who never had a sexual relationship, who married in adolescence in order to escape the household, and who have become pregnant in order to try to form a loving relationship with someone. Moreover, adult sexual relationships are negatively affected in a variety of ways. The ability to communicate with the sexual partner, to feel secure in expressing the limits of one's sexual comfort, and even to experience sexual arousal may be interfered with due to a lack of mutuality in the survivor's first sexual experiences. One client, a woman who was an executive secretary in a Fortune 500 firm, reported that she was compelled to control men through her sexuality; each time she met a wealthy man through her work, she would seduce and than abandon him, taking pleasure in her dominion over men.

Tendencies toward impulsiveness, lack of insight, and lack of self-respect can easily promote revictimization. The formation of close, intimate relationships is difficult because healthy adult relationships rely on trust, a secure sense of self in relation to another, the ability to regulate oneself in emotional conflicts, and sufficient knowledge of one's partner. Marriage and parenthood, in particular, test the self-boundaries an individual has established and likely create more stress than satisfaction for many incest victims.

On the other hand, adulthood does afford the opportunity to leave the home, to form new relationships, and eventually to reflect upon and resolve the conflictual patterns of one's life. Physical distance can promote psychological distance and pave the path for the ability to reflect upon and to reason about the childhood sexual experience. Moreover, having one's own children and parenting those children, particularly during the ages when one's own abuse occurred, may serve as a stimulus for reawakening forgotten or unresolved aspects of the abuse. In our experience, the average age of the adult incest survivor in retrospective studies other than college samples, approximately 32–38 years, suggests that incest victims too enter a period of adulthood self-reflection. Interestingly, many incest survivors enter therapy with presenting problems other than a history of child sexual abuse, and a sizable number do not recall the abuse until later in the therapy relationship. Thus, the therapy process, including the availability of a secure relationship with an adult, may stimulate the recollection process and lead to resolution of the trauma (Herman & Schztzow, 1987).

CONCLUSION

Our developmental analysis has contrasted typical emotional development with the atypicalities of incestuous families that promote dissociative disorder. There is a growing belief that such disorders emerge as a result of early childhood trauma such as father–daughter incest. We offer a transactional model by which normative dissociative phenomena in early childhood may be converted into disorders as a function of (1) predisposing qualities of the parent–child relationship that may increase the chance of incest occurring, (2) the developmental status of the child during the time the trauma is occurring, and (3) the capabilities and coping styles of the family once the incest has stopped. Many of our ideas have had to rely more on clinical experience than empirical evidence, but we are encouraged that a developmental framework provides a means of conceptualizing typical and atypical dissociative phenomena.

There is an acute need for comparative research on the relation between typical and atypical dissociation. This research requires attention to developmental theory in order to assess the degree to which atypicalities are qualitatively different from typical dissociativelike phenomena. The fluidity with which young children switch roles, their propensities for experiencing imaginary friends and internal voices, the ease with which they shift states and appear to forget distress, and their suggestibility or even hypnotizability are all characteristics that can be examined in typical preschoolers and contrasted with same-age children who have experienced intense trauma such as incest.

It is necessary and possible to understand how challenges to normative processes and deviations at a given point in time relate to the development of a clinical condition. Developmental psychology offers theoretical perspectives on the course of children's psychological growth that allow the use of age as a marker for cognitive or socioemotional capacities and that permit cross-sectional comparisons of nonrisk and high-risk children within specific age groups using measures that are developmentally sensitive. However, questions addressing individual differences in early childhood patterns of regulating emotion and the etiology of a dissociative disorder require longitudinal research. Such work is expensive, time-consuming, and difficult, and therefore requires careful conceptualization. Ideally, longitudinal work using high- and low-risk samples would address the nature of the child's coping prior to trauma, at the time of trauma or its disclosure, and periodic assessment of functioning over time. Developmental psychology offers a framework for identifying which elements of early childhood and family functioning predict later outcome.

Developmental psychology also offers many procedures for studying social and emotional functioning in children. In clinical research, there tends to be an exclusive reliance on symptom checklists and diagnostic interviews. Although these are valuable toward certain ends, it is also important to recognize that self-report and parental report data are limited by factors such as a child's age or a family member's clinical condition. The problems associated with dissociative disorder, for example, are likely to interfere with the ability to make accurate observations regarding one's own or other's behavior in emotionally challenging situations. As can be gleaned from our chapter, developmental research offers a wide variety of observational methods for studying children and families. Although most have been used to study normative patterns or individual differences within unselected populations, many are sensitive to clinically relevant aspects of functioning and can be used to compare risk and nonrisk groups. One fruitful approach is to assess functioning under emotionally challenging conditions. For example, the research on attachment in early childhood suggests that there are distinct ways of coping with separation from a parent that may be directly comparable to coping with other distressing situations.

Dissociation is such a fascinating intrapsychic phenomenon that it is easy to lose sight of the familial context in which dissociative disorders develop. Qualities of parents in dysfunctional families may promote and sustain abnormal dissociative styles that not only accompany but may actually precede the onset of extreme trauma to offspring as in the case of incest. Unfortunately, there is a dearth of research on the families of individuals with a dissociative style or disorder. Again, such research needs to include observational techniques including those that present emotional challenges that access dissociation-related phenomena rather than relying solely on self-report. A developmental perspective can guide research on understanding "dissociation-generating" families, which could provide a subsequent basis for the prevention and treatment of dissociative disorder in the at-risk child.

ACKNOWLEDGMENT. We wish to thank Frank Putnam for his constructive critique of an earlier draft of this chapter.

REFERENCES

Adams-Tucker, C. (1985). Defense mechanisms used by sexually abused children. *Children Today, 14*, 8-12.

Ainsworth, M., Blehar, M. C., Waters, E., & Wall, S. (1978). *Patterns of attachment: A psychological study of the strange situation*. Hillsdale, NJ: Erlbaum.

Alexander, P. C. (1992). The application of attachment theory to the study of sexual abuse. *Journal of Consulting and Clinical Psychology, 60*, 185-195.

Alexander, P. C., & Schaeffer, C. M. (1994). A typology of incestuous families based on cluster analysis. *Journal of Family Psychology, 8*, 458-470.

Alexander, P. C., Anderson, C., Schaeffer, C. M., Brand, B., Zachary, B., & Kretz, L. (1995). Attachment as a mediator of long-term effects in survivors of incest. Manuscript submitted for review.

Alexander, P. C., & Schwartz, K. (1995). *The family characteristics of dissociative individuals.*

Anderson, C. L., & Alexander, P. C. (1995). The relationship between dissociation and fearful-avoidant attachment in adult women survivors of incest. Manuscript submitted for review.

Back, K. W., & Gergen, K. J. (1968). The self through the latter span of life. In C. Gordon & K. Gergen (Eds.), *The self in social interaction* (pp. 101-143). New York: Wiley.

Beeghly, M., & Cicchetti, D. (1994). Child maltreatment, attachment, and the self system: Emergence of an internal state lexicon in toddlers at high social risk. *Development and Psychpathology, 8*, 5-30.

Berndt, T. (1981). Relations between social cognition, nonsocial cognition, and social behavior: The case of friendship. In J. H. Flavell & L. D. Ross (Eds.), *Social cognitive development* (pp. 176-199). New York: Cambridge University Press.

Bliss, E. L. (1988). A re-examination of Freud's basic concepts from studies of multiple personality disorder. *Dissociation, 1*, 36-40.

Bloom, L. (1991). *Language development: From two to three* New York: Cambridge University Press.

Bowlby, J. (1969). *Attachment and loss* (Vols. 1 & 2). New York: Basic Books.

Bowlby, J. (1985). Violence in the family as a function of the attachment system. *American Journal of Psychoanalysis, 44*, 9-27.

Braun, B. G. (1984). The role of the family in the development of multiple personality disorder. *International Journal of Family Psychiatry, 5*, 303-313.

Braun, B. G. (1989). Psychotherapy of the survivor of incest with a dissociative disorder. *Psychiatric Clinics of North America, 12*, 307-325.

Braun, B. G., & Sachs, R. (1987). The development of multiple personality disorder: Predisposing, precipitating, and perpetuating factors. In R. P. Kluft (Ed.), *Childhood antecedents of multiple personality* (pp. 38-64). Washington, DC: American Psychiatric Press.

Bretherton, I. J., Fritz, C., Zahn-Waxler, C., & Ridgeway, D. (1986). Learning to talk about emotions: A functionalist perspective. *Child Development, 57*, 529-548.

Carlson, V., Cicchetti, D., Barnett, D., & Braunwald, K. (1989). Disorganized/disoriented attachment relationships in maltreated infants. *Developmental Psychology, 25*, 525-531.

Cicchetti, D., & Beeghly, M. (1990). *The self in transition: Infancy to adulthood.* Chicago: University of Chicago Press.

Cole, P. M., & Putnam, F. W. (1992). Effect of incest on self and social functioning: A developmental psychopathology perspective. *Journal of Consulting and Clinical Psychology, 60*, 174-184.

Cole, P. M., Woolger, C., Power, T. P., & Smith, K. D. (1992). Parenting difficulties in incest survivors. *Child Abuse and Neglect, 16*, 239-249.

Connell, J. P. (1990). Context, self, and action: A motivational analysis of self-system processes across the life span. In D. Cicchetti & M. Beeghly (Eds.), *The self in transition: Infancy to adulthood* (pp. 61-67). Chicago: University of Chicago Press.

Cowan, P. A. (1991). Individual and family life transitions: A proposal for a new definition. In P. A. Cowan & E. M. Hetherington (Eds.), *Family transitions* (pp. 3-30). Hillsdale, NJ: Erlbaum.

Cramer, P. (1991). *The development of defense mechanisms: Theory, research, and assessment.* New York: Springer-Verlag.

Damon, W. A. (1983). *Social and personality development.* New York: Norton.

Damon, W. A., & Hart, D. (1982). The development of self-understanding from infancy through adolescence. *Child Development, 53*, 831-857.

Dix, T. (1991). The affective organization of parenting: Adaptive and maladaptive processes. *Psychological Bulletin, 110*, 3-25.

Dodge, K. A., Pettit, G. S., & Bates, J. E. (1994). Effects of physical maltreatment on the development of peer relations. *Development and Psychopathology, 8*, 43-56.

Douglas, V. (1965). Children's responses to frustration: A developmental study. *Canadian Journal of Psychiatry, 19*, 161-168.

Downs, W. R. (1993). Developmental considerations for the effects of childhood sexual abuse. *Journal of Interpersonal Violence, 8*, 331-345.

Dunn, J. (1988). *The beginnings of social understanding*. London: Basil Blackwell.
Dunn, J., & Kendrick, C. (1982). *Siblings: Love, envy, and understanding*. Cambridge, MA: Harvard University Press.
Elder, G. H. (1991). Family transitions, cycles, and social change. In P. A. Cowan & E. M. Hetherington (Eds.), *Family transitions* (pp. 31-58). Hillsdale, NJ: Erlbaum.
Everett, C., Halperin, S., Volgy, S., & Wissler, A. (1989). *Treating the borderline family: A systemic approach*. New York: Harcourt Brace Jovanovich.
Ferguson, T. J., Stegge, H., & Damhuis, I. (1991). Children's understanding of guilt and shame. *Child Development, 62*, 827-839.
Fischer, K. W. (1980). A theory of cognitive development: The control and construction of hierarchies of skills. *Psychological Review, 87*, 477-531.
Fischer, K. W., & Ayoub, C. (1994). Affective splitting and dissociation in normal and maltreated children: Developmental pathways for self in relationships. In D. Cicchetti & S. Toth (Eds.), *Psychopathology and the development of self* (pp. 149-222). Rochester, NY: Rochester University Press.
Fischer, K. W., & Pipp, S. L. (1984). Development of the structures of unconscious thought. In K. Bowers & D. Meichenbaum (Eds.), *The unconscious reconsidered* (pp. 88-148). New York: Wiley.
Fischer, K. W., Shaver, P. R., & Carnochan, P. (1990). How emotions develop and how they organize development. *Cognition and Emotion, 4*, 81-127.
Fraiberg, S. (1959). *The magic years*. New York: Scribner.
Freud, A. (1966). *The ego and the mechanisms of defense*. New York: International Universities Press.
Gardner, G. G., & Olness, K. (1981). *Hypnosis and hypnotherapy with children*. New York: Grune & Stratton.
Garvey, C. (1977). *Play*. Cambridge, MA: Harvard University Press.
Gelinas, D. J. (1983). The persisting negative effects of incest. *Psychiatry, 46*, 312-332.
Harris, P. L. (1983). Infant cognition. In M. M. Haith & J. J. Campos (Eds.), *Handbook of child psychology: Vol. 2. Infancy and developmental psychobiology* (pp. 689-782). New York: Wiley.
Harter, S. (1982). Children's understanding of multiple emotions: A cognitive-developmental approach. In W. F. Overton (Ed.), *The relationship between social and cognitive development* (pp. 147-194). Hillsdale, NJ: Erlbaum.
Harter, S. (1983). Developmental perspectives on the self-system. In E. M. Hetherington (Ed.), *Handbook of child psychology* (4th ed.). *Socialization, personality, and social development* (pp. 275-386). New York: Wiley.
Harter, S., & Monsour, A. (1992). A developmental analysis of conflict caused by opposing attributes in the adolescent self-portrait. *Developmental Psychology, 28*, 251-260.
Herman, J. L., & Schatzow, E. (1987). Recovery and verification of memories of childhood sexual trauma. *Psychoanalytic Psychology, 4*, 1-14.
Izard, C. E. (1979). *Emotions in personality and psychopathology*. New York: Plenum Press.
Kagan, J. (1981). *The second year: The emergence of self-awareness*. Cambridge, MA: Harvard University Press.
Kendall-Tackett, M. A., & Simon, A. F. (1988). Molestation and the onset of puberty: Data from 365 adults molested as children. *Child Abuse and Neglect, 12*, 73-81.
Kluft, R. P. (1984). Treatment of multiple personality disorder. *Psychiatric Clinics of North America, 7*, 9-30.
Kluft, R. P. (1985). Childhood multiple personality disorder: Predictors, clinical findings, and treatment results. In R. P. Kluft (Ed.), *Childhood antecedents of multiple personality disorder*. Washington, DC: American Psychiatric Press.
Kluft, R. P., Braun, B. G., & Sachs, R. (1984). Multiple personality, intrafamilial abuse, and family psychiatry. *International Journal of Family Psychiatry, 5*, 283-301.
Kobak, R., & Hazan, C. (1991). Attachment in marriage: Effects of security and accuracy of working models. *Journal of Personality and Social Psychology, 60*, 861-869.
Kopp, C. B. (1982). Antecedents of self-regulation: A developmental perspective. *Developmental Psychology, 18*, 199-214.
Levenson, D. J. (1978). *The seasons of a man's life*. New York: Ballantine.
Liotti, G. (1992). Disorganized/disoriented attachment in the etiology of the dissociative disorders. *Dissociation, 5*, 196-204.

Main, M., & Cassidy, J. (1988). Categories of response to reunion with the parent at age 6: Predictable from infant attachment classifications and stable over a 1-month period. *Developmental Psychology, 24*, 415-426.

Main, M., & Goldwyn, R. (1984). Predicting rejection of her infant from mother's representation of her own experience: Implications for the abused-abusing intergenerational cycle. *Child Abuse and Neglect, 8*, 203-217.

Main, M., & Hesse, E. (1990). Parents' unresolved traumatic experiences are related to infant disorganized attachment status: Is frightened and/or frightening parental behavior the linking mechanism? In M. Greenberg, D. Cicchetti, & E. M. Cummings (Eds.), *Attachment in the preschool years* (pp. 161-182). Chicago: University of Chicago Press.

Main, M., & Hesse, E. (1992). Attaccamento disorganizato/disorientato nell infanzia e stati mentali dissociati nei genitori [Disorganized/disoriented infant behavior in the Strange Situation, lapses in the monitoring of reasoning and discourse during the parents' Adult Attachment Interview, and dissociative states: In support of Liotti's hypothesis.] [Translated (into Italian) by V. Chiarini.] In M. Ammaniti & D. Stern (Eds.), *Attaccamento e psicoanalici* (pp. 86-140). Bari, Italy: Laterza.

Main, M., & Solomon, J. (1986). Discovery of an insecure-disorganized attachment pattern. In T. B. Brazelton & M. W. Yogman (Eds.), *Affective development in infancy* (pp. 95-124). Norwood, NJ: Ablex Publishing.

Main, M., & Solomon, J. (1990). Procedures for identifying infants as disorganized/disoriented during the Ainsworth strange situation. In M. Greenberg, D. Cicchetti, & E. M. Cummings (Eds.), *Attachment in the preschool years* (pp. 121-160). Chicago: University of Chicago Press.

Main, M., Kaplan, N., & Cassidy, J. (1985). Security in infancy, childhood, and adulthood: A move to the level of representation. In I. Bretherton & E. Waters (Eds.), *Growing points of attachment theory and research: Monographs of the Society for Research in Child Development, 50*, (1-2, Serial No. 209), 66-104.

Malatesta, C. Z. (1990). The role of emotions in the development and organization of personality. In R. A. Thompson (Ed.), *Socioemotional development: Nebraska Symposium on Motivation, 1988* (pp. 1-56). Lincoln: University of Nebraska Press.

McCrone, E. R., Egeland, B., Kalkoske, M., & Carlson, E. A. (1994). Relations between early maltreatment and mental representations of relationships assessed with projective storytelling in middle childhood. *Development and Psychopathology, 8*, 99-120.

Nemiah, J. C. (1989). Dissociative disorders. In H. Kaplan & B. J. Saddock (Eds.), *Comprehensive textbook of psychiatry* (5th ed., pp. 1028-1044). Baltimore, MD: Williams & Wilkins.

Peterson, G. (1991). Children coping with trauma: Diagnosis of "dissociation identity disorder." *Dissociation, 4*, 152-164.

Putnam, F. W. (1984). The study of multiple personality disorder: General strategies and practical considerations. *Psychiatric Annals, 14*, 58-62.

Putnam, F. W. (1985). Dissociation as an extreme response to trauma. In R. P. Kluft (Ed.), *Childhood antecedents of multiple personality* (pp. 66-97). Washington, DC: American Psychiatric Press.

Putnam, F. W. (1989). *Diagnosis and treatment of multiple personality disorder*. New York: Guilford.

Putnam, F. W. (1991). Dissociative disorders in children and adolescents: A developmental perspective. *Psychiatric Clinics of North America, 14*, 519-531.

Rothbart, M. K., & Ahadi, S. A. (1994). Temperament and the development of personality. *Journal of Abnormal Psychology, 103*, 55-66.

Rothbart, M. K., Ziaie, H., & O'Boyle, C. G. (1992). Self-regulation and emotion in infancy. In N. Eisenberg & R. A. Fabes (Eds.), *Emotion and its regulation in early development* (pp. 7-24). San Francisco: Jossey-Bass.

Ruble, D. N., Boggiano, A. K., Feldman, N. S., & Loebl, J. H. (1980). A developmental analysis of the role of social comparison in self-evaluation. *Developmental Psychology, 16*, 105-115.

Rutter, M., & Garmezy, N. (1983). Developmental psychopathology. In E. M. Hetherington (Ed.), *Handbook of child psychology* (4th ed.). *Socialization, personality, and development* (pp. 775-911). New York: Wiley.

Sachs, R. G., Frischolz, E. J., & Wood, J. I. (1988). Marital and family therapy in the treatment of multiple personality disorder. *Journal of Marital and Family Therapy, 14*, 249-259.

Sanders, B., McRoberts, G., & Tollefson, C. (1989). Childhood stress and dissociation in a college population. *Dissociation, 2*, 17-23.

Schibuk, M., Bond, M., & Bouffard, R. (1989). The development of defenses in childhood. *Canadian Journal of Psychiatry, 34*, 581-588.
Selman, R. L. (1980). *The growth of interpersonal understanding*. New York: Academic Press.
Sexton, M., Harralson, T., Hulsey, T., & Nash, M. (1988). *Sexual abuse and hypnotic susceptibility: Correlates in adult women*. Paper presented to Society for Clinical and Experimental Hypnosis, Special Invited Symposium: Dissociation and Trauma.
Spiegel, D. (1986). Dissociation, double binds, and posttraumatic stress in multiple personality disorder. In B. Braun (Ed.), *Treatment of multiple personality disorder* (pp. 63-77). Washington, DC: American Psychiatric Press.
Sroufe, L. A., & Fleeson, J. (1988). The coherence of family relationships. In R. A. Hinde & J. Stevenson-Hinde (Eds.), *Relationships within families: Mutual influences* (pp. 27-47). Oxford, England: Clarendon Press.
Sroufe, L. A., & Rutter, M. (1984). The domain of developmental psychopathology. *Child Development, 55*, 1184-1199.
Stifter, C. A., & Moyer, D. (1991). The regulation of positive affect: Gaze aversion activity during mother-infant interaction. *International Journal of Behavioral Development, 14*, 111-123.
Stipek, D. J., Gralinski, J. H., & Kopp, C. B. (1990). Self-concept development in the toddler years. *Developmental Psychology, 26*, 972-977.
Trad, P. V. (1989). *The preschool child*. New York: Wiley.
Trickett, P. K., MacBride-Chang, C., & Putnam, F. W. (1994). The classroom performance and behavior of sexually abused females. *Development and Psychopathology, 6*, 183-194.
van der Kolk, B. (1987). The psychological consequences of overwhelming life experiences. In B. van der Kolk (Ed.), *Psychological trauma* (pp. 1-30). Washington, DC: American Psychiatric Press.
Waterman, J. (1986). Developmental considerations. In K. MacFarlane & J. Waterman (Eds.), *Sexual abuse of young children*, (pp. 15-29). New York: Guilford.
Waters, E., Wippman, J., & Sroufe, L. A. (1979). Attachment, positive affect, and competence in the peer group: Two studies in construct validation. *Child Development, 50*, 821-829.
Watson, D., & Clark, L. A. (1984). Negative affectivity: The disposition to experience aversive emotional states. *Psychological Bulletin, 96*, 465-490.
Wolf, D. P. (1990). Being of several minds: Voices and versions of the self in early childhood. In D. Cicchetti & M. Beeghly (Eds.), *The self in transition: Infancy to childhood* (pp. 183-212). Chicago: University of Chicago Press.
Wolff, P. H. (1987). *The development of behavioral states and the expression of emotion in early infancy*. Chicago: University of Chicago Press.
Wyatt, G. E., & Newcomb, M. (1990). Internal and external mediators of women's sexual abuse in childhood. *Journal of Consulting and Clinical Psychology, 58*, 758-767.
Zahn-Waxler, C., Radke-Yarrow, M., & King, R. A. (1979). Child-rearing and children's prosocial initiations toward victims of distress. *Child Development, 50*, 319-330.

5

Child Abuse in the Etiology of Dissociative Disorders

Jean M. Goodwin and Roberta G. Sachs

A growing body of literature, both case reports and surveys, links dissociative symptoms and disorders to childhood experiences of severe abuse. Several surveys (Bliss, 1980, 1984; Braun & Sachs, 1985; Kluft, 1984a; Putnam, Gurof, Silberman, Barbar, & Post, 1986) report that 97% of patients with multiple personality disorder (MPD; also known as dissociative identity disorder, or DID, since the publication of the *Diagnostic and Statistical Manual of Mental Disorders*, Fourth Edition [DSM-IV; American Psychiatric Association, 1994]) report some history of abuse during childhood. Since the early 1980s, the hypothesis that this high frequency of prior abuse is somehow intrinsically related to the development of dissociative symptoms has become central to theory and research in the field. The present chapter analyzes in detail this proposed etiologic association between childhood abuse and MPD. We review case histories and case surveys in which adults and children describe sadistically assaultive and soul-murdering childhood environments and the depersonalization phenomena and fantasy absorption that took place during moments when this environment became overwhelming. We examine the problem of corroborating histories of child abuse, which remains a major objection to the hypothesis. We also review similarities between dissociative disorder patients and other child abuse survivors. Similarities in family characteristics, victim symptoms, and community response indicate that dissociative disorder patients may represent some of the more severely abused and severely symptomatic of a continuum of survivors of child abuse (Braun, 1990). Both abuse and dissociation were denied by

Jean M. Goodwin • Department of Psychiatry, University of Texas Medical Branch, Galveston, Texas 77555-0428. **Roberta G. Sachs** • Highland Park Psychological Resources, 660 LaSalle Place, Highland Park, Illinois 60035.

Handbook of Dissociation: Theoretical, Empirical, and Clinical Perspectives, edited by Larry K. Michelson and William J. Ray. Plenum Press, New York, 1996.

professionals in the first half of the twentieth century, probably as part of the same historical process (Goodwin, 1985b). Comprehensive biopsychosocial understanding of these disorders requires integration of the child abuse hypothesis with data about genetics, physiology, psychology, comorbidity, and natural history, including treatment responses in patients who dissociate.

PRIOR CHILD ABUSE IN CASE HISTORIES AND SURVEYS OF PATIENTS WITH DISSOCIATIVE DISORDERS

Books detailing the case histories of patients with MPD have a predictable rhythm leading to the recovery of the memory of childhood trauma. In *Sybil* (Schrieber, 1983) we read about how the patient's mother hanged her upside down by the feet and then inserted an enema tube into the child's urethra. *The Minds of Billy Milligan* (Keyes, 1981) describes a similarly chilling scene: Billy is sodomized by his stepfather and later buried in the barn for telling his mother; a breathing tube is left in his mouth, but his father urinates into it. The details are excruciating and seemingly endless.

Rosenbaum and Weaver (1980) reviewed all cases of multiple personality published between 1934 and 1978 and found that the majority report incest or other brutal sexual abuse in childhood, often by a psychotic adult. Saltman and Solomon (1982) added six more such cases and suggested that much of the symptomatology of multiplicity can be understood as a particular defensive reaction to sadistic sexual trauma in childhood.

Bliss (1980), too, saw MPD as a sequel to childhood abuse in individuals capable of responding to trauma with deep levels of self-hypnosis that can lead to dreamlike confusion about reality and about the self. Nine of his 14 patients reported childhood rapes; three others responded to the item with question mark.

Putnam and co-workers (1986) surveyed therapists treating 100 patients diagnosed as having MPD. He found that 97% of these patients described traumatic childhoods; 83% described childhood sexual abuse; 75% reported physical abuse; 61% reported extreme neglect or abandonment; and 41% had witnessed extreme violence. The number of types of childhood trauma undergone was significantly correlated with the number of alternate personalities. Coons and Milstein (1984) found a prior history of sexual or physical abuse in 85% of patients with MPD. Four other large surveys find prior child abuse in 95 to 98% of such patients (Braun, 1990). These 80 to 100% frequencies of self-report of prior child abuse by MPDs seem significantly different from the percentage of 42% found in unselected psychiatric inpatients (Carmen, Rieker, & Mills, 1984).

In addition, there seemed to be qualitative differences in the nature of the prior abuse described by MPDs. Cornelia Wilbur (1984a) has detailed the planned, bizarre, sadistic, multifaceted assaults on the child's self-esteem, of which physical damage may be the least destructive element. These are not families who abuse out of lack of impulse control in moments of crisis. In these families the child may be partially buried in a backyard grave as the standard mode of discipline. Family rituals may include several adults genitally instrumentating a preschool child, using bottles or icepicks, the locking of children in closets for days (then punishing them for having inevitably soiled themselves), and family participation in ritual tortures, which may involve actual or threatened mutilations of animal or human victims (Putnam, 1989). Children are physiologically assaulted with forced fasts, forced feeding, forced enemas and cathartics, and forced alcohol intoxication. They are denied medical attention. Within any category of abuse, the abuse experienced by the future dissociative disorder patient is extreme. For example, in the sexual abuse cases, these patients seem more likely to have experienced incest pregnancies, instrumentation with physical damage to genitalia, involvement of multiple sexual abusers, involvement of siblings and other children as covictims, threats of death or threats with weapons, and beating or bondage associated with the sexual contact (Goodwin, 1993a).

In the realm of emotional abuse, the dissociative patients are likely to have been openly ridiculed and humiliated by multiple family members and insulted when most hurt and vulnerable, such as being called a whore while the father is attempting anal intercourse. Humiliating emotional abuse often takes place around presents and holidays. In one family, the father always bought and wrapped presents for all the children and left them under the tree, but on Christmas morning he burned all the presents. Another dissociative patient, as a young boy of 8, had a group of boys arrive for his birthday party. His alcoholic mother opened the door to greet them stark naked. Subsequently, he was ostracized by neighbors in his upper-class suburb. Braun (1984a,b) has discussed the mixed messages that are given to the child. For example, the child may be burned and then hugged. The child can be told, "I love you," and a few seconds later is psychologically devalued, being told by the same parent, "You're no good" or "I hate you." When the abuser is sadistic, there is emphasis on acquiring total control over the child through terrorized obedience and the induction of the child into violence as a coperpetrator (Goodwin, 1993a).

Again and again one hears these patients describe a chronic family pattern of emotional neglect and abuse with chronic unresolved conflict, resentment, and blaming of the children, confusion with miscommunication and misinformation, and an inability to mobilize care or protection in crisis. This chronic state is then punctuated by traumatic episodes—severe emotional abuse, a traumatic abandonment such as being locked in a closet, a physical beating, or, most often, a rape (Braun, 1984b).

DISSOCIATION AS A DEFENSE AGAINST CHILDHOOD TRAUMA

The kinds of trauma described by patients with severe dissociative disorders share characteristics with the kinds of trauma described by shell-shocked combat veterans (Goodwin, 1985a). In the traumatic situation the abused child (1) feared for his/her own life, (2) feared for the life of a loved person, (3) was in a state of blurred consciousness due to fatigue, pain, illness, or substance ingestion, (4) experienced some sort of moral confusion, at times related to secrecy or actual "brainwashing," and (5) had no available support (Kluft, 1984a). The 5-year-old raped during sleep and told that she and her mother will be killed if she tells experiences the same five traumatogenic factors as does the adult in heavy combat who is wounded, whose buddy is killed, and whose family does not want to talk about the war (van der Kolk,

1984). Moral confusion and dilemmas characterize both situations, as the subject is ordered to obey commands to disobey the usual prohibitions against overt violence or sexuality.

There is a body of data linking a variety of dissociative symptoms to the experience of stress—derealization, depersonalization, fugue, and amnesia. All of these can occur in combat situations, panic attacks, and posttraumatic disorders (APA, 1987, 1994; Spiegel, 1984). Bliss (1980, 1984) would link these symptoms to the occurrence in extreme stress of spontaneous deep trance states, which are, he hypothesizes, an emergency defense system in humans and other animals. When the attacked animal lapses into deep trance, the attacker may believe the prey is dead and abandon the attack. The animal is protected by trance from overwhelming anxiety and its somatic consequences, which can result in death. The trance-induced permeability between psychological and somatic states may be lifesaving by producing anesthesia or feats of extraordinary endurance and strength (Ross, 1989). If the animal subsequently survives, posttrance amnesias and distortions protect against crippling residual phobias (Volgyesi, 1963). The absorption and suggestibility of the trance state allow intense concentration on the problem of survival and automatic obedience, which is often adaptive in the presence of the attacker. (Later, however, this lack of critical capacity may transform the attacker's emotional abuse into unquestioned tenets of the victim's poor self-esteem.) The "hidden observer" phenomenon allows the traumatized individual objectivity and emotional distance despite the panic-producing death threat.

Folklore and literature support the concept that dissociation protects against death threat. In Jewish tradition there is a custom that when a child is very ill, on the brink of death, one changes the child's name in the hope that the Angel of Death will go away empty-handed if the child it has come to collect does not answer to the old name (Arlow, 1966).

Many clinicians view the severe dissociative disorders as a maladaptive use of dissociation in the face of the chronic stress of physical, emotional, or sexual abuse (Putnam, 1985; Spiegel, 1984; Stern, 1984). A child who is continuously beaten by his/her parents may defend against an attack by dissociating. Where abuse is continuous, dissociation occurs repeatedly. Gradually, these dissociated states may begin to take on a life history of their own, and if the process progresses, different "personalities" or different "realities" may begin to develop as split-off experiential worlds.

One source of supporting data for this hypothesis comes from studies of general population samples reporting significant correlations between severity of remembered child abuse and elevations of measures of dissociation (DiTomasso and Routh, 1993). Not all victims, however, even of the most severe child abuse, develop dissociative disorders. The most plausible explanation seems to be that there are wide constitutional differences in the ability to dissociate. Clinical observation and research conducted over the last 25 years have clearly documented a range of individual differences in response to a hypnotic induction (Frischholz, 1985; Hilgard, 1970; Spiegel & Spiegel, 1978). Those hypnotic phenomena that are most similar to dissociative symptoms, such as posthypnotic amnesia and the "hidden observer," are significantly correlated with high hypnotizability. In other words, only the most hypnotizable subjects evidence dissociative phenomena (Hilgard,

1977). Abused children with limited capacities to dissociate may handle their terror in other ways—through impulsive action, psychosomatic symptoms, obsessions or compulsions, creative sublimation, or other mechanisms.

There may also be individual differences in the ability or tendency to create fantasy figures who can substitute for the dissociated self during abuse incidents, or who can remain untouched by the abuse in a fantasy world. The extraordinary imaginative capacity of some dissociative patients has been noted (Wilbur, 1984b). There may be another population of abuse survivors who are able to dissociate, but do not elaborate alternative imaginative realities. Such individuals may be hampered by depersonalization, uncontrolled trance phenomena, and dense childhood amnesia, but may not develop fantasy identities.

CORROBORATIVE EVIDENCE FOR PATIENTS' ACCOUNTS OF CHILDHOOD ABUSE

How valid is the patient's self-report? Since many consider patients with dissociative disorders to be overly histrionic, they also question whether some of their reported incidents of child abuse are elaborated by the patient in order to self-dramatize. Freud came to view his patients' accounts of prior seductions as verbalized fantasies; events that the patient wished or imagined had happened but never did (Goodwin, 1985b, 1993b). Some therapists are extremely cautious about accepting the bizarre and grotesque accounts of family life recounted by patients with multiple personality disorder with the same degree of certitude with which they accept a patient's accounts of allergies or prior hospitalization.

Some of this caution is based on resistance to confronting a world in which such horrors are commonplace. Some caution, however, is justified. The basic therapeutic stance in reconstructing childhood memories requires an openness to possible additions, to shifts of emphasis, to new emotional coloring, to restructuring. In reconstructing an episode from a dissociative patient's past, therapist and patient must face: (1) sometimes total forgetting and amnesia; (2) splitting of the event into multiple memories or memory fragments held by different parts of the self that were present or nearby at times of overwhelming stress; (3) distorted or partial memories deliberately introduced by an alter who is trying to conceal something worse than this "cover memory"; (4) memory that exists only as overwhelming emotion, reenactment, somatic sensations, or dream material; and (5) memories of dreams or fantasies derived from traumatic nightmares in childhood, or from daydreams during trance states self-induced to protect the patient from his/her overwhelming fear during abusive episodes. However, when corroborative data have been available, time and again the therapeutic conclusion has been that the end result of these distortions had led to minimization, rather than exaggeration, of the extent of the childhood abuse (Putnam, 1989).

The search for corroborative and documentary evidence about the patient's often totally forgotten childhood is an important part of treatment. School and pediatric records can be helpful, and the patient may be ready for this kind of documentation before family contact. Protective service or psychiatric records may be available for the patient, for a sibling, or for a parent. Death or suicide of a sibling is not infrequent in these disturbed families, and death certificates and autopsy records are helpful here. Criminal and civil court records may also contain pertinent data.

Parents, parent figures, and siblings can sometimes be interviewed or reached by telephone or letter. In interviewing family members it helps to know that most abusive parents deny abuse and that most require intensive individual and group therapy before they can profit from family therapy. Siblings are often more open. Like the parents, they may deny abuse; but if asked specifically about violent behaviors, they may describe witnessing violence or experiencing or perpetrating abuse.

The task in interviews is the simple, almost journalistic one of rediscovering details about life history that have been lost in the patient's dissociative amnesia and confusion. Where did the family live and when? What were the major family events? Illnesses? Deaths? Job changes? Did the patient have extrafamilial caretakers? Reviewing a parent's childhood history may be useful for both the parent and the patient, in illuminating the nature of the parent's own emotional impoverishment. Collateral interviews with family members should be done gently and with informed consent, as paranoid or depressive breaks or suicidal attempts are possible. With the dissociative patient, as with the abused child in foster or group home care, it may be helpful to make a "life book" where documents, photographs, memories, and information from collateral sources (including dissociated self-states) can be integrated.

A current physical examination of the dissociative patient can also provide data about fragmentary childhood memories. There may be radiological evidence of fractures or genital mutilation or other scarring. It should be noted that the absence of physical evidence does not disprove childhood abuse (Goodwin, 1982). In some cases the patient will decide to involve a trained investigator, by informing protective service or law enforcement authorities about memories of crimes a parent may have committed, or by hiring counsel to bring suit for damages against a parent or parent figure.

Experienced therapists report that when corroboration was attempted, this could be achieved in more than two thirds of patients (Braun, 1984b; Kluft, 1984b; Kluft, Braun, & Sachs, 1984). For example, in one case the patient claimed that when she was a little girl she had suffered a ruptured appendix and had been forced by her mother to walk to the hospital. Hospital records confirmed her account. In another case, a male dissociative patient claimed that his mother had inserted pearls into his penis and pushed them up the urethra with a thermometer. When kidney stones later prompted urologic consultation, considerable scar tissue was noted in the patient's urethra and the passage was so dilated that a large stone passed with little difficulty. Other kinds of convincing corroborative data include eyewitnessing of abusive events by siblings, parents, adult or child acquaintances, or the identification of other victims of physical or sexual violence either among family members or neighbors or acquaintances who name the same abuser.

Neurophysiological evidence for prior child abuse can be clinically observed during the course of therapy in some patients as they describe child abuse. For example, one patient reported being repeatedly burned with a cigarette by her mother. When she described this, the therapist noted red spots like burn marks appearing on the patient's skin. In another case, as the patient was describing how she had been choked by her mother, her voice changed abruptly to become hoarse and raspy. When a patient shows extreme physical pain or panic during a reconstruction, it may be helpful to obtain a pulse rate. When physiological changes are present, the patient's narrative may have to be interrupted to avoid retraumatization.

Other types of neurophysiological evidence can be seen in the patient's current response to touch or other contact. One patient reported that whenever anyone started to hug her she would hold her breath. When asked why, the patient said, "Because that's the way I begin to go away." She described rapes by her father when she was a child. She habitually dissociated from these attacks by holding her breath and trying to disappear into the wall.

Such phenomena are instances of the "truth of abreaction" experienced by many therapists. When a 3-year-old ego state describes a sexual assault by her father in the language of a chronological 3-year-old and using similar kinds of drawing, one is hard put to disbelieve her account in the midst of an abreactive storm that may include the destruction of the father doll and long episodes of sobbing. The reenactments of traumata that occur in these patient's lives can also be emotionally convincing: for example, the mother who does not recall her own rape at age 4 until her daughter is raped at that exact age or the patient raped in adulthood by a policeman as a prelude to recalling an identical childhood rape by a similar authority figure.

More research is needed about the collection and assessment of accounts of childhood trauma. Available data indicate that automatic dismissal of such accounts as fantasy is not warranted, even (or perhaps especially) when the account includes amnestic gaps. Herman and Schatzow (1987) found in a sample of 53 female patients who gave sexual abuse histories that two thirds experienced dissociative or amnestic gaps in their narratives, and three quarters were able to obtain corroborative data about their sexual abuse. Williams (1993) interviewed 100 adult women whose child sexual abuse had been substantiated by medical records 17 years before. Thirty eight percent denied any memory of sexual abuse.

These phenomena are consistent with laboratory research. Memory for events ebbs and flows with time. Memory for traumatic events and memories from childhood are particularly fragile (Loftus, 1993). Procedural memory can persist, producing physiological and emotional effects when narrative memory has faded (Erdelyi, 1989). Because highly hypnotizable subjects are capable of experiencing both negative and positive hallucinations and can misfile these as memory, either with or without specific external suggestions, these phenomena, too, must be factored into the reconstructive process.

DATA FROM CHILDREN WITH DISSOCIATIVE DISORDERS

Since children and adolescents with dissociative disorders are closer in time to childhood trauma, reconstruction with eyewitness or other evidentiary corroboration is sometimes easier. Kluft (1984a) found that four of five children with MPD had been physically abused and that abusive incidents had precipitated new personality splits. He also reported the case of a mother–child pair, both of whom had dissociative disorders with the elaboration of alter personalities. Both host personalities denied that physical abuse was a problem, even when this occurred in the psychiatrist's office. It became apparent that both mother and child switched to other personalities during abusive incidents. Fagan and McMahon (1984) also reported four cases of childhood MPD, all of which involved severe child abuse.

Braun (1985) has reported that dissociative disorders may be transgenerational. In a study of 17 MPD cases where family history data were available, several patients with MPD were found to have mothers who suffered from this disorder. The dissociative mothers were also abusive to their children. Braun estimates that 10% of the children of patients with MPD are abused, often by violent alters. Such children may carry a genetic vulnerability to high hypnotizability as well as being exposed to a parent who displays sudden and extreme shifts in behavior and emotion, as well as coping with incidents of traumatic abuse. These factors may contribute to the transgenerational transmission of dissociative disorders in some families (Kluft et al., 1984).

When dissociation develops in childhood, the defensive function against the situational stress may be quite clear (Goodwin, 1985a), as illustrated by the following case:

> A 13-year-old girl complained to her mother of sexual abuse by her brother. When mother ignored these complaints, the girl began to hear a named voice inside her head telling her to criticize and rebel against her mother.

The case is reminiscent of Despine's 1836 description of 11-year-old Estelle, whose alter personality could not tolerate her mother, although the host personality was a devoted daughter (Ellenberger, 1980). Despine was unable to identify the reality factors associated with his child patient's hatred of the mother.

PATTERNS IN CHILD ABUSE EPIDEMIOLOGY WHICH SUGGEST LINKS WITH THE DISSOCIATIVE DISORDERS

Like MPD (DID) child abuse tends to run in families with as many as 80% of abusers having been emotionally, physically, or sexually abused in childhood (Goodwin, 1982; Helfer, McKinney, & Kempe, 1976; Oliver, 1993). As noted in the previous section, some child victims of abuse present with dissociative symptoms. Some abusive parents also are observed to dissociate (Brown, 1983). When a child abuse victim describes the abusive parent as "two different" people, this may represent accurate reality testing rather than the emergence of primitive splitting (Lesnik-Oberstein, 1983). The following case illustrates the kind of problems protective service workers face in treating perpetrators who dissociate:

> Six-year-old Jennifer was referred to protective services because of severe tantrums at school during which she threw off her clothes and shouted obscenities. Physical examination showed a slack vagina, a broken hymen, and many bruises. She said "Daddy squashes me when he lies on top of me and hurts my wee-wee." She played repetitive games in therapy in which she was pursued and tortured

by a monster. Her father, Victor, met confrontation with a blank denial, although he said he had had a precognition that his child might be sexually abused. He suggested a séance to identify the abuser. He had two prior convictions for pedophilia. He was usually soft-spoken and articulate, but exhibited sudden violent behavior changes: on one occasion he strangled the family dog, on another, he attempted to run over the social worker. He described his mother as evil and his father as a tyrant. His twin brother had been psychiatrically hospitalized after trying to knife the mother. The only treatment Victor would accept was sex change surgery so that he could become the named female alter who had cross-dressed since childhood.

Parental dissociative disorder should be considered in those child abuse cases where (1) the abuse is bizarre or severe, (2) the abuser denies all memory of the abusive incident, (3) the abuser has multiple names or ways of presenting himself, and (4) the violence in the abuser's family was extreme.

A review of the child abuse literature provides convincing evidence that severely disturbed families of the type described by patients with dissociative disorders exist, and that they account for a substantial minority of cases—15 to 50%, depending on the type of abuse substantiated. Even with mandated reporting and treatment of child abuse, it is estimated that at least 30% of abused children will be reabused (Gabinet, 1983). As many as 15% of battered babies die and 50% suffer serious damage (Smith, 1978). Faller (1991) estimates that 16% of incest cases involve "polyincestuous" families in which the average number of perpetrators is three and the average number of victims about the same. In most of these polyincestuous cases, extrafamilial perpetrators and group sexual activity are also present. Recent data indicate that concepts from the 1970s and earlier describing the "gentle" incest offenders were naive (Goodwin, 1993a). Such perpetrators may have multiple sexual victims outside as well as inside the home, multiple other sexual paraphilias, and other criminal offenses including property crimes and physical assaults (Weinrott & Saylor, 1991). The work of Dorothy Lewis and her collaborators (1979) indicates that antisocial syndromes may be frequent not only among the perpetrators but also among the victims of child abuse.

Data about abusive parents broaden our questions about constitutional factors. Antisocial personality, alcoholism and addictions, paraphilia, and mood disorders (bipolar and unipolar) can all lead to severe parenting failures. For many of these conditions there is also evidence of genetic transmission. There may be several different kinds of familial pathways associated with intergenerational severe abuse.

Data from general population surveys confirm the existence of severe sexual abuse. About 7% of women in the general population have experienced sexual abuse by a father or stepfather. Sexual abuse by brothers is often extremely violent (Finkelhor, 1979; Goodwin, 1982; Russell, 1983). Three percent of parents admit to having kicked, punched, or bitten a child in the previous year (Gelles, 1979). Three percent of college men admit to having molested a child (Fromuth, Burkhart, & Jones, 1991). We know from physical examinations and autopsies of child victims and from interviews with abusive parents that beatings, burning, knifing, tying down, biting, and genital mutilation may accompany the sexual abuse of children. Indeed, it has been suggested that Freud's seduction theory was based in part on his having witnessed the autopsies of raped and murdered children while studying in Paris (Masson, 1984).

SIMILARITY OF SYMPTOM PATTERNS IN ABUSED CHILDREN AND PATIENTS WITH DISSOCIATIVE DISORDERS

In MPD, the child personalities who still carry the affectively charged memories of abuse display many symptoms that are similar to those seen in abused children and particularly similar to those seen in victims of intrafamilial sex abuse or incest (Gelinas, 1983; Goodwin, 1982). In latency-age incest victims, one sees headaches, stomachaches, and, more rarely, elective mutism, or globus hystericus (difficulty swallowing) or hysterical blindness. School failure or erratic school performance may become a problem and the school may complain that the child is lying, sexually acting out, or fighting. In adolescence, the most symptomatic victims present with runaways, promiscuity, suicide attempts, and pseudoseizures. Partial amnesia for the sexual abuse may be reinforced by drug use or other compulsive behavior such as eating disorders or sexual addictions. There may be deep confusion about sexual identity, sexual orientation, and pleasure.

The dissociative identity disorder patient seems to represent a layered composite of all these symptom complexes. Indeed, in treating some of the most severely affected multiple personalities, one seems to be dealing with a human encyclopedia of all possible sequelae of sexual abuse in childhood. One can see in the various alters (1) the adaptation of denying the abuse and maintaining a childlike asexual innocence, (2) the adaptation of rebelling against an authority perceived as corrupt by rule-breaking and open, sometimes violent, defiance, (3) the adaptation of becoming a sexual expert and using one's sexual experience to advantage in promiscuity or prostitution, (4) the adaptation of exonerating the perpetrator by taking all guilt upon oneself and abandoning oneself to suicidal regret and self-blame, and (5) the adaptation of feeling chosen and special and above society's rules. Each of these positions can be seen in members of an incest victim' group as well as in the internal group of some dissociative patients (Goodwin, 1989).

SIMILARITIES IN HISTORICAL RESPONSES TO CHILD ABUSE AND DISSOCIATIVE DISORDERS

Both child abuse and MPD (DID) (the most complex dissociative syndrome) are ancient syndromes well-described in folklore and mythology. For example, an ancient Egyptian legend describes Helen of Troy as having two selves, one of which stayed in Egypt throughout the years of the Trojan War (Green, 1967). According to this tale, it was her "Ka," or double, that went with Paris to Troy to be raped and to endure the siege. The myth alleges that it was the true, unwearied, unsullied Helen that Menelalus reclaimed in Egypt after the years of war. Our patients, too, tell us about the longing to send someone else to endure the pain and the desire to preserve the potential of the self as it was before it was traumatized. One patient described the death of her only supportive family member at age 4; she recalls thinking, "I'll stop right here and I'll wait ... and part of me stopped ... part of me decided to wait for him" (Confer & Ables, 1983, p.66).

However, neither child abuse nor MPD achieved a place in the scientific literature until the late nineteenth century when Janet and Freud, respectively, laid the framework for the modern understanding of multiple personality and of the traumatic effects of child abuse. The use of dissociation as a heuristic mechanism for understanding clinical symptomatology is usually credited to Janet (1889), who believed that consciousness consisted of several streams that did not necessarily flow together. His theory explained why material that entered consciousness via one stream might not necessarily be accessible to another stream. This is exemplified in MPD (DID) in situations where one or more ancillary personalities carry affectively charged memories of child abuse about which the host personality may be totally amnestic.

Although Freud is not remembered primarily as an investigator of child abuse and its effects, in the 1880s he was developing his seduction theory, which postulated that all neurotic symptoms represented either unconscious repetition of childhood sexual abuse, as in conversion seizures (Goodwin, Bergman, & Simms, 1979), or remnants of tactics used by the child to protect against the traumatic impact of abuse, such as obsessional thought (Masson, 1984). Had Freud's and Janet's observations been brought together at that time, the present chapter might have been written in 1890. However, both multiple personality and child abuse were destined virtually to vanish from the psychiatric literature from the turn of the century to 1970.

Rosenbaum (1980) has noted that the diagnosis of MPD fell into disrepute around 1910. He hypothesized that one reason for this decline was the introduction of the term *schizophrenia* by Bleuler. Rosenbaum goes on to argue that many true MPD patients were instead given a diagnosis of schizophrenia. This explanation may account for the sharp decline in reports of MPD listed in the *Index Medicus* from 1903 to 1978. Freud's disenchantment with hypnosis as a technique and his quarrels with Janet may have reinforced the decline into obscurity of Janet's (1889) ideas.

Another aspect of the rapid decline of interest in MPD is that many psychiatrists started to believe that it was an artifact of hypnotic suggestion and hence not a real diagnostic entity (Braun, 1984c; Kluft, 1982). These practitioners incorrectly asserted that investigators from Despine to Prince had been unknowingly shaping the very behavior they were observing (Laramore, Ludwig, & Cain, 1977). Research that has focused on using hypnosis to "create" multiple personalities (Kampman, 1976) is a fallacious extension of this kind of logic. The current diagnostic criteria for DID stress the importance of differential diagnosis, including schizophrenia and other possibilities and balancing concerns about underdiagnosis due to lack of professional awareness with concerns about overdiagnosis due to the suggestibility of highly hypnotizable dissociative patients.

During this same era, Freud's rejection of the seduction theory on grounds that patients were recounting sexual fantasies rather than real events created a scientific mythology that for generations resisted all assaults by the realities brought to therapists by the numerous victims of incest and their families. Not until 20 years after the pediatrician, Henry Kempe, advocated the concept that babies with broken bones might have been battered by their parents (Goodwin, 1985b) were psychiatrists able to entertain the idea that children who recounted sexual contacts with parents might have been sexually abused.

Many professionals and the public at large continue to resist both the idea that dissociation exists and that abused children develop symptoms, perhaps because both multiple personality patients and incest victims require us to believe things about parents that we would prefer not to know (Miller, 1984). Humanistic, post-Christian Western society finds bizarre and sadistic torture incomprehensible. We have difficulty assimilating data that tell us that among certain schoolmasters, certain elite secret police, certain religious cults, or sex rings, physical abuse and torture are encouraged and condoned (Benthall, 1991; Goodwin, 1993a). It often has been easier to blame or diagnose the victim rather than to try to confront or empathize with the adult who has abused. Also, therapists are often all too willing to focus on present-day somatic complaints or impending psychosis rather than working to fill in the traumatic realities behind a patient's childhood amnesia. Fortunately, since 1975, understanding, case identification, and treatment efficacy have progressed in both the field of child abuse and dissociation.

CONCLUSIONS

This chapter has reviewed evidence that MPD (DID) is etiologically related to dissociative responses to severe childhood abuse. Therapeutic reconstruction of the life histories of patients like "Sybil" and Billy Milligan has revealed multimodal childhood torture as a central reality of the patient's life. When larger series of cases have been studied, childhood abuse has been found to be a factor in 80 to 100% of cases. The abusive environment usually includes several types of abuse: physical, sexual, emotional, abandonment, witnessed violence, and severe neglect, often related to parental alcoholism or other illness. There is also often a special quality of deliberate, cruel persecution of the child, with parental attempts to maximize the child's physical and mental pain alternating with periods of normal parenting. Contrary to some clinician's expectations, when corroborative evidence for prior abuse is diligently sought, it can almost always be obtained. The physiological and emotional changes exhibited by the client during trauma narration are convincing to clinicians but require further study. The many distortions of memory and communication in DID appear designed to minimize and conceal prior abuse, not to exaggerate it. When children with DID are evaluated, they are almost always undergoing abuse, and the splitting off of alters can readily be traced to recent abusive incidents. The study of children with the syndrome has also provided evidence that some of the parents sadistically abusing these children also have DID. A review of the child abuse literature indicates that protective service workers are also seeing bizarre and sadistic child abuse, which is a demographic fact of our society, not an invention of patients with DID. The transgenerational transmission of child abuse parallels patterns of transgenerational transmission seen in dissociative disorders. Patients with DID seem to demonstrate a composite of the symptoms seen in incest and child abuse victims generally.

The centrality of child abuse in the etiology of dissociative disorders does not imply unimodal causation, but rather opens the field to genetic studies of hypnotizability, antisocial behavior, mood disorders, and addictions and to biological data about the developmental physiology of trauma, learned helplessness, traumatic memory, traumatic anxiety, state change, and "kindling" effects (Erdelyi, 1989; van der Kolk, 1987; Post, Weiss, & Post, 1988).

REFERENCES

American Psychiatric Association, (1987). *Diagnostic and statistical manual of mental disorders* (3rd ed., rev.). Washington, DC: Author.

American Psychiatric Association, (1994). *Diagnostic and statistical manual of mental disorders* (4th ed.). Washington, DC: Author.

Arlow, J. A. (1966). Depersonalization and derealization. In R. M. Loewenstein, L. M. Newman, M. Schur, & A. J. Solnit (Eds.), *Psychoanalysis: A general psychology* (pp. 456-478). New York: International Universities Press.

Benthall, J. (1991). Invisible wounds: Corporal punishment in British schools as a form of ritual. *Child Abuse and Neglect, 15*, 377-388.

Bliss, E. L. (1980). Multiple personalities: A report of 14 cases with implications for schizophrenia and hysteria. *Archives of General Psychiatry, 37*, 1388-1397.

Bliss, E. L. (1984). Spontaneous self-hypnosis in multiple personality disorder. *Psychiatric Clinics of North America, 7*, 135-148.

Braun, B. G. (1984a). Towards a theory of multiple personality and other dissociative phenomena. *Psychiatric Clinics of North America, 7*, 171-193.

Braun, B. G. (1984b). The role of the family in the development of multiple personality disorder. *International Journal of Family Psychiatry, 5*(4), 303-312.

Braun, B. G. (1984c). Hypnosis creates multiple personality: Myth or reality. *International Journal of Clinical and Experimental Hypnosis, 32*, 191-197.

Braun, G. (1985). The transgenerational incidence of dissociation and multiple personality disorder: A preliminary report. In R. Kluft (Ed.) *Childhood antecedents of multiple personality* (pp. 127-150). Washington, DC: American Psychiatric Association.

Braun, B. (1990). Dissociative disorders as a sequel to incest. In R. P. Kluft (Ed.), *Incest-related syndromes of adult psychopathology* (pp. 227-246). Washington, DC: American Psychiatric Association Press.

Braun, B., & Sachs, R. (1985). The development of multiple personality disorder: Predisposing, precipitating, and perpetuating factors. In R. Kluft (Ed.), *Childhood antecedents of multiple personality* (pp. 37-64). Washington, DC: American Psychiatric Association Press.

Brown, G. W. (1983). Multiple personality disorder in a perpetrator of child abuse. *Child Abuse and Neglect, 7*, 123-126.

Carmen, E. H., Rieker, P. P., & Mills, T. (1984). Victims of violence and psychiatric illness. *American Journal Psychiatry, 141*, 378-383.

Confer, W., & Ables, B. (1983). *Multiple personality: Etiology, diagnosis and treatment*. New York: Human Sciences Press.

Coons, P. M., & Milstein, V. (1984). Rape and posttraumatic stress in multiple personality. *Psychological Reports, 55*, 839-845.

DiTomasso, M. J., & Routh, D. K. (1993). Recall of abuse in childhood and three measures of dissociation. *Child Abuse and Neglect, 17*, 477-485.

Ellenberger, H. F. (1980). *The discovery of the unconscious*. New York: Basic Books.

Erdelyi, M. H. (1989). Repression, reconstruction and defense: History and integration of the psychoanalytic and experimental frameworks. In J. L. Singer (Ed.), *Repression and dissociation* (pp. 1-33). Chicago: University of Chicago.

Fagan, J., & McMahon, P. (1984). Incipient multiple personality in children: Four cases. *Journal of Nervous and Mental Disease, 172*, 26-36.

Faller, K. C. (1991). Polyincestuous families. An exploratory study. *Journal of Interpersonal Violence, 6*, 310-322.

Finkelhor, D. (1979). *Sexually victimized children*. New York: Free Press.

Frischholz, E. (1985). The relationship among dissociation, hypnosis, and child abuse in the development of multiple personality disorder. In R. Kluft (Ed.), *Childhood antecedents of multiple personality* (pp. 99-126). Washington, DC: American Psychiatric Association Press.

Fromuth, M. E., Burkhart, B. R., & Jones, C. W. (1991). Hidden child molestation: An investigation of adolescent perpetrators in a non-clinical sample. *Journal of Interpersonal Violence, 6*, 376-384.

Gabinet, L. (1983). Child abuse treatment failures reveal need for redefinition of the problem. *Child Abuse and Neglect*, 7, 395-402.

Gelinas, D. (1983). The persisting negative effects of incest. *Psychiatry, 46*, 312-332.

Gelles, R. J. (1979). *Family violence*. Beverly Hills, CA: Sage.

Goodwin, J. (1982). *Sexual abuse: Incest victims and their families*. Boston: John Wright/PSG.

Goodwin, J. (1985a). Post-traumatic symptoms in incest victims. In S. Eth & R. S. Pynoos (Eds.), *Post-traumatic stress disorders in children* (pp. 155-168). Washington, DC: American Psychiatry Association Press.

Goodwin, J. (1985b). Credibility problems in multiple personality disorder patients and abused children. In R. Kluft (Ed.), *Childhood antecedents of multiple personality* (pp. 1-20). Washington, DC: American Psychiatry Association Press.

Goodwin, J. (1989). Recognizing multiple personality disorder in adult incest victims. In *Sexual abuse* (2nd ed., pp. 160-168). Chicago: Yearbook.

Goodwin, J. (1993a), *Rediscovering childhood trauma*. Washington, DC: American Psychiatric.

Goodwin, J. (1993b). The seduction hypotheses. 100 years after. In P. Paddison (Ed.), *Treatment of adult survivors of incest* (pp. 139-145). Washington, DC: American Psychiatric Press.

Goodwin, J., Bergman, R., & Simms, M. (1979). Hysterical seizures: A sequel to incest. *American Journal of Orthopsychiatry, 49*, 698-703.

Green, R. L. (1967). *Tales of ancient Egypt*. New York: Penguin.

Helfer, R. E., McKinney, J. P., and Kempe, R. (1976). Arresting or freezing the developmental process. In *Child abuse and neglect, the family and community* (pp. 64-73). R. E. Helfer & C. H. Kempe (Eds.), Cambridge: Ballinger.

Herman, J. (1992). *Trauma and recovery*. New York: Basic Books.

Herman, J., & Schatzow, E. (1987). Recovery and verification of memories of childhood sexual trauma. *Psychoanalytic Psychology, 4*, 1-14.

Hilgard, E. R. (1970). *Personality and hypnosis: A study of imaginative involvement*. Chicago: University of Chicago Press.

Hilgard, E. R. (1977). *Divided consciousness: Multiple controls in human thought and action*. New York: John Wiley.

Janet, P. (1889). *L'Automatisme psychologique*. Paris: Felix Alcan.

Kampman, R. (1976). Hypnotically induced multiple personality: An experimental study. *International Journal of Clinical and Experimental Hypnosis, 24*, 215-227.

Keyes, D. (1981). *The minds of Billy Milligan*. New York: Random House.

Kluft, R. (1984a). Multiple personality in childhood. *Psychiatric Clinics of North America*, 7, 121-134.

Kluft, R. P. (1984b). Treatment of multiple personality disorder. *Psychiatric Clinics of North America*, 7, 9-29.

Kluft, R. P. (1982). Varieties of hypnotic interventions in the treatment of multiple personality. *American Journal of Clinical Hypnosis, 24*, 230-240.

Kluft, R. P., Braun, B. G., & Sachs, R. (1984). Multiple personality, intrafamilial abuse, and family psychiatry. *International Journal of Family Psychiatry*, 5(4), 283-301.

Laramore, K., Ludwig, A., & Cain, R. (1977). Multiple personality: An objective case study. *British Journal of Psychiatry, 131*, 35-40.

Lesnik-Oberstein, M. (1983). Denial of reality: A form of emotional child abuse. *Child Abuse and Neglect*, 7, 123-126.

Lewis, D. O., Shanok, S., & Balla, D. (1979). Perinatal difficulties, head and face trauma, and child abuse in the medical histories of serious youthful offenders. *American Journal of Psychiatry, 136*, 419-423.

Loftus, E. (1993). The reality of repressed memories. *American Psychologist, 48*, 518-537.

Masson, J. (1984). *The assault on truth: Freud's suppression of the seduction theory*. New York: Farrar, Straus, & Giroux.

Miller, A. (1984). *Thou shalt not be aware: Society's betrayal of the child*. New York: Farrar, Straus, & Giroux.

Oliver, J. E. (1993). Intergenerational transmission of child abuse: Rates, research and clinical implications. *American Journal of Psychiatry, 150*, 1315-1324.

Perry, B. D. (1994). Neurobiological sequelae of childhood trauma: PTSD in children. In M. M. Murburg (Ed.), *Catecholamine function in posttraumatic stress disorder: Emerging concepts* (pp. 233-256). Washington, DC: American Psychiatric Press.

Post, R. M., Weiss, S. R. B., & Post, A. (1988). Cocaine-induced behavioral sensitization and kindling: Implications for the emergence of psychopathology and seizures. *Annals of the New York Academy of Science, 537*, 292-308.

Putnam, F. (1985). Dissociation as a response to extreme trauma. In R. Kluft (Ed.), *Childhood antecedents of multiple personality* (pp. 65-98). Washington, DC: American Psychiatric Press.

Putnam, F. W. (1989). *Diagnosis and treatment of multiple personality disorder*. New York: Guilford.

Putnam, F. W., Gurof, J. J., Silberman, E. K., Barbar, L., & Post, R. M. (1986). The clinical phenomenology of multiple personality disorder. A review of 100 recent cases. *Journal of Clinical Psychiatry, 47*, 285-293.

Rosenbaum, M. (1980). The role of the term schizophrenia in the decline of diagnoses of multiple personality. *Archives of General Psychiatry, 37*, 1383-1385.

Rosenbaum, M., & Weaver, G. (1980). Dissociated state: Status of a case after 38 years. *Journal of Nervous and Mental Diseases, 168*, 597-603.

Ross, C. A. (1989). *Multiple personality disorder*. New York: John Wiley.

Russell, D. (1983). The incidence and prevalence of intrafamilial and sexual abuse of female children. *Child Abuse and Neglect*, 7(2), 133-146.

Saltman, V., & Solomon, R. S. (1982). Incest and multiple personality. *Psychological Reports, 40*, 1137-1141.

Schrieber, F. (1983). *Sybil*. Chicago: Henry Regnery.

Smith, S. (1978). *The Maltreatment of children*. Baltimore: University Park Press.

Spiegel, D. (1984). Multiple personality as a post-traumatic stress disorder. *Psychiatric Clinics of North America, 7*, 101-110.

Spiegel, D. (1993). Multiple post-traumatic personality disorder. In R. P. Kluft & C. G. Fine (Eds.), *Clinical perspectives on multiple personality disorder* (pp. 87-100). Washington, DC: American Psychiatric Press.

Spiegel, H., Spiegel, D. (1978). *Trance and treatment: Clinical uses of hypnosis*. New York: Basic Books.

Stern, C. R. (1984). The etiology of multiple personalities. *Psychiatric Clinics of North America, 7*, 149-159.

van der Kolk, B. A. (1984). *Post-traumatic stress disorders: psychological and biological sequelae*. Washington, DC: American Psychiatric Press.

van der Kolk, B. A. (1987). *Psychological trauma*. Washington, DC: American Psychiatric Press.

Volgyesi, F. A. (1963). *Hypnosis of man and animals*. Baltimore: Williams and Wilkins.

Weinrott, M., & Saylor, M. (1991). Self-report of crimes committed by sex offenders. *Journal of Interpersonal Violence, 6*, 286-300.

Wilbur, C. (1984a). Multiple personality and child abuse. *Psychiatric Clinics of North America, 7*, 3-8.

Wilbur, C. B. (1984b). Treatment of multiple personality. *Psychiatric Annals, 14*, 27-31.

Williams, L. M. (1992). Adult memories of childhood sexual abuse: Preliminary findings from a longitudinal study. *The Advisor, 5*, 19-21.

6

Disorganization and Disorientation in Infant Strange Situation Behavior

Phenotypic Resemblance to Dissociative States

Mary Main and Hillary Morgan

The Ainsworth Strange Situation is a brief, structured observational procedure in which one-year-old infants are exposed to two brief separations from the parent in an unfamiliar laboratory environment (Ainsworth & Wittig, 1969). The infant's response to this moderately stressful experience appears to reflect the history of the caregiving it has experienced, and three traditional patterns of infant-mother "attachment organization" have been identified, each related to a particular pattern of maternal[1] care (Ainsworth, Blehar, Waters & Wall, 1978). Infants who explore the room and the toys in the parent's presence, show signs of missing the parent on separation, seek proximity and contact on reunion, and then return to play are termed *secure*. The mothers of these infants have repeatedly been observed to be

[1]Ainsworth's Baltimore study involved infant-mother dyads only. While many investigators have now observed father-infant dyads within the Strange Situation, mothers and infants remain the principle focus in attachment research. While we refer to observations of infant-mother interaction and use the feminine form in references to the attachment figure, the reader should be aware that infants are usually attached to the father as well as to the mother, and that investigations of the influence of the early attachment to the father have been undertaken by several laboratories (as see Suess, Grossmann, & Sroufe, 1992).

Mary Main • Department of Psychology, University of California at Berkeley, Berkeley, California 94720. **Hillary Morgan** • Department of Psychology, University of California at Davis, Davis, California 95616.

Handbook of Dissociation: Theoretical, Empirical, and Clinical Perspectives, edited by Larry K. Michelson and William J. Ray. Plenum Press, New York, 1996.

relatively "sensitive and responsive" to their signals and communications across the first year of life. Infants who focus almost exclusively on the toys, actively avoiding and ignoring the parent on reunion, are termed ***insecure-avoidant***, a response linked to the mother's consistent rejection of infant attachment behavior. Finally, infants who seem distressed, angry, and preoccupied with the mother throughout the procedure, and fail to settle by the end of the final reunion episode are termed *insecure-resistant/ambivalent* (hereafter, *insecure-resistant*). This behavior pattern has been found linked to inconsistent and unpredictable maternal responsiveness. Each of these three traditional patterns of attachment are considered to represent organized strategies for dealing with the stress of separation from the parent in a strange environment (Main, 1990), although attachment to the mother has repeatedly been found to predict less favorable outcomes than does secure attachment in later childhood (see Cassidy & Berlin, 1994, and Main, 1995, for an overview of the foregoing studies).

In the last decade, a fourth, *insecure-disorganized/disoriented* attachment category has been identified (Main & Solomon, 1986, 1990). This category was developed following the observation that some infants suffer one or several disruptions in behavioral integration during the Strange Situation, as shown in markedly disorganized and/or disoriented behavior exhibited in the parent's presence. While home observations of disorganized infants and their parents have yet to be completed, Main and Hesse (1990, 1992) have proposed that disorganized and disoriented behavior may result from frightened and/or frightening behavior on the part of the parent. In general, these infants are currently expected to be at greater risk for psychopathology than those falling in the "organized" insecure attachment categories (Zeanah & Emde, 1993), and Liotti (1992) has proposed that disorganized-disoriented infants may be more vulnerable than other infants to developing dissociative disorders in later life.

The overall aim of the present chapter is to examine Liotti's hypothesis in the light of what is presently known regarding behavioral and representational processes in disorganized-disoriented children and their parents. While not all disorganized-disoriented behaviors have a clear relation to dissociative phenomena, some infants have been observed, for example, in postures which bear a strong resemblance to dissociative trance.[2] Thus, a number of one-year-olds have been observed freezing all movement for as long as 45 seconds, sometimes with hands in air. During this period the infant appears unresponsive to changes in the environment, with eyes unmoving and half-closed. Additionally, the Strange Situation behavior of a subset of disorganized-disoriented (hereafter, disorganized) infants is suggestive of the intrusion of dissociated actions (and/or of brief changes in executive control) as described by Hilgard (1977/1986). For example, one 12-month-old responded to the first seconds of reunion with her father as follows:

> Creeping rapidly forward to father as though to greet him in the doorway, the infant suddenly stops and turns her head 90 degrees to the side. Gazing blankly

[2]The most recent version of the *Diagnostic and Statistical Manual of Mental Disorders* (DSM-IV) identifies "dissociative trance" as a "narrowing of awareness of immediate surroundings or stereotyped behaviors or movements that are experienced as being beyond one's control" (American Psychiatric Association, 1994, p. 490).

at the wall with face expressionless and eyes half-closed, she slaps her hand on the floor three times. These gestures appear aggressive, yet they have a ritualistic quality. The baby then looks forward again, smiles, and resumes her approach to father, seeking to be picked up.

Main and Hesse (1990, 1992) have proposed that disorganized-disoriented infant attachment status may result from frightened and/or frightening behavior on the part of the parent. Specifically, they suggest that because the attachment figure is the primate infant's haven of safety in times of alarm, the infant *frightened by* the attachment figure should experience simultaneous tendencies to approach and to take flight. Conditions of this kind present an attached infant with a paradox which cannot be resolved in behavioral terms, and a collapse of behavioral and attentional strategy is therefore expectable.

Since maltreated infants will frequently have been directly threatened by the attachment figure, this theory accords well with the fact that the great majority (about 80%) of parentally maltreated infants in high-risk samples have been found disorganized (Carlson, Cicchetti, Barnett, & Braunwald, 1989; Lyons-Ruth, Repacholi, McLeod, & Silva, 1991). Disorganized behavior also appears, however, in about 20% of infants in low-risk samples, where it has repeatedly been found associated with parental lapses in the monitoring of reasoning or discourse during discussions of traumatic experiences—most often the death of a significant person. These lapses have been observed during the Adult Attachment Interview (George, Kaplan, & Main, 1985/1995) where, when asked to describe a significant loss experience the parent of a disorganized infant may fall silent; may exhibit contradictions and confusions regarding the time at which the loss occurred; or may subtly indicate that the dead person is in some way considered still alive in the physical sense (Main & Hesse, 1990). Lapses of this kind suggest momentary disorganization and disorientation in reasoning and language processes and may, like infant disorganized attachment status, also fit to a dissociative model (Main & Hesse, 1992). Main and Hesse have proposed that parents suffering such lapses within the interview context may also sporadically exhibit frightened, dissociated behavior in the presence of their infants, and hence at times be frightening. Under these conditions, the parent's experience of trauma is presumed to be reflected in frightened-dissociated behavior which, while sufficiently frightening to yield behavioral disorganization in infancy, is not directly threatening. In such cases, the infant's disorganized attachment status may be seen as a *second-generation effect* of the parent's own directly traumatic experiences (Main & Hesse, 1990).

A relation between disorganized attachment status as observed with the primary caregiver in infancy and increased vulnerability to dissociative disorder was first proposed by Liotti (1992). Because frightened-frightening parental behavior arouses contradictory tendencies in the attached infant, Liotti suggested that disorganized behaviors may represent a semihypnotic response to the "paradoxical behavioral injunction" presented by the frightened-frightening parent. Liotti's (1993) hypothesis has been elaborated in a case study involving a dissociative adult patient, who focused obsessively on anomalous fears regarding the fate of her infant and was later found likely to have been disorganized with her mother during infancy. Additionally, utilizing a relatively large clinic population, Liotti has found evidence that a high proportion of patients suffering specifically from dissociative (as compared to other) disorders may have been disorganized with mother during infancy (Liotti, 1992, in press). Further support for Liotti's hypothesis comes from a recently completed prospective longitudinal study of adolescents originally observed in the Strange Situation in infancy. In this study, dissociative behavior observed by teachers in the high school setting was found predictable from disorganized attachment status with the mother (Carlson, submitted manuscript).

If the essential feature of the dissociative disorders is "a disruption in the usually integrated functions of consciousness, memory, identity or perception of the environment" (American Psychiatric Association, 1994), disorganized and disoriented behavior as it appears in the 12-month-old infant can at present only provide intriguing parallels to dissociative experiences described by adults and by older children. Moreover, although some lapses in reasoning and discourse observed in the parents of disorganized infants seem compatible with a dissociative model, these individuals have yet to be systematically queried regarding any accompanying sense of disruption in consciousness, memory, identity, or perception.

In this chapter, we refer therefore to a *phenotypic* resemblance between disorganized behavior observed in infants, lapses in the monitoring of reasoning or discourse observed in adults during the discussion of traumatic experience, and dissociative states. The term phenotypic is selected for the purpose of reminding the reader that we are dealing with appearances only. We do not know whether the causes and antecedents of these phenomena are similar (homologous), and we have as yet no satisfactory assessments of the subjective experiences of individuals exhibiting the behaviors described. Indeed, whether early disorganized attachment status in fact increases vulnerability to dissociative states, experiences, and disorders is an empirical question which is only now beginning to be addressed in prospective longitudinal studies.

In the conclusion to this chapter, we suggest that disorganized attachment status in infancy is likely to increase vulnerability to a number of unfavorable outcomes, including not only dissociative disorders, but also phobias, anxiety, and heightened aggressiveness. In keeping with Lyons-Ruth's (in press) recent analysis of the relations between hostile-aggressive behavior in the school setting and infant disorganized attachment in a poverty sample, we speculate that there may be an asymmetry of relation between disorganized attachment and dissociative disorder dependent on whether we are looking forwards from infancy (few disorganized infants in Lyons-Ruth's sample showed clinical levels of hostile-aggressive behavior) or looking backward (the great majority of those exhibiting above normal levels of hostile-aggressive behavior had been disorganized as infants). Looking forward, then, we may find that only a small proportion of previously disorganized individuals suffer from dissociative disorder in later life. Looking backward from those already suffering from such disorders, we may find that a substantial majority had been disorganized with the primary caregiver during infancy. We examine some of the reasons why this asymmetry of relations may be expected; we suggest that there may be a general heightening of suggestibility and hypnotizability in some previously disorganized infants; and we offer some suggestions for future studies.

ATTACHMENT, FEAR, AND THE MAINTENANCE OF BEHAVIORAL ORGANIZATION WITHIN THE STRANGE SITUATION: BOWLBY'S THEORY AND AINSWORTH'S THREE TRADITIONAL ATTACHMENT CATEGORIES

In order to understand the import of both organized and disorganized responses to the mother's leavetaking in an unfamiliar environment, it is necessary to turn to the theory of attachment as developed by Bowlby (1969, 1973, 1980). Drawing on evolutionary theory, anthropology, and observations of ground-living primates, Bowlby called attention to the functioning of an attachment behavioral system which, having evolved in man's original environment of evolutionary adaptedness, still acts to lead the infant to continually monitor the physical and psychological accessibility of parental figures, termed attachment figures (Bowlby, 1958, 1969, 1982). Behaviors having the predictable outcome of increasing proximity between infant and attachment figure (such as crying, calling, pursuing, and clinging) are termed attachment behaviors, and are ascribed to the activity of this complex, instinctively guided but environmentally influenced control system. For ground-living primates attachment behavior, i.e., behavior assisting the infant in maintaining proximity to a protective, older individual represents the primary behavioral mechanism regulating infant safety and survival. Although at present the survival of human infants is usually assured even during substantial separations from attachment figures, the infant's behavioral and emotional repertoire—i.e., its response to threat of separation, to separation itself, and to reunion—is still considered to be influenced by its evolutionary heritage (Bowlby, 1973, 1980). Although less readily activated at older ages, the system is presumed to function throughout the lifetime, and variations in the physical and psychological accessibility of attachment figures occurring during adulthood are still considered to account for central aspects of an individual's mental state.

The selection of the first attachment figure (usually, but not necessarily, the infant's biological parent) normally takes place between about 6 and 9 months of age, and virtually all infants become attached. Attachments are presumed to be formed on the basis of contingent social interactions (Ainsworth, 1969), but there is no evidence that these interactions need be positive and infants unquestionably take insensitive and maltreating parents as attachment figures. Once an attachment figure has been selected, the infant closely monitors his or her whereabouts, preserving proximity even under non-stressful conditions. If threatening conditions arise, the system becomes highly activated, and the infant is led immediately to seek close proximity and contact. In quiescent conditions where the attachment figure is readily accessible, the infant's exploratory system is often activated, and the infant then engages in play.

The import of the attachment figure to primate infants may be better understood by considering the fact that while for some species a den or other dwelling is sought in times of danger, for the ground-living, nomadic primates the attachment figure is the single location which the infant must seek in times of alarm (Bowlby, 1969). For purposes of the present chapter, it is critical to note that the attachment behavioral system is intimately related to fear, intensively focused upon the location and accessibility of specific individuals, and heightened by frightening conditions of any kind.

The Strange Situation and the Three Traditional Patterns of Infant–Parent Attachment: Organized Responses Observed when the Parent (Sensitive or Insensitive) Is Not Directly Frightening

The Strange Situation was designed to illustrate the functioning of the attachment behavioral system in 1-year-old human infants by exposing them to two "natural clues" to the increased likelihood of danger (Bowlby, 1973), namely, (1) an unfamiliar environment, in which (2) the parent briefly departs (Ainsworth et al., 1978). The 15- to 20-minute procedure is conducted in a comfortable laboratory room filled with toys. Each episode is designed to last for 3 minutes, while separation episodes are terminated within 30 seconds or less if the infant is distressed. In the first episode, the infant and mother are alone for three minutes, during which time most infants explore the room and the toys. A stranger enters at the opening of the second episode, and gradually attempts to engage the infant in play. In the next episode, the mother departs and the infant is left with the stranger, after which the mother returns. Three minutes later, the parent departs again, and the infant is left entirely alone. The stranger then returns, attempting to comfort the infant if necessary, and the mother returns again for the second and final reunion episode. At the onset of each reunion the parent calls the child's name from outside the door, and then pauses in the door to greet the infant. The procedure is videotaped in order to permit extensive study of the infant's behavior.

The Strange Situation procedure was originally used in conjunction with an intensive short-term longitudinal study of infant–mother dyads observed in the home throughout the first year of life (Ainsworth & Wittig, 1969). At the outset of this Baltimore study, Ainsworth expected almost all infants to use mother as a "secure base" for exploration and play when she was present during the Strange Situation; to show increasing signs of missing her during her absences (crying, calling, searching); to greet her actively on reunion, usually demanding proximity and/or contact; and to return to play once her continuing presence was assured. As the reader can infer, this is the secure response pattern, and it is the behavioral sequence to be expected on the basis of Bowlby's description of the normal functioning of the attachment behavioral system.

Ainsworth discovered, however, that only two-thirds (13/23) of the infants in her study exhibited this secure response pattern. This pattern was later found associated with maternal sensitivity and responsiveness to the infant's signals and communications, with mothers of secure infants being found more accepting, cooperative, and accessible than the mothers of insecure infants. Succeeding Strange Situation studies, now conducted worldwide, have continued to show that about 55% to 65% of infants in low-risk samples are secure with their mothers as determined by these behavioral criteria (see Van IJzendoorn & Kroonenberg, 1988). Ainsworth selected letter-names for each "pattern" or "organization" of attachment to a particular parent as represented in Strange Situation behavior, with the secure behavioral response being designated as pattern B (Ainsworth et al., 1978).

Because the parent of the secure infant is relatively prompt and dependable in responding to its signals, for secure infants the primary problem posed by the Strange Situation is one of changes in caregiver location and additional anxieties arising regarding the caregiver's likely responsiveness are unlikely to be present. Sroufe, Egeland and others have demonstrated that children showing this response pattern to the mother during infancy later exhibit more positive affect, greater concentration, greater social competence and greater ego-resilience than insecure infants at 6, 10, and even 15 years of age (see especially Grossmann & Grossmann, 1991; Main, 1995; Urban, Carlson, Egeland, & Sroufe, 1991). Moreover, outcomes appear to be most favorable when a child has been judged secure with father as well as mother (Suess, Grossmann & Sroufe, 1992).

The reader will recall, however, that in Ainsworth's original study (N = 23), only two-thirds of infants showed the secure response pattern. Unexpectedly, six infants showed little or no distress during separation from the mother, focused on exploring the toys during her absence and, failing to exhibit attachment behavior, actively avoided and ignored the mother on reunion. As noted earlier, Ainsworth's home records indicated that the mothers of these insecure-avoidant ("pattern A") infants were rejecting of attachment behavior in the home, turning the infant away in response to bids for access (see Main, 1995; and Main & Stadtman, 1981, for overview). In continuing studies of low-risk samples, this pattern of Strange Situation response has been exhibited by about 20% to 30% of infants.

Main has argued that infants whose caregivers have been persistently rejecting may be facing a more complex problem in the Strange Situation than are secure infants (Main, 1990). More specifically, the response of avoidant infants may be influenced by the caregiver's consistent rejection of expressions of distress and efforts to gain proximity, leading these infants to minimize the display of attachment behavior relative to the probable high state of activation of the attachment behavioral system. The high heart-rate of these infants during the separation episodes of the Strange Situation suggests experiences of distress comparable to or even greater than that of secure infants, providing some support for the hypothesis that, despite the absence of overt display of attachment behavior, the attachment behavioral system remains activated (Sroufe and Waters, 1977; Spangler & Grossmann, 1993). The persistent attention to toys appearing under these conditions has been seen as enabling the infant to maintain an "organized shift of attention" away from the potentially stressful elements of the procedure.[3]

Four infants in Ainsworth's Baltimore sample were highly distressed by the Strange Situation, with some showing heightened apprehension even prior to the first separation. These insecure-resistant infants became markedly upset upon separation from the mother, yet appeared unable to obtain comfort from her when she returned. Reunions were marked by continued displays of distress, intermittent displays of anger, and an apparent inability to return to exploration and play. Home observations of these infants showed that, while not notably rejecting, their mothers were discouraging of autonomy, insensitive, and unpredictable

[3]Several hypotheses regarding the function of avoidance have been advanced, including the possibility that avoidance not only assists in the maintenance of behavioral organization, but also facilitates the infant in refraining from the display of attachment behavior toward a caregiver who has persistently rebuffed both approach and expressions of distress (Main, 1981; Main & Weston, 1982).

(Ainsworth et al., 1978; Cassidy & Berlin, 1994). In succeeding studies of low-risk samples, this "C" pattern of infant behavior has been displayed by about 5% to 15% of infants.

Elsewhere, Main has suggested that infants of parents who are unpredictable, and therefore potentially undependable in an emergency, may need to exaggerate displays of attachment behavior in circumstances indicating even minimal cues to danger (Main, 1990). In light of a history of unpredictability on the part of the caregiver, then, resistant infants may respond to the stress of the Strange Situation by *maximizing* the display of attachment behavior relative to the likely state of the behavioral system and the environment. This latter pattern is displayed by about 5% to 15% of infants.

Issues of the stability of attachment organization, contributions from the constitutional characteristics of the child, and cultural relativism have been pursued at length elsewhere (see Main, 1995, for a recent overview), but may be summarized as follows. First, in low-risk samples, reunion behavior following a one-hour separation from mother at age six has been found predictable from ABC attachment status at one year of age (Main & Cassidy, 1988; Wartner, Grossmann, Fremmer-Bombik & Suess, 1994). Overall distributions of ABC attachment patterning show some variation between countries, but the secure response pattern is shown by the majority of infants worldwide, and there are greater differences in ABC distributions within than between countries (Van IJzendoorn & Kroonenberg, 1988). Maternal characteristics appear to influence Strange Situation behavior to a greater extent than do child characteristics (Van IJzendoorn, Goldberg, Kroonenberg & Frenkel, 1992), but the role of child characteristics remains intriguing. To date there are no published studies of behavior genetics as related to infant Strange Situation behavior, although several such studies are currently under way.

DISORGANIZED-DISORIENTED INFANT ATTACHMENT BEHAVIOR: A COLLAPSE OF BEHAVIORAL AND ATTENTIONAL STRATEGIES RESULTING FROM THE PARADOX PRESENTED BY FRIGHTENED/ FRIGHTENING PARENTAL BEHAVIOR?

The disorganized infant attachment category was developed following the increasingly widespread recognition that responses to the Strange Situation procedure in a number of infants observed in both low-risk (Main & Weston, 1981) and high-risk-maltreatment samples were "unclassifiable" within the traditional ABC system. In high-risk-maltreatment samples, a peculiar and unclassifiable mix of avoidant (A) and resistant (C) behaviors had been frequently observed, leading to the use of an "A-C" attachment category identified somewhat differently across investigations (e.g., Crittenden, 1985; Radke-Yarrow, Cummings, Kuczinski & Chapman, 1985; see Main & Solomon, 1990, for review).

With the aim of better understanding "unclassifiable" attachment status in infants 12 to 18 months of age, Main and Solomon examined videotapes of the Strange Situation behavior of 55 infants judged difficult to classify (Main & Solomon, 1986). The consistency in patterning of Strange Situation behavior called for by Ainsworth's original directions had been absent in about 13% of infants in Main's Bay Area sample (Main & Weston, 1981), and during the initial review of these videotapes, the possibility that further coherent organizations or patternings of response would be identified was held open. Despite this approach, however, no new patterns of organization comparable in coherence to Ainsworth's secure, avoidant and resistant patterns emerged.

What unclassifiable infants were instead found to share in common was the display of a diverse array of inexplicable, odd, disorganized, disoriented or overtly conflicted behaviors in the parent's presence. Many of these behaviors were suggestive of an underlying experience of distress or even fright without solution, and many could be most readily interpreted if it was presumed that the infant was experiencing distress, apprehension or fright while having nowhere to turn.

One unclassifiable infant, for example, responded with apprehension to the stranger's entrance but, moving away from rather than to the parent, leaned her forehead on the wall, sobbing. Another rose to greet the parent on reunion, then fell prone to the floor, with head hidden in arms. In other examples, unclassifiable infants began crying shortly following reunion, then backed away from the parent, turning in circles in the corner of the room; approached the parent with head averted; rocked on hands and knees following an abortive approach; screamed for the parent by the door on separation, then moved silently away as the parent entered; raised hand to mouth in an apprehensive gesture immediately on the parent's entrance; and slowly struck the parent's face with a trancelike expression, while apparently in a good mood. Many of these behaviors appeared to be of a type ethologists term conflict behaviors, that is, behaviors that result from the simultaneous activation of incompatible behavioral systems (see, e.g., Hinde, 1970).

The most striking theme running through the list of behaviors observed in unclassifiable infants was that of ***disorganization***, or an observed contradiction in movement pattern, corresponding to an inferred contradiction in intention or plan. Some infants, for example, approached the parent in anomalous ways that contained signs of inhibition (as creeping sideways toward the parent with head averted). The term ***disorientation*** was also used to describe behavior which, while not overtly disorganized, nonetheless indicated a lack of orientation to the present environment, such as immobilized behavior accompanied by a dazed expression.

Following their initial review of videotapes taken from the Bay Area sample, Main and Solomon expanded their data base to include 200 difficult-to-classify Strange Situation videotapes collected in their own and other laboratories, half taken from low-risk, and half from high-risk and/or maltreatment samples (Main & Solomon, 1990). The directions for identifying disorganized behavior were then formalized, and interjudge agreement was obtained with several laboratories. While by definition no exhaustive list of disorganized behaviors could be created, seven thematic headings were identified. Infants are now judged to fit the disorganized (D) category when, in the presence of the caregiver, they display behaviors fitting to one or more of the following headings:

1. Sequential display of contradictory behavior patterns, e.g., calling loudly for parent at door followed by avoidance at parent entrance;
2. Simultaneous display of contradictory behavior patterns, e.g., clinging to the parent while arching the body away;
3. Undirected, misdirected, incomplete and interrupted movements and expressions, e.g., turning around and greeting the stranger brightly, arms raised, as parent enters the room;

4. Stereotypies, asymmetrical movements, mistimed movements and anomalous postures, e.g., rocking vigorously on hands and knees, or assuming an awkward, uninterpretable posture;
5. Freezing, stilling and slowed movements and expressions, e.g., suddenly stopping movement and freezing, hands in air, for 25 seconds or more; or moving toward parent in extremely slow motion, as though resisting forward movement;
6. Direct indices of apprehension regarding the parent, e.g., fear-smile or hand-to-mouth gesture at parent entrance; and
7. Direct indices of disorganization and disorientation, e.g., raising hand to mouth upon return of the parent, accompanied by a confused expression.

Bouts of disorganized-disoriented behavior sufficient for assignment to the category are often brief, not infrequently consisting of just one episode lasting 10 to 30 seconds. The disorganized category is always assigned together with a best-fitting, alternate avoidant, secure, resistant, or cannot classify (previously "unclassifiable" or sometimes "A-C") category. An infant whose behavior is, for example, otherwise well-fitting to the secure attachment category can be designated disorganized-alternate secure (D-B) on the basis of less than a minute of "freezing" with a trancelike expression in the mother's presence.

The nature of many disorganized behaviors is such that it is natural to look for neurological or other forms of impairment. Some disorganized behavior patterns (such as stereotypies) are found in impaired infants (for example, those suffering from autism or Downs' syndrome) but there is little evidence to date that disorganized attachment status is substantially influenced by constitutional factors in low-risk samples. If constitutional deficiencies were a substantial influence on the development of disorganized behavior, then the behavior would normally be expected to appear with both the parents.[4,5] In a Bay Area sample containing 34 infants classified as disorganized with one parent, however, only three infants were also judged "disorganized" with a second parent (Main & Solomon, 1990). Similarly, Krentz found no relationship between unclassifiable (disorganized) attachment status with mother and with daycare caregiver (Krentz, 1982) and in a recent study

[4]The only way of determining the role of heritable genetic factors in vulnerability to developing disorganized-disoriented behavior patterns is through the methodologies established by behavior genetics. Newborn behavior patterns are occasionally used as estimates of temperament, however, and by combining two independent, low-risk samples of infants and mother in Germany, Spangler and his colleagues (Spangler, Fremmer-Bombik, & Grossmann, 1995) have uncovered a modest but significant ($p < .05$) association between disorganized attachment status at one year and behavioral dysregulation during the newborn period as assessed by the Brazelton examination. As Spangler and his colleagues point out, this finding could implicate intrauterine experiences, interactions in the earliest days of life, heritable characteristics, or some combination of these factors. A recent study of a large (> 130) poverty sample conducted in Minnesota found no relation between disorganized attachment and newborn responses to the Brazelton, maternal medical problems, maternal history of drug or alcohol use, medical complications during pregnancy or delivery, infant anomalies at birth, or Carey temperament ratings at 3 months (Carlson, submitted manuscript). It is not clear, however, whether these investigators undertook an analysis of the Brazelton specific to indications of "dysregulation" as identified in the German samples.

[5]This reasoning holds unless the pattern is heritable through mother only, a possibility which cannot be completely ruled out given recent findings in genetics.

of 90 families conducted in London, no infant was judged disorganized with both mother and father (Steele, Steele, & Fonagy, in press).

Finally, infant disorganized attachment status does not appear *sui generis*, but rather is well predicted from (1) parental maltreatment and (2) lapses in reasoning and discourse observed when the parent attempts to discuss traumatic experiences during the Adult Attachment Interview. Moreover, where infants are observed independently in separate Strange Situation procedures with each parent, disorganization appears specifically and exclusively with the parent who has exhibited these reasoning-discourse lapses. None of these results exclude the possibility of a modest role played by heritable genetic factors, of course, and a study of pre-adopt parents in which the parent is administered the Adult Attachment Interview prior to the birth of the first child would be of considerable interest.

Characteristics of the Parents of Disorganized-Disoriented Infants

Studies of parent-infant interaction in disorganized dyads are now in progress, but published reports are not yet available. As noted, however, two correlates of infant disorganized attachment status are at present known. First, two studies have compared the Strange Situation behavior of infants with maltreating parents with that of well-matched controls. About 80% of the infants in maltreating families in each study were judged disorganized, as compared to between 20% and 40% of the controls (Carlson et al., 1989; Lyons-Ruth et al., 1991). This finding is in keeping with the Main-Hesse hypothesis (discussed below), since the maltreated infant is directly exposed to threatening and inherently frightening behavior on the part of the primary attachment figure. The finding is also in keeping with the hypothesized link between disorganized infant attachment status and dissociative phenomena, since dissociation is frequently believed to result from abuse in childhood (Malinosky-Rummell & Hoier, 1991; Sanders & Giolas, 1991; Sandberg & Lynn, 1992), and indeed to follow on a wide variety of directly traumatic experiences (Putnam, 1985; Spiegel, 1990). Retrospective studies of adults with dissociative disorders find dissociative symptoms originating in childhood, and Kluft (1985), who conceptualized these disorders as a defense against severe child abuse, found patients reported becoming multiple at a median age of 3. If dissociative disorders are related to early abuse experiences, and disorganized attachment is linked to these disorders, it is in keeping with Liotti's hypothesis that a very high proportion of abused infants should be found disorganized.

Infant Disorganized Attachment Status as Predicted from Parental Lapses in Monitoring during the Discussion of Potentially Traumatic Experiences. The association between indices of disorganized mental states with respect to major loss experiences and infant disorganized attachment status was first uncovered in conjunction with a sixth-year follow-up study of Main's Bay Area sample (Main, Kaplan & Cassidy, 1985). In this study, transcripts of a parent's discussion of his or her attachment history during the Adult Attachment Interview (George et al., 1985) were compared with the child's Strange Situation behavior towards that parent five years earlier. This hour-long interview focuses initially upon the description and evaluation of the adult's relationship to each parent during childhood. Adults are later asked whether they had experienced the death of a parent or parental figure, any close family member, or other person who was especially important to them; how they reacted to the loss at the time; how they thought the loss had affected their adult personalities; and how it may have affected their responses to their child. The interview is transcribed verbatim, and following the application of several detailed scoring systems, each subject is assigned a single overall classification for his or her "state of mind with respect to attachment" (Main & Goldwyn, 1985-1995). The classification system focuses upon discourse usage during the description and evaluation of relationship history, rather than upon relationship history in itself.

In keeping with the Ainsworth tripartite system, transcripts obtained from the parents in the Bay Area study were first placed in one of three categories equivalent to the infant classifications: secure (corresponding to secure infant attachment status), preoccupied with past attachment experiences (corresponding with resistant attachment status), and dismissing of attachment (corresponding with avoidant attachment status). A substantial match was found between a parent's attachment status, as identified within the Adult Attachment Interview, and infant attachment status, as assessed within the Strange Situation. Thus, secure parents were observed to have had secure infants; preoccupied parents to have had resistant infants; and dismissing parents to have had avoidant infants. This association between adult security, as assessed utilizing the Adult Attachment Interview, and infant security, as assessed in the Strange Situation, has been replicated in 16 succeeding samples (Van IJzendoorn, 1995).

The systematic nature of the relation between the three "organized" infant and adult attachment categories suggested additionally that the Adult Attachment Interview might be analyzed in ways which could serve to predict the infant's disorganized classification. Somewhat astonishingly, during the discussion of loss experiences, language and reasoning processes appearing in the parents of disorganized infants were found to reflect the Strange Situation behavior exhibited by their infants, in being suggestive of momentary disorganization and disorientation (Main et al., 1985). Thus, in this Bay Area study a strong association was found between infant disorganized attachment status and lapses in the monitoring of reasoning or discourse during the parent's discussion of potentially traumatic events (in this sample, the death of significant persons). A replication study undertaken by Ainsworth and Eichberg demonstrated that parents who had suffered a significant loss, but did *not* show lapses in reasoning or discourse during the discussion of this occurrence did not have disorganized infants (Ainsworth & Eichberg, 1991). Shortly thereafter, infant disorganized attachment status was shown to be linked as well with discourse/reasoning lapses occurring during the discussion of abuse (Carlson, 1990; Ward & Carlson, 1995).

A system was then developed for scoring indices of disorganized mental processes surrounding the discussion of potentially traumatic experiences in verbatim Adult Attachment Interview transcripts (Main & Goldwyn, 1985-1995; Main & Hesse, 1990). Where discourse or reasoning lapses were marked, the speaker was classified as unresolved-disorganized/disoriented (hereafter, unresolved-disorganized) with respect to the experience being described. As was the case with disorganized behavior in infants, no exhaustive list of indicators of disorganization in language and reasoning processes could be compiled. Thematic headings were, however, identified and an Adult Attachment Interview transcript is now classified as unresolved-disorganized if speech surrounding the discussion of a potentially traumatic event appears consonant with examples such as the following:

1. Lapses in the monitoring of reasoning during discussion of the experience. These include indications of incompatible beliefs, often suggesting that the lost person is considered simultaneously dead and alive in a physical, rather than a religious-metaphysical sense, e.g., "It was actually better when he was dead, because then he could get on with being dead and I could get on with my schoolwork;" or "My father thinks I should go to law school." Indications of a belief in having been causal in the death where no material cause was present are also understood to be lapses in the monitoring of reasoning, e.g., "He died that night because I forgot to pray for him." Similar principles are extended to identifying unresolved-disorganized responses to the discussion of abuse experiences.
2. Lapses in the monitoring of discourse during discussion of the experience. These are identified through, e.g., alterations in the form (register) of discourse during the discussion of a potentially traumatic experience, suggesting that the individual has entered into a special state of mind. These alterations include several different kinds of disoriented changes in speech, such as sudden attention to extreme details surrounding a death, an abrupt shift into a eulogistic style of speech ("She was young, she was lovely, and she was torn from us by that most dreaded of diseases, tuberculosis, and I remember, even now, the funeral, the weeping of her mother and sisters, the smell of the flowers ..."), or suddenly raising the discussion of a traumatic experience in a completely unrelated context ("We used to play dodge ball during recess. My mother died when I was 20").[6] Again, similar principles are extended to the discussion of abuse experiences.

Just as infant disorganized attachment status can be assigned from only a few seconds of behavior, adult unresolved attachment status is often assigned on the basis of only a few sentences. This given, it is especially striking that the association between parental discourse lapses and infant disorganized attachment uncovered in the Bay Area sample (Main & Hesse, 1990) has been replicated in six succeeding samples, including two poverty samples and four samples in which the Adult Attachment Interview had been administered prior to the birth of the child (Ainsworth & Eichberg, 1991; Benoit & Parker, 1994; Carlson, 1990; Radojevic, 1992;

[6]Main and Goldywn (1985-1995) also required judges to place an Adult Attachment Interview transcript in the unresolved attachment category on the basis of reports of extreme behavioral reactions in response to the trauma. These include reports of displacement of grief reactions, such as extreme reactions to the death of public figures following absence of reaction to the death of a parent, and reports of suicide attempts. If the speaker convincingly indicates that her mental organization is now entirely different than at the time of the reaction, such reports would not be included as indicative of unresolved-disorganized status. Both our own experience and those of other investigators informally queried have indicated that assignment to the unresolved-disorganized adult attachment category on the basis of reports of extreme behavioral reactions is very rare, perhaps comprising under 5% of cases of unresolved-disorganized category assignment.

Steele, Steele & Fonagy, in press; Ward & Carlson, 1995).[7] In a recent meta-analysis the effect size representing the overall relation between the unresolved-disorganized adult attachment category and the disorganized infant attachment category was found to be d = .65 (Van IJzendoorn, 1995).

The reader should note that certain indications of affective states which might appear clinically suggestive of incomplete resolution of a traumatic experience are *not* considered unresolved in this context. These include reports of lingering grief, crying during the discussion of the experience, expressions of continuing regret for experiences missed with the lost person or (in the case of abuse) expressions of continuing hatred for the perpetrators. Instead, assignment to the unresolved-disorganized category is based solely on the above-described lapses in discourse and reasoning.

The Paradox Presented by a Frightening/Frightened Attachment Figure: Disorganized-Disoriented Behavior as Indicative of a Collapse of Behavioral/Attentional Strategies. Above, we discussed the ways in which infants of parents who are rejecting or unpredictable, but not frightening, maintain behavioral and attentional organization in stressful circumstances. Since the attachment figure provides the infant with its only solution to conditions of danger, however, both behavioral and attentional organization are likely to break down if something about the attachment figure herself is frightening. A parent who is frightening is, paradoxically, at once a haven of safety and a source of alarm, compelling the infant to simultaneously approach and to take flight (Main, 1981). Because conditions of this kind are, of course, not resolvable in behavioral terms, they should lead to the collapse of behavioral strategy observed in disorganized behavior. A collapse of attentional strategy as observed in disorientation may also be expected, since the infant will be too frightened to manage the "organized" shift of attention associated with avoidance, while also being unable to focus its attention upon the frightening parent (Main & Hesse, 1992).

This approach to the understanding of infant disorganized-disoriented behavior is well illustrated in the study of battered infants, discussed above. It was also noted, however, that disorganized infant attachment occurs in a substantial proportion of infants in low-risk samples, where it has been linked to discourse-reasoning lapses on the part of the parent. While maltreatment of course occurs in low-risk samples, it seems reasonable to consider other patterns of behavior which may be associated with parental unresolved-disorganized attachment status.

[7]As of the present writing, we are aware of only two failures of replication. Steele et al. (in press) did not find an association between unresolved/disoriented adult attachment status and disorganized infant attachment status in a London prebirth sample of 90 fathers and infants. In contrast to Radojevic's (1992) recent study, in which a high proportion of infants were judged disorganized with father and a marked relation to the unresolved category was found, in the London sample only four infants had been judged disorganized with father. Kolar and her colleagues (Kolar, Vondra, Friday, & Valley, 1993) found no association between unresolved adult attachment status and infant disorganized attachment status in a very low socioeconomic status sample of mothers and infants. Their suggested explanation of the overall failure of match between Adult Attachment Interview classification and infant Strange Situation classification in this sample was a lack of comprehension of the interview questions in some of the mothers.

Elsewhere, Main and Hesse have made the preliminary interpretation that discourse/reasoning lapses occurring during the Adult Attachment Interview may result from the intrusion of frightening ideation which is normally at least partially dissociated (Main & Hesse, 1992). From this point of view, parents suffering from unresolved experiences of trauma may be expected on occasion to exhibit fright (alarm) in the presence of the infant, in response to traumatic memories, or to aspects of the environment somehow associated with those memories (when, for example, the memories themselves are not fully accessible to consciousness). Under these conditions, the parent's frightened-alarmed behavior will not have an external referent (as when the infant reaches for a dangerous object or when a potentially dangerous object is observed), but rather will be untraceable as to experimental source (Hesse & Main, submitted). Because of its potentially alarming nature, parental behavior of this kind may place the infant in a conflict situation not unlike the one created by a parent whose behavior is directly frightening.

In keeping with a more general hypothesis examined earlier, then, Main and Hesse have proposed that frightened (alarmed) as well as frightening (maltreating) behavior may be a mechanism linking the parent's traumatized state of mind to the infant's disorganized/disoriented behavior in stressful situations. Children as young as 2½ months can in fact discriminate and respond to adult emotional expressions (Tronick, 1989), and by 9 months of age infants are able to identify objects that elicit adults' emotional responses (see Bretherton, 1992, for review). We may therefore speculate that by nine months infants could well become confused and frightened if unable to identify the source of the parents' distress.

LIOTTI'S HYPOTHESIS: LINKING INFANT DISORGANIZED ATTACHMENT STATUS TO INCREASED VULNERABILITY TO DISSOCIATIVE STATES

Liotti has suggested that some disorganized infants may enter hypnotic states as a defense against the kinds of frightened-frightening behavior described by Main and Hesse, and that repeated experiences of this kind may make a child vulnerable to developing dissociative disorders in response to succeeding trauma (Liotti, 1992, in press). This line of reasoning is based on the link between dissociation and hypnotic (trancelike) states, and on the fact that paradoxical behavioral injunctions are known to constitute one technique for inducing hypnotic states. Paradoxical injunctions are seen in the "confusion techniques" of hypnotic induction, in which the hypnotist may, for example, rapidly urge the subject to engage in contradictory movements which cannot be carried out at the same time (Erickson, 1964). Liotti links these paradoxical confusion techniques to the experience of the infant who, interacting with a frightening and/or frightened attachment figure, is repeatedly exposed to the simultaneous and contradictory impulses of approach and flight.

While there is as yet only limited evidence that individuals suffering from dissociative disorder were disorganized as infants (see Carlson, submitted manuscript, discussed below), there is some preliminary support for a link between this specific disorder and mothers' experience of loss around the time of the offspring's birth. Among 46 patients seen in a Rome clinic, 62% reported that their mothers had experienced the loss of a significant relative within two years before to two years after their birth. In contrast, only 13% of the 119 patients with other psychiatric disorders reported that their mothers had experienced a loss during this period of time (Liotti, 1992). Although these data are anamnestic, the potentially traumatic impact of major loss occurring at this time could imply an increased likelihood that the mothers of many of the dissociative patients were frightened/frightening in the patient's earliest years, and hence that these patients may have been disorganized in infancy.

Dissociative Responses to a Parent's Traumatic Memories: The Case of Lisa

Above, we suggested that, like overtly threatening behavior, frightened behavior untraceable as to a direct experiential source may be frightening to the infant, and could therefore be the mechanism linking the parent's traumatic experiences to the infant's disorganized behavior (Main & Hesse, 1990, 1992). Specifically, when a parent reacts with fright to traumatic memories, or to otherwise benign aspects of the immediate environment which are idiosyncratically associated with those memories, the infant may find the parent's behavior alarming, become frightened by the parent, and hence, be placed in the behavioral/attentional paradox described above. Liotti (1993) further suggested that such behavior may also inadvertently lead to the intergenerational transmission of dissociated fears and memories, since experiences occurring while the child is in a trancelike state may enter memory in altered form, and later be especially difficult to retrieve (cf. the description of Anna O.'s "hypnoid states" as described by Breuer & Freud, 1893).

In support of this hypothesis, Liotti has described a 44-year-old patient, Lisa, who presented with a history of failed psychotherapies and complex disturbances (Liotti, 1993). Lisa's difficulties included frequent thoughts of committing suicide, flickering attention, perceptual distortions and bizarre trancelike states (blank spells during which she seemed to lose the ability to think and feel). These difficulties were accompanied by a peculiar obsessive-compulsive disturbance, triggered whenever glass was broken in the home. At such times, she became obsessed with the idea that tiny fragments of glass could escape her attention, be inhaled or ingested by her daughter, and cause her death.

This obsessive-compulsive pattern had its onset about one year after the birth of her daughter, who was hospitalized for pneumonia at that time. Thereafter, Lisa became panicked when she observed her daughter's difficulty breathing. This panic was followed by an emerging concern that fragments of glass might be a source of danger to her daughter, and at this time her blank spells, paralysis and obsessive-compulsive behavior began. Lisa now engaged in meticulous cleaning, spending hours searching every corner of the house for minute, barely visible pieces of glass. The search was executed under the pressure of mounting anxiety, which often ended in frenzied paralysis of gaze and movement. As Liotti describes it, under these conditions the surface of a table, glinting beneath a ray of light, could become a trap, forcing Lisa to remain motionless for an hour or more, staring at the table in a desperate effort to make certain that no fragment of glass was present.

During one of her blank spells, Lisa's therapist asked whether Lisa's mother had ever appeared frightened or frightening. Asking "How could you know?", Lisa replied with what she termed "a terrible story." When Lisa was about 18 months old, her sister was born, and her mother had taken the newborn infant to the beach. Her mother had then suffered a fit of dizziness, whereupon the baby fell from her arms, and lay with her face in the sand. The next day the infant developed a high fever and died within the week. In Lisa's earliest years, her mother would frequently recount this story, looking guilty and frightened and speaking in a highly incoherent, fragmented and disorganized fashion. Lisa described herself as suffering from an uncanny feeling of impending disaster while she listened to her mother's rehearsal of her sister's illness and death.

Lisa's therapist reviewed the details of this story in the following sessions, and asked whether she saw any similarity between grains of sand and fragments of glass. Lisa acknowledged that grains of sand and fragments of glass were both tiny, shining, barely visible things. Moreover, as Liotti recounts, she then noted that her mental representation of both glass and sand was related to the danger of death if a baby inhaled or ingested them. Lisa had never previously made this connection between the death of her newborn sister (lying face down in the sand, to which her mother had attributed the infant's fatal illness) and the imagined death of her own child (if she did not succeed in clearing away all broken glass). Once her therapist had assisted her in finding the parallels between her mother's experiences and her fears, Lisa's blank spells disappeared for several months. After two years both her blank spells and her obsessive fears appeared to be gone completely.

As noted above, Lisa recalled feeling "uncanny" when her mother would tell the story of her newborn sister's death. Liotti suggested that this feeling might indicate that Lisa had entered trancelike states during the many retellings of this story, and that Lisa may have failed to make the connection between her mother's story and her own fears because she had encoded the story while in an altered state of consciousness.

Disorganized Attachment Status in Infancy, Childhood, and Adulthood: Reconsidered in the Light of Liotti's Hypothesis

Following Liotti's analysis, Main and Hesse reconsidered the phenomena of disorganized attachment noting (1) that some behaviors leading to disorganized category placement bear a phenotypic resemblance to behaviors that would be expectable had the infant entered a dissociative state, and (2) that some lapses in the monitoring of reasoning or discourse observed during the attempted discussion of traumatic experiences are compatible with behavior which is expectable when an individual either enters into or reveals the existence of a dissociative state (Main & Hesse, 1992). Like Main (1991), Liotti has suggested that children disorganized with mother in infancy may be more vulnerable than other children to creating multiple, conflicting and rapidly shifting representations of self, other and relationships (Liotti, 1992, 1993, in press), and we provide support for this contention.

Reconsideration of Infant Disorganized–Disoriented Attachment Status. As noted, Main and Solomon had used the term disorientation to describe behavior which, while not overtly disorganized, nonetheless indicated a lack of orientation to the present environment, such as immobilized behavior accompanied by a dazed expression (Main & Solomon, 1990, p. 133). This description of disorientation is in itself indicative of an alteration of consciousness, and Main and Solomon present numerous examples suggestive of such alterations, as, freezing all movement with a trancelike expression, arms held out waist-high as though in arrested motion. Judges are also instructed to consider assigning disorganized attachment status when noting disorganized wandering accompanied by a disoriented expression (observed in one infant whose mother was unresolved-disorganized), and when noting any markedly disoriented facial expression, as seen in a sudden "blind" look where the infant has previously used her eyes normally (observed in one infant whose parent was later suspected of abuse).

If trancelike states can indeed be compared to early self-hypnotic experiences, and if early self-hypnotic experiences are in fact causally linked to later dissociation (which is contested by some investigators, see Ross, 1989), then an ability to dissociate may indeed develop in some individuals disorganized with the primary caregiver during infancy. According to Putnam (Putnam, 1993), "the single best predictor of a dissociative disorder [in children] is frequent trancelike behavior ... The child is usually amnesic for these episodes and on termination of the trance state may resume an interrupted task as if nothing had happened" (p. 42). One of the primary signs of infant disorganized attachment status is behavior resembling the dissociative trance, and Putnam's description can be compared with the following observations of disorganized infants in the Strange Situation:

> An infant sitting on the floor appears to be playing happily with her mother during their second reunion. She suddenly slumps forward, her upper body collapsed between her legs, and her torso falling flat on the floor. After three seconds of stillness, she rises back to a sitting position and resumes playing.
>
> Upon reunion, a mother picks up her very active son and sits down with him on her lap. He sits still and closes his eyes. His mother calls his name but he does not stir. Still calling his name, she bounces him on her knee and gently shakes him, but he remains limp and still. After several seconds he opens his eyes, slides off her lap, and darts across the room to retrieve a toy.

Main and Solomon defined disorganization as an observed contradiction in movement pattern suggesting an inferred contradiction in intention or plan. Such contradictions in movement do not inevitably imply dissociative processes, and dissociative processes need not be inferred when, for example, an abused infant shows signs of fear in smiling at the parent, or makes awkward, repeated stop-start approach movements toward her. These movements and expressions indicate conflict between approach and flight and, like indications of uncertainty or indesiveness in general, need not involve an accompanying lapse in consciousness (Main & Hesse, 1992).

As the reader is no doubt aware, however, the phenomena of hypnosis (and dissociation) include complex and purposeful actions undertaken outside of the awareness of the actor. In Hilgard's "neodissociation" theory, it is not considered unreasonable to attribute these actions to dissociated systems, operating either alongside or outside of the principal system usually associated with consciousness. From this point of view, each system may produce relatively coherent patterns of behavior with sufficient complexity to represent some degree of internal organization (Hilgard, 1977/1986; see also Bowlby, 1980). We may term the manifestations of these secondary systems dissociated actions, and some disorganized infant behavior does appear in this form (Main & Hesse, 1992). One candidate for dissociated action consists in an episode of distress or angry behavior which appears without explanation or warning in the middle of a long period of contented play, and then ceases as abruptly as it began. In addition, some infants have been observed raising arms to the stranger (with whom they have already spent several minutes) with a bright greeting ("Hi!") as the parent enters the room. They have also been observed following the parent to the door crying, then smiling at the door as though in greeting as it closes. The disorientation implied in each of these latter behavior patterns is marked enough to imply a lapse in awareness of the immediate surround.

One example of a seemingly dissociated action was given at the onset of this presentation, where an infant was observed interrupting a bright approach to the parent with aggressive slapping of the floor. A number of other infants in an apparently good mood have been observed assuming a dazed or trancelike expression, reaching slowly to strike at the parent's face or eyes, and then resuming affectionate behavior or play behavior. The intrusion of aggressive actions while in apparent good mood provides a striking parallel to behavior to be expected as a result of temporary changes in executive control.

In sum, not all disorganized behavior patterns fit readily to the phenomena of dissociation. Trancelike states and seemingly dissociated actions observed in a subset of disorganized infants would, however, seem highly compatible with a dissociative model (Main & Hesse, 1992).

A Reexamination of Lapses in Monitoring Observed in the Parents of Disorganized-Disoriented Infants: Fit to a Dissociative Model? In response to Liotti's theorizing, Main and Hesse reconsidered the instructions for identifying lapses in the monitoring of reasoning or discourse during the Adult Attachment Interview (Main & Hesse, 1992). Dissociation has been traditionally considered associated with traumatic experiences (Spiegel, 1990), and is identified through alterations in consciousness and behavior. This given, it is especially intriguing that the directions for identifying unresolved-disorganized attachment status require focus upon alterations in the patterning of discourse occurring specifically during the attempted discussion of traumatic experiences. Many of the unresolved parents of disorganized infants are otherwise good speakers, and lapses in reasoning and discourse occur only in these specific passages.

Lapses in the monitoring of discourse have been described as indicating that the speaker has entered a state of mind in which she or he is no longer appropriately conscious of the interview situation, and has in fact "lost awareness of the discourse context ... [suggesting] an encapsulation or segregation of the event from normal consciousness" (Main & Goldwyn, 1985-1995/1991 edition). Strikingly, some adult discourse lapses directly parallel disoriented infant behavior. Just as infants may halt all behavior and freeze for several seconds, only to resume movement, some adults fall silent in the middle of a sentence discussing loss or trauma, and then complete the sentence, 20 seconds or more later, as if no time had passed. Others may never complete the sentence, as, "He died, and his face [52 second pause]. I guess I was just finishing high school."

Other examples of lapses compatable with a dissociative model include sudden shifts into differing registers of speech (discussed above); sudden, inappropriate intrusions into the interview of information regarding a loss or other traumatic experience; and changes into childlike speech forms while discussing early traumatic experiences (e.g., "If I didn't tell my mom about my report card then she'd be really mad, *'cause I'd hided it from*, you know, I hid it from her, and um ... that's when the punishment came, you know ..."). Although grammatically corrected ("I hided ... I hid"), this lapse suggests that in retelling the story of an abusive episode, the speaker had become sufficiently absorbed that her usage of the past tense became that of a very young child.

The Main and Goldwyn (1985–1995) directions for identifying lapses in the monitoring of reasoning also appear compatible with directions which might be used to identify (1) efforts to dissociate memories from awareness, (2) current interference from partially dissociated memories, and (3) co-existing but incompatible and dissociated memories. For example, some unresolved speakers describe themselves as putting bad memories in special places in their minds, or making their minds "just go away" during an abuse experience. Others seem to suffer an intrusion of visual-sensory images which interfere with correct speech, such as, "Yes, well what he did was hit me, stick, stick, hurts ... brown stick." Finally, as noted earlier, some lapses have suggested the simultaneous existence of incompatible systems of memory and consciousness, indicating that a lost person is simultaneously believed dead and alive.

If lapses in monitoring such as those outlined above are indicative of at least microdissociative states, then individuals exhibiting such lapses in the interview context may enter altered states in other contexts as well. In keeping with this expectation, several parents of disorganized infants have informally been observed in what appear to be dissociative states during the Ainsworth Strange Situation (Main & Hesse, 1990). Several mothers of disorganized infants have exhibited abrupt changes in vocal quality, especially when greeting their infants after separation. In two cases, the mother's voice dropped to the male range as she called to her infant; in other cases, the mother's "Hi" took on a "haunted" quality ("Hiiiiiii") through simultaneous voicing and devoicing. One mother made a similar "eerie" or "haunted" sound as she reached for her infant's hand, although this time the underlying sound ("Huuuuunh") was not part of a greeting. Another mother, who had suffered chronic sexual abuse by her father throughout her childhood, bent over her seated infant and lapsed into low, haunted, frightening and incomprehensible non-language sounds in a deep register. Some mothers of disorganized infants have been observed sitting immobilized with eyes half closed or blankly staring into space. In two of these cases, the infant immediately exhibited disoriented behavior.

Difficulties Contingent on Multiple Models of Self, Other, and Relationships: A Special Vulnerability for Former Disorganized Infants? If disorganized attachment is rooted in frightened–frightening parental behavior, disorganized children may not only develop more frightening and rapidly shifting representations of self, other, and relationships than other children, but may at times have difficulty in accessing any representation at all (as may be the case when the child suffers a "blank spell," or is lost in a trancelike state). Liotti (1993, in press) suggests that some children disorganized as infants may feel that the self is all powerful (frightening to the parent) yet also completely vulnerable (helpless to the parent's aggression). Similarly, the parent may be represented as both good (for the infant to survive the caretaker must at least be minimally attentive) and frightening (frightened by traumatic memories, or possibly even abusive to the infant). These incompatible models may contribute to dissociative experiences in children who have been disorganized as infants. Thus:

> If the structures of propositional self-knowledge are fragmented rather than coherent, competing rather than harmoniously orchestrated, and mutually incompatible rather than reciprocally integrated, the serial organization of information may be hindered. Simultaneous or rapidly alternating incompatible, dissociated actions may then be observed, while altered states of consciousness will be subjectively experienced. (Liotti, 1992, p. 200)

Our sixth-year follow-up studies of a Bay Area sample of infants seen in the Strange Situation with both parents (Main et al., 1985), as well as succeeding studies by other investigators (e.g., Solomon & George, 1995) provide some support for Liotti's contention (see also Main, 1991). First, children judged disorganized with a particular parent in infancy often show controlling (role-reversing) responses to reunion with that parent at age six, being either punitive toward the parent or inappropriately solicitous and caregiving (Main & Cassidy, 1988; replicated in a South German sample by Wartner et al., 1994; see also Jacobsen et al., 1992). While this suggests that the previously disorganized infant tends in part to "solve" the paradox presented by the frightened-frightening attachment figure by stepping into the role of the parent, and out of the role of attached child (Main & Cassidy, 1988), a 6-year-old cannot in fact avoid also remaining in the "role" of the child. We must therefore presume that at least two, or possibly even three contradictory roles (child, punitive parent, solicitous-caregiving parent) may be developing with respect to this primary relationship.

Representational as well as behavioral processes were investigated in the 6-year-olds involved in the Bay Area study, and disorganized attachment status with mother in infancy predicted drawings, responses to a family photograph, and Separation Anxiety Test responses suggestive of fear, disorientation, contradiction, and absorption. The family drawings made by previously disorganized children frequently had bizarre, distressing elements, and have been discussed at length elsewhere (see Main, 1995, for overview). Responses to presentation of a family photograph were also anomalous, suggesting that visual presentation of the family had an overwhelming and/or absorbing quality, which drew attention away from the immediate situation (Main et al., 1985). One child, for example, stared into the photograph for several seconds, then murmured "where are you, mama?", while another handled the photograph tenderly, then set it on the table and patted it. Several appeared depressed when presented with the photograph, and some seemed "lost" when gazing at it.

Kaplan (1987) administered Hansburg's Separation Anxiety Test (Hansburg, 1972; adapted for younger children by Klagsbrun & Bowlby, 1976) to the children in the Bay Area follow-up study. In this procedure, each six-year-old was presented with a series of six photographs of parent-child separations, and then asked what the pictured child might feel, and what the pictured child might do. Kaplan described the responses of previously disorganized-disoriented infants as fearful-disorganized/disoriented, since the children appeared inexplicably afraid and yet unable to do anything about it. Some children remained silent throughout the task, whispering their answers, shrugging excessively, or falling silent for long periods. Kaplan compared these responses to the stilling and freezing responses observed in disorganized infants in the Strange Situation.

Other children seen in Kaplan's study engaged in catastrophic fantasies, suggesting that the attachment figure would be seriously hurt or killed. One described the pictured girl as feeling afraid, because "her dad might die and then she would be all by herself," since her mother had died. Another suggested that the child would lock himself up in a closet, and kill himself. Additionally, some previously disorganized children implied that actions occurred without an agent, that is, that things occurred or were done to them without knowing who the actor was. For example, asked what would happen after the parents left the child alone in the house the child might answer, "the light might go out." Such statements had an eerie quality, suggesting the presence of unknown, invisible actors (Kaplan, 1987).

Note that statements of the latter kind are consonant with a history of interactions with a traumatized parent repeatedly experiencing fright untraceable as to source. Moreover, in many of these narratives the child imagines a situation which Main and her colleagues had described as the essential experience of the disorganized infant—an experience of fright, without solution (Main & Hesse, 1990; Main & Solomon, 1990). Kaplan's findings were replicated in a Berlin study conducted by Teresa Jacobsen (Jacobsen, Ziegenhain, Muller, Rottmann, Hofmann, & Edelstein, 1992). Later, Jacobsen discovered that Icelandic children exhibiting Kaplan's fearful/disorganized response to separation stories at seven experienced marked difficulties with verbally presented tests of formal reasoning in adolescence (Jacobsen, Edelstein & Hofmann, 1994).[8]

Solomon and her colleagues used controlling reunion behavior toward the mother to identify 6-year-olds likely to have been disorganized with mother in infancy (Main & Cassidy, 1988), studying the responses of these children to parent-child separations as presented in doll play (Solomon, George & De Jong, 1995). In this study, a judge blind to the 6-year-old's reunion behavior found that the majority of the controlling children depicted the self and caregivers as both frightening and unpredictable, or frightened and helpless, a result consistent with a previous study in which the mothers of controlling children had described themselves as helpless or unable adequately to protect the child (George & Solomon, in press). All eight of the controlling children (and only 1 of the remaining 36 children) were judged frightened, either entering into fearful/violent and catastrophic "nightmare" fantasies,[9] or else, like Kaplan's "silent" children, being constricted, inhibited, and silent. In a catastrophic fantasy, for example, the house might catch fire while the parents are gone. The child runs to a hill for safety, only to see the parents die below him on the road in a car accident. Finally, the child himself might die, thrown from the hill in an earthquake (cf. Solomon & George, 1991). Following repeated prompts from

[8]The fearful-disorganized children in Jacobsen's study were also described as exceptionally low in observed self-confidence, a finding which accords well with Cassidy's report of an association between the controlling category and negative self-concept (Cassidy, 1988).

[9]In a London study of first-born children in 100 middle-class families, themes of hurt and violence also appeared in the doll-play of five-year-olds disorganized with mother in infancy (Steele et al., 1995). In this sample, the Adult Attachment Interview had been administered prior to birth, and mother's unresolved/disorganized attachment status predicted these themes as well.

the examiner, some of the silent (constricted-inhibited) controlling children also offered catastrophic fantasies.

Among the controlling children, fantastic disasters frequently arose without warning, and some of the children quickly gave post-hoc explanations as though they themselves were surprised or disturbed by the direction the story had taken. Solomon and her colleagues suggest that disorganization at the representational level is consistent with models of segregated or unintegrated systems of representation (Bowlby, 1980; Spiegel, 1990), and that the abrupt shift from constricted to chaotic doll-play shown by some of the children in the study implied that a "system which is parallel and segregated from consciousness" (Bowlby, 1980, p. 59) had suddenly become disinhibited (Solomon et al., 1995).

CONCLUSIONS AND SUGGESTIONS FOR FUTURE STUDIES

We began this chapter with a description of the close tie between fear and attachment, emphasizing the way in which the attachment figure normally provides an infant with the solution to situations which are frightening. We suggested that the "organized" (avoidant and resistant) patterns of insecure attachment represent strategies for responding to frightening situations available to infants whose parents are insensitive but not directly frightening, and that the behavioral manifestations of these strategies may follow on alterations in the patterning of attention (Main, 1990).

Infant behavioral organization should, however, be expected to break down if something about the attachment figure becomes directly frightening. This is a condition that is too alarming and confusing for behavioral organization to be maintained through an "organized shift in attention" away from the caregiver (the avoidant response pattern). At the same time, since the attachment figure is in this case the source of the alarm, organization cannot be maintained by increasing proximity to the caregiver (the secure and resistant response patterns), nor indeed can the attached infant safely take flight. Under these conditions the collapse of attentional and behavioral strategies observed in disorganized/disoriented behavior will be expectable. This outcome can be expected in response either to direct maltreatment or to frightened parental behavior related to the parent's own history of trauma (Main & Hesse, 1990, 1992).

Liotti pointed to the phenotypic resemblance between hypnotic states and some kinds of disorganized/disoriented behavior observed in infancy, and suggested that frightened/frightening behavior on the part of an attachment figure may constitute a paradoxical behavioral injunction of the kind yielding hypnotic states (Liotti, 1992). On this basis, he argued that individuals disorganized/disoriented with mother in infancy may be more vulnerable than others to dissociative disorders (Liotti, 1992). Liotti's hypothesis was supported by a case study, and by an anamnestic study of dissociative versus other clinic patients. We provided further partial support for this proposal with a description of trancelike expressions and dissociated actions considered indicative of disorganized attachment. An analysis of some lapses observed in the narratives of the parents of disorganized infants during discussions of traumatic events also appeared to fit to a dissociative model.

In keeping with the developmental pathways analysis proposed by Bowlby (Bowlby, 1988), and recently elaborated by Carlson and Sroufe (Carlson & Sroufe,

1995), Liotti has suggested that dissociative disorder would be most likely to develop in disorganized infants later exposed to intervening trauma (Liotti, 1992, 1993). We would point to the possibility that this intervening trauma could be quite specific, as the case of Lisa illustrates. Lisa's first year with her infant had been uneventful, and she described herself as having enjoyed caring for the baby. Her trancelike states and her fears for her infant did not appear until her infant had developed severe pneumonia. At that time, observation of the infant's breathing difficulties led to the onset of panic. This "stressor" is specific to Lisa's history (i.e., to Lisa's mother's story), and other more general intervening life-stressors (as, loss of a significant person) might not have led to the onset of this disorder.

As this chapter goes to press, the first prospective longitudinal study focusing on disorganized attachment status as related to dissociative behavior and overall psychopathology in adolescence has been completed by Elizabeth Carlson (submitted manuscript), utilizing Sroufe and Egeland's large Minnesota poverty sample. Disorganized attachment in infancy significantly predicted dissociative behavior in both the elementary and highschool setting, as indicated by a dissociative sub-scale for the Achenbach devised by Carlson (Achenbach & Edelbrock, 1986). Additionally, the K-SADS (Kiddie Schedule for Affective Disorders and Schizophrenia) was administered to more than 130 of these subjects at 17½ years, and the adolescent's overall history of psychopathology was rated on a 7-point Likert-type scale. Disorganized attachment status with mother in infancy was significantly related to overall psychopathology as determined from this interview schedule. Additionally, the only adolescents diagnosed as having experienced dissociative episodes according to K-SADS criteria (n = 3) had been classified as disorganized with mother during infancy.

Increased vulnerability to the dissociative disorders is not the only unfavorable sequelae which has been considered in relation to early disorganized attachment status. Hesse and Main have proposed that children disorganized as infants may develop anxiety, and may be more vulnerable than other individuals to phobias (Hesse & Main, submitted manuscript). This suggestion is compatible with a recent report in which a strong majority of mothers with anxiety disorders were found unresolved-disorganized within the Adult Attachment Interview (Manassis et al., 1994). Additionally, Lyons-Ruth (in press) has suggested that elevated levels of aggressive/disruptive behavior such as are observed in antisocial conduct disorder may be expected in some formerly disorganized/disoriented infants. Lyons-Ruth's hypothesis is supported by the finding that 83% of seven-year-olds in a high-risk, poverty sample exhibiting levels of hostility outside of normal range had been judged disorganized in infancy. Elevated levels of aggressive behavior in the school setting were also found significantly and specifically associated with the controlling sixth-year attachment category in a recent study of 44 middle-class mother-child dyads[10] (Solomon et al., in press).

[10]Despite present theorizing regarding vulnerabilities to be uncovered in previously disorganized infants, many can be expected to function competently in later life. Using a Charlottesville sample, Cohn (1990) found that the overall social competence of controlling 6-year-olds was indistinguishable from that of secure 6-year-olds, while in a German sample including several 6-year-olds who had been disorganized with mother in infancy some were considered socially competent (most were socially incompetent, see Wartner et al., 1994). As Wartner suggests, the successful outcomes for some of these children may stem from the fact that in her middle-class sample, the majority of children judged disorganized as infants had alternatively fit to a secure Strange Situation response pattern.

Among disorganized infants whose development follows an unfavorable course a variety of outcomes are, then, expected. With respect specifically to the dissociative disorders, it would seem reasonable to presume that looking backward from an existing dissociative disorder in childhood or adulthood, we may find the expected relation to infant disorganized attachment status with mother or another primary caregiver. Forward-looking prediction will necessarily be limited, since those unfavorable life events later contributing to development of the disorder cannot be known in advance, and since a substantial proportion of infants are disorganized, while only a small percentage of individuals are dissociative. Forward-looking prediction could conceivably be somewhat enhanced, however, through an examination of sub-types of disorganization and disorientation. Among the likeliest candidates to be predictive of the dissociative disorders are trancelike stilling and freezing, dissociated actions, and simultaneous or rapidly alternating exhibition of avoidance and resistance (see Main & Hesse, 1992, for an extensive discussion of "A-C" attachment status in relation to dissociative identity disorder). Additionally, forward-looking prediction may be enhanced where attachment to both parents is known, and disorganized attachment status with both parents in infancy may increase vulnerability to disorder by exacerbating the child's experience of "fright without solution."

To date, we are not aware of any finalized reports other than Carlson's regarding dissociation in individuals disorganized with one or both parents in infancy. Many developmental investigators, however, now have longitudinal samples available which include videotaped observations of infant-mother (and not infrequently, infant-father) Strange Situations. The children in these samples presently range to 19 years of age, and further assessments of dissociative capacities and any existing evidence for dissociative disorders can now be undertaken. The most straightforward test of Liotti's hypothesis would be to utilize an extensive Dissociative Disorders Interview Schedule with a selected subsample of adolescents, comparing those who had been, for example, disorganized with both parents in infancy with those who had been disorganized with neither. In such studies, cooperation between clinical investigators and developmental investigators is advisable, with investigators undertaking the Strange Situation assessments being highly skilled and reliable[11] in use of the Main and Solomon coding system (Main & Solomon, 1990).

Putnam (1988, 1989) has suggested that personality switches in dissociative identity disorder may be based on the highly discrete, rapidly changing behavioral states observed in newborns (Wolff, 1987). While switching, adults often appear to enter trancelike states with blank, unseeing eyes, facial twitching, upward rolls of the eyes, and sudden shifts in affect. Main and Hesse (1992) have pointed out that these adult behaviors are similar to infant disorganized behaviors, and may reflect a temporary lapse in the serial processing of information contingent on exposure to

[11]It should be noted that the coding system for identifying disorganized/disoriented behavior in the Strange Situation is complex, and that in a meta-analysis of the overall relation between parental unresolved/disorganized and infant disorganized attachment status, Van IJzendoorn found a strong relation between the extent of training coders had had in the infant system and the strength of relation between unresolved/disorganized parental and disorganized infant attachment status reported for a given sample (Van IJzendoorn, 1995). A list of individuals trained in the infant coding system should be available by winter 1996. Similarly, training is necessary to identifying controlling behavior at age six, and to identifying unresolved-disorganized adult attachment status.

an attentional/behavioral paradox. In order to determine the overall similarity between the behaviors described by Putnam and those observed in infancy, an examination of adults undergoing changes in identity states could be undertaken by investigators skilled in application of the system for identifying disorganized behavior during infancy. In addition, a modification of the infant system could be applied to videotapes of the Adult Attachment Interview as individuals respond to queries regarding loss or abuse experiences. If lapses in the monitoring of reasoning or discourse are indicative of partially dissociative experiences and/or of state shifts, then behavioral indices of disorganization and disorientation during the discussion of traumatic events may occur primarily in these individuals.

If disorganized infant attachment is in fact associated with dissociative states, it may correlate with other variables known to be related to dissociative capacity. Cooper and London found that children's hypnotic ability increased with longer resting EEG alpha durations (Cooper & London 1976), and a study of attachment in relation to brain-wave activity is presently in progress. Dissociative capacity has been found associated with family enmeshment (Mann, 1992), and there is preliminary evidence that adults whose overall description and evaluation of family history is placed in the preoccupied-enmeshed adult attachment category are more likely than others to be judged unresolved/disorganized on the basis of their discussions of trauma (Adam, Sheldon-Kellar & West, in press). Finally, dissociative capacity has been found associated with being fantasy-prone (Lynn & Rhue, 1988), and with belief in the paranormal (Nadon & Kihlstrom, 1987). Similarly, unresolved-disorganized attachment status during adolescence has been found associated with paranormal beliefs, including spiritualism, astrology, and ideas of possession (Main, 1993), and a modest relation to absorption has recently been uncovered (Hesse & VanIJzendoorn, unpublished data).

Hypothalamic-pituatary-adrenal axis dysregulation has recently been found in sexually abused girls (see DeBellis et al., 1994), who as a population are not infrequently reported to suffer from dissociative episodes. In this context, it is especially intriguing to note a report regarding significantly elevated adrenocortisol activity following the Strange Situation in disorganized (as opposed to secure and avoidant) infants observed in a low-risk sample in Germany (Spangler and Grossmann, 1993). In this study, ABCD infants did not differ significantly in cortisol output prior to the onset of the Strange Situation, but cortisol output was found to be increasing 15 minutes and even 30 minutes following the procedure specifically in disorganized infants[12] (cortisol output for secure infants was falling). These results were recently replicated by Gunnar and her colleagues in a high-risk sample studied at Minnesota, where cortisol was again significantly and specifically found elevated in disorganized infants following the Strange Situation (Hertsgaard et al., 1995). A similar rise in cortisol specific to disorganized infants has been observed

[12]The results of this German study are especially striking given that the great majority of the disorganized infants were alternatively assigned to the secure attachment category. This means that only a few seconds of (disorganized-disoriented) behavior distinguished infants showing the greatest rise in post-Strange Situation cortisol activity from those whose cortisol (following expectable diurnal rhythms) was falling.

in a third sample (Spangler & Schieche, 1994). In this sample, immunogobulin was observed to decrease as well.

Perhaps the broadest-ranging outcome expectable for children and adults disorganized with the primary caregiver in infancy is elevated hypnotic ability and overall dissociative capacity, including increased vulnerability to suggestion. Both controlling children, and adults or adolescents disorganized with one or both parents in infancy could be directly tested for hypnotizability, and these variables could also be explored in unresolved adolescents and adults. Conceivably, the catastrophic fantasies observed in many disorganized children may be reflective (if not directly representative) of the parent's traumatic experiences, and disorganized children may not only be more suggestible than other children, but may also experience a heightened vulnerability to false memory (Main, 1993, in press).

SUMMARY AND IMPLICATIONS FOR RECENT CONTROVERSIES

Trancelike states and seemingly dissociated actions appear in moderately stressful laboratory separation and reunion procedures as early as 12 months of age. They are considered indicative of disorganized/disoriented attachment status with respect to the parent with whom the infant is observed. At this age period, dissociative responses are unlikely to be due to the effects of suggestion, and the very high proportion of maltreated infants found disorganized/disoriented may bear upon current controversies concerning relations (usually only retrospectively reported) between dissociation and abuse. In several low-risk samples, disorganized infant attachment has been found predictable from seemingly micro-dissociative lapses in discourse or reasoning occurring as the parent attempts to respond to close querying regarding potentially traumatic experiences (such as abuse by attachment figures and/or the death of significant persons). Main and Hesse have theorized that the link between parental discourse/reasoning lapses and infant disorganization may lie in episodes of frightened/frightening parental behavior in which the parent responds to partially dissociated memories for traumatic experiences during interactions with the infant. Parental behavior of this kind presents the attached infant with a paradox in which the collapse of behavioral and attentional strategies seen in disorganized/dissociative behavior is expectable. Additionally, the traumatic memories occasioning frightened/frightening behavior in parents may for some children later become confused with personal (albeit "false") memory for similar catastrophes (Main, in press), since the child's consciousness while observing frightened/frightening parental behavior may be altered.

ACKNOWLEDGMENTS. This chapter was completed while Dr. Main was sponsored as a Visiting Professor by the Center for Child and Family Studies and by the Institute for the Study of Education and Human Development at Leiden University, the Netherlands. Dr. Morgan's preparation of this chapter was supported in part by a grant from the National Institute of Mental Health, T32MH18931, to the Postdoctoral Training Program in Emotion Research (Paul Ekman, Director). The authors are grateful to Erik Hesse for his assistance in the final preparation of this manuscript.

REFERENCES

Adam, Kenneth, S., Sheldon-Kellar, Adrienne E., & West, M. (in press). Attachment organization and history of suicidal behavior in adolescents. *Journal of Clinical and Consulting Psychology*.

Ainsworth, M. D. S. (1967). *Infancy in Uganda: Infant care and the growth of love*. Baltimore: Johns Hopkins University.

Ainsworth, M. D. S. (1969). Object relations, dependency and attachment: A theoretical review of the infant-mother relationship. *Child Development, 40*, 969-1025.

Ainsworth, M. D. S., Blehar, M. C., Waters, E., & Wall, S. (1978). *Patterns of attachment: A psychological study of the Strange Situation*. Hillsdale, NJ: Erlbaum.

Ainsworth, M. D. S., & Eichberg, C. (1991). Effects on infant-mother attachment of mother's unresolved loss of an attachment figure, or other traumatic experience. In C. M. Parkes, J. Stevenson-Hinde, & P. Marris (Eds.), *Attachment across the life cycle* (pp. 160-183). New York: Routledge.

Ainsworth, M. D. S., & Wittig, B. A. (1969). Attachment and exploratory behavior of one-year-olds in a strange situation. In B. M. Foss (Ed.), *Determinants of infant behavior IV*. London: Methuen.

American Psychiatric Association (1994). Diagnostic and statistical manual of mental disorders (4th ed.). Washington, D.C.: American psychiatric association.

Benoit, D., & Parker, K. C. H. (1994). Stability and transmission of attachment across three generations. *Child Development, 65*, 1444-1456.

Bretherton, I. (1992). Social referencing, intentional communication, and the interfacing of minds in infancy. In S. Feinman (Ed.), *Social referencing and the social construction of reality* (pp. 57-77). New York: Plenum Press.

Breur, J., & Freud, S. (1893-1898). *Studies in hysteria*. Standard Edition, Vol. 2. London: Hogarth.

Bowlby, J. (1969). *Attachment* (Vol. 1 of *Attachment and loss*, 2nd edition). London: Hogarth Press.

Bowlby, J. (1973). *Separation: Anxiety and anger* (Vol. 2 of *Attachment and loss*). London: Hogarth Press.

Bowlby, J. (1979). *The making and breaking of affectional bonds*. London: Tavistock.

Bowlby, J. (1980). *Loss: Sadness and depression* (Vol. 3 of *Attachment and loss*). London: Hogarth Press.

Bowlby, J. (1988). *A secure base: Parent-child attachment and health human development*. New York: Basic Books.

Carlson, E. A. (1990). *Individual differences in quality of attachment organization in high-risk adolescent mothers*. Unpublished doctoral dissertation. Columbia University.

Carlson, E. A. (submitted). *A prospective longitudinal study of disorganized/disoriented attachment*.

Carlson, E. A., & Sroufe, L. A. (1995). Contribution of attachment theory to developmental psychopathology. In D. Cicchetti & D. Cohen (Eds.), *Developmental Psychopathology: Theory and Methods* (Vol. 1, pp. 581-617). New York: Wiley.

Carlson, V., Cicchetti, D., Barnett, D., & Braunwald, K. (1989). Disorganized/disoriented attachment relationships in maltreated infants. *Developmental Psychology, 25*, 525-531.

Cassidy, J. (1988). The self as related to child-mother attachment at six. *Child Development, 59*, 121-134.

Cohn, D. A. (1990). Child-mother attachment of 6-year-olds and social competence at school. *Child Development, 61*, 152-162.

Cooper, L. M., & London, P. (1976). Children's hypnotic susceptibility, personality, and EEG patterns. *International Journal of Clinical and Experimental Hypnosis, 24*, 140-148.

Crittenden, P. M. (1985). Maltreated infants: Vulnerability and resilience. *Journal of Child Psychology and Psychiatry, 26*, 85-96.

DeBellis, M. D., Chrousos, G. P., Dorn, L. D., Burke, L., Helmers, K., Kling, M. A., Trickett, P. K., & Putnam, F. P. (1994). Hypothalamic-pituitary-adrenal axis dysregulation in sexually abused girls. *Journal of Clinical Endocrinology and Metabolism, 78*(2), 249-254.

Egeland, B., & Sroufe, L. A. (1981). Developmental sequelae of maltreatment in infancy. In R. Rizley & D. Cicchetti (Eds.), *Developmental perspectives in child maltreatment* (pp. 77-92). San Francisco: Jossey-Bass.

Erickson, M. (1964). The confusion technique in hypnosis. *American Journal of Clinical Hypnosis, 6*, 183-207.

Fox, N. A., Kimmerly, N. L., & Schafer, W. D. (1991). Attachment to mother/attachment to father: A meta-analysis. *Child Development, 62*, 210-225.

George, C., Kaplan, N., & Main, M. (1985/1995). *An adult attachment interview: Interview protocol.* Unpublished manuscript, University of California, Berkeley, Department of Psychology, Berkeley, CA.

George, C., & Solomon, J. (1989). Internal working models of caregiving and security of attachment at age six. *Infant Mental Health Journal, 10*(3), 222-237.

George, C., & Solmon, J. (in press). Representational models of relationships: Links between caregiving and attachment. *Infant Mental Health Journal.*

Grossmann, K. E., & Grossmann, K. (1991). Attachment quality as an organizer of emotional and behavioral responses in a longitudinal perspective. In C. M. Parkes, J. Stevenson-Hinde & P. Marris (Eds.), *Attachment across the life cycle* (pp. 93-114). London: Tavistock/Routledge.

Hansburg, H. G. (1972). *Adolescent separation anxiety*. Springfield, IL: Charles C Thomas.

Hertsgaard, L., Gunnar, M., Erickson, M. F., & Nachmias, M. (1995). Adrenocortical responses to the Strange Situation in infants with disorganized/disoriented attachment relationships. *Child Development, 66,* 1100-1106.

Hesse, E., & Main, M. (submitted). *Frightened behavior in traumatized but non-maltreating parents: Potential risk factor with respect to anxiety*. Submitted manuscript.

Hilgard, E. R. (1977/1986). *Divided consciousness: Multiple controls in human thought and action.* New York: Wiley.

Hinde, R. A. (1970). *Animal behavior: A synthesis of ethology and comparative psychology* (2nd ed.). New York: McGraw-Hill.

Jacobsen, T., Edelstein, W., & Hofmann, V. (1994). A longitudinal study of the relation between representations of attachment in childhood and cognitive functioning in childhood and adolescence. *Developmental Psychology,* 30(1), 112-124.

Jacobsen, T., Ziegenhain, U., Muller, B., Rottmann, U., Hofmann, V., & Edelstein, W. (1992, September). *Predicting stability of mother-child attachment patterns in day-care children from infancy to age 6*. Poster presented at the Fifth World Congress of Infant Psychiatry and Allied Disciplines, Chicago.

Kaplan, N., & Main, M. (1985). *A system for the analysis of children's drawings*. Unpublished manuscript, Department of Psychology, University of California at Berkeley, Berkeley, CA.

Kaplan, N. (1987). *Individual differences in 6-year-olds' thoughts about separation: Predicted from attachment to mother at age 1.* Unpublished doctoral dissertation, Department of Psychology, University of California, Berkeley, Berkeley, CA.

Kihlstrom, J. F. (1987). The cognitive unconscious. *Science, 237,* 1445-1452.

Klagsbrun, M., & Bowlby, J. (1976). Responses to separation from parents: A clinical test for young children. *British Journal of Projective Psychology, 21,* 7-21.

Kluft, R. P. (Ed.) (1985). *Childhood antecedents of multiple personality*. Washington, DC: American Psychiatric Press.

Kolar, A. B., Vondra, J. I., Friday, P. W., & Valley, C. (March, 1993). *Intergenerational concordance of attachment in a low-income sample*. Poster presented at the 60th Meeting of the Society for Research in Child Development, New Orleans, LA.

Krentz, M. S. (1982). *Qualitative differences between mother-child and caregiver-child attachments of infants in family daycare*. Unpublished doctoral dissertation, California School of Professional Psychology, Berkeley, Berkeley, CA.

Liotti, G. (1992). Disorganized/disoriented attachment in the etiology of the dissociative disorders. *Dissociation, 4,* 196-204.

Liotti, G. (1993). Disorganized attachment and dissociative experiences: An illustration of the developmental-ethological approach to cognitive therapy. In H. Rosen & K. T. Kuehlwein (Eds.), *Cognitive therapy in action* (pp. 213-239). San Francisco, CA: Jossey-Bass.

Liotti, G. (in press). Disorganized/disoriented attachment in the psychotherapy of the dissociative disorders. In S. Goldberg, R. Muir & J. Kerr (Eds.), *Attachment theory: Historical, developmental and clinical significance*. Hillsdale, NJ: Analytic Press, Inc.

Lynn, S. J., & Rhue, J. W. (1988). Fantasy proneness: Hypnosis, developmental antecedents, and psychopathology. *American Psychologist, 43,* 35-44.

Lyons-Ruth, K. L. (in press). Attachment relationships among children with aggressive behavior problems: The role of disorganized early attachment strategies. *Journal of Consulting and Clinical Psychology*.

Lyons-Ruth, K., Repacholi, B., McLeod, S., & Silva, E. (1991). Disorganized attachment behavior in infancy: Short-term stability, maternal and infant correlates, and risk-related subtypes. *Development and Psychopathology*, *3*, 397–412.

Main, M. (1981). Avoidance in the service of attachment: A working paper. In K. Immelmann, G. Barlow, L. Petrinovitch, & M. Main (Eds.), *Behavioral development: The Bielefeld interdisciplinary project* (pp. 651–693). New York: Cambridge University Press.

Main, M. (1990). Cross-cultural studies of attachment organization: Recent studies, changing methodologies and the concept of conditional strategies. *Human Development*, *33*, 48–61.

Main, M. (1991). Metacognitive knowledge, metacognitive monitoring, and singular (coherent) vs. multiple (incoherent) models of attachment: Findings and directions for future research. In C. M. Parkes, J. Stevenson-Hinde, & P. Marris (Eds.), *Attachment across the life cycle* (pp. 127–159). New York: Routledge.

Main, M. (1993, October). *Implications of recent studies in attachment for three issues in psychoanalysis: Treatment outcomes, "false" memories and the hermeneutic controversy*. Paper presented at the Hincks Institute Conference on Attachment, University of Toronto, Toronto, Canada.

Main, M. (1995). Recent studies in attachment: Overview, with selected implications for clinical work. In S. Goldberg, R. Muir & J. Kerr, *Attachment Theory: Historical, developmental and clinical significance* (pp. 407–470). Hillsdale, NJ: Analytic Press, Inc.

Main, M. (in press). Attachment: An overview. *Journal of Consulting and Clinical Psychology*.

Main, M., & Cassidy, J. (1988). Categories of response to reunion with the parent at age 6: Predictable from infant attachment classification and stable over a 1-month period. *Developmental Psychology*, *24*, 415–426.

Main, M., & Goldwyn, R. (1985–1995). *Adult attachment scoring and classification system*. Unpublished manuscript, Department of Psychology, University of California at Berkeley, Berkeley, CA.

Main, M., & Hesse, E. (1990). Parents' unresolved traumatic experiences are related to infant disorganized attachment status: Is frightened and/or frightening parental behavior the linking mechanism? In M. T. Greenberg, D. Cicchetti, & E. M. Cummings (Eds.), *Attachment in the preschool years: Theory, research, and intervention* (pp. 161–182). Chicago: University of Chicago Press.

Main, M., & Hesse, E. (1992). Disorganized/disoriented infant behavior in the Strange Situation, lapses in the monitoring of reasoning and discourse during the parent's Adult Attachment Interview, and dissociative states. In M. Ammaniti & D. Stern (Eds.), *Attachment and psychoanalysis* (pp. 86–140). Rome: Gius, Laterza, and Figli. (Translated into Italian.)

Main, M. (1993, April). *Adolescent attachment organization: Findings from the BLAAQ self-report inventory and relations to dissociation and absorption*. Symposium presented at the biennial meeting of the Society for Research in Child Development, New Orleans, LA.

Main, M., Kaplan, N., & Cassidy, J. (1985). Security in infancy, childhood, and adulthood: A move to the level of representation. In I. Bretherton & E. Waters (Eds.), *Growing points of attachment theory and research. Monographs of the Society for Research in Child Development*, *50*(1–2, Serial No. 209), 66–104.

Main, M., & Solomon, J. (1986). Discovery of an insecure-disorganized/disoriented attachment pattern. In T. B. Brazelton & M. Yogman (Eds.), *Affective development in infancy* (pp. 95–124). Norwood, NJ: Ablex.

Main, M., & Solomon, J. (1990). Procedures for identifying infants as disorganized/disoriented during the Ainsworth Strange Situation. In M. T. Greenberg, D. Cicchetti, & E. M. Cummings, *Attachment in the preschool years: Theory, research, and intervention* (pp. 121–160). Chicago: University of Chicago Press.

Main, M., & Weston, D. (1981). The quality of the toddler's relationship to mother and father. *Child Development*, *52*, 932–940.

Main, M., & Weston, D. (1982). Avoidance of the attachment figure in infancy: Descriptions and interpretations. In C. M. Parkes & J. Stevenson-Hinde (Eds.), *The place of attachment in human behavior*. New York: Basic Books.

Malinosky-Rummell, R. R., & Hoier, T. S. (1991). Validating measures of dissociation in sexually abused and nonabused children. *Behavioral Assessment*, *13*, 341–357.

Manassis, K., Bradley, S., Goldberg, S. Hood, J., & Swinson, R. P. (1994). Attachment in mothers with anxiety disorders and their children. *Journal of the American Academy of Child and Adolescent Psychiatry*, *33*, 1106–1113.

Mann, B. J. (1992). Family process and hypnotic susceptibility: a preliminary investigation. *The Journal of Nervous and Mental Disease*, *180*, 192-196.

Nadon, R., & Kihlstrom, J. F. (1987). Hypnosis, psi, and the psychology of anomalous experience. *Behavioral and Brain Sciences*, *10*, 597-599.

Putnam, F. W. (1985). Dissociation as a response to extreme trauma. In R. P. Kluft (Ed.), *The childhood antecedents of multiple personality*. Washington, DC: American Psychiatric Press.

Putnam, F. W. (1988). The switch process in multiple personality disorder and other state-change disorders. *Dissociation*, *1*, 24-32.

Putnam, F. W. (1989). *Diagnosis and treatment of multiple personality disorder*. New York: Guilford.

Putnam, F. W. (1993). Dissociative disorders in children: Behavioral profiles and problems. *Child Abuse and Neglect*, *17*, 39-45.

Radke-Yarrow, M., Cummings, E. M., Kuczynski, L., & Chapman, M. (1985). Patterns of attachment in two- and three-year-olds in normal families and families with parental depression. *Child Development*, *56*, 884-893.

Radojevic, M. (July, 1992). *Predicting quality of infant attachment to father at 15 months from prenatal paternal representations of attachment: An Australian contribution*. Paper presented at the 25th International Congress of Psychology, Brussels, Belgium.

Ross, C. (1989). *Multiple personality disorder: Diagnosis, clinical features and treatment*. New York: Wiley.

Sandberg, D. A., & Lynn, S. J. (1992). Dissociative experiences, psychopathology and adjustment, and child and adolescent maltreatment in female college students. *Journal of Abnormal Psychology*, *101*, 717-723.

Sanders, B., & Giolas, M. H. (1991). Dissociation and childhood trauma in psychologically disturbed adolescents. *American Journal of Psychiatry*, *148*, 50-54.

Solomon, J., & George, C. (1991, April). *Working models of attachment of children classified as controlling at age six: Disorganization at the level of representation*. Paper presented at the biennial meeting of the Society for Research in Child Development, Seattle, WA.

Solomon, J., George, C., & DeJong, A. (1995). Children classified as controlling at age six: Evidence of disorganized representational strategies and aggression at home and at school. *Development and Psychopathology*, *7*, 447-463.

Spangler, G., & Grossmann, K. E. (1993). Biobehavioral organization in securely and insecurely attached infants. *Child Development*, *64*, 1439-1450.

Spangler, G. & Schieche, M. (1994). Biobehavioral organization in one-year-olds: Quality of mother-infant attachment and immunological and adrenocortisol regulation. *Psychologische Beitrage*, *36*, 30-35.

Spiegel, D. (1990). Hypnosis, dissociation, and trauma: Hidden and overt observers. In J. L. Singer (Ed.), *Repression and dissociation: Implications for personality theory, psychopathology, and health* (pp. 121-142). Chicago: University of Chicago Press.

Spieker, S. J., & Booth, C. (1985, April). Family risk typologies and patterns of insecure attachment. In J. Osofsky (chair), *Interventions with infants at risk: Patterns of attachment*. Symposium conducted at the biennial meeting of the Society for Research in Child Development, Toronto, Ontario, Canada.

Steele, M., Fonagy, P., Yabsley, S., Woolgar, M., & Croft, C. (1995, March), *Maternal representations of attachment during pregnancy predict the quality of children's doll-play at five years of age*. Presented at the biennial meeting of the Society for Research in Child Development, Indianapolis, IN.

Steele, H., Steele, M., & Fonagy, P. (in press). Associations among attachment classifications of mothers, fathers and infants: Evidence for a relationship-specific perspective. *Child Development*.

Suess, G. J., Grossmann, K. E., & Sroufe, L. A. (1992). Effects of infant attachment to mother and father on quality of adaptation in preschool: From dyadic to individual organization of self. *International Journal of Behavioral Development*, *15*, 43-65.

Tronick, E. Z. (1989). Emotions and emotional communication in infants. *American Psychologist*, *44*, 112-119.

Urban, J., Carlson, E., Egeland, B., & Sroufe, A. (1991). Patterns of individual adaptation across childhood. *Development and Psychopathology*, *3*, 445-460.

Van IJzendoorn, M. H. (1995). Adult attachment representations, parental responsiveness and infant attachment: A meta-analysis on the predictive validity of the Adult Attachment Interview. *Psychological Bulletin*, *117*, 3, 387-403.

Van IJzendoorn, M. H., Goldberg, S., Kroonenberg, P. M. & Frenkel, O. J. (1992). The relative effects of maternal and child problems on the quality of attachment: A meta-analysis of attachment in clinical samples. *Child Development*, *63*: 840-858.

Van IJzendoorn, M. H., & Kroonenberg, P. M. (1988). Cross-cultural patterns of attachment: A meta-analysis of the Strange Situation. *Child Development*, *59*: 147-156.

Ward, M. J., & Carlson, E. A. (1995). The predictive validity of the adult attachment interview for adolescent mothers. *Child Development*, *66*, 69-79.

Wartner, U. G., Grossmann, K., Fremmer-Bombik, E., & Suess, G. (1994). Attachment patterns at age six in south Germany: Predictability from infancy and implications for preschool behavior. *Child Development*, *65*, 1014-1027.

Wolff, P. H. (1987). *The development of behavioral states and the expression of emotions in early infancy*. Chicago: University of Chicago Press.

7

Dissociative Disorders in Children and Adolescents

Nancy L. Hornstein

INTRODUCTION

The clinical evolution of the recognition and treatment of dissociative disorders occurring during childhood and adolescence owes a debt of gratitude to several bodies of research and clinical literature that have accumulated over the last two decades, including posttraumatic stress, the psychological sequelae of trauma and child abuse, child development, and the study of dissociative disorders in adults. The complexities of symptomatic presentation and underlying deficits that accompany overt "dissociation" are perhaps nowhere as remarkable as they are during the process of ongoing development in children. The evolution of knowledge in these overlapping areas of investigation has created a framework for the conceptualization and recognition of childhood dissociative disorders among those suffering from the psychological sequelae of trauma.

Among the complexities facing diagnosticians and treating clinicians alike are the variety of symptomatic disturbances that are part and parcel of the phenomenology of dissociative disorders in both children and adults, such as disturbances in identity (splitting, fragmentation), affect regulation (depression, mood swings, feelings isolated-dissociated from experience), autohypnotic phenomenon (trances, misperceptions, time distortions, psychogenic numbing), memory disturbances (psychogenic amnesia, fugue), revivification of traumatic experiences (flashbacks, hallucinations), behavioral disturbances (inattention, poor impulse

Nancy L. Hornstein • Department of Psychiatry, Child Division, University of Illinois at Chicago and Institute for Juvenile Research, Chicago, Illinois 61612.

Handbook of Dissociation: Theoretical, Empirical, and Clinical Perspectives, edited by Larry K. Michelson and William J. Ray. Plenum Press, New York, 1996.

control), and self-injury and suicidality (Albini & Pease, 1989; Barach, 1991; Bliss, 1984; Bowman, 1990; Bowman, Blix, & Coons, 1985; Braun & Sachs, 1985; Braun, 1985; Brierre & Runtz, 1988; Chu & Dill, 1990; Conte & Schuerman, 1988; Coons, Bowman, & Milstein, 1988; Coons, Cole, Pellow, & Milstein, 1990; Dell & Eisenhower, 1990; Ensink, 1992; Fagan & McMahon, 1984; Famularo, Kinscherff, & Fenton, 1992; Fink & Golinkoff, 1990; Fink, 1988; Fraiberg, 1982; Goodwin, 1990; Greaves, 1980; Horevitz & Braun, 1984; Hornstein & Tyson, 1991; Hornstein & Putnam, 1992, 1994; Kluft, 1984, 1985a,b, 1986, 1987a,b, 1991; Kramer, 1990; Loewenstein, 1990; Ludwig, 1983; Malenbaum & Russel, 1987, McLeer, Deblinger, Henry, & Orvaschel, 1992; Peterson, 1990; Putnam, Guroff, Silberman, Barban, & Post, 1986; Putnam, 1985, 1989, 1990, 1991, 1993; Ross, Miller, Bjornson, Reagor, Fraser, & Anderson, 1991; Ross, Miller, Bjorson, Reagor, Fraser, & Anderson, 1990; Ross, Norton, & Wozney, 1989; Russel, Bott, & Sammons, 1989; Schetky, 1990; Schulz, Braun, & Kluft, 1989; Shengold, 1989; Sherkow, 1990; Stein, Goldring, Siegel, Burman, & Sorenson, 1988; Steinberg, Rounsaville, & Cicchetti, 1990; van der Kolk & Kadish, 1987; Venn, 1984; Vincent & Pickering, 1988; Weiss, Sutton, & Utecht, 1985).

The theoretical model behind the diagnosis of dissociative identity disturbance has contributed further to our clinical understanding of the patient's symptomatic presentation and his/her subjective experience. It is also helpful for developing effective therapeutic approaches toward both adults (Barach, 1991; Braun & Sachs, 1985; Chu & Dill, 1990; Coons et al., 1988, 1990; Ensink, 1992; Fink & Golinkoff, 1990; Greaves, 1980; Horevitz & Braun, 1984; Kluft, 1987a,b, 1991; Loewenstein, 1990; Lovinger, 1983; Putnam, 1985, 1989, 1990; Putnam et al., 1986; Ross et al., 1989, 1990; Schulz et al., 1989; Shengold, 1989; Sherkow, 1990; Spiegel, 1990, 1991; van der Kolk & Kadish, 1987) and children (Bowman 1990; Bowman et al., 1985; Brierre & Runtz, 1988; Dell & Eisenhower, 1990; Donovan & McIntyre, 1990; Fagan & McMahon, 1984; Famularo et al., 1992; Fine, 1988; Fink, 1988; Fraiberg, 1982; Goodwin, 1990; Hornstein & Tyson, 1991; Hornstein & Putnam, 1992; Kluft 1984, 1985a,b, 1986, 1987a,b, 1991; Malenbaum & Russel, 1987; Peterson, 1990; Putnam, 1990, 1991, 1993; Sherkow, 1990; Terr, 1990; Vincent & Pickering, 1988; Weiss et al., 1985).

Although child and adolescent dissociative disorders were described in nineteenth- and early twentieth-century clinical reports (Bowman, 1990; Fine, 1988), they later disappeared from clinical focus (along with their adult counterparts) for much of the twentieth century. The sudden increase in reports of patients with dissociative disorders caused initial controversy in modern psychiatry, with questions about the validity of the observers' perceptions in light of a century passing with few reports of these phenomenon. Reasons for this historical dearth of clinical interest and reports on these disorders have been postulated (Putnam, 1985, 1989). Among the limiting factors described were theoretical adherence to a model emphasizing repression rather than dissociation as a means of excluding information from conscious awareness.

Today, social scientists and historians have eloquently ruptured the myth of "pure scientific truth," showing how we are vulnerable to fashions and trends and how "what we see" is profoundly influenced by our theoretical constructs. My own impression is that the advent of powerful antipsychotic medications led researchers to focus eagerly on the biogenetics of psychiatric illness, temporarily stalling investigations into the role environmental influences play in the development of psychiatric disorders (not to mention their impact on "bioendocrinologic" and immune functioning), of which trauma and child abuse are but examples. Interest in psychiatric sequelae related to stress and trauma is enjoying a resurgence as other areas of psychiatric investigation reach limitations in their explanatory power.

Efforts to understand dissociative disorders are best served by a recognition that we do not need to choose between our "theoretical truths," which seem to compete with and contradict each other; rather, we can recognize that each of them attempts to capture and cognitively organize some element of observable reality, facilitating our understanding, investigation, and clinical work. The challenge then becomes searching for ways to integrate conflictual observations and theoretical understandings that threaten our current understanding and signal us to defensively reject, repress, or even dissociate them.

This chapter will present current research on dissociative disorders in children and adolescents, highlighting the relationship between dissociative disorders and childhood experiences of trauma/abuse, and will include clinical illustrations of the role dissociation plays in the complex symptomatic presentation of these young patients and the consequent differential diagnostic dilemma presented to the clinician. An important but too often underemphasized point that will enhance understanding of the material to follow is that dissociation is a defense that is integral (by definition) to the symptomatic presentations in the dissociative disorders, yet it is only one aspect of these patients' complex developmental adjustment to their experiences. The real utility of identifying dissociative symptoms lies in the recognition that the variety of disturbances in identity, affect modulation, behavioral control, and attention that are present in these children are integrally related to their past traumatic experiences. Thus, correct identification of dissociative symptoms has a tremendous impact on later diagnostic and treatment formulations in these cases and has implications for psychosocial intervention to prevent further trauma as well.

DISSOCIATION AND DISSOCIATIVE DISORDER

In order to meaningfully discuss a topic, in this case dissociation, one should have a clear definition or description of the phenomenon. In the *Diagnostic and Statistical Manual of Mental Disorders*, 4th Edition (DSM-IV) (American Psychiatric Association, 1994), a dissociative disturbance is defined as "a disturbance or alteration in the normal integrative functions of identity, memory or consciousness" (Armstrong, Putnam, & Carlson, 1994). These include dissociative identity disturbance (DID), psychogenic fugue, psychogenic amnesia, depersonalization disorder, and dissociative disorder not otherwise specified (DDNOS). Dissociative identity disturbance (formerly multiple personality disorder) involves alterations in all three areas: identity, memory, and consciousness. One immediately runs into problems defining such constructs as "identity" and "consciousness" and in differentiating the alterations in memory that represent dissociation versus those present in repression. A truly cogent discussion of this topic would require at the very least it's own chapter, if not an entire book, so interested readers are referred to two excellent discussions of this topic by Ensink (1992) and by Putnam (1989).

An abbreviated discussion should clarify the nature of the phenomenon being described. One conceptualization of dissociation, evolved from work with adult patients, emphasizes a "disturbance in consciousness." In this conceptualization, persons vary in the frequency and intensity of disturbances in the continuity of conscious awareness. There is a continuum from minor dissociations of everyday life, such as driving past your exit on the freeway, to the major forms of psychopathology involving dissociation, such as multiple personality disorder (Putnam et al., 1986; Putnam, 1989). All patients with a dissociative disorder suffer from a variety of dissociative experiences such as amnesia, daze states, depersonalization, derealization, and fugue states (Putnam, 1989). Putnam et al. (1986) found that experiences of amnesia or time loss (time gaps) were the single most commonly reported symptom in patients receiving the diagnosis of multiple personality disorder. Ensink (1992, p. 52) provides useful criteria for differentiating dissociative "time-gaps" from other disturbances in consciousness. She writes:

> [R]eports can be considered time-gaps only if they meet these criteria:
>
> 1. The person reports to have had no consciousness of the environment or her/his behavior.
> 2. The person can not describe any focus of attention. This differentiates experience [sic] of time-gaps from daydreaming, being absorbed in thoughts, or events excluded from awareness because the focus of attention was on another event.
> 3. The person has no conscious or voluntary control of behavior (like speaking, reading, writing), normally guided by consciousness. This criterion differentiates extensive time-gaps from passive behavior such as staring or sitting down and from complex but skilled acts normally not selectively attended such as driving a car.
> 4. Other people tend not to notice any difference in functioning of the person: This criterion differentiates extensive time-gaps from immediate [sic] evident disturbances in consciousness, such as coma, fainting, pseudo-epileptical attacks or more subtle changes in consciousness, such as staring, daydreaming, sleepwalking, etc.

This "operational description" of the dissociative symptom of time gaps is included because it helps distinguish the kind of dissociative experiences that clearly differentiate patients with dissociative disorders from those with other disturbances.

The child clinician or researcher has a difficult job in trying to use adult descriptions of dissociative experiences when attempting to interview children about similar phenomena. The clinician immediately encounters developmental limitations in elucidating dissociative experiences in children. These limitations include children's immature cognitive systems, which necessitates concretizing questions about their "dissociative experiences"; immature speech and language, which make dissociative identity disturbance impossible to diagnose before a child has achieved certain milestones in their acquisition of language skills; the gradual evolution of the child's internally held and integrated identity construct or subjective sense of identity over the primary school years; and the developmentally driven changes in the capacity for and the frequency of the child's use of dissociative defenses. Again, an adequate treatment of these considerations would require a chapter in itself, although aspects of these issues are touched on in other chapters in this volume.

In light of the difficulties in evaluating children for dissociative disorders, a clinical rule of thumb is to look for subjective experiences in children that are corollaries to those of their adult counterparts, but with a level of organization, "form of expression," and limitations in the child's capacity to report them that is influenced greatly by the child's age and acquisition of developmental milestones. As children with dissociative disorders approach adolescence, the overt manifestations of their diagnosis are increasingly similar to those of adults. In children younger than school age, dissociation can be recognized; but the diagnosis of dissociative identity disturbance is very difficult and should include consultation with experts experienced with this age group. Frequently, a diagnosis of DDNOS must suffice in combination with clinical descriptions that elaborate on the areas of disturbance present relative to norms for children of that age and developmental level.

Dr. Gary Peterson has proposed a diagnostic category of "Dissociative Disorder of Childhood" in recognition of these limitations (Peterson, 1990). In his working copy for consideration by the Dissociative Disorders Study Group of the Task Force on DSM-IV, he describes the "essential features of this disorder" as: "(1) the experience by the child of having amnestic periods and/or trancelike states and (2) the child showing marked changes in behavior and functioning. In addition, the child must exhibit an array of behaviors and/or emotional states which would usually be considered to be symptoms of other disorders." His articles and the text of the remainder of the DMS-IV proposal are additional sources for discussion of the diagnostic issues referred to above.

IDENTIFYING DISSOCIATIVE SYMPTOMS IN CHILDREN

There are several diagnostic screening tools available for use with children that aim to detect the presence of dissociative symptoms. The most well-developed and tested is the Childhood Dissociation Checklist (CDC) (Putnam, 1993), which can be used in school-age children. For adolescents, the Adolescent Dissociative Experiences Scale (Armstrong et al., 1994) and, for older adolescents, the Structured Clinical Interview for the DSM-III-R Dissociative Disorders (SCID-D) Steinberg, Rounsaville, & Cicchetti, 1990) can be used.

Ultimately, there is no available diagnostic substitute for the clinical interview and evaluation. In order to better illustrate the clinical manifestations of dissociative disorders in childhood, I'll turn to examples from some contemporary research. (A portion of the following is a reworking of information from earlier publications [Hornstein & Putnam, 1992, 1994].) The children who will be described were part of a previously published study delineating the clinical profile of dissociative disorders in childhood and adolescence (Hornstein & Tyson, 1991). In that study, behavioral and symptomatic presentations of two independently collected case series of children with dissociative disorders (64 cases), 44 with multiple personality disorder (MPD; now dissociative identity disturbance) in DSM-IV, and 20 with DDNOS were compared with each other to test the construct validity of these diagnoses in children and adolescents.

The first series, collected by Nancy Hornstein (NH), was largely composed of children seen for evaluation and treatment in an inpatient unit at the University of

California at Los Angeles. The second series, collected by Frank Putnam was largely composed of outpatients seen either as part of a longitudinal research project on the psychobiological effects of sexual abuse conducted by the Laboratory of Developmental Psychology, National Institute of Mental Health, or in consultation either with other NIH research projects or at Children's Hospital National Medical Center, Washington, DC. The diagnoses of MPD or DDNOS were made using DSM-III-R (American Psychiatric Association, 1987) criteria augmented by NIMH criteria based on clinical interviews of the children and their guardians, protective service caseworkers, teachers, and therapists, and in the case of inpatients included extended observation on the ward. Standard psychological testing was obtained on the majority of children. Parents or guardians also completed the CDC (Putnam, 1993). The mean ages in these two series (NH) followed by (FP) were 9.55 ± 3.36 years and 10.84 ± 3.63 years, respectively; there were 14 females and 16 males (NH) and 28 females and 6 males (FP). The number diagnosed as having MPD versus DDNOS were 22 versus 8 (NH) and 22 versus 12 (FP).

These children reported and/or were observed to have a variety of dissociative symptoms, such as trance or daze states, depersonalization, involuntary movements, passive influence experiences, and so forth and identity problems such as alter personalities, spontaneous age regression, rapid changes in personality, and so forth. Additionally, all children with MPD had demonstrable time gaps that would have met the operational criteria described previously, as did many of the children who received diagnoses of DDNOS.

As previously alluded to, gathering interview data on amnestic experiences or time gaps in children is more difficult than gathering similar data from adult patients. The reasons for this include that children's development of adult time perception does not occur until late childhood, and a child's report of "not remembering" behavior often represents "motivated forgetting" of their behavior to escape consequences or uncomfortable feelings. Identifying time gaps often requires interviewing strategies that take into account the child's developmental level supplemented with observational data obtained in a variety of settings that suggest discontinuities in the child's conscious experience.

Anchoring inquiry in the events of the child's daily life is the best approach for obtaining information about dissociative experiences in preadolescent youngsters. The interviewer may ask about gaps in the child's memory for common everyday experiences, such as times he's been told that he already ate lunch when he thought it was still morning, or times she is confused in class because she last remembered the teacher going over math problems on the board and now the other kids are all working on social studies. The child is asked to recount in his or her own words experiences they have had that are similar to this. The interviewer may also ask about experiences when the child requests to do an activity only to be told, "but, you already did that."

To differentiate between dissociative experiences and lying, or motivated forgetting, it is useful to inquire whether the child ever got thanked for doing a chore he or she doesn't recall doing. An 11-year-old girl brightened when asked this question, replying, "Oh yes, all the time. Just last night my Mom said 'thanks for doing the dishes.' I thought she was teasing me because I didn't do them, but when I looked in the kitchen they were all done and my Mom was happy. I know she didn't do them either, so I can't guess who did because we were the only people at home." This child was previously assumed to be a chronic liar because of her disavowals of negative behaviors that had been observed by others.

Observing the child for incongruous or unusual behaviors during the interview and inquiring about these, as well as inquiring "what just happened?" when a child stares blankly, seems to change the subject, or seems suddenly confused about a question the interviewer asked can reveal dissociative time gaps that occur during the interview itself. The child is asked to describe his observed behaviors to ascertain possible gaps in recall.

Emotionally laden experiences are often occasions in which time gaps occur for dissociative children. Inquiry into experiences such as explosive outbursts, schoolyard fights, or intense family sessions can lead to discovery of dissociative processes. When a child seems to remember superficially, pressing him for whether he actually remembers the occurrence or remembers only what he was later told happened and has "blank periods" during the experience can help him describe his subjective experience. Children who do not dissociate revel in this chance to give detailed descriptions of what they feel and experience. Children who dissociate may describe control-influence phenomenon or other aspects of their subjective awareness of dissociative experiences. An 8-year-old boy responded to requests for the details of his actual experiences during the frequent fights he was having by saying, "You know, the bad me just takes over. (How?) It kind of comes out my nose, and mouth and ears. (And then what happens?) Well, that bad me, it's got a hold on my arm, and it's running my legs too. I'm saying inside 'no! stop!' but my legs just keep going, and then my arm is striking the other boy and I can't stop it. I also get a voice in my mind telling me to 'mind my own business'."

In adopting an approach that asks for details of a patient's subjective experiences, numerous misleading assumptions are avoided, as well as the danger of supplying information about symptoms which the child assents to for the sake of simplicity, giving the interviewer a false sense of knowing what is going on with the patient. Initially, there is no shortcut for experience in gaining access to this information from children, along with a sense of developmentally typical versus unusual responses deserving of more detailed follow-up. With children who have been abused, gaining this access can be difficult and time consuming, since often a level of trust must be built with them before they will talk openly. In some ways, dogged attempts to understand their unique experiences, rather than to impose preconceived notions on them, enhances the trust-building process.

Observational or historical data that lead the experienced clinician to consider a dissociative disorder in a child's differential diagnosis include behavioral manifestations of dissociative time gaps. These include disavowal of witnessed behavior, amnesia, fluctuations in apparent attentional ability, concentration, knowledge, or performance, entrance into spontaneous "trancelike" states in which the child is oblivious to external stimuli (often leading to evaluation for seizure activity), and learning or reading difficulties.

In children with DID, there are "switches" between different states of consciousness or subjective senses of self that are not integrated into conscious awareness; these can be referred to as alternate personalities (alters). As in their adult counterparts, these alters in children with DID manifest relatively stable patterns of behavior, affect, gestures, speech patterns (tone, pitch, complexity of language etc.), manner of relating, and aspects of identity (gender and role identifications, name, age, etc.) that differ from each other.

The first clue that a child inpatient had DID came when an ordinarily ultra-feminine girl, calling herself Joanne, suddenly became rough and tomboyish, exhibiting differences in mannerism and voice tone during a baseball game. She insisted upon being called "Jo" in this setting. By the time she returned to the unit, she again was feminine, calling herself Joanne. When asked about the boyish "uniform" she still wore and why she asked to be called "Jo" earlier, she initially stared blankly, then she said, "Oh, I'm never really there when I have to do that boy stuff." When asked what she meant, she shrugged, later elaborating "Oh, I think that some boy Jo that talks to me takes my place." She was asked how this works. Her reply, "I don't know really, I don't remember it well," preceded her entry into a state in which she appeared dazed, then had an abrupt change in manner, saying "I don't want to talk about this s ... t, Doc. Joanne don't bother anybody. This ain't really none of your concern." Needless to say, this was the first dissociative "change in personality" that was witnessed in her.

In children, these "switches" between alternate personality states are frequently observable as rapid age regression, sudden shifts in demeanor or personality characteristics, or marked variations in ability and skill level. The younger the child, the less elaborated these alters are relative to the often extensive elaboration of separate "personality characteristics" seen in the alters of adult MPD patients. Kluft (1984, 1985a,b, 1986) has pointed out that children have relatively fewer resources through which alters can express separateness. In fact, children may be very subtle and resourceful in the ways their "alters" attempt to assert their separate identities, requiring close attention to detail on the part of the clinician.

A 9-year-old boy reported having three separate selves: a good, a bad, and a regular Larry. In the process of trying to understand whether or not these "selves" represented dissociative phenomenon, he was asked if it would be possible for others to identify which self he was at a given moment. He smiled slyly and said, "Yes, but they'd have to know how to." (What would they have to know?) "Well, the good Larry is all in white and is a good Larry fairy, and the bad Larry is in red like a devil. The regular Larry is just plain skin." (Well, which Larry is speaking now?) A broad smile: "Well, I'm the bad Larry, since you're asking about all the problems. I'm wearing a red shirt and you're wearing red too." Further interviewing made clear that this boy had MPD.

Children's alters similarly have less investment in the "separateness" of their identities, and there tend to be less rigid amnestic barriers between the different personality states. Despite these differences, all of the children who received a diagnosis of multiple personality disorder did meet full DSM-III-R criteria for the diagnosis.

None of the children in the inpatient series came with open revelations about "having different personalities." At most they complained of "hearing voices" or behaving in ways they "couldn't explain" or "couldn't remember." They were unanimous in their secretiveness and fear that talking about their subjective experiences of dissociative phenomenon made them "weirdos." They were fearful of what other children and adults would think of them if they knew about this, and in all cases one basis of the treatment alliance was their expectation that their therapist would help them have more control so that these phenomenon could be even more "private" than they were initially. There was relatively no observable secondary gain through "dramatics" or attention seeking for the disorder. In several of the children, observations of dissociative symptomatology were present for some time before a diagnosis of DID could be made. For two of the children, the diagnosis became apparent only on subsequent hospitalizations. This is in contrast to some cases seen in consultation in the private sector where aspects of the treatment the children were receiving seemed to "reinforce" dramatic displays of symptomatology. In these cases, diagnosis was complicated by a style of "treatment" that included an inordinate amount of suggestion and gratification for displays of "dissociative alter's behavior." In those cases it was only after a washout period of appropriate treatment that the child could be adequately evaluated.

There are ongoing questions about the role of development in the elaboration and organization of dissociative experience into alternate personalities during childhood. In the cases above where there was a time gap antedating the emergence of the DID diagnosis, retrospective accounts of the children argued in favor of the increasing trust in the therapeutic relationship, rather than developmental variables, playing a role in their eventual diagnosis. It is important to maintain a high index of suspicion in children with extensive abuse histories and the presence of some dissociative symptoms before DID is ruled out, especially when symptoms suggestive of other disorders do not respond to the usual treatment approaches. Some instances of DDNOS seem clinically to represent a traumatic dissociative disorganization that is so severe that no real sense of self has been able to emerge. These cases may initially present as reactive attachment disorders, atypical psychosis, or even autism. In several of these, the provision of a stable nurturing environment and treatment led the children to gradually organize a poorly integrated identity diagnosable then as DID prior to forming an integrated sense of self. Further research is needed on this group of children and on identifying subtypes of DDNOS.

CLINICAL PRESENTATION OF CHILDHOOD DISSOCIATIVE DISORDERS

All of the children with dissociative disorders in our sample, whether MPD or DDNOS, had a plethora of affective, anxiety, attention-concentration problems, and behavioral and learning difficulties that were suggestive of other diagnoses and frequently played a role in their presentation for psychiatric treatment (Hornstein & Putnam, 1992). Suicidal ideation was also frequently present in both groups, as were auditory hallucinations. The average child had received close to three psychiatric diagnoses prior to the diagnosis of a dissociative disorder. The most common prior diagnoses were major depression or depressive psychosis (45.3%), posttraumatic stress disorder (29.6%), oppositional defiant disorder (17%), conduct disorder (14%), and attention deficit hyperactivity disorder (12.5%).

The presenting symptoms of depression, suicidality, auditory hallucinations, and behavioral problems parallel symptom presentations reported for adult dissociative disorder patients (Bliss, 1984; Chu & Dill, 1990; Coons et al., 1988; Fink & Golinkoff, 1990; Greaves, 1980; Horevitz & Braun, 1984; Kluft, 1987a,b, 1991; Loewenstein, 1990; Putnam et al., 1986; Putnam, 1989; Ross et al., 1989, 1990, 1991; Schulz et al., 1989; Steinberg, 1991; Steinberg et al., 1990) and for previously reported individual child cases and small clinical series (Bowman et al., 1985; Dell & Eisenhower, 1990; Fagan & McMahon, 1984; Hornstein & Tyson, 1991; Hornstein & Putnam, 1992; Kluft, 1984, 1985a,b, 1986; Malenbaum & Russel, 1987; Peterson, 1990; Putnam, 1993; Riley & Mead, 1988; Vincent & Pickering, 1988; Weiss et al., 1985), supporting a common syndromal pattern of symptoms present in child, adolescent, and adult MPD cases. The children's dissociative symptoms were reviewed earlier in this chapter, so the manifestations of the most frequent symptoms other than dissociation will be discussed.

Affect

A majority of the children had symptoms such as irritability, affect lability, depression, hopeless feelings, low self-esteem, self-blame, and so on. Many had suicidal ideation and some had attempted suicide. The children with MPD differed in having made more serious suicide attempts. In observing these children over time, some had chronic dysphoria, which was typically unresponsive to antidepressant medication, but most had a very reactive mood. They were up when things were going well, but had an exquisite sensitivity to slights, frustrations, alterations in the mood-attentiveness of caregivers, and extreme rejection sensitivity. Following a perceived injury to their self-esteem, their mood would plummet, suicidal ideation might emerge, and they might remain dysphoric for days.

In some of the children, there were identifiable alternate personalities who were sad, hopeless, and full of self-blame for the abuse they had experienced. Environmental "triggers" that in some way reminded the children of their abuse frequently precipitated a "switch" into one of these alternate personalities. It was typical of these children that they held themselves responsible for abusive, neglectful behavior of others toward them and for other difficulties they experienced in relationships. Their feelings of hopelessness and worthlessness, while transitory, could nevertheless lead to quite serious suicide attempts such as running out in front of cars, or in the case of one young girl an attempt at self-electrocution via a knife in a light socket.

Anxiety–Posttraumatic Symptoms

All of these children could be described as "sick with worry"; often this related to realistic or at worst understandable concerns about the stability of their relationships, the endurance of the regard in which others held them, the well-being of their caregivers, and their own adequacy. Most had all the classic posttraumatic stress disorder symptoms of hypervigilance, hyperstartle, fears, flashbacks, avoidant behaviors, intrusive thoughts related to traumatic experiences, and traumatic nightmares.

The hours before bedtime were associated for many of the children with the emergence of intrusive thoughts about abuse that frequently occurred at home during these hours and were often a period in which dissociative symptoms such as spontaneous age regressions, amnesias, "switches" in personality, and so forth occurred. For other children, use of the bathroom facilities brought on sudden reactions of terror, flashbacks, or dissociative phenomenon as well. An 11-year-old boy with MPD first showed signs of dissociation when he was discovered huddled in a corner of the bathroom, disoriented to location and the identity of a familiar caregiver. Later, it was discovered that this child had been repeatedly and violently sodomized, continued to experience pain with bowel movements related to his injuries, and had severe flashbacks whenever he attempted to use the toilet.

Conduct–Behavioral Problems

Many of these children had explosive temper outbursts, oppositional or disruptive behavior, and problems with aggression and fighting. Although often accused of lying, they frequently had at least partial amnesia for their explosive, aggressive, and disruptive behaviors. These behaviors were often sudden, unpredicted, and out of keeping with the child's usual demeanor. Absent from these cases was the triad of enuresis, cruelty to animals, and fire-setting.

The child's frequent misperceptions of interactions, perceived threats, as well as rejection hypersensitivity played a role in producing these problems. Often these abrupt behavior changes were preceded by a switch in personality in those children with MPD. The children with DDNOS had similar alterations in perception and cognition during their explosions, although they retained conscious recall and some ability to integrate these behaviors.

These kinds of behavior problems were frequently the reason for referral to inpatient treatment. Usually, when the dissociative aspect of the child's explosions was recognized, the child could be assisted to gain better control of these behaviors. Caregivers who were made aware of the kinds of perceptual and cognitive distortions that occurred when these children entered a state of defensive upset were also more effective at providing appropriate reassurance to these children, preventing the familiar eruption into aggressive behavior.

The conflicts around autonomy, identity, separation, and individuation that are focal during adolescence make work with adolescent patients with dissociative disorders particularly challenging in terms of managing acting-out behavior, even though their presentation was otherwise similar to that of adult patients.

Sexualized Play, Inappropriate Sexual Behavior

Compulsive masturbation and promiscuity are frequent and 15% of the children, including some very young children, had perpetrated sexual assaults or abuse on other children. Most of the children were troubled by a variety of issues related to sexuality and their sexual identity. For some, sexual acting out was a way of compulsively reenacting their own experiences, and for others it served as a reassurance that "they were normal," allaying fears of homosexuality in boys who were molested by male perpetrators, or attempting to affirm their attractiveness and control over relationships. For a few, there was sexual excitement in the victimization of others, and many were vulnerable to revictimization by adults or other children.

Attention–Concentration, Learning Problems

These children's high level of anxiety, posttraumatic symptoms, and their dissociative trance states, amnesias, and so forth frequently manifested themselves through difficulty attending to lessons and concentrating on school work. In some children there were significant auditory processing difficulties, learning problems, or difficulty with reading. Again, those children who have been followed through their course of treatment have had remarkable amelioration of these difficulties as their internal disruption has decreased. This is all the more surprising given the past history of intrauterine exposure to alcohol and/or drugs and past head trauma to which some of these children were exposed. Comorbid diagnoses are, of course, possible, but even when assumed present and treated as such, the better part of clinical wisdom is served through reevaluation as treatment progresses.

Dissociative episodes in childhood may be evident at times as perplexing variations in the child's knowledge, skill level, and performance. Different alters may have differing abilities and knowledge, or may have no conscious recall of having learned something when another alter is present. Marked variations on psychological tests assessing similar abilities may be seen, or there can be enormous variations on the same test on different days as the child experiences switches in personality.

The most striking example of this was a young girl who had evidence of nerve deafness on two subsequent but different examinations, but in different ears. Neurologically, her hearing was perfectly intact in both ears, but when she dissociated she had two different alters, each experiencing deafness in opposite ears; the deafness was a conversion symptom related to two separate traumatic incidents.

Hallucinations–Thought Process Disturbances

Auditory hallucinations were present in most of the dissociative children. In the majority of cases the child heard a voice or voices experienced as arising internally and having distinctive characteristics such as age, gender, and personal attributes, e.g., the voice of my father telling me I'm no good. These are similar to descriptions by adults with MPD of their auditory hallucinations. Other types of hallucinations were also experienced, such as seeing "ghosts," having visual hallucinations of alters, and less commonly a variety of somatic and tactile hallucinations, often representing hallucinated reexperiences of a somatic or sensory element of dissociated traumas.

Frequent dissociation can cause a child to appear confused or disorganized at times and tends to occur in stressful or emotion-laden situations. Apparent tangentiality can be the efforts of the patient experiencing time gaps to cover up his or her symptoms. Many of the children routinely confabulated to cover up memory gaps, both to others and themselves. None of the children had a persistent thought disorder, as frequent dissociation responded to safety, structure, and treatment. Dissociative experiences of having thoughts removed or put into the mind were present in some children with MPD, representing a statistically nonsignificant trend. These experiences are commonly reported by adult MPD patients, in addition to those with schizophrenic and bipolar illnesses (Fink & Golinkoff, 1990; Kluft, 1987a; Ross et al., 1990). Passive influence experiences, e.g., made thoughts and feelings, complex bodily movements not felt to be voluntarily initiated, automatic writing, and so forth are also commonly reported in adult MPD patients (Fink & Golinkoff, 1990; Kluft, 1987a; Ross et al., 1990). In child MPD cases, the experience of involuntarily initiated body movements distinguished them from children with DDNOS. An example of a child's description of this type of dissociative phenomenon is present in the section on identifying dissociative symptoms in children.

A number of clinical variables assist the clinician to differentiate between childhood dissociation and childhood schizophrenia; of note, however, much lower rates of control and influence experiences are reported in schizophrenic children compared to those with MPD, along with much higher rates of delusional phenomenon (Russel et al., 1989).

Overall Clinical Picture

Children with dissociative disorders have a complicated symptomatic picture related to the interaction between their use of dissociative defenses, the symptoms from past traumatic experiences, and the problems they experience in regulating their affect and behavior, as well as establishing a coherent experience of self and others.

DIFFERENTIAL DIAGNOSIS

The complex symptomatic picture phenomenologically associated with dissociative disorders in children often suggests or mimics more commonly diagnosed childhood psychiatric disorders. Table 1 briefly describes symptoms frequently found in dissociating children that may superficially appear to represent other diagnoses (Hornstein & Tyson, 1991).

The presence of a dissociative disorder is no protection against seizures, developmental learning disorders, or other diagnoses. The most important initial diagnostic step is often, nevertheless, the recognition of dissociative symptoms. A trial of treatment for dissociative disorder frequently leads to reduction or resolution of "seizures" in the presence of a normal electroencelphologram, affective, attentional, thought-disordered, and learning disability symptoms.

CHILDHOOD TRAUMA AND DISSOCIATION

Other chapters in this volume will no doubt adumbrate the relationship between childhood trauma and dissociative disorders in the adult dissociative disorder and trauma literatures. In our series (Hornstein & Putnam, 1992), an overwhelming majority of the children had experienced some identifiable trauma. In those with MPD, over 80% had documented histories of sexual abuse and in 60% of the cases this was combined with physical abuse as well. Documentation of neglect was

Table 1. **Dissociative Symptoms Mistakenly Attributed to Other Diagnoses**

Dissociative symptom	Behavioral appearance	Misdiagnosis
Brief amnestic periods	"Trancelike," odd behavior, explosive outbursts	Absence/psychomotor seizures
	Poor attention, concentration, hyperarousal	Attention deficit with hyperactivity
	Disavowal of witnessed behavior	Conduct disorder
Switching between alternate personalities	Aggressive alters, running away, truancy	Conduct disorder
	Alters differ in task performance, academic achievement, other skills	Developmental learning disorder
Affect disturbances	Different alters may have different moods, depressed-suicidal and excited alters not uncommon. Symptoms of posttraumatic stress disorder, including problems sleeping related to hyperarousal/nightmares common	Affective disorder
Thought process disturbances	Alters experienced as hallucinated voices; visual hallucinations of past trauma; alters, partial control by alter similar to passive influence. Rapid switching causes discontinuity in stream of thought.	Psychotic illness
Somatoform symptoms	Headaches commonly accompany switching.	Somatoform disorders Tic disorders
	Parasthesias, somatic hallucinations, conversion symptoms, odd movements, etc.	
Anxiety Posttraumatic stress disorder	A high level of anxiety or accompanying posttraumatic stress disorder is common in dissociating children.	Primary anxiety disorder

available in 80% of the cases. The percentages were only slightly lower in those cases with DDNOS. Additionally, over 70% of the children witnessed family violence.

The high percentage of documented abuse, neglect, witnessed violence, and other trauma in this large clinical series of children with dissociative disorders provides validation for the already-existing literature linking traumatic, and particularly abusive, experiences in early childhood with the development of dissociative disorders (Bowman et al., 1985; Braun & Sachs, 1985; Braun, 1990; Chu & Dill, 1990; Coons et al., 1988; Ensink, 1992; Fraiberg, 1982; Greaves, 1980; Hornstein & Tyson, 1991; Hornstein & Putnam, 1992, 1994; Kluft, 1984, 1985a,b, 1986, 1987a,b, 1991; Kramer, 1990; Loewenstein, 1990; Lovinger, 1983; Ludwig, 1983; Putnam et al., 1986; Putnam, 1985, 1989, 1990; Rao, DiClemente, & Ponton, 1992; Rao, Hornstein, & Stuber, 1994; Ross et al., 1991; Schetky, 1990; Shengold, 1989; Sherkow, 1990; Spiegel, 1990, 1991; Stein et al., 1988; Stern, 1984; van der Kolk & Kadish, 1987; Venn, 1984). It also weighs the "fact versus fantasy" debate regarding the validity of adult recollections of childhood abusive experiences in patients with dissociative disorders toward acceptance of there being some basis in reality for their reports, however the passage of time may have altered, coalesced, or elaborated on the representation of "vertical truth" in contemporary memory of past subjective experiences.

TREATMENT CONSIDERATIONS

What statistics and phenomenological descriptions cannot capture is the big picture of how early in life many of these children (especially those with DID) experienced neglect and abuse, the extent, severity, and chronicity of their trauma, the chaotic and/or sadomasochistic nature of the relationships with caregivers that was a reality for them, and the psychological impact of this past on their ongoing experience of self and self with other. These children's clinical presentation becomes clearer when grasped in light of the children's efforts to adapt to, survive in, and relate to a world populated by unpredictable significant others and replete with traumatic experiences. These children could never rely on having basic needs for nurture and protection met, and many experienced overt abandonment in addition to combinations of physical, sexual, and emotional abuse, domestic violence, exploitation, and sadism. The extent of the abuse, it's age of onset, the degree of neglect, and the presence or absence of some stable adult relationship figure prominently in the degree of psychological disturbance each individual child has, as do the child's strengths, intellect, creativity, and disposition.

The child may have initially used dissociation to manage an overwhelming trauma. With repeated trauma and neglect in the early years, it is not only the specific traumas that are psychologically overwhelming. Many aspects of relationships become highly conflictual, dependency needs are in and of themselves overwhelming in this milieu, and affects become sources of danger and conflict. The child's internalization of these highly conflictual experiences produces within the child conflicts with aspects of their own identity. To integrate these conflicting identifications, with their associated affects and traumatic memories, would cause overwhelming anxiety. As a result, the child dissociates.

An aspect of the usual DID child's adaptation is the organization of the dissociated selves or alters around the extremes of response that must be readily available to allow continued development in the face of repeated traumas. Fantasy assists the child in coping with overwhelming realities. Often each alter has a different fantasied representation of the child and the characteristics of the caregiver. With an environment that demands constant vigilance and self-protective responses, there is little time to focus on the development of internal regulation of affect and behavior. An excellent adaptation to a world of repeated trauma becomes a handicap when called upon to develop trusting, intimate relationships, focus on learning in school, or behave in a predictable, consistent manner. The longing to trust in the caring response of another, to develop true intimacy, is at odds with the terror that past trauma may be repeated.

The role of the therapist is to assist these children's development of increasing capacities for trust and intimacy, build internal capabilities for managing affect and behavior, develop defenses that aid in resolution of internal conflicts and past traumatic experiences without being overwhelmed, and finally to integrate the dissociated aspects of his or her personality. The treatment of childhood dissociative disorders can be conceptualized as involving six tasks. These tasks are not discrete, but to some extent they assume relative temporal predominance. They are (1) the establishment of a safe, nurturing environment; (2) the formation of a therapeutic alliance; (3) the improvement of overall ego functioning and containment of disruptive-destructive behaviors; (4) a systematic uncovering of dissociated aspects of identity, broadening the scope of tolerable affect, increasing the range of coping strategies, decreasing dissociative barriers, abreaction and working through of traumatic memories and conflict laden issues; (5) integration of alters; and (6) Postintegration therapy and follow-up at regular intervals through adolescence.

Prognosis depends on the establishment, first and foremost, of a nontraumatic environment for the child, and the ability of the child and therapist to develop a working therapeutic relationship. Ensuring a safe, nontraumatic, nurturing environment can be daunting in an age of decreasing social and mental health services. Without this, however, treatment can only be palliative; an attempt to remove the child's dissociative defenses is destructive and likely to fail. A number of refractory treatments, on closer inspection, failed to address this issue adequately (Hornstein & Tyson, 1991). What about the child who has a loving and stable foster family who lives in the heart of gang warfare in the inner city? What about the child whose needs for food, clothing, and shelter are met in an institution that provides little nurture? The therapist of the MPD child must be willing to roll up his sleeves and attempt to address these issues realistically. Creative partial solutions can be beneficial.

The degree of overall psychiatric disturbance in the child, his or her age, past experiences, strengths, and support systems become factors that influence the child's ability to develop a working therapeutic alliance and how quickly the therapy proceeds. Reports of individual and small case series have been optimistic about the rapidity to which childhood MPD can respond to treatment (Kluft, 1985a,b, 1986, 1987a; Riley & Mead, 1988; Vincent & Pickering, 1988; Weiss et al., 1985). Making the correct diagnosis is helpful for designing interventions that bring about improvements in the child's functioning. The child experiences unintegrated aspects of themself as separate, alien, difficult to understand, or completely abhorrent. This is true even when the dissociation is incomplete and the child retains some awareness of these feelings and behaviors. Accepting the child's subjective experience enhances the therapeutic alliance. It is important to treat dissociative experiences in an empathic and matter-of-fact fashion, getting to know the child's subjective and/or dissociated experiences of themselves, us, and their "world." If the child has ways of subjectively identifying dissociated aspects of self as separate, it is helpful to know these and respond to preferences of the child's regarding communication with these alters. Understanding the child's inner experience and the importance it holds alleviates much of the anxiety that previously undiagnosed children with DID have. They seem to feel, "If you can understand and accept this, then perhaps so can I," and their ability to grasp that alternate personalities are actually parts of themselves rather than "someone else" is thus enhanced. One must assume that an aspect of a child's need to dissociate is a conviction that some feelings and/or behaviors are unacceptable and will lead to rejection or abuse. Seemingly paradoxically, willingness to accept these alters in a matter-of-fact fashion actually decreases the child's pressure to use dissociative defenses in the presence of a focus on establishing age-appropriate behavioral functioning. It is important that the therapist, family, and others in contact with the child avoid the voyeuristic fascination that can accompany an introduction to DID. Being overly enthusiastic about meeting all the alters, "getting them to switch," and so forth can be exploitative and also can provide a secondary reinforcement of the illness where the child feels his/her value depends on their interest to the psychiatric community.

Effective therapeutic intervention often includes the development of individualized, psychodynamically informed, behavioral interventions that the family and school use to assist the child maintain function when threatened. Therapeutic interventions, which may or may not include dynamic interpretations, should be judged by their ability to produce lasting effects on the child's behavior and ability to have relationships. If an intervention is unsuccessful, assume the problem is with the intervention, not the child: Reexamine the understanding and design of the intervention. The goal of early interventions is to help the child to effectively meet conflicting needs in relationships while maintaining age-appropriate functioning and remaining as free as possible of dissociative episodes. For the child with DID, this requires creating an awareness and understanding in the child of the presence of dissociative experiences and working to alleviate undermining conflicts.

The child is often taught new coping strategies and ways of gaining attention and other forms of positive reinforcement for more functional behaviors. A focus on positive reinforcement that seeks to avoid punitive consequences for problematic behaviors is most effective behaviorally with traumatized children. Limits should be set on destructive behaviors through redirection or brief time-outs. The use of seclusion or physical restraint should be limited to situations where this is absolutely necessary to contain behaviors that would be physically damaging to the child or others. Care should be taken so that the use of these measures is neither punitive nor inadvertently reinforcing. Specific interventions that are particularly useful for children with DID include continual reassurance of physical safety. Often dissociative episodes are triggered by fear, resulting in the emergence of aggressive alters. Reassurance of safety decreases the frequency of this kind of switching. Misinterpretation of their physical and social environment is also common in these children. They often require verbal assistance in order to clarify misconceptions and decrease dissociative episodes.

Children can be taught to explore feelings and thoughts in the safety of the therapy session, where a variety of relaxation techniques and careful pacing may be used to provide "containment" of anxiety and affect during, at the close of, and between sessions. The child is helped to achieve a sense of mastery over his/her dissociation and switching by identifying the thoughts and feelings that occur at those times. Dissociative barriers are decreased by encouraging the child to tolerate and explore feelings and thoughts that are present in dissociated parts of himself. Additionally, children are encouraged and reinforced for learning to call on previously dissociated aspects of self to help them in difficult situations. For example, the child is encouraged to see if there is "someone inside" who can help to soothe when she or he is upset or aggressive. Integration of this soothing capacity into the child's developing self-definition follows over time. When indicated, it helps to speak to all the alters collectively. Particularly when there is a need to deescalate aggressive or nonverbal alters. Acknowledgment of the alters as a collective encourages cooperation, decreases dissociative barriers, and helps set the stage for ultimate integration.

In the event of assaultive or destructive behaviors, especially at home or in school, a consequence (time-out, etc.) should be required regardless of whether the alter that "acted like that" is still present. After the consequence the child may be told, "You are all responsible for what happens. Maybe there are some ways that you can all help each other with feelings so that none of you have to take a time-out." When emergent feelings and/or traumatic memories have created difficulties in the child's ability to function, intervention is focused on restoring functional behavior so the child can resume age-appropriate activity as soon as possible.

All of the child's alters must be validated and their individual and collective strengths identified and discussed with the child. They should be viewed as equally desirable and important and allowed to exist without criticism. This helps the child to achieve greater acceptance of the alters as valuable aspects of himself, which are to be integrated rather than disavowed. These interventions help the child attain an improved ability to function in all settings, increased self-acceptance, and an awareness of his/her use of dissociative defenses. The child's growing capacity to tolerate a variety of feelings, memories, and experiences results in a diminution of the need to dissociate, as well as increased mastery over his/her behavior.

In cases where there is a favorable, nurturing environment, resources for intensive treatment, and a child with considerable resiliency and capacity for developing intimacy despite having a severe dissociative disorder, treatment can indeed be rapid and successful. Integration generally is the natural outcome of a decreased need for dissociative defenses as treatment resolves traumatically induced conflicts and improves ego functioning. Often, there is some anxiety about "losing the ability to dissociate" that emerges as integration begins. Active discussion of the changes taking place, reinforcement of emerging strengths, and encouragement to proceed help at this time, as does an openness to creative understandings the child develops in order to cognitively master these occurrences and provide self-reassurance.

Many cases do not fit this hopeful picture, however. In them, there has been some success, but measured in small increments over greater lengths of time (Hornstein & Putnam, 1994). In all children who have had a dissociative disorder, follow-up at intervals after integration is essential, even after postintegration therapy has ensured stabilization. We do not know the impact of developmental challenges and future traumas on these children, and inevitably they encounter some conflict that threatens their new integration when their continuing development brings about the need to achieve new levels of mastery in areas of previous conflict—such as the emergence of sexuality, separation-individuation, independence, and intimacy in love—relationships through adolescence into young adulthood.

There is a need for further research on treatment outcomes, prognostic indicators, which approaches work best with which children, and so forth. An effective therapeutic approach relies on the bedrock of dynamically oriented therapy, supplemented with an understanding of dissociative processes that allows for limited hypnotic interventions that help the child contain overwhelming affects and memories, occasional cognitive and behavioral interventions, family work, and intervention with the school when necessary. A more extensive review of treatment approaches would require it's own chapter, but the skills of most experienced child therapists do nicely with some added supervision by someone familiar with childhood dissociative disorders. There is also a need for longitudinal follow-up of childhood dissociative cases to ascertain course and outcome, the stability of integration as the child enters adolescence and adulthood, and their vulnerability to new traumas.

REFERENCES

Albini, T. K., & Pease, T. E. (1989). Normal and pathological dissociations of early childhood. *Dissociation, 2*, 14?-150.

American Psychiatric Association. (1987). *Diagnostic and statistical manual of mental disorders* (3rd ed., rev.). Washington, DC: Author.

American Psychiatric Association. (1994). *Diagnostic and statistical manual of mental disorders* (4th ed.). Washington, DC: Author.

Armstrong, J., Putnam, F., & Carlson, E. (1994). Adolescent Dissociative Experiences Scale. *Dissociation*,

Barach, P. M. (1991). Multiple personality disorder as an attachment disorder. *Dissociation, 3*, 117-123.

Bernstein, E. L., & Putnam, F. W. (0000) Development, reliability, and validity of the dissociation scale. *Journal of Nervous and Mental Disease, 174*, 727-735.

Bliss, E. (1984). A symptom profile of patient with multiple personalities, including MMPI results. *Journal of Nervous and Mental Disease, 174*, 197-202.

Bowman, E. S. (1990). Adolescent multiple personality disorder in the nineteenth and early twentieth century. *Dissociation, 3*, 179-187.

Bowman, E. S., Blix, S., & Coons, P. M. (1985). Multiple personality in adolescence: Relationship to incestual experiences. *Journal of American Academy of Child Adolescent Psychiatry, 24*, 109-114.

Braun, B. G. (1990). Dissociative disorders as a sequelae to incest. In R. P. Kluft (Ed.), *Incest-related syndromes of adult psychopathology* (pp. 227-252). Washington, DC: American Psychiatric Press.

Braun, B. G., & Sachs, R. G. (1985). The development of multiple personality disorder: Predisposing, precipitating, and perpetuating factors. In R. P. Kluft (Ed.), *Childhood antecedents of multiple personality* (pp. 37-64). Washington, DC: American Psychiatric Press.

Brierre, J., & Runtz, M. (1988). Post sexual abuse trauma. In G. E. Wyatt & G. J. Powell (Eds.), *Lasting effects of child sexual abuse* (pp. 85-99). Newbury Park, CA: Sage.

Chu, J. A., & Dill, D. L. (1990). Dissociative symptoms in relation to childhood physical and sexual abuse. *American Journal of Psychiatry, 147*, 887-892.

Conte, J. R., & Schuerman, J. R. (1988). The effects of sexual abuse on children: A multidimensional view. In G. E. Wyatt & G. J. Powell (Eds.), *Lasting effects of child sexual abuse* (pp. 135-154). Newbury Park, CA: Sage.

Coons, P., Bowman, E., & Milstein, V. (1988). Multiple personality disorder: A clinical investigation of 50 cases. *Journal of Nervous and Mental Disease, 176*, 519-527.

Coons, P. M., Cole, C., Pellow, T. A., & Milstein, V. (1990). Symptoms of posttraumatic stress and dissociation in women victims of abuse. In R. P. Kluft (Ed.), *Incest-related syndromes of adult psychopathology* (pp. 205-226). Washington, DC: American Psychiatric Press.

Dell, P. F., & Eisenhower, J. W. (1990). Adolescent multiple personality disorder. *Journal of the American Academy of Child Adolescent Psychiatry, 29*, 359-366.

Donovan, D. M., & McIntyre, D. (1990). *Healing the hurt child*. New York: Norton.

Ensink, B. J. (1992). *Confusing realities: A study on child sexual abuse and psychiatric syndromes*. Amsterdam, Netherlands: VU University Press.

Fagan, J., & McMahon, P. P. (1984). Incipient multiple personality in children: Four cases. *Journal of Nervous and Mental Disease, 172*, 26-36.

Famularo, R., Kinscherff, R., & Fenton, T. (1992). Psychiatric diagnoses of maltreated children: Preliminary findings. *Journal of the American Academy of Child Adolescent Psychiatry, 31*, 863-867.

Fine, C. G. (1988). The work of Antoine Despine: The first scientific report on the diagnosis and treatment of a child with multiple personality disorder. *American Journal of Clinical Hypnosis, 32*, 33-39.

Fink, D., & Golinkoff, M. (1990). Multiple personality disorder, borderline personality disorder and schizophrenia: A comparative study of clinical features. *Dissociation, 3*, 127-134.

Fink, D. L. (1988). The core self: A developmental perspective on the dissociative disorders. *Dissociation, 1*, 43-47.

Fraiberg, S. (1982). Pathological defenses in infancy. *Psychoanalytic Quarterly, 51*, 612-635.

Goodwin, J. M. (1990). Applying to adult incest victims what we have learned from victimized children. In R. P. Kluft (Ed.), *Incest related syndromes of adult psychopathology* (pp. 55-74). Washington, DC: American Psychiatric Press.

Greaves, G. B. (1980). Multiple personality: 165 years after Mary Reynolds. *Journal of Nervous and Mental Disease, 168*, 557-596.

Horevitz, R. P., & Braun, B. G. (1984). Are multiple personalities borderline? *Psychiatric Clinics of North America, 7*, 69-88.

Hornstein, N. L., & Putnam, F. W. (1992). Clinical phenomenology of child and adolescent dissociative disorders. *Journal of American Academy of Child Adolescent Psychiatry, 31*, 1077-1085.

Hornstein, N. L., & Putnam, F. W. (1994). Abuse and the development of dissociative symptoms and multiple personality disorder. In C. Pfeffer (Ed.), *Intense stress and mental disturbance in children* (pp. 000-000). Washington, DC: American Psychiatric Press.

Hornstein, N. L., & Tyson, S. (1991). Inpatient treatment of children with multiple personality/dissociative disorders and their families. *Psychiatric Clinics of North America, 14*, 631-638.

Kluft, R. P. (1984). Multiple personality in childhood. *Psychiatric Clinics of North America, 7*, 121-134.

Kluft, R. P. (1985a). Childhood multiple personality disorder: Predictors, clinical findings, and treatment results. In R. P. Kluft (Ed.), *Childhood antecedents of multiple personality* (pp. 167-196). Washington, DC: American Psychiatric Press.

Kluft, R. P. (1985b). Hypnoptherapy of childhood multiple personality disorder. *American Journal of Clinical Hypnosis, 27*, 201-210.

Kluft, R. P. (1986). Treating children who have multiple personality disorder. In B. G. Braun (Ed.), *Treatment of multiple personality disorder* (pp. 81-105). Washington, DC: American Psychiatric Press.

Kluft, R. P. (1987a). First-rank symptoms as a diagnostic clue to multiple personality disorder. *American Journal of Psychiatry, 144*, 293-298.

Kluft, R. P. (1987b). An update on multiple personality disorder. *Hospital Community of Psychiatry, 144*, 293-298.

Kluft, R. P. (1991). Clinical presentations of multiple personality disorder. *Psychiatric Clinics of North America, 14*, 605-630.

Kramer, S. (1990). Residues of incest. In H. B. Levine (Ed.), *Adult analysis and childhood sexual abuse* (pp. 149-170). Hillsdale, NJ: Analytic Press.

Loewenstein, R. J. (1990). Somatoform disorders in victims of incest and child abuse. In R. P. Kluft (Ed.), *Incest related syndromes of adult psychopathology* (pp. 75-111). Washington, DC: American Psychiatric Press.

Lovinger, S. L. (1983). Multiple personality: A theoretical view. *Psychotherapy: Theory, Research and Practice, 20*, 425-434.

Ludwig, A. M. (1983). The psychological functions of dissociation. *American Journal of Clinical Hypnosis, 26*, 93-99.

Malenbaum, R., & Russel, A. J. (1987). Multiple personality disorder in an 11-year-old boy and his mother. *Journal of American Academy of Children's Adolesent Psychiatry, 26*, 436-439.

McLeer, S. V., Deblinger, E., Henry, D., Orvaschel, H. (1992). Sexually abused children at high risk for post-traumatic stress disorder. *Journal of American Academy of Children's Adolescent Psychiatry, 31*, 875-879.

Peterson, G. (1990). Diagnosis of childhood multiple personality. *Dissociation, 3*, 3-9.

Putnam, F., Guroff, J., Silberman, E., Barban, L., & Post, R. (1986). The clinical phenomenology of multiple personality disorder: Review of 100 recent cases. *Journal of Clinical Psychiatry, 47*, 285-293.

Putnam, F. W. (1985). Dissociation as a response to extreme trauma. In R. P. Kluft (Ed.), *Childhood antecedents of multiple personality* (pp. 66-97). Washington, DC: American Psychiatric Press.

Putnam, F. W. (1989). *Diagnosis and treatment of multiple personality disorder*. New York: Guilford Press.

Putnam, F. W. (1990). Disturbances of "self" in victims of childhood sexual abuse. In R. P. Kluft (Ed.), *Incest related syndromes of adult psychopathology* (pp. 000-000). Washington DC: American Psychiatric Press.

Putnam, F. W. (1991). Dissociative disorders in children and adolescents: A developmental perspective. *Psychiatric Clinics of North America, 14*, 519-531.

Putnam, F. W. (1993). Dissociative disorders in children: Behavioral profiles and problems. *Child Abuse and Neglect, 17*, 39-45.

Rao, K. DiClemente, R. J., & Ponton, L. E. (1992). Child sexual abuse of Asians compared with other populations. *Journal of American Academy of Child Adolescent Psychiatry, 341*, 880-886.

Rao, K., Hornstein, N. L., & Stuber, M. (1994). Dissociative symptoms in child and adolescent cancer survivors. Unpublished data.

Riley, R. L., & Mead, J. (1988). The development of symptoms of multiple personality in a child of three. *Dissociation, 1*, 41-46.

Ross, C. A., Norton, G. R., & Wozney, K. (1989). Multiple personality disorder: An analysis of 236 cases. *Canadian Journal of Psychiatry, 34*, 413-418.

Ross, C. A., Miller, S. D., Bjornson, L., Reagor, P., Fraser, G. A., & Anderson, G. (1990). Structured interview data on 102 casees of multiple personality disorder from four centers. *American Journal of Psychiatry, 147*, 596-601.

Ross, C. A., Miller, S. D., Bjornson, L., Reagor, P., Fraser, G. A., & Anderson, G. (1991). Abuse histories in 102 cases of multiple personality disorder. *Canadian Journal of Psychiatry, 36*, 97-101.

Russel, A. T., Bott, L., & Sammons, C. (1989). Phenomenology of schizophrenia occurring in childhood. *Journal of the American Academy of Child Adolescent Psychiatry, 23*, 399-407.

Schetky, D. H. (1990). A review of the literature on long-term effects of childhood sexual abuse. In R. P. Kluft (Ed.), *Incest related syndromes of adult psychopathology* (pp. 35-54). Washington, DC: American Psychiatric Press.

Schulz, R., Braun, B. G., & Kluft, R. P. (1989). Multiple personality disorder: Phenomenology of selected variables in comparison to major depression. *Dissociation, 2*, 45-51.

Shengold, L. (1989). *Soul murder*. New Haven, CT: Yale University Press.

Sherkow, S. P. (1990). Consequences of childhood sexual abuse on the development of ego structure: A comparison of child and adult cases. In H. B. Levine (Ed.), *Adult Analysis and Childhood Sexual Abuse* (pp. 93-115). Hillsdale, NJ: The Analytic Press.

Spiegel, D. (1990). Trauma, dissociation and hypnosis. In R. P. Kluft (Ed.), *Incest related syndromes of adult psychopathology* (pp. 247-261). Washington, DC: American Psychiatric Press.

Spiegel, D. (1991). Dissociation and trauma. In A. Tasman & S. M. Goldfinger (Eds.), *American psychiatric press review of psychiatry* (pp. 261-275). Washington, DC: American Psychiatric Press.

Stein, J. A., Goldring, J. M., Siegel, J. M., Burman, A., & Sorenson, S. B. (1988). Long-term psychological sequelae of child sexual abuse: The Los Angeles epidemiologic catchment area study. In G. E. Wyatt & G. J. Powell (Eds.), *Lasting effects of child sexual abuse* (pp. 135-154). Newbury Park, CA: Sage.

Steinberg, M. (1991). The spectrum of depersonalization: Assessment and treatment. In A. Tasman & S. M. Goldfinger (Eds.), *American psychiatric press review of psychiatry*. Washington, DC: American Psychiatric Press.

Steinberg, M., Rounsaville, B., & Cicchetti, V. (1990). The structured clinical interview for DSM-III-R dissociative disorders: Preliminary report on a new diagnostic instrument. *American Journal of Psychiatry, 147*, 76-81.

Stern, C. R. (1984). The etiology of multiple personality. *Psychiatric Clinics of North America*, 7, 149-160.

Terr, L. (1990). *Too scared to cry*. New York: Harper & Row.

van der Kolk, B., & Kadish, W. (1987). Amnesia, dissociation, and the return of the repressed. In B. A. van der Kolk (Ed.), *Psychological trauma* (pp. 173-190). Washington, DC: American Psychiatric Press.

Venn, J. (1984). Family etiology and remission in a case of psychogenic fugue. *Family Process, 23*, 429-435.

Vincent, M., & Pickering, M. R. (1988). Multiple personality disorder in childhood. *Canadian Journal of Psychiatry, 33*, 524-529.

Weiss, M. Sutton, P. J., & Utecht, A. J. (1985). Multiple personality in a 10-year-old girl. *Journal of the American Academy of Child Adolescent Psychiatry, 24*, 495-501.

III
THEORETICAL MODELS

Although there exist a plethora of models and metaphors that have been applied to dissociative phenomena, our understanding of the theoretical processes involved is still at an initial stage. In this section, three important perspectives are presented to help clarify the construct of dissociation. First, dissociation is examined from a neurobiological perspective; second, dissociation is discussed in terms of hypnosis; and third, dissociation is discussed in terms of an information-processing perspective.

In examining dissociation from a neurobiological perspective, Krystal and his colleagues make an important contribution, since this area has not received extensive development. The researchers initially review pharmacological methods of inducing dissociative-like conditions in both patients and healthy individuals and then move on to cortical areas such as the frontal cortex and limbic structures involved in various aspects of dissociative processes. Chapter 8 concludes with an examination of therapeutic implications. Although not directly, this chapters offers some insights as to the classification of PTSD, which is currently described by DSM-IV as an anxiety disorder, and its relationship to dissociative disorders.

Given that historically dissociation and hypnosis have been described in similar ways, the chapter by Whalen and Nash helps to delineate the relationship between the two constructs. First, it is clear that under hypnosis, individuals can display dissociative-like processes such as alternations in perception, sensation, emotion, and cognition. Second, hypnosis has been used successfully to treat dissociative disorders. Third, subjective experiences described within the hypnotic state such as "feeling unreal" or "things happening automatically" appear similar to descriptions of dissociative experiences. And fourth, in the clinical literature there has been an implicit connection between sexual trauma, dissociation, and hypnosis since the nineteenth century. In fact, Janet saw dissociation as underlying both psychopathology and real hypnotic processes. However, the research reviewed in this chapter leads one to the conclusion that as an individual trait, there is little if any overlap between hypnotic susceptibility and dissociative experiences. Further, although there is evidence to suggest that early trauma leads to dissociative experiences, the empirical evidence does not lead one to the same conclusion with trauma and hypnotic susceptibility. An open research question remains as to whether hypnosis, as useful as it is, carries a special relationship for the treatment of dissociative disorders over and above other forms of therapy.

Based on their work with trauma victims, Foa and Hearst-Ikeda examine the construct of dissociation from an information processing perspective. Chapter 10 begins by differentiating the construct of dissociation into various aspects and examines its relationship to stress and trauma. For example, based on the animal literature, it is suggested that avoidance and numbing involve different mechanisms. These differentiations are then considered in terms of abuse, assault, and trauma victims and implications for treatment. If dissociation prevents the activation of a traumatic memory, then successful treatment would require techniques such as exposure therapy, which would repeatedly access the traumatic memory.

8

Recent Developments in the Neurobiology of Dissociation

Implications for Posttraumatic Stress Disorder

John H. Krystal, Alexandre Bennett, J. Douglas Bremner, Steven M. Southwick, and Dennis S. Charney

There is a growing recognition by researchers and clinicians that dissociative states are an integral component of traumatic stress response. The term *dissociation* has been employed to describe a spectrum of subjective experiences in which perceptual, affective, memory, and identity functions are altered. Particular symptoms or syndromes associated with dissociative states include distorted sensory perceptions, altered time perception, amnesia, derealization, depersonalization, conversion symptoms, fugue states, and multiple personality (Freud & Breuer, 1953; Mayer-Gross, 1935; Hilgard, 1977; Spiegel & Cardeña 1991; Bremner et al., 1992). Despite the broad array of symptoms associated with dissociative states in posttraumatic stress disorder (PTSD), some recent data suggest that these symptoms may be expressed across individuals as a single symptom cluster, rather than as independent clusters of symptoms (Bremner et al., in review).

There is now ample documentation that dissociation occurs at the time of traumatization, particularly in those individuals who progress to develop PTSD (Janet, 1889; Fischer, 1945; Krystal, 1968, 1988; Spiegel & Cardeña 1991; Carlson & Rosser-Hogan 1991; Bremner et al., 1992, 1993). Dissociative states and increased

John H. Krystal, Alexandre Bennett, J. Douglas Bremner, Steven M. Southwick, and Dennis S. Charney • Department of Psychiatry, Yale University School of Medicine, and National Center for PTSD, Department of Veterans Affairs Medical Center, West Haven, Connecticut 06516.

Handbook of Dissociation: Theoretical, Empirical, and Clinical Perspectives, edited by Larry K. Michelson and William J. Ray. Plenum Press, New York, 1996.

hypnotizability also develop as ongoing sequelae of traumatization (Spiegel, Hunt, & Dondershine, 1988; Bernstein & Putnam, 1986; Loewenstein & Putnam, 1988; Bremner et al., 1992, 1993). While dissociated, acutely traumatized individuals may appear confused, emotionally dulled, or even catatonic, giving rise to descriptive phrases such as "shell shock" (Kardiner, 1941; Grinker & Spiegel, 1945; Krystal, 1968). Decades following traumatization, while recalling their traumatic experiences, individuals may experience time as being slowed, have altered sensory perceptions, and have feelings of unreality (Bremner et al., in review). Less frequently, adult traumatization may produce fugue states, conversion reactions, or multple personality as ongoing symptoms of PTSD (Grinker & Spiegel, 1945; McDougle & Southwick, 1990).

Childhood psychological traumatization is also associated with dissociative symptoms. In one study, approximately 60% of 450 adults traumatized as children had periods in their lives when they had no memory of their abuse (Briere & Conte, 1993). Dissociative symptoms arising from childhood traumatization continue in adulthood (Putnam, Guroff, Silberman, Barban, & Post, 1986; Hermann, Perry, & van der Kolk, 1989). For example, psychiatric inpatients with histories of childhood trauma have higher levels of dissociative symptoms than nontraumatized inpatients (Chu & Dill, 1992).

Flashbacks, perhaps the most distinctive PTSD symptom, appear to represent the convergence of dissociative states, intrusive traumatic memories, and hyperarousal. During flashbacks, patients vividly reexperience aspects of the traumatic response while feeling detached from their surrounding environment. Ongoing sensory processing may be altered or disrupted and patients may report that they are in a fog or that they blacked out (Bremner et al., 1993). Flashbacks involving the recollection of traumatic experiences are frequently associated with intense emotional responses and paniclike states (Mellman & Davis, 1985). Most flashbacks are brief, lasting only a few minutes. However, some flashbacks may last several hours or several days. Some flashbacks are accurate depictions of a traumatic situation and others have unreal or distorted qualities, similar to dreams.

Despite progress in identifying, characterizing, and quantitatively assessing dissociative states, there has been surprisingly little study of their neurobiology in adults and no published studies, to our knowledge, of the developmental neurobiology of dissociation. Associated with the failure to elucidate a unique neurobiology for dissociative states, there have been few placebo-controlled pharmacotherapy trials for dissociative disorders and no specific antidissociative drugs developed. The absence of antidissociative pharmacotherapies contrasts with the development of anxiolytics, antiobsessionals, antipsychotics, mood-stabilizing agents, and antidepressants. In light of the paucity of research in this area, the commonly held view—that the core features of dissociative disorders are unresponsive to pharmacotherapy—is not surprising (Kluft, 1987).

This chapter will review recent progress made in studying the neurobiology of dissociative states in PTSD patients. In particular, it will focus on studies that have produced dissociative states in healthy individuals and patients with PTSD or other neurological disorders. In doing so, this chapter will attempt to highlight bridges between the neurobiology and treatment of PTSD.

BARBITURATES AND GUIDED RECOLLECTION: "NARCOSYNTHESIS"

The medical facilitation of traumatic memory recall and flashbacks in traumatized individuals began in World War II as part of a therapeutic approach called *narcosynthesis* or, more recently, the *amytal interview*. This approach combined barbiturates and guided recollection of traumatic memories (Sargent & Slater, 1940; Bartemeier, Kubie, Menninger, Romano, & Whitehorn, 1946; Grinker & Spiegel, 1945). The use of barbiturates to facilitate traumatic memory recall was illustrated by a case reported by Grinker (1944, pp. 142–143):

> That afternoon I gave him 0.25 gm of pentothal sodium intravenously. He was then told that he was up in the air on a strafing mission and that the man on his wing was aflame.... Immediately he [shouted] to his friend ... pull up and bail out. Why doesn't he pull up and bail out?... he went over and over the traumatic situation, crying and sobbing. As this reaction subsided he was allowed to close his eyes and sleep ... [upon awakening] He stated I must have been asleep. I had a dream about [my friend] ...

The facilitation of traumatic memories by barbiturates and benzodiazepines creates the appearanace of a paradox: drugs with prominent amnestic effects improving memory function. These drugs impair attention, learning, and memory in humans (Kirk, Roache, & Griffiths, 1990; Krystal et al., in review). However, their amnestic effects arise primarily through interfering with memory encoding rather than memory storage or retrieval (Ghoneim & Mewaldt, 1990). Mechanisms through which barbiturates facilitate the recollection of traumatic memories and flashbacks are poorly understood. Barbiturates enhance the actions of gamma-aminobutyric acid (GABA) at the $GABA_A$ receptor (Olsen, 1981) and they block the actions of glutamate at non-*N*-methyl-D-aspartic acid (NMDA) receptors (Collins & Anson, 1987; Morgan, Bermudez, & Chang, 1991). However, barbiturates are not specific in their capacity to facilitate recollection of traumatic memories in that ether, ethanol, nitrous oxide, and scopolamine–morphine combinations also appear to facilitate the recall of inaccessible memories (Erickson, 1945; Rosen & Meyers, 1947).

The prodissociative effects of these drugs are indirect. Benzodiazepines, for example, do not increase scores on scales measuring dissociation in healthy individuals (Krystal et al., in review). Clinical observations suggest that the sedating and anxiolytic medications employed in narcosynthesis reduce anxiety and thus may lessen the resistance to recalling anxiety-associated memories (Grinker & Spiegel, 1945). This view is consistent with a patient who experienced flashbacks during relaxation training (Fitzgerald & Gonzalez, 1994). Alternatively, these medications, viewed as "truth sera" by the popular press, may suppress involuntary mechanisms responsible for reducing voluntary access to traumatic memories (Kardiner & Spiegel, 1947). Related to this hypothesis, recent physiological research has provided additional evidence of a neural basis for directed forgetting and other processes associated with reduced voluntary access to established memories (Geiselman, Bjork, & Fishmann, 1983; Paller, 1990).

Flashbacks have been precipitated in Vietnam veterans with chronic PTSD following the intravenous administration of sodium lactate (Rainey et al., 1987), yohimbine (Southwick et al., 1993), and m-chlorophenylpiperazine (MCPP) (Southwick et al., 1991). Administration of each of these substances produces panic attacks in a significant proportion of patients with either panic disorder (Pitts & McClure, 1967; Charney, Heninger, & Breier, 1984; Charney, Woods, Goodman, & Heninger, 1987) or PTSD (Rainey et al., 1987; Southwick et al., 1991, 1993), but not other patients groups. However, PTSD patients are the first group studied to experience flashbacks following administration of these substances.

Rainey and his associates (1987) compared the response to intravenous sodium lactate, isoproterenol, and a dextrose placebo in seven Vietnam combat veterans, six of whom also met criteria for panic disorder. All seven patients experienced flashbacks following lactate, two patients also experienced flashbacks after isoproterenol infusion, and one patient experienced a flashback during placebo infusion. The authors described these flashbacks as similar to those occurring naturally as part of PTSD. Dissociative experiences that accompanied flashbacks included depersonalization, derealization, and auditory and visual sensory perceptions. Six of the seven lactate-induced flashbacks, both isoproterenol flashbacks, and the dextrose flashback were followed by paniclike states. However, the absence of reported anxiety ratings makes it impossible to determine whether subpanic increases in anxiety preceded the flashbacks. The overlap of panic disorder and PTSD in the patients in this study was another limitation of this study, because it raised concerns that lactate-induced flashbacks were a property of panic disorder and not independently associated with PTSD. Little is known about the mechanisms through which lactate produced panic attacks and flashbacks in PTSD patients.

The precipitation of flashbacks and panic attacks in PTSD patients by yohimbine linked noradrenergic systems, implicated in fear and arousal regulation, to the symptoms of PTSD (Southwick et al., 1993). Yohimbine activates central noradrenergic neurons through blockade of α-2 receptors located on noradrenergic neurons. These α-2 receptors mediate, in part, feedback inhibition of noradrenergic neurons (Starke, Borowski, & Endo, 1975). Following yohimbine, 40% (8/20) of patients experienced flashbacks and 70% (14/20) of patients experienced panic attacks. No panic attacks and only one flashback emerged following placebo administration. Although 45% of the patients in this study also met *Diagnostic and Statistical Manual of Mental Disorders*, 3rd edition, revised (DSM-III-R) (American Psychiatric Association, 1987) criteria for panic disorder, 43% of the yohimbine-induced panic attacks occurred in individuals without panic disorder. The risk of a yohimbine-induced panic attack was increased in patients with panic disorder relative to those without comorbid panic disorder (89 vs. 43%). However, history of panic disorder did not appear to influence the likelihood of experiencing a yohimbine-induced flashback. The following vignette illustrates features of a yohimbine-induced flashback:

10:00 AM: [Initiation of yohimbine infusion]
10:05 AM: Subject reports hot and cold flashes, goose bumps, palpitations.

10:10 AM: Subject reports clammy hands; he asked the nurse to move away from him ... in case he felt like running. "I feel like I'm picking up dead bodies; the centrifuge sounds like a helicopter ... A chopper is shooting at us; we're trying to shoot back at it! One of the guys' head is shot off! Brains are coming at me! I smell burnt flesh ... I feel scared, I can't hear what's going on....

The operational definition for flashback employed in this study led to the exclusion of many dissociative states produced by yohimbine in the PTSD patients. The following criteria were employed to define a drug-induced flashback: (1) reexperiencing of a past traumatic event during drug infusion, (2) the reexperiencing must involve one or more sensory modalities, and (3) for patients with a history of flashbacks, the drug-induced state must be similar to naturally occurring flashbacks. Despite the expedient characterization of flashbacks as being present or absent, yohimbine actually produced a continuum of dissociative phenomena. Patients experienced varying degrees of derealization and depersonalization that were often accompanied by other dissociative symptoms. Yohimbine also elicited a range of altered perceptual experiences, some of which were fragmentary or vague. For example, one patient perceived the shadow produced by a sink in the testing facility to be the shadow made by a tank turret. In addition to stimulating flashbacks, yohimbine significantly increased the recall of traumatic memories. Although yohimbine produced symptoms of autonomic arousal in many patients, these symptoms were not the sole predictor of flasbacks within a session. Yohimbine also significantly increased the recall of traumatic memories. In some cases, symptoms of autonomic arousal followed or were coincident with the reported retrieval of traumatic memories (Southwick, personal communication). Thus, it appeared that noradrenergic systems might be involved in the elicitation of dissociative symptoms as a direct consequence of its central pharmacological actions on neural circuitry contributing to dissociation and memory retrieval. These data contrasted with models in which noradrenergic contributions to PTSD symptoms were entirely mediated by peripheral autonomic systems.

The yohimbine study suggested that activation of noradrenergic systems by yohimbine produced panic attacks and flashbacks in a subset of PTSD patients. One question raised by this study was whether the elicitation of flashbacks by yohimbine reflected a specific response to α-2 receptor blockade or whether all anxiogenic drugs produce flashbacks in PTSD patients. In order to investigate this question, yohimbine and MCPP effects were compared in this population (Southwick et al., 1991). This study found that both MCPP and yohimbine produced flashbacks and other dissociative states in veterans with combat-related PTSD. Preliminary analyses indicated that patients tended to experience panic attacks following yohimbine or MCPP, but not both medications. As with the initial study, drug-induced traumatic memories, autonomic activation, and anxiety states could be associated with the induction of flashbacks, although no single response preceded flashbacks in all cases. These observations raised the possibility that yohimbine and MCPP caused flashbacks by modulating a final common pathway that has yet to be identified or that multiple mechanisms might lead to the induction of flashbacks.

In order to to continue the search for key neurotransmitter systems involved in dissociation in PTSD patients, we studied the effects of the benzodiazepine antagonist, flumazenil, in PTSD patients. This drug failed to precipitate flashbacks or panic attacks in PTSD patients (Randall et al., in press). As with lactate, yohimbine, and MCPP, this agent has been reported to produce panic attacks in patients with panic disorder (Woods, Charney, Silver, Krystal, & Heninger, 1991). The absence of flumazenil-induced panic attacks and flashbacks indicates that PTSD is not associated with the overproduction of an endogenous benzodiazepine inverse agonist, such as diazepam-binding inhibitor, that might contribute to anxiety symptoms in other disorders (Costa & Guidotti, 1987). Future studies will be needed to determine whether benzodiazepine inverse agonists, such as FG-7142 or iomazenil, which precipitate anxiety in healthy subjects (Dorow, Horowski, Paschelke, Amin, & Braestrup, 1983; Randall, Bremner, Southwick, Krystal, & Charney, personal communication), will produce flashbacks in PTSD patients.

Case reports suggest that alcohol and opiate withdrawal may increase PTSD symptoms, including flashbacks (Kosten & Krystal, 1988; Salloway, Southwick, & Sadowsky, 1990; Seibyl, personal communication). Central noradrenergic systems are activated during alcohol and opiate withdrawal, suggesting a possible parallel between yohimbine- and withdrawal-induced flashbacks (Kosten & Krystal, 1988).

INDUCTION OF DISSOCIATIVE STATES IN HEALTHY INDIVIDUALS

Pathophysiological models that hypothesize a "final common pathway" for the neurobiology of dissociation presuppose that modulation of the activity of this pathway might produce dissociative states in healthy individuals. To date, three classes of drugs commonly produce dissociativelike states in healthy subjects: (1) antagonists of the *N*-methyl-D-aspartate (NMDA) subtype of glutamate receptor, (2) cannabinoids, and (3) serotonergic hallucinogens.

The noncompetitive NMDA receptor antagonist anesthetics, phencyclidine and ketamine, produce a derealized and depersonalized state characterized by marked perceptual alterations and psychosis at subanesthetic doses (Luby, Cohen, Rosenbaum, Gottlieb, & Kelley, 1959; Domino, Chodoff, & Corsson, 1965; Yamakura, Mori, Masaki, Shimoji, & Mishina, 1993; Javitt & Zukin, 1991). The capacity of ketamine to produce dissociativelike states in healthy subjects has been rigorously evaluated in a series of studies (Krystal et al., 1994a,b, in review). In these studies, dissociative symptoms were rated using the Clinician-Administered Dissociative States Scale (CADSS) (Bremner et al., in review). At low blood levels, ketamine produced a light-headed feeling. At higher blood levels, subjects reported the slowing of time and alterations in the vividness, form, and context of sensory experiences. For example, subjects noted that objects appeared brighter or duller than expected, larger or smaller than usual, distorted in shape, or with altered proximity. Also, some subjects had difficulty hearing someone speaking close to them, while reporting that a radio playing quietly in the next room sounded unusually loud. Altered proprioceptive experiences were reported by subjects, who felt that their limbs changed form or were floating in air.

Cognitive effects of ketamine were also prominent. Subjects reported constriction of their field of attention, resulting in the sensation of tunnel vision or the feeling that they were surrounded by fog. As ketamine blood levels rose, the circumference of their field of attention was increasingly constricted. For example, subjects attending to a computer keyboard lost track of events happening on the computer monitor. Ketamine also produced learning and memory impairments. Its effects increased proportionately to the dose administered and the duration of delay between stimulus presentation and testing. Ketamine also interfered with executive functions such as abstraction, assessed by proverb interpretation, and problem solving, evaluated by the Wisconsin Card Sorting Test. Although subjects felt that they had lost control of their thought processes, with effort they could focus on tasks. Ketamine also produced emotional and identity-related responses. At low doses, it had mild anxiolytic properties, while larger doses generally produced euphoria and anxiety. Anxiety stimulated by ketamine tended to follow perceptual alterations and thought disorganization and to be related to their degree of comfort with the drug-induced disturbances in thought and perception. Some subjects found the perceptual alterations produced by ketamine quite pleasurable, analogous to a ride in an amusement park, while others found ketamine effects frightening.

Ketamine-induced insight impairments may have contributed to the elicitation of anxiety. Following drug infusion, some subjects lost the perspective that their mental status change was produced by ketamine and they became concerned that they had contracted a mental illness. Transient identity alterations were also observed with ketamine. For example, a subject who received ketamine (0.26 mg/kg intravenous bolus followed by 0.65 mg/kg per hr) stated "at first it seemed that I didn't exist, I couldn't process information; after a while, I was convinced that I was an organism; then I realized I was a human being; then after a longer while I remembered that I was a medical student." Ketamine did not lead to the emergence of multiple personalities, flashbacks, or vivid intrusive memories in research subjects. However, symptoms associated with psychosis, including delusions and thought disorder, were observed during ketamine infusion.

Two ongoing studies have attempted to pharmacologically alter ketamine-induced dissociative states by pretreating healthy subjects with lorazepam or haloperidol (Krystal et al., in review). Preliminary data from these studies suggested that 2 mg lorazepam administered orally 2 hours prior to ketamine administration tended to reduce altered environmental perceptions, but had no effects on other dissociative symptoms or psychotic states produced by ketamine. Haloperidol failed to reduce dissociative symptoms, vigilance impairments, or amnestic effects produced by ketamine, but reduced ketamine-induced distractibility, abstraction impairments, and bizarreness of thought processes. These data suggested that, at the doses tested, neither agent is a true ketamine antidote. They are also consistent with the literature suggesting that neuroleptics have limited efficacy in treating dissociative symptoms (Kluft, 1987).

Dissociative states have also been produced by psychoactive cannabinoids, such as tetrahydrocannabinol the principal psychoactive component of marijuana and hashish. Cannabinoids bind to a specific G-protein-coupled reeptor (Herkenham et al., 1990) through which they alter cellular functions including blockade of N-type calcium channels, inhibition of cyclic AMP accumulation, and stimulation of arachidonic acid and intracellular calcium release (Felder et al., 1993). Some cannabinoid effects may be mediated by stimulation of glucocorticoid receptors

(Eldridge & Landfield, 1990) and blockade of NMDA receptors (Feigenbaum et al., 1989). At high doses, cannabinoid intoxication produces depersonalization, derealization, perceptual alterations, and insight impairments (Bromberg, 1939; Melges, Tinklenberg, Hollister, & Gillespie, 1970; Dittrich, Battig, & von Zeppelin, 1973). Cannabis has been reported to produce flashbacks in the drug-free state that resemble cannabis intoxication (Hollister, 1986). In one study (Stanton, Mintz, & Franklin, 1976), 3% (1/31) of habitual marijuana users and 1% (3/348) of nonhabitual users reported flashbacks when drug-free, suggesting that flashbacks were not a frequent consequence of cannabis use. However, this study suggested that marijuana use also enhanced the likelihood of experiencing flashbacks following ingestion of the serotonergic hallucinogens.

Serotonergic hallucinogens, such as lysergic acid diethylamide (LSD), mescaline, and dimethyltryptamine (DMT), also produce dissociative symptoms. These agents stimulate serotonin-2 (5-HT_2) receptors (Rasmussen, Glennon, & Aghajanian, 1986; Titeler, Lyon, & Glennon, 1988). These drugs produce pronounced visual hallucinations, illusions, synesthesia, and expansive or portentious emotional responses (Freedman, 1968). Following ingestion of these psychedelics, feelings of derealization or depersonalization may also be prominent. Environmental stimuli may be experienced in a fragmented manner, body image may be distorted, and individuals may feel detached from their surroundings (Savage, 1955; Liebert, Werner, & Wapner, 1958; Klee, 1963; Rodin & Luby, 1966; Freedman, 1968). Some clinicians also have reported that LSD may facilitate the recall of repressed memories (Freedman, 1968), although this capacity has never been rigorously evaluated. Relative to the phencyclidine or ketamine experience, psychedelic hallucinogens tend to produce perceptual effects that predominate over dissociative effects and impairments in higher cognitive functions.

Flashbacks have been reported in healthy individuals following serotonergic hallucinogen use. Freedman (1968) and Horowitz (1969) suggested that LSD intoxication was traumatic for some users because it diminished control over awareness, resulting in intense emotional states experienced as beyond their control. In such cases, LSD flashbacks might have a traumatic etiology. However, some LSD-like experiences, such as synesthesia, may be reexperienced long after drug ingestion by individuals who find such experiences pleasant. These effects do not easily fit a trauma model, suggesting that sensitization, conditioning, or state-dependent learning might also apply (Freedman, 1968, 1984; Horowitz, 1969; McGee, 1984). Subject expectancy may also play a role in druglike flashbacks. One study found that flashbacks may be produced in healthy subjects following placebo administration, if subjects are coached to anticipate that a placebo will to produce flashbacks (Heaton, 1975). Heaton suggested that the expectancy of flashbacks led subjects to mislabel and selectively attend to aspects of normal experience that are consistent with a flashbacklike experience.

LESSONS FROM BRAIN STIMULATION STUDIES

Flashbacks are common to PTSD and conditions associated with local activation of cortical and limbic structures. Hughlings Jackson first described the complex polysensory reexperiencing of events that occurred in association with temporal lobe epilepsy as memory flashbacks (Taylor, 1931). Patients wtih clinical and encephalographic evidence of temporal lobe epilepsy exhibited a range of dissociative symptoms including depersonalization, derealization, auditory and visual hallucinations, and multiple personalities (Mesulam, 1981). Sacks (1985) also described a patient with seizure foci in her medial temporal structures that produced repetitive reexperiencing of Irish folk melodies. Anticonvulsant treatment eliminated the intrusive musical reexperiencing, but also eliminated her ability to recall the melodies.

Penfield and his colleagues elicited dreamlike states, memories, and complex experiential phenomena through direct electrical stimulation of structures in the temporal lobe, temporoparietal association areas, hippocampus, and amygdala (Penfield & Perot, 1963). Temporal lobe stimulation resulted in some individuals reexperiencing frightening events in a polysensory fashion, such as a possible thwarted kidnapping. However, neutral or pleasant experiences were also produced, such as hearing a choir sing White Christmas. The amygdala and hippocampus appear to be implicated in the experiential phenomena associated with temporal lobe activation. Gloor, Olivier, Quesney, Andermann, and Horowitz (1982) found that experiential phenomena were associated with direct stimulation of the amygdala and the hippocampus. Moreover, memories, dreamlike states, or other complex experiential phenomena were only produced when temporal cortical stimulation was followed by after-discharges in the amygdala or hippocampus. Results of this study were consistent with an earlier one that produced complex experiential phenomena through electrical stimulation of the hippocampus and amygdala (Halgren Walter, Cherlow, & Crandall, 1978).

The brain stimulation studies suggest that the hippocampus and amygdala control the retrieval of memory in a highly specific manner, much as a program might control access to information stored on a computer. However, this interpretation appears overly simple. Complex experiential phenomena are usually associated with high-intensity stimuli or after-discharges, suggesting that fairly large cortical areas must be activated (Halgren et al., 1978). Also, stimulation of the same location over several trials does not reliably reproduce experiential phenomena, while stimulation of disparate cortical regions may produce identical experiences (Halgren et al., 1978; Horowitz, Adams, & Rutkin, 1968). In addition, surgical excision of an area that produces a memory when directly stimulated does not eliminate the memory (Baldwin, 1960). A more circumspect interpretation of these data is that memory is stored within distributed networks and that the amygdala and hippocampus stimulations bias the retrieval of memories in a more general fashion, such as facilitating access to an associative network.

One of the striking similarities of flashback associated with PTSD and the brain stimulation studies are the inflexible nature of memory retrieval under these conditions. Dreams and memories often replay traumatic scenes in their entirety rather than being retrieved with the cognitive flexibility characteristic of declarative memory. The neurobiology underlying the loss of retrieval flexibility and efficiency associated with traumatic memory retrieval, limbic stimulation studies, and the developmental disorders are currently unclear. However, reduced mnemonic flexibility has been reported to characterize memory retrieval under conditions where the hippocampus is activated independently of the frontal cortex (Moscovitch, 1992). Memory encoding by the hippocampus is modular and organizing links between memories arise largely through cue association, as occurs during conditioning (Moscovitch, 1992). Retrieval strategies involving the hippocampus are cue-dependent and not strategic. In other words, the hippocampus cannot efficiently scan stored memories to retrieve a particular memory, even though it is involved in memory encoding. The organizing and strategizing component of memory retrieval appears to be dependent on the frontal cortex (Moscovitch, 1989, 1992). Thus, flashbacks may share the qualities of memory retrieval exhibited by individuals during hippocampal stimulation because these conditions involve retrieval strategies that bypass the frontal component of memory retrieval in the face of relative preservation of the hippocampal component of memory retrieval.

Recollective processes that bypass frontal executive mechanisms controlling the strategic recollection of information may also share the quality of being reexperienced rather than recalled. Flashbacks produced in seizure patients by electrical stimulation (Penfield & Perot, 1963) and those occurring in PTSD (Bremner et al., 1992; Southwick et al., 1991) were both described in this manner. Frontal cortical networks have been implicated in executive functions related to the control of memory retrieval (Baddeley, 1986). Frontal lobe lesions, unlike hippocampal lesions, impair retrieval of autobiographical information (Baddeley & Wilson, 1988). The frontal cortex has also been implicated in the prioritization of responses, the generation of mental representations within working memory, self-monitoring, and editing of thought (Stuss, 1992; Goldman-Rakic, 1987; Baddeley, 1986). The frontal cortex is nested within networks involving the amygdala, mediodorsal thalamic nucleus, the hippocampus, and other regions that provide access to input regarding the nature and meaning of memories that are formed (Goldman-Rakic, 1987). Sedative-hypnotic agents produce impairments on tests sensitive to frontal cortical impairment, as does ketamine (Krystal et al., 1994b, in review).

THALAMIC NETWORKS AND DISSOCIATIVE STATES

Dissociative states occur normally in individuals without dissociative disorders at extremely low or high levels of sensory processing. Reductions in the intensity or variability of sensory stimulation, associated with hypnosis, sleep deprivation, and sensory deprivation, may produce altered states of consciousness with dissociative features (Freud & Breuer, 1953; Bexton, Heron, & Scott, 1954; Lilly, 1956; Cappon & Banks, 1960; Krystal, 1988). As an extreme illustration of this point, sensory polyneuropathies may cause marked depersonalization and derealization associated with feelings of being disembodied (Sacks, 1985). Heightened sensory stimulation or arousal may also produce altered sensory processing. Significant levels of arousal and anxiety heighten the salience and vividness of environmental stimuli. Under stress, attention is narrowed to the most salient aspects of the environment, consistent with the need to focus on the danger at hand. Thus, individuals fixate faster and longer on unusual or highly informative objects, such as weapons (Brown & Kulik, 1977; Burke et al., 1992; Christianson & Loftus, 1991), while less critical but important information about the context of the trauma may not receive much attention

(Kramer, Buckhout, & Eugenio, 1990). At extremely high levels of arousal, coherent integration of sensory information breaks down and dissociative symptoms emerge, even in individuals without dissociative disorders (Cappon & Banks, 1961; Ludwig, 1972; Krystal, Woods, Hill, & Charney, 1988, 1991).

The thalamus plays a critical role in modulating responsivity to environmental stimuli associated with sleep and dreaming and may play a similar role in the genesis of dissociative states. As illustrated in Figure 1, the thalamus serves as a sensory gate or filter that directly and indirectly modulates the access of sensory information to the cortex, amygdala, and hippocampus (Amaral & Cowen, 1980; McCormick, 1992; Steriade & Llinas, 1988; Turner & Herkenham, 1991). During slow wave sleep, for example, thalamic nuclei exhibit slow spindle oscillations that disrupt the transmission of sensory information to cortical and limbic structures (Steriade & Deschenes, 1984). During wakefulness, thalamic neurons fire in a relay mode that facilitates transmission of sensory information to cortical regions. Rapid eye move-

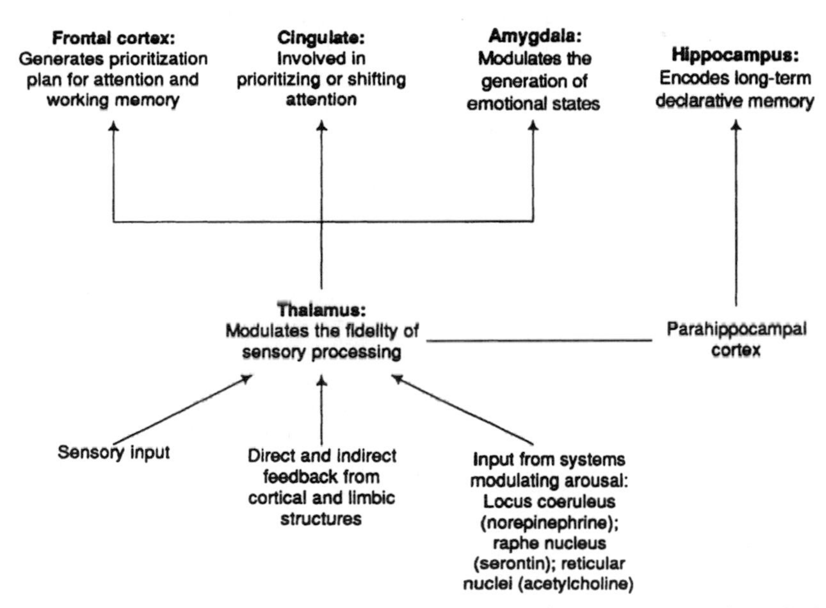

Figure 1. This schematic illustrates the position of the thalamus within networks that may be involved in the generation of dissociative states. Sensory information reaches the thalamus and is transmitted to limbic and cortical regions responsible for modulating thought, attention, learning and memory, and emotion. The thalamus receives input from limbic regions, such as the amygdala, and brainstem regions involved in stress-related arousal. It also receives direct and indirect feedback from cortical regions involved in prioritizing attention. When functioning in relay mode, the thalamus facilitates the accurate transmittal of sensory information. However, when slow oscillatory firing patterns predominate, the thalamus impedes the flow of sensory information to cortical and limbic regions associated with the predominate focus on internally generated thought processes and sensory experiences associated with dreaming, night terrors, and perhaps dissociation (from Krystal, Bennett, Bremner, Southwick, & Charney, in press).

ment (REM) sleep, associated with dreaming, is characterized by phasic enhancement of the activity of glutamatergic thalamocortical cells (Steriade, Datta, Paré, Oakson, & Curró Dossi, 1990; Steriade & McCarley, 1990). In this model, dreams and other sleep-related internally generated experiences may arise as thalamocortical or other direct cortical projections from the amygdala and hippocampus bypass the oscillatory thalamic processes that disrupt the flow of sensory information to the cortex (Swanson, 1981; Llinás & Paré, 1991). Thus, like dissociative states, sleep states may neurobiologically preserve associative and mnemonic functions while interrupting sensory processing. Sensory processing alterations associated with dissociative states could indicate the intrusion of sleep-related disturbances in sensory processing into the waking state. If so, then alterations in thalamic activity might link a spectrum of altered states of consciousness such as hypnosis, dreaming, and other conditions in which there is a combination of the features of sleep and waking states (Mahowald & Schenck, 1991; Llinás & Paré, 1991). Dissociative states might also be related to night terrors in which features of waking behavior intrude upon sleep (Fischer, Kahn, Edwards, & Davis, 1973; Kales et al., 1980; Oswald & Evans, 1985). Evidence for a thalamic role in maintaining the boundary of sleeplike behavior and wakefulness is provided by patients with paramedian thalamic infarctions. These patients exhibit a profound sense of detachment, reduced responsivity to sensory stimuli, and sleeplike posturing throughout the circadian cycle without the electrophysiological correlates of non-REM sleep (Guilleminault, Quera-Salva, & Goldberg, 1993).

A thalamic role in dissociation is suggested by its distinctive role in modulating the onset of night terrors as opposed to nightmares. Posttraumatic nightmares occur within REM sleep and are not generally associated with motor behaviors, although they may repetitively review aspects of the trauma (Fisher, Byrne, Edwards, & Kahn, 1970; Fisher et al., 1973; Greenberg, Pearlman, & Bampel, 1972). In contrast, posttraumatic night terrors bear a closer resemblance to flashbacks occurring in the waking state. Night terrors are associated with confusion upon awakening, reduced responsivity to environmental stimuli, displays of intense emotion, significant autonomic activation, increased sleep motility, complex motor activity, and somnambulism (Lavie & Hertz, 1979; Hafez, Metz, & Lavie, 1987; van der Kolk, Blitz, Burr, Sherry, & Hartmann, 1984; Fisher et al., 1970, 1973). Despite behavioral evidence that traumatic incidents are being reexperienced during night terrors, such as calls for help and appearing to act out physical struggles, individuals are generally amnestic for the content of their experiences. As with flashbacks and nightmares, night terrors may be precipitated in PTSD patients by reminders of the trauma or environmental stress (Krystal, 1968; Fisher et al., 1970). Unlike nightmares, night terrors occur during deep sleep, particularly stage 4, and generally within the first hour after falling asleep (Fisher et al., 1973; Kales et al., 1980). Nightmares and night terrors may be further distinguished by the effects of paramedian thalamic lesions. These lesions eliminate the stages of sleep that contain night terrors, but do not alter REM sleep and dreaming (Guilleminault et al., 1993).

Sensory distortions associated with stress may develop, in part, as a consequence of the thalamic role in modulating sensory processing. Thalamic nuclei appear to work both in series and in parallel with brain regions involved in traumatic stress response. One region that may be critical for fear learning and traumatic stress response is the central nucleus of the amygdala (LeDoux, 1987; Davis, 1992; Charney, Deutch, Krystal, Southwick, & Davis, 1993). Once activated by uncontrollable stressors, the central nucleus of the amygdala facilitates the thalamic relay of sensory information to cortical and limbic structures (Clugnet & LeDoux, 1990; McDonald, 1982; Steriade et al., 1990).

Central noradrenergic systems are also activated by signfiicant uncontrollable stressors and have been linked to traumatic stress response (van der Kolk, Greenberg, Boyd, & Krystal, 1985; Krystal et al., 1989). Stress-induced noradrenergic activation would be expected to facilitate thalamic transduction of sensory information by stimulating thalamic α-1 adrenoceptors that increase thalamic activity associated with wakefulness and to inhibit slow thalamic oscillations (Buzsáki, Kennedy, Solt, & Ziegler, 1990; McCormick & Wang, 1991). Postsynaptic α-2 receptors promote thalamic slow oscillations. Thus yohimbine, an α-2 antagonist, could incease thalamic bursting by increasing norepinephrine release and blocking the stimulation slow oscillations produced by postsynaptic α-2 receptors (Buzsáki et al., 1990).

Serotonergic systems, linked to PTSD symptoms by the MCPP study described above (Southwick et al., 1993), also heighten sensory processing via the 5-HT_2 receptor (McCormick & Wang, 1991). Both MCPP and the serotonergic hallucinogens stimulate subtypes of this receptor (Sheldon & Aghajanian, 1991). Perceptual alterations associated with extreme or uncontrollable stress suggest that the massive activation of monoamine systems under these conditions may modulate thalamic function in a fashion that results in interference rather than enhancement of the fidelity of sensory transmission.

Alterations in thalamic glutamatergic function also could contribute to sensory gating disturbances. Glutamate is the primary excitatory neurotransmitter within the thalamus (McCormick, 1992) and the neurotransmitter involved with thalamic afferents from the amygdala, cerebral cortex, and hippocampus (Aggleton & Mishkin, 1984; Aggleton, Desimone, & Mishkin, 1986; Giguere & Goldman-Rakic, 1988; LeDoux & Farb, 1991; McCormick, 1992). Indirect cortical thalamic modulation also occurs via a circuit involving the striatum, globus pallidus, subthalamic nucleus, and thalamus (Carlsson & Carlsson, 1990). Both NMDA and non-NMDA glutamate receptors are localized to the thalamus, where they have complementary functions (McCormick, 1992). Previous reviews have suggested that alterations of the sensory filter function of the thalamus via blockade of NMDA receptors could contribute to the psychotomimetic effects of the NMDA antagonists (Carlsson & Carlsson, 1990). Given the prominent role of non-NMDA glutamate receptors in corticostriato-thalamic circuitry, subanesthetic doses of selective NMDA antagonists might be predicted to produce distortions rather than complete blockade of thalamic sensory gating functions. This prediction is consistent with clinical observations, suggesting that ketamine produces a state of detachment or withdrawal rather than sleep. Also, ketamine produces sensory distortions and illusions rather than blockade of sensory perceptions or pure hallucinatory experiences (Krystal et al., 1994a). The capacity of sensory deprivation to reduce rather than augment the behavioral effects of phencyclidine further suggests that NMDA antagonists alter, rather than block, sensory processing (Cohen, Luby, Rosenbaum, & Gottlieb, 1960). Future research is needed to clarify the extent of thalamic contributions to dissociative states.

The thalamus is a heterogenous structure and component thalamic nuclei have distinctive cortical afferents and efferents and different patterns of synaptic organization (M. L. Schwartz, Dekker, & Goldman-Rakic, 1991). For example, the reticular nuclei of the thalamus fucntion in some ways as an extension of brainstem and midbrain reticular activating systems (Steriade & Llinás, 1988). However, other thalamic nuclei, such as the anteroventral and mediodorsal nuclei, appear to be involved in associative processes, such as learning (Orona & Gabriel, 1983; Gabriel, Sparenborg, & Stolar, 1987; Gabriel, Vogt, Kubota, Poremba, & Kang, 1991).

Sensory processing alterations and changes in attention may be linked in dissociative states. Clinically, the bridge between sensory gating and attention modulation is evident in the reduced responsivity to environmental stimuli exhibited by dissociated individuals and their reported focus on peripheral sensory stimuli or internal mental processes (Carlson & Putnam, 1989). This connection also is suggested by the convergence of corticolimbic networks upon the anterior cingulate gyrus, a brain region implicated in the capacity to shift and focus attention (Pardo, Pardo, Janer, & Raichle, 1990; Bench et al., 1993). Anterior cingulate lesions may produce symptoms reminiscent of thalamic, limbic, and cortical lesions including confusion, vivid daydreaming, apathy, impairments in sustained attention, and learning impairments (Whitty & Lewin, 1957; Laplane, Degos, Baulac, & Gray, 1981). Direct projections to the anterior cingulate gyrus from midline and intralaminar thalamic nuclei suggest that the cingulate gyrus is responsive to shifts in thalamic sensory processing functions (Vogt, Rosene, & Pandya, 1979). As suggested by the clinical case reports of patients wtih cingulate lesions, the cingulate gyrus may also be involved in the attribution of salience and the acquisition and retrieval of learned information (Gabriel et al., 1991; Gaffan, Murray, & Fabre-Thorpe, 1993). The contributions of the cingulate gyrus to sensory processing, emotional regulation, and learning are facilitated by its connectivity to other brain regions. For example, hippocampal and anteroventral thalamic inputs converge upon the anterior cingulate gyrus via the posterior cingulate gyrus (Gabriel et al., 1987; Gabriel & Sparenborg, 1987). Similarly, the anterior cingulate gyrus is an important point of convergence for a network involving the amygdala, prefrontal cortex, and mediodorsal thalamic nucleus (Aggleton & Mishkin, 1984; Goldman-Rakic & Porrino, 1985; Gaffan & Murry, 1990; Gaffan et al., 1993; Orona & Gabriel, 1983).

CORTICAL DISCONNECTIVITY AND DISSOCIATION

Geschwind (1980, p. 191) wrote, "there is no evidence for the existence of any all-purpose computer in the brain." Consistent with this view, cortical functions are highly distributed across several cortical regions that require integration in order to generate coherent conscious experience. For example, frontoparietal interactions help to locate memories or mental representations in space, while frontohippocampal interactions appear to contribute contextual information regarding these memories (Goldman-Rakic, 1987). Also, the frontal cortex itself contains many functionally heterogeneous regions. Distinct frontal cortex loci mediate the generation of iconic or working memories for the location and features of environmental stimuli. Brain lesions of one region of the frontal cortex results in memory gaps for spatial features, while lesions of the other region produce an inability to recall faces (Goldman-Rakic, 1987; Wilson, Scalaidhe, & Goldman-Rakic, 1993). If corticocortical interactions were disturbed or disrupted, experiences and cognitive functions dependent on integrated cortical activity might be distorted. For example, if frontal cortical regions processing features of objects and their spatial attributes were interacting dysfunctionally, one might generate mental representations for stimuli in which features were not correctly matched to their spatial locations, i.e., objects could be experienced out of context or in bizarre or incoherent ways. Disturbances in function arising from abnormal integration of cortical function may be similar, by analogy, to conduction aphasias. In conduction aphasias, both comprehension and fluency are preserved, but speech is paraphasic because information cannot be effectively transmitted from association to motor cortices (Geschwind, 1970).

Drugs that produce dissociative states disturb cortical integration at several levels. The key output neurons of the cortex are pyramidal neurons that utilize glutamate as their primary neurotransmitter. These neurons are regulated locally by modulatory GABAergic neurons. Pyramidal neurons also receive distant input from subcortical monoaminergic, glutamatergic, and peptidergic systems and glutamatergic input from pyramidal neurons in other cortical areas (Goldman-Rakic, 1987; Lewis, Hayes, Lund, & Oeth, 1992). In the piriform cortex, serotonergic hallucinogens inhibit pyramidal neuronal activity by stimulating GABAergic interneurons via the 5-$HT_{2A/2B}$ receptors. However, these drugs also activate pyramidal neurons through stimulating 5-HT_{2C} receptors (Sheldon & Aghajanian, 1991). Electrophysiological data suggest that ketamine distorts the functional connectivity within the cortex by blocking the NMDA receptor-mediated component of glutamatergic corticocortical connectivity. One study, for example, suggested that blockade of NMDA receptors allowed sensory information to reach the cortex, but interfered with the coherent transmission of this information from receptive areas to association cortices (Corssen & Domino, 1966). Barbiturates, which preferentially block non-NMDA glutamate receptors (Collins & Anson, 1987; Morgan et al., 1991), might also interfere with cortical integration, although the human psychopharmacology of non-NMDA glutamate receptors has received little direct study.

SUMMARY: ALTERATION IN GLUTAMATERGIC FUNCTION, A FINAL COMMON PATHWAY FOR DISSOCIATION?

Clinical studies related to the neurobiology of dissociative states are summarized in Table 1. Yohimbine and MCPP produce dissociative states only in PTSD patients, who are prone to have these experiences. These drugs primarily produce dissociative states while stimulating anxiety or traumatic recollections. Thus, yohimbine and MCPP may not directly induce dissociation, but rather contribute to the activation of networks resulting in a dissociative state in vulnerable individuals. In the amygdala, hippocampus, thalamus, and cortex, noradrenergic and serotonergic systems serve to modulate the activity of glutamatergic neurons (Goldman-Rakic, 1987; Lewis et al., 1992). Given the central role of glutamate in corticocortical, thalamocortical, amygdalocortical, and hippocampocortical connectivity, glutamatergic systems in the brain may be considered the framework on which

Table 1. Summary of Pharmacologically Facilitated Dissociative States

Substance	Healthy subjects[a]	PTSD patients[a]
Yohimbine	−	+
MCPP	−	+
Lactate	−	+
Sedative-hypnotics	−	+[b]
Benzodiazepine antagonists	−	−
NMDA antagonists	+	?
Cannabinoids	+	?
Serotonergic hallucinogens	+	?

[a]+, Associated with dissociative state; −, not associated with dissociative state; ?, unclear association with dissociative state; not formally evaluated in patients with PTSD.
[b]Facilitation of dissociation during guided recollection.

higher cognitive functions rest. Thus, it may not be surprising that a drug, such as ketamine, that alters glutamatergic neurotransmission produces dissociative states in healthy individuals. The possibility that glutamate systems might be fundamentally involved in generating dissociative states is consistent with the observation that dissociative states produced by ketamine in healthy people arise as a direct consequence of drug administration and are not dependent on generating intense emotional responses or memories. The direct evocation of dissociative states by an NMDA antagonist raises the possibility that reductions in NMDA receptor function contribute to dissociative states in humans. If so, then pharmacological agents that enhance NMDA receptor function might have antidissociative properties (Jones, Wesnes, & Kirby, 1991; Saletu, Grünberger, & Linzmayer, 1986; Schwartz et al., 1991; Nicholls, 1993).

IMPLICATIONS FOR THE TREATMENT OF PTSD

Dissociative phenomena, traumatic memories, and affective regulation are highly interrelated in PTSD patients. As reviewed earlier, traumatic memories and intense emotions may trigger dissociative phenomena in PTSD patients. Similarly, dissociative states and particular emotional states make the recall of traumatic memories more accessible. Completing the triangle, traumatic memories and dissociative phenomena may precipitate strong emotional responses. Thus, reducing the incidence of flashbacks and the intrusiveness and distress related to traumatic memories must be understood in the context of treating each of the three interactive processes.

The first step in treating dissociative states in traumatized individuals is to alleviate the marked depersonalization, derealization, and extreme emotional arousal. Barbiturates and benzodiazepines may be useful for this purpose (Kluft, 1987). The long-term benefits of acute anxiolysis are currently unclear. However, Kardiner (1941) emphasized the importance of the peritraumatic period in creating a long-lasting appraisal of traumatic events. Acute anxiolysis may be helpful in reducing negatively valenced cognitive distortions. Thus, in the context of supportive therapy, benzodiazepine treatment may facilitate the development of a more adaptive appraisal of the traumatic stress. Acute anxiolysis might alter the pairing of emotions and memories. Anxiolysis may also reduce or prevent the development of dissociative states, thus facilitating reflective reevaluation of information related to the trauma.

Once hyperarousal is controlled, a second challenge faced by clinicians is to reduce amnesia for traumatic events. Almost every psychotherapeutic strategy for treating acute psychological trauma has as a goal the integration of the traumatic experience within the conscious life of patients (Freud & Breuer 1953; Horowitz, 1976; Krystal, 1988). This task is difficult if the patient is amnestic for the trauma. Several guided recollection strategies have been employed to facilitate patients' access to traumatic memories including relaxation training, free association, dream interpretation, hypnosis, and narcosynthesis (Grinker & Spiegel, 1943; Bartemeier et al., 1946; Krystal, 1988; Keane, Fairbank, Caddell, & Zimering, 1989). Each of these processes takes advantage of an altered state of consciousness associated with increased suggestibility in which there is a reduction in functions usually associated with the frontal cortex, such as reflection, self-monitoring, and editing of thought (Stuss, 1992).

A potential risk associated with conducting guided recollection in a compromised state is that ideas introduced by the clinician may be more readily incorporated into the memories of the patient. For example, under hypnosis or during cannabis intoxication, subjects may not be able to accurately monitor the source or validity of recalled memories (Laurence & Perry, 1983; Pfefferbaum, Darley, Tinklenberg, Roth, & Kopell, 1977). This concern is particularly relevant to narcosynthesis or other techniques in which the therapist recreates the roles of people within the patient's traumatic memory in order to facilitate memory retrieval (Grinker & Spiegel, 1943, 1945). Further, the use of pharmacological agents, such as amytal, in narcosynthesis may produce amnesia for remembered information (Ghoneim, Hinrichs, & Mewaldt, 1984). Because patients may not fully recall information produced during narcosynthesis at later times (Grinker, 1944), narcosynthesis may be best viewed as an information-gathering procedure.

Once an individual has access to memories of the trauma, what can the patient–clinician dyad do with them to reduce the incidence of intrusive memories or flashbacks? Most patients are tormented by the intrusion of traumatic memories, and for these individuals, merely reviewing them an additional time is not necessarily therapeutic. Freud and Breuer (1953) initially suggested two strategies for reducing dissociative or conversion symptoms associated with hysteria: abreaction and the formation of new associations to the traumatic memories. By abreaction, Freud and Breuer meant the discharge, during therapy, of stored feelings that could not be adequately expressed at the time of the trauma. This hydraulic view of emotions has largely been abandoned (Krystal, 1978). Alternatively, modern cognitive, behavioral, and insight-oriented therapies focus on altering cognitive, affective, and identity-related associations to the trauma (Krystal, 1988; Keane et al., 1989; Foa, Steketee, Olasov, & Rothbaum, 1989). Psychotherapy may help to reduce the intrusiveness and distress related to traumatic memories by altering associations to the traumatic events, essentially changing the meaning of the trauma to the individual.

Managing the recollection of traumatic memories, dissociative states, and intense affects in patients is a tremendous clinical challenge facing the clinician treating PTSD. Guided reexperiencing of the trauma could evoke dissociative states that interfere with associative learning and interfere with generalizing therapeutic gains beyond the clinical setting. Intense emotions evoked during such recollections could reinforce the association between traumatic memories and intolerable intense emotions, sensitizing individuals to reminders, promoting a sense of helplessness or other negative appraisals of the trauma, and making the individual more reluctant or unable to review traumatic material in subsequent therapy sessions (Pitman et al., 1991). Further, by stimulating intense emotional responses and negative association in some individuals, flooding may exacerbate depression or provoke impulsive behavior, including substance abuse (Pitman et al., 1991). These potential problems help to explain the need for extensive relaxation training prior to the initiation of guided reexposure therapies, such as flooding (Keane et al., 1989). This step is probably a useful adjunct to all psychotherapies for PTSD patients (Hickling, Sison, & Vanderploeg, 1986). Further, one might predict that care must be taken to titrate the level of arousal associated with guided recollection of traumatic memories to the patient's capacity to process information. When, in the course of a therapy session, patients provide clinical data consistent with the induction of dissociative states, further efforts to encourage them to process traumatic material seem unlikely to be fruitful.

The concern that interference with higher cognitive functions limits the clinical utility of altered states of consciousness applies equally to proposed pharmacological adjuvants to psychotherapy such as the serotonergic hallucinogens (cf., Freedman, 1968) and NMDA antagonists (cf., Krystal et al., 1994a). Particularly in patients with chronic PTSD who have been in many years of treatment, there seems to be little benefit in guiding them to reexperience the trauma at the expense of repeated dissociative episodes. Carefully conducted flooding therapy, preceded by relaxation training, may reduce intrusive symptoms of PTSD, but have no beneficial impact on numbing or avoidance (Keane et al., 1989). These authors highlight significant psychological and social deficits that impair treatment response in patients with chronic PTSD. Thus, treatments aimed at reevaluating traumatic memories may have important, but focused, roles in their therapy. Also, research is needed to characterize optimal strategies for integrating pharmacotherapy approaches with these cognitive and behavioral psychotherapies.

If, analogous to relaxation training, pharmacological strategies were developed that preserved cognitive functions in the face of strong affects and traumatic memories, the formation of new associations to traumatic memories might proceed more effectively and rapidly. Benzodiazepines, reportedly useful in some PTSD symptoms in patients with dissociative disorders (Loewenstein, Hornstein, & Farber, 1988) might help by reducing the affective distress, although their amnestic properties might be counterproductive at high doses. Alternatively, one could evaluate pharmacological approaches to enhancing the cognitive processing. In this regard, drugs that facilitate NMDA receptor function via enhancement of the glycine site, such as cycloserine or milacemide (B. L. Schwartz, Hashtroudi, Herting,

Handerson, & Deutsch, 1991; Saletu et al., 1986), should be evaluated for anti-dissociative and other cognitive enhancing properties in PTSD patients.

Antidepressants are the best-studied pharmacotherapy for PTSD, and research suggests that they provide a moderate degree of relief from flashbacks and intrusive memories. Case reports suggest that tricyclic antidepressants may reduce flashbacks, night terrors, and distress related to intrusive memories of the trauma (Marshall, 1975; Burnstein, 1983). Similar findings have been reported in open label trials of monoamine oxidase inhibitors (Hogben & Cornfield, 1981; Lerer et al., 1987) and serotonin reuptake blockers (McDougle, Southwick, Charney, & St. James, 1991; Davidson, Roth, & Newman, 1991; Nagy, Morgan, Southwick, & Charney, 1993). Placebo-controlled trials of tricyclic antidepressants and monoamine oxidase inhibitors have supported the findings from the open label trials, although variability between studies and small effect sizes have limited the optimism regarding the efficacy of these agents (Kosten, Frank, Dan, McDougle, & Giller, 1991; Davidson et al., 1990; Reist et al., 1989; Lerer et al., 1987). The few studies that reported reexperiencing symptoms individually indicated that antidepressants were most effective in reducing the intrusion of traumatic memories and nightmares and less effective in reducing dissociative phenomena such as flashbacks and amnesia (Lerer et al., 1987; Nagy et al., 1993). The disparity between dissociative and other intrusive symptoms may indicate that antidepressants reduce flashbacks as a secondary consequence of the other effects of these drugs. One mechanism possibly related to the efficacy of these agents is their capacity to prevent or reduce the consequences of noradrenergic hyperreactivity in PTSD patients (Krystal et al., 1989). This hypothesis is consistent with the capacity of fluoxetine treatment to block yohimbine-induced panic attacks in patients with panic disorder (Goddard, Charney, Heinger, & Woods, 1990). The limited efficacy of agents based on monoaminergic transmission suggests that a new direction is need in the development of pharmacotherapies for dissociative disorders. This new direction may be based in the pharmacology of excitatory amino acid neurotransmission implicated in the genesis of dissociative states.

Carbamazepine has also shown utility in reducing hyperarousal, sleep disturbance, and flashbacks in some PTSD patients (Lipper et al., 1986). Despite limited investigation, carbamazepine has received particular attention due to its capacity to suppress a form of neural sensitization, kindling, that may provide a cellular model for the sensitization to repeated stressors (Post & Weiss, 1989). Further studies with anticonvulsant agents appear warranted.

Cognitive-enhancing pharmacotherapies, such as arginine vasopressin, have been suggested as treatments for memory deficits associated with PTSD (Pitman, 1988; Pitman et al., 1993). Cognitive-enhancing pharmacotherapeutic strategies might be beneficial in reducing encoding deficits associated with short-term memory impairment in PTSD patients. Drugs that might be evaluated for this purpose include ones that facilitate glutamate and acetylcholine function, such as the glycine partial agonist, cycloserine (Jones et al., 1991), and the cholinesterase inhibitor, tacrine (Davis et al., 1992). Vasopressin has been used to facilitate memory retrieval in patients with PTSD (Pitman, Orr, & Lasko, 1993), based on preclinical studies suggesting that vasopressin may enhance memory consolidation and retrieval in animals. However, the preclinical foundation of the vasopressin studies has been questioned because subsequent studies have suggested that the promnestic effects of exogenous administration of this hormone are attributable to its enhancement of arousal (Dawson, Heyes, & Iverson, 1992).

Cognitive-enhancing agents do not appear to be the appropriate pharmacotherapeutic approach for reducing amnesia for the trauma. As noted earlier, posttraumatic amnesia appears to arise from the suppression of retrieval rather than from an ongoing memory encoding deficit. There is no evidence to suggest that tacrine or cycloserine reduce the integrity of memory repression. Agents that do appear to facilitate the recollection of traumatic memories, such as lactate, yohimbine, vasopressin, and MCPP, appear to reduce posttraumatic amnesia via facilitating state-dependent retrieval. However, the sedative-hypnotic agents are the most commonly employed agents for this purpose, when combined with some form of guided recollection, such as the amytal interview.

IMPLICATIONS

Dissociative states have received relatively little attention from neurobiologists. However, the initial pharmacological challenge studies suggest that many neurotransmitter systems play important modulatory roles in the pathological development of dissociative states, as in PTSD. Glutamate systems are critically involved in cortical and limbic circuitry involved in sensory processing, attention regulation, and strategic memory retrieval. Recent studies, employing ketamine, suggest that deficits in NMDA receptor function may produce dissociationlike states in healthy individuals. Further characterization of the neurobiology of these functions may facilitate the development of antidissociative pharmacotherapies.

ACKNOWLEDGMENTS. This work was supported by funds from the Department of Veterans Affairs to the National Center for Posttraumatic Stress Disorder, the VA-Yale Alcoholism Research Center, and the Merit Review Grant Program (J.H.K.).

REFERENCES

Aggleton, J. P., Mishkin, M. (1984). Projection of the amygdala to the thalamus in the cynomologous monkey. *Journal of Comparative Neurology, 222*, 56-68.

Aggleton, J. P., Desimone, R., & Mishkin, M. (1986). The origin, course and termination of the hippocampothalamic projections in the macaque. *Journal of Comparative Neurology, 243*, 409-421.

American Psychiatric Association. (1987). *Diagnostic and statistical manual of mental disorders* (3rd ed., rev.). Washington, DC: Author.

Baddeley, A. D. (1986). *Working memory*. New York: Oxford University Press.

Baddeley, A., & Wilson, B. (1988). Frontal amnesia and the dysexecutive syndrome. *Brain and Cognition*, 7, 212-230.

Baldwin, M. (1960). Electrical stimulation of the mesial temporal region. In: E. R. Ramey & D. S. O'Doherty (Eds.), *Electrical studies on the unanesthetized brain* (pp. 159-176). New York: Hoeber.

Bartemeier, L. H., Kubie, L. S., Menninger, K. A., Romano, J., Whitehorn, J. C. (1946). Combat exhaustion. *Journal of Nervous and Mental Disease, 104*, 489-525.

Bench, C. J., Frith, C. D., Grasby, P. M., Friston, K. J., Paulesu, E., Frackowiak, R. S. J., & Dolan, R. J. (1993). Investigations of the functional anatomy of attention using the Stroop test. *Neuropsychologia, 31*, 907-922.

Bernstein, E., & Putnam, T. (1986). Development, reliability, and validity of a dissociation scale. *Journal of Nervous and Mental Disease, 174*, 727-735.

Bexton, W. H., Heron, W., & Scott, T. H. (1954). Effects of decreased variation in the sensory environment. *Canadian Journal of Psychology, 8*, 70-76.

Bremner, J. D., Southwick, S., Brett, E., Fontana, A., Rosenheck, R., & Charney, D. S. (1992). Dissociation and posttraumatic stress disorder in Vietnam combat veterans. *American Journal of Psychiatry, 149*, 328-332.

Bremner, J. D., Steinberg, M., Southwick, S. M., Johnson, D. R., & Charney, D. S. (1993). Use of the Structured Clinical Interview for DSM-IV Dissociative Disorders for systematic assessment of dissociative symptoms in posttraumatic stress disorder. *American Journal of Psychiatry, 150*, 1011-1014.

Bremner, J. D., Mazure, C. M., Putnam, F. W., Southwick, S. M., Marmar, C., Hansen, C., Lubin, H., Roach, L., Freeman, G., Krystal, J. H., & Charney, D. S. (In review). Measurement of dissociative states with the Clinician-Administered Dissociative States Scale (CADSS).

Briere, J., & Conte, J. (1993). Self-reported amnesia for abuse in adults molested as children. *Journal of Traumatic Stress, 6*, 21-31.

Bromberg, W. (1939). Marihuana: A psychiatric study. *Journal of the American Medical Association, 113*, 4-12.

Brown, R., & Kulik, J. (1977). Flashbulb memories. *Cognition, 5*, 73-99.

Burke, A., Heuer, F., & Reisberg, D. (1992). Remembering emotional events. *Memory and Cognition, 20*, 277-290.

Burnstein, A. T. (1983). Treatment of flashbacks by imipramine. *American Journal of Psychiatry, 140*, 509.

Buzsáki, G., Kennedy, B., Solt, V. B., & Ziegler, M. (1990). Noradrenergic control of thalamic oscillation: The role of $\alpha 2$ receptors. *European Journal of Neuroscience, 3*, 222-229.

Cappon, D., & Banks, R. (1960). Studies in perceptual distortion. *AMA Archives of Neurology and Psychiatry, 10*, 99-104.

Cappon, D., & Banks, R. (1961). Orientational perception: A review and preliminary study of distortion in orientational perception. *Archives of General Psychiatry, 5*, 380-392.

Carlson, E. B., & Putnam, F. W. (1989). Integrating research on dissociation and hypnotizability: Are there two pathways to hypnotizability? *Dissociation, 2*, 32-38.

Carlson, E. B., & Rosser-Hogan, R. (1991). Trauma experiences, posttraumatic stress, dissociation, and depression in Cambodian refugees. *American Journal of Psychiatry, 148*, 1548-1552.

Carlsson, M., & Carlsson, A. (1990). Schizophrenia: A subcortical neurotransmitter imbalance syndrome? *Schizophrenia Bulletin, 16*, 425-432.

Charney, D. S., Heninger, G. R., & Breier, A. (1984). Noradrenergic function in panic anxiety: Effects of yohimbine in healthy subjects and patients with agoraphobia and panic disorder. *Archives of General Psychiatry, 41*, 751-763.

Charney, D. S., Woods, S. W., Goodman, W. K., & Heninger, G. R. (1987). Serotonin function in anxiety. II. Effects of the serotonin agonist MCPP in panic disorder patients and healthy subjects. *Psychopharmacology, 92*, 14-24.

Charney, D. S., Deutch, A. Y., Krystal, J. H., Southwick, S. M., & Davis, M. (1993). Psychobiologic mechanisms of posttraumatic stress disorder. *Archives of General Psychiatry, 50*, 294-305.

Christianson, S. A., & Loftus, E. F. (1991). Remembering emotional events: The fate of detailed information. *Cognition and Emotion, 5*, 81-108.

Chu, J. A., & Dill, D. L. (1990). Dissociative symptoms in relation to childhood physical and sexual abuse. *American Journal of Psychiatry, 147*, 887-892.

Clugnet, M. C., & LeDoux, J. (1990). Synaptic plasticity in fear conditioning circuits: Induction of LTP in the lateral nucleus of the amygdala by stimulation of medial geniculate body. *Journal of Neuroscience, 10*, 2818-2824.

Cohen, B. D., Luby, E. D., Rosenbaum, G., & Gottlieb, J. S. (1960). Combined sernyl and sensory deprivation. *Comprehensive Psychiatry, 1*, 345-348.

Collins, G. G. S., & Anson, J. (1987). Effects of barbiturates on responses evoked by excitatory amino acids in slices of rat olfactory cortex. *Neuropharmacology*, *26*, 161-171.
Corssen, G., & Domino, E. F. (1966). Dissociative anesthesia: Further pharmacologic studies and first clinical experience with phencyclidine derivative CI-581. *Anesthesia and Analgesia*, *45*, 29-40.
Costa, E., & Guidotti, A. (1987). Neuropeptides as cotransmitters: Modulatory effects at GABAergic synapses. In H. Y. Meltzer (Ed.), *Psychopharmacology: The Third Generation of Progress* (pp. 425-435). New York: Raven Press.
Davidson, J. R. T., Kudler, H. S., Smith, R. D., Mahorney, S., Lipper, S., Hammett, E. B., Saunders, W. B., & Cavenar, J. O. (1990). Treatment of post traumatic stress disorder with amitriptylinie and placebo. *Archives of General Psychiatry*, *47*, 259-266.
Davidson, J., Roth, S., & Newman, E. (1991). Fluoxetine in post-traumatic stress disorder. *Journal of Traumatic Stress*, *4*, 419-423.
Davis, K. L., Thal, L. J., Gamzu, E. R., Davis, C. S., Woolson, R. F., Gracon, S. I., Drachman, D. A., Schneider, L. S., Whitehouse, P. J., Hoover, T. M., & The Tacrine Study Group. (1992). A double-blind, placebo-controlled multicenter study of tacrine for Alzheimer's disease. *New England Journal of Medicine*, *327*, 1253-1259.
Davis, M. (1992). The role of the amygdala in fear-potentiated startle: Implications for animal models of anxiety. *Trends in Pharmacological Sciences*, *13*, 35-41.
Dawson, G. R., Heyes, C. M., & Iverson, S. D. (1992). Pharmacological mechanisms and animal models of cognition. *Behavioral Pharmacology*, *3*, 285-297.
Dittrich, A., Battig, K., & von Zeppelin, I. (1973). Effects of $(-)\Delta^9$—*trans*-tetrahydrocannabinol (Δ^9-THC) on memory, attention and subjective state: A double blind study. *Psychopharmacology (Berlin)*, *33*, 369-376.
Domino, E. F., Chodoff, P., & Corssen, G. (1965). Pharmacologic effects of CI-581, a new dissociative anesthetic, in man. *Clinical Pharmacology and Therapeutics*, *6*, 279-291.
Dorow, R., Horowski, R., Paschelke, G., Amin, M., & Braestrup, C. (1983). Severe anxiety induced by FG7142, a β-carboline ligand for the benzodiazepine receptor. *Lancet*, *2*, 98-99.
Eldridge, J. C., & Landfield, P. W. (1990). Cannabinoid interactions with glucocorticoid receptors in rat hippocampus. *Brain Research*, *534*, 135-141.
Erickson, M. H. (1945). Hypnotic treatment techniques for the therapy of acute psychiatric disturbances in war. *American Journal of Psychiatry*, *101*, 668-672.
Feigenbaum, J. J., Bergmann, F., Richmond, S. A., Mechoulam, R., Nadler, V., Kloog, Y., & Sokolovsky, M. (1989). Nonpsychotropic cannabinoid acts as a functional *N*-methyl-D-aspartate receptor blocker. *Proceedings of the National Academy of Science USA*, *86*, 9584-9587.
Felder, C. C., Briley, E. M., Axelrod, J., Simpson, J. T., Mackie, K., & Devane, W. A. (1993). Anandamide, an endogenous cannabimmetic eicosanoid, binds to the cloned human cannabinoid receptor and stimulates receptor-mediated signal transduction. *Proceedings of the National Academy of Science USA*, *90*, 7656-7660.
Fisher, C. (1945). Amnesic states in war neurosis: The psychogenesis of fugues. *Psychoanalytic Quarterly*, *14*, 437-458.
Fisher, C., Byrne, J., Edwards, A., & Kahn, E. (1970). A psychophysiological study of nightmares. *Journal of the American Psychoanalytic Association*, *18*, 747-782.
Fisher, C., Kahn, E., Edwards, A., & Davis, D. M. (1973). A psychophysiological study of nightmares and nightterrors. I. Physiological aspects of the stage 4 night terror. *Journal of Nervous and Mental Disorders*, *157*, 75-98.
Fitzgerald, S. G., & Gonzalez, E. (1994). Dissociative states induced by relaxation training in a PTSD combat veteran: Failure to identify trigger mechanisms. *Journal of Traumatic Stress*, *7*, 111-116.
Foa, E. B., Steketee, G., & Olasov Rothbaum, B. (1989). Behavioral/cognitive conceptualizations of posttraumatic stress disorder. *Behavioral Therapeutics*, *20*, 155-176.
Freedman, D. X. (1968). On the use and abuse of LSD. *Archives of General Psychiatry*, *18*, 330-347.
Freedman, D. X. (1984). LSD: The bridge from human to animal. In B. L. Jacobs (Ed.), *Hallucinogens: Neurochemical, behavioral, and clinical perspectives* (pp. 203-226). New York, Raven Press.
Freud, S., & Breuer, J. (1953). On the psychical mechanism of hysterical phenomena. In E. Jones (Ed.), *Sigmund Freud, M.D., LL.D. Collected papers* (Vol. 1, pp. 24-41). London: Hogarth Press.
Gabriel, M., & Sparenborg, S. (1987). Posterior cingulate cortical lesions eliminate learning-related unit activity in the anterior cingulate cortex. *Brain Research*, *409*, 151-157.

Gabriel, M., Sparenborg, S. P., & Stolar, N. (1987). Hippocampal control of cingulate cortical and anterior thalamic information processing during learning in rabbits. *Experimental Brain Research, 67*, 131-152.

Gabriel, M., Vogt, B. A., Kubota, Y., Poremba, A., & Kang, E. (1991). Training-stage related neuronal plasticity in limbic thalamus and cingulate cortex during learning: A possible key to mnemonic retrieval. *Behavioral Brain Research, 46*, 175-185.

Gaffan, D., & Murray, E. A. (1990). Amygdalar interaction with the mediodorsal nucleus of the thalamus and the ventromedial prefrontal cortex in stimulus-reward associative learning in the monkey. *Journal of Neuroscience, 10*, 3479-3493.

Gaffan, D., Murray, E. A., & Fabre-Thorpe, M. (1993). Interaction of the amygdala with the frontal lobe in reward memory. *European Journal of Neuroscience, 5*, 968-975.

Geiselman, R. E., Bjork, R. A., & Fishman, D. L. (1983). Disrupted retrieval in directed forgetting: A link with posthypnotic amnesia. *Journal of Experimental Psychology, 112*, 58-72.

Geschwind, N. (1970). The organization of language and the brain. *Science, 170*, 940-944.

Geschwind, N. (1980). Neurological knowledge and complex behaviors. *Cognitive Science, 4*, 185-193.

Ghoneim, M. M., & Mewaldt, S. P. (1990). Benzodiazepines and human memory: A review. *Anesthesiology, 72*, 926-938.

Ghoneim, M. M., Hinrichs, J. V., & Mewaldt, S. P. (1984). Dose-response analysis of the behavioral effects of diazepam: I. learning and memory. *Psychopharmacology, 82*, 291-295.

Giguere, M., & Goldman-Rakic, P. S. (1988). Mediodorsal nucleus: Areal, laminar, and tangential distribution of afferents and efferents in the frontal lobe of Rhesus monkeys. *Journal of Comparative Neurology, 277*, 195-213.

Gloor, P., Olivier, A., Quesney, L. F., Andermann, F., & Horowitz, S. (1982). The role of the limbic system in experiential phenomena of temporal lobe epilepsy. *Annals of Neurology, 12*, 129-144.

Goddard, A., Charney, D. S., Heinger, G. R., & Woods, S. W. (1990). Effects of the 5-HT reuptake blocker on anxiety induced by yohimbinie. *Society of Neuroscience Abstracts, 16*, 1177.

Goldman-Rakic, P. S. (1987). Circuitry of primate prefrontal cortex and regulation of behavior by representational memory. In F. Plum (Ed.), *Handbook of physiology. Section I: Higher functions of the brain* (pp. 373-417). New York, Oxford University Press.

Goldman, Rakic, P. S., & Porrino, L. J. (1985). The primate mediodorsal (MD) nucleus and its projections to the frontal lobe. *Journal of Comparative Neurology, 242*, 535-560.

Greenberg, R., Pearlman, C. A., & Bampel, D. (1972). War neuroses and the adaptive function of REM sleep. *British Journal of Medical Psychology, 45*, 27-33.

Grinker, R. R. (1944). Treatment of war neuroses. *Journal of the American Medical Association, 126*, 142-145.

Grinker, R. R., & Spiegel, J. P. (1943). *War Neuroses in North Africa*. New York: Josiah Macy Jr Foundation.

Grinker, R. R., & Spiegel, J. P. (1945). *War neuroses*. Philadelphia: Blakiston.

Guilleminault, C., Quera-Salva, M.-A., & Goldberg, M. P. (1993). Pseudo-hypersomnia and pre-sleep behavior with bilateral paramedian thalamic lesions. *Brain, 116*, 1549-1563.

Hafez, A., Metz, L., & Lavie, P. (1987). Long-term effects of extreme situational stress on sleep and dreaming. *American Journal of Psychiatry, 144*, 344-347.

Halgren, E., Walter, R. D., Cherlow, D. G., & Crandall, P. H. (1978). Mental phenomena evoked by electrical stimulation of the human hippocampal formation and amygdala. *Brain, 101*, 83-117.

Heaton, R. K. (1975). Subject expectancy and environmental factors as determinants of psychedelic flashback experiences. *Journal of Nervous and Mental Disorders, 161*, 157-165.

Herkenham, M., Lynn, A. B., Little, M. D., Johnson, M. R., Melvin, L. S., De Costa, B. R., & Rice, K. C. (1990). Cannabinoid receptor localization in brain. *Proceedings of the National Academy of Science USA, 87*, 1932-1936.

Hermann, J. K., Perry, J., & van der Kolk, V. A. (1989). Childhood trauma in borderline personality disorder. *American Journal of Psychiatry, 148*, 490-495.

Hickling, E. J., Sison, G. F. P. Jr., & Vanderploeg, R. D. (1986). Treatment of posttraumatic stress disorder with relaxation and biofeedback training. *Biofeedback and Self Regulation, 11*, 125-134.

Hilgard, E. R. (1977). *Divided consciousness: Multiple controls in human thought and action*. New York: Wiley.

Hogben, G. L., & Cornfield, R. B. (1981). Treatment of war neurosis with phenelzine. *Archives of General Psychiatry, 38*, 440-445.

Hollister, L. E. (1986). Health aspects of cannabis. *Pharmacological Reviews, 38*, 2-20.

Horowitz, M. J. (1969). Flashbacks: Recurrent intrusive images after the use of LSD. *American Journal of Psychiatry, 126*, 565-569.

Horowitz, M. J., Adams, J. E., & Rutkin, B. B. (1968). Visual imagery on brain stimulation. *Archives of General Psychiatry, 19*, 469-486.

Jackson, A., Koek, W., & Colpaert, F. C. (1992). NMDA antagonists make learning and recall state-dependent. *Behavioral Pharmacology, 3*, 415-421.

Janet, P. (1889). *Automatisme psychologique*. Paris: Balliere.

Javitt, D. C., & Zukin, S. R. (1991). Recent advances in the phencyclidine model of schizophrenia. *American Journal of Psychiatry, 148*, 1301-1308.

Jones, R. W., Wesnes, K. A., & Kirby, J. (1991). Effects of NMDA modulation in scopolamine dementia. *Annals of the New York Academy of Science, 640*, 241-244.

Kales, J. D., Kales, A., Soldatos, C. R., Caldwell, A. B., Charney, D. S., & Martin, E. D. (1980). Night terrors: Clinical characteristics and personality patterns. *Archives of General Psychiatry, 37*, 1413-1417.

Kardiner, A. (1941). *The traumatic neuroses of war*. Psychosomatic Monograph II-III. Washington, DC: National Research Council.

Kardiner, A., & Spiegel, H. (1947). *War stress and neurotic illness*. New York, Hoeber.

Keane, T. M., Fairbank, J. A., Caddell, J. M., & Zimering, R. T. (1989). Implosive (flooding) therapy reduces symptoms of PTSD in Vietnam combat veterans. *Behavior Therapy, 20*, 245-260.

Kirk, T., Roache, J. D., & Griffiths, R. R. (1990). Dose-response evaluation of the amnestic effects of triazolam and pentobarbital in normal subjects. *Journal of Clinical Psychopharmacology, 10*, 160-167.

Klee, G. D. (1963). Lysergic acid diethylamide (LSD-25) and ego functions. *Archives of General Psychiatry, 8*, 57-70.

Kluft, R. F. (1987). An update on multiple personality disorder. *Hospital and Community Psychiatry, 38*, 363-373.

Kosten, T. R., & Krystal, J. H. (1988). Biological mechanisms in post traumatic stress disorder: Relevance for substance abuse. In M. Galanter (Ed.), *Recent developments in alcoholism* (Vol. 6, pp. 49-68). New York: Plenum Press.

Kosten, T. R., Frank, J. B., Dan, E., McDougle, C. J., & Giller, E. L. Jr. (1991). Pharmacotherapy for posttraumatic stress disorder using phenelzine or imipramine. *Journal of Nervous and Mental Disorders, 179*, 366-370.

Kramer, T. H., Buckhout, R., & Eugenio, P. (1990). Weapon focus, arousal, and eyewitness memory: Attention must be paid. *Law and Human Behavior, 14*, 167-184.

Krystal, H. (1968). *Massive psychic trauma*. New York: International Universities Press.

Krystal, H. (1978). Trauma and affects. *Psychoanalytic Study of the Child, 33*, 81-116.

Krystal, H. (1988). *Integration and self-healing: Affect, trauma, alexithymia*. Hillsdale, NY: Analytic Press.

Krystal, J. H., Woods, S. W., Hill, C. L., & Charney, D. S. (1988). Characteristics of self-defined panic attacks. In *1988 new research program and abstracts*. Washington, DC: American Psychiatric Association.

Krystal, J. H., Kosten, T. R., Perry, B. D., Southwick, S., Mason, J. W., & Giller, E. L. Jr. (1989). Neurobiological aspects of PTSD: Review of clinical and preclinical studies. *Behavior Therapy, 20*, 177-198.

Krystal, J. H., Woods, S. W., Hill, C. L., & Charney, D. S. (1991). Characteristics of panic attack subtypes: Assessment of spontaneous panic, situational panic, sleep panic, and limited symptom attacks. *Comprehensive Psychiatry, 32*.

Krystal, J. H., Karper, L. P., Seibyl, J. P., Freeman, G. K., Delaney, R., Bremner, J. D., Heninger, G. R., Bowers, M. B. Jr., & Charney, D. S. (1994a). Subanesthetic effects of the NMDA antagonist, ketamine, in humans: Psychotomimetic, perceptual, cognitive, and neuroendocrine effects. *Archives of General Psychiatry, 51*, 199-214.

Krystal, J. H., Karper, L. P., Bennett, A., Abi-Dargham, A., D'Souza, D. C., Gil, R., Charney, D. S. (1994b). Modulation of frontal cortical function by glutamate and dopamine antagonists in healthy subjects and schizophrenic patients: A neuropsychological perspective. Neuropsychopharmacology *10*(3S), 230S.

Krystal, J. H., Bennett, A., Bremner, J. D., Southwick, S. M., & Charney, D. S. (in press). Toward a cognitive neuroscience of dissociation and altered memory functions in post-traumatic stress disorder. In M. Friedman, D. S. Charney, & A. Y. Deutch (Eds.), *Neurobiological consequences of stress from adaptation to PTSD*. New York: Raven Press.

Krystal, J. H., Karper, L. P., D'Souza, D. C., Morrissey, K., Bennett, A., Abi-Dargham, A., Bremner, J. D., Heninger, G. R., Bowers, M. B., Charney, D. S. (in review). Interactive effects of subanesthetic ketamine and lorazepam in humans: Psychotomimetic, dissociative, cognitive, and neuroendocrine responses.

Laplane, D., Degos, J. D., Baulac, M., & Gray, F. (1981). Bilateral infarction of the anterior cingulate gyri and the fornices. Report of a case. *Journal of the Neurological Sciences*, *51*, 289-300.

Laurence, J.-R., & Perry, C. (1983). Hypnotically created memory among highly hypnotizable subjects. *Science*, *222*, 423-524.

Lavie, P., & Hertz, G. (1979). Increased sleep motility and respiration rates in combat neurotic patients. *Biological Psychiatry*, *14*, 983-987.

LeDoux, J. E. (1987). Emotion. In F. Plum (Ed.), *Handbook of physiology: The nervous system V*. (pp. 419-459). Washington, DC: American Physiological Society.

LeDoux, J. E., & Farb, C. R. (1991). Neurons of the acoustic thalamus that project to the amygdala contain glutamate. *Neuroscience Letters*, *134*, 145-149.

Lerer, B., Bleich, A., Kotler, M., Garb, R., Hertzberg, M., & Levin, B. (1987). Post-traumatic stress disorder in Israeli combat veterans: Effect of phenelzine treatment. *Archives of General Psychiatry*, *44*, 976-981.

Lewis, D. A., Hayes, T. L., Lund, J. S., & Oeth, K. M. (1992). Dopamine and the neural circuitry of primiate prefrontal cortex: Implications for schizophrenia research. *Neuropsychopharmacology*, *6*, 127-134.

Liebert, R. S., Werner, H., & Wapner, S. (1958). Studies on the effects of lysergic acid diethylamide (LSD-25). *AMA Archives of Neurology and Psychiatry*, *79*, 580-584.

Lilly, J. C. (1956). Mental effects of reduction of ordinary levels of physical stimuli on intact healthy persons. *Psychiatry Research Reports*, *5*, 1-9.

Lipper, S., Davidson, J. R. T., Grady, T. A., Edinger, J., Hammett, E. B., Mahorney, S. L., & Cavenar, J. O. (1986). Preliminary study of carbamazepine in post traumatic stress disorder. *Psychosomatics*, *27*, 849-854.

Llinás, R. R., & Paré, D. (1991). Of dreaming and wakefulness. *Neuroscience*, *44*, 521-535.

Loewenstein, R. J., & Putnam, F. (1988). A comparison study of dissociative symptoms in patients with partial-complex seizures, MPD, and PTSD. *Dissociation*, *1*, 17-23.

Loewenstein, R. J., Hornstein, N., & Farber, B. (1988). Open trial of clonzaepam in the treatment of posttraumatic stress symptoms in multiple personality disorder. *Dissociation*, *1*, 3-12.

Luby, E. D., Cohen, B. D., Rosenbaum, G., Gottlieb, J. S., & Kelley, R. (1959). Study of a new schizophrenomimteic drug—sernyl. *AMA Archives of Neurology and Psychiatry*, *81*, 363-369.

Ludwig, A. M. (1972). "Psychedelic" effects produced by sensory overload. *American Journal of Psychiatry*, *128*, 1294-1297.

Mahowald, M. W., & Schenck, C. H. (1991). Status dissociatus a perspective on states of being. *Sleep*, *14*, 69-79.

Marshall, J. R. (1975). The treatment of night terrors associated with the posttraumatic syndrome *American Journal of Psychiatry*, *132*, 293-295.

Mayer-Gross, W. (1935). On depersonalization. *British Journal of Medical Psychology*, *15*, 103-126.

McCormick, D. A. (1992). Neurotransmitter actions in the thalamus and cerebral cortex and their role in the neuromodulation of thalamocortical activity. *Progress in Neurobiology*, *39*, 337-388.

McCormick, D. A., & Wang, Z. (1991). Serotonin and noradrenaline excite GABAergic neurones of the guinea pig and cat nucleus reticularis thalami. *Journal of Physiology*, *442*, 235-255.

McDonald, A. J. (1982). Organization of amygdaloid projections to the mediodorsal thalamus and prefrontal cortex: A fluorescence retrograde transports study in the rat. *Journal of Comparative Neurology*, *62*, 46-58.

McDougle, C. J., & Southwick, S. M. (1990). Emergence of an alternate personality in combat-related posttraumatic stress disorder. *Hospital and Community Psychiatry*, *41*, 554-556.

McDougle, C. J., & Southwick, S. M., Charney, D. S., & St. James, R. L. (1991). An open trial of fluoxetine in the treatment of posttraumatic stress disorder. *Journal of Clinical Psychopharmacology, 11*, 325-327.

McGee, R. (1984). Flashbacks and memory phenomena: A comment on "flashback phenomena—clinical and diagnostic dilemmas. *Journal of Nervous and Mental Disorders, 172*, 273-278.

Melges, F. T., Tinklenberg, J. R., Hollister, L. E., & Gillespie, H. K. (1970). Temporal disintegration and depersonalization during marihuana intoxication. *Archives of General Psychiatry, 23*, 204-210.

Mellman, T. A., & Davis, G. C. (1985). Combat-related flashbacks in post-traumatic stress disorder: Phenomenology and similarity to panic attacks. *Journal of Clinical Psychiatry, 46*, 379-382.

Morgan, W. W., Bermudez, J., & Chang, X. (1991). The relative potency of pentobarbital in suppressing the kainic acid or the *N*-methyl-D-aspartic acid-induced enhancement of cGMP in cerebellar cells. *European Journal of Pharmacology, 204*, 335-338.

Moscovitch, M. (1989). Confabulation and the frontal systems: Strategic versus associative retrieval in neuropsychological theories of memory. In H. L. Roediger III & F. M. Craik (Eds.), *Varieties of memory and consciousness: Essays in honour of Endel Tulving* (pp. 133-160). Hillsdale, NJ: Lawrence Erlbaum.

Moscovitch, M. (1992). Memory and working-with-memory: A component process model based on modules and central system. *Journal of Cognitive Neuroscience, 4*, 257-267.

Nagy, L. M., Morgan, C. A. III, Southwick, S. M., & Charney, D. S. (1993). Open prospective trial of fluoxetine for posttraumatic stress disorder. *Journal of Clinical Psychopharmacology, 13*, 107-113.

Nicholls, D. G. (1993). The glutamatergic nerve terminal. *European Journal of Biochemistry, 212*, 613-631.

Olsen, R. W. (1981). GABA-benzodiazepine-barbiturate receptor interactions. *Journal of Neurochemistry, 37*, 1-13.

Orona, E., & Gabriel, M. (1983). Multiple-unit activity of the prefrontal cortex and mediodorsal thalamic nucleus during acquisition of discriminative avoidance behavior in rabbits. *Brain Research, 263*, 295-312.

Oswald, I., & Evans, J. (1985). On serious violence during sleep-walking. *British Journal of Psychiatry, 147*, 688-691.

Paller, K. A. (1990). Recall and stem-completion priming have different electrophysiological correlates and are modified differentially by directed forgetting. *Journal of Experimental Psychology, 16*, 1021-1032.

Pardo, J. V., Pardo, P. J., Janer, K. W., & Raichle, M. E. (1990). The anterior cingulate cortex mediates processing selection in the Stroop attentional conflict paradigm. *Proceedings of the National Academy of Science USA, 87*, 256-259.

Penfield, W., & Perot, P. (1963). The brain's record of auditory and visual experience. A final summary and discussion. *Brain, 86*, 595-696.

Pfefferbaum, A., Darley, C. F., Tinklenberg, J. R., Roth, W. T., & Kopell, B. S. (1977). Marijuana and memory intrusions. *Journal of Nervous and Mental Disorders, 165*, 381-386.

Pitman, R. K. (1988). Posttraumatic stress disorder, conditioning and network theory. *Psychiatric Annals, 18*, 182-189.

Pitman, R. K., Altman, B., Greenwald, E., Longpre, R. E., Macklin, M. L., Poire, R. E., & Steketee, G. S. (1991). Psychiatric complications during flooding therapy for posttraumatic stress disorder. *Journal of Clinical Psychiatry, 52*, 17-20.

Pitman, R. K., Orr, S. P., & Lasko, N. B. (1993). Effects of intranasal vasopressin and oxytocin on physiologic responding during personal combat imagery in Vietnam veterans with posttraumatic stress disorder. *Psychiatry Research, 48*, 107-117.

Pitts, F. N., & McClure, J. N. (1967). Lactate metabolism in anxiety neurosis. *New England Journal of Medicine, 277*, 1329-1336.

Post, R. M., & Weiss, S. R. B. (1989). Sensitization, kindling, and anticonvulsants in mania. *Journal of Clinical Psychiatry, 59*(suppl.), 23-30.

Putnam, F. W., Guroff, J. J., Silberman, E. K., Barban, L., & Post, R. M. (1986). The clinical phenomenology of multiple personality disorder: Review of 100 recent cases. *Journal of Clinical Psychiatry, 47*, 285-293.

Rainey, J. M. Jr., Aleem, A., Ortiz, A., Yeragani, V., Pohl, R., & Berchou, R. (1987). A laboratory procedure for the induction of flashbacks. *American Journal of Psychiatry, 144*, 1317-1319.

Randall, P. K., Bremner, J. D., Krystal, J. H., Heninger, G. R., Nicolaou, A. L., & Charney, D. S. (In press). Effects of the benzodiazepine antagonist, flumazenil, in PTSD. *Biological Psychiatry*. in review.

Rasmussen, K., Glennon, R. A., & Aghajanian, G. K. (1986). Phenethylamine hallucinogens in the locus coeruleus: Potency of action correlates with rank order of 5-HT_2 binding affinity. *European Journal of Pharmacology, 132*, 79-82.

Reist, C., Kauffmann, C. D., Haier, R. J., Sangdahl, C., DeMet, E. M., Chicz-DeMet, A., & Nelson, J. N. (1989). A controlled trial of desipramine in 18 men with posttraumatic stress disorder. *American Journal of Psychiatry, 146*, 513-516.

Rodin, E., & Luby, E. (1966). Effects of LSD-25 on the EEG and photic evoked responses. *Archives of General Psychiatry, 14*, 435-441.

Rosen, H., & Myers, H. J. (1947). Abreaction in the military setting. *AMA Archives of Neurology and Psychiatry, 57*, 161-172.

Sacks O. (1985). *The man who mistook his wife for a hat*. New York: Summitt Books.

Saletu, B., Grüberg, J., & Linzmayer, L. (1986). Acute and subacute CNS effects of milacemide in elderly people: Double-blind placebo-controlled quntitateive EEG and psychometric investigations. *Archives of Generontology and Geriatrics, 5*, 165-181.

Salloway, S., Southwick, S., & Sadowsky, M. (1990). Opiate withdrawal presenting as posttraumatic stress disorder: A case of malingering following the L'Ambiance Plaza Building disaster. *Hospital and Community Psychiatry, 41*, 666-667.

Sargent, W., & Slater, E. (1940). Acute war neuroses. *Lancet, 2*, 1-2.

Savage, C. (1955). Variations in ego feeling induced by D-lysergic acid diethylamide (LSD-25). *Psychoanalytic Review, 42*, 1-16.

Schwartz, B. L., Hashtroudi, S., Herting, R. L., Hnaderson, H., & Deutsch, S. I. (1991). Glycine prodrug facilitates memory retrieval in humans. *Neurology, 41*, 1341-1343.

Schwartz, M. L., Dekker, J. J., & Goldman-Rakic, P. S. (1991). Dual mode of corticothalamic synaptic termination in the mediodorsal nucleus of the rhesus monkey. *Journal of Comparative Neurology, 309*, 289-304.

Shapiro, M. L., & O'Connor, C. (1992). *N*-methyl-D-aspartate receptor antagonist MK-801 and spatial memory representation: Working memory is impaired in an unfamiliar environment but not in a familiar environment. *Behavioral Neuroscience, 106*, 604-612.

Sheldon, P. W., & Aghajanian, G. K. (1991). Excitatory responses to serotonin (5-HT) in neurons of the rat piriform cortex: Evidence for mediation by 5-HT_{1C} receptors in pyramidal cells and 5-HT_2 receptors in interneurons. *Synapse, 9*, 208-218.

Southwick, S. M., Krystal, J. H., Morgan, A., Nagy, L. M., Dan, E., Johnson, D., Bremner, D., & Charney, D. S. (1991). Yohimbine and *m*-chlorophenylpiperazine in PTSD. *1991 new research program and abstracts: American Psychiatric Association, 144th annual meeting*.

Southwick, S. M., Krystal, J. H., Morgan, C. A., Johnson, D. R., Nagy, L. M., Nicolau, A., Heninger, G. R., & Charney, D. S. (1993). Abnormal noradrenergic function in post traumatic stress disorder. *Archives of General Psychiatry, 50*, 266-274.

Spiegel, D., & Cardeña, E. (1991). Disintegrated experience: The dissociative disorders revisited. *Journal of Abnormal Psychology, 100*, 366-378.

Spiegel, D., Hunt, T., & Dondershine, H. E. (1988). Dissociation and hypnotizability in posttraumatic stress disorder. *American Journal of Psychiatry, 145*, 301-305.

Stanton, M. D., Mintz, J., & Franklin, R. M. (1976). Drug flashbacks. II. Some additional findings. *International Journal of Addiction, 11*, 53-69.

Starke, K., Borowski, E., & Endo, T. (1975). Preferential blockade of presynaptic α-adrenoceptors by yohimbine. *European Journal of Pharmacology, 34*, 385-388.

Steriade, M., & Deschenes, M. (1984). The thalamus as a neuronal oscillator. *Brain Research Review, 8*, 1-63.

Steriade, M., & Llinás, R. R. (1988). The functional states of the thalamus and the associated neuronal interplay. *Physiological Reviews, 68*, 649-741.

Steriade, M., & McCarley, R. W. (1990). *Brainstem control of wakefulness and sleep*. New York: Plenum Press.

Steriade, M., Datta, S., Paré, D., Oakson, G., & Curró Dossi, R. (1990). Neuronal activities in brain-stem cholinergic nuclei related to tonic activation in thalamocortical systems. *Journal of Neuroscience, 19*, 2541-2559.

Stuss, D. T. (1992). Biological and psychological development of executive function. *Brain and Cognition, 20*, 8-23.

Swanson, L. W. (1981). A direct projection from Ammon's horn to prefrontal cortex in the rat. *Brain Research, 21*, 150-154.

Taylor, J. (Ed.). (1931). *Selected writings of John Hughlings Jackson on epilepsy and epileptiform convulsions*. London: Hodder and Stroughton.

Titeler, M., Lyon, R. A., & Glennon, R. A. (1988). Radioligand binding evidence implicates the brain 5-HT_2 receptor as a site of action for LSD and phenylisopropylamine hallucinogens. *Psychopharmacology, 94*, 213-216.

Turner, B. H., & Herkenham, M. (1991). Thalamoamygdaloid projections in the rat: A test of the amygdala's role in sensory processing. *Journal of Comparative Neurology, 313*, 295-325.

van der Kolk, B., Blitz, R., Burr, W., Sherry, S., & Hartmann, E. (1984). Nightmares and trauma: A comparison of nightmares after combat with lifelong nightmares in veterans. *American Journal of Psychiatry, 141*, 187-190.

van der Kolk, B., Greenberg, M., Boyd, H., & Krystal, J. (1985). Inescapable shock, neurotransmitters, and addiction to trauma: Toward a psychobiology of posttraumatic stress. *Biological Psychiatry, 20*, 314-325.

Vogt, B. A., Rosene, D. L., & Pandya, D. N. (1979). Thalamic and cortical afferents differentiate anterior from posterior cingulate cortex in the monkey. *Science, 204*, 205-207.

Whitty, C. W. M., & Lewin, W. (1957). Vivid day-dreaming an usual form of confusion following anterior cingulectomy. *Brain, 80*, 72-76.

Wilson, F. A. W., Scalaidhe, S. P. O., & Goldman-Rakic, P. S. (1993). Dissociation of object and spatial processing domains in primate prefrontal cortex. *Science, 260*, 1955-1958.

Woods, S. W., Charney, D. S., Silver, J. M., Krystal, J. H., & Heninger, G. R. (1991). Benzodiazepine receptor responsivity in panic disorder. II. Behavioral, biochemical, and cardiovascular responses to the benzodiazepine receptor antagonist flumazenil. *Psychiatry Research, 36*, 115-127.

Yamakura, T., Mori, H., Masaki, H., Shimoji, K., & Mishina, M. (1993). Different sensitivities of NMDA receptor channel subtypes to non-competitive antagonists. *Neuroreport, 4*, 687-690.

9

Hypnosis and Dissociation

Theoretical, Empirical, and Clinical Perspectives

Jonathan E. Whalen and Michael R. Nash

The term *association* is used to describe the binding or linking together of ideas. For over a century now, it has been invoked to explain various aspects of learning, attitude change, and motivation (Skinner, 1953; Watson, 1930). In the later part of the nineteenth century, Janet described an opposing phenomenon of the separation of certain mental operations from the main body of consciousness with various degrees of autonomy (West, 1967). He termed this symptomatology *desagregation* (translated from the French as disaggregation), later referred to as dissociation. Since the inception of dynamic psychiatry and experimental psychopathology in the late nineteenth century, spontaneously occurring dissociative symptomatology has been linked to hypnosis, with theorists positing the two phenomena to have similar (and sometimes even identical) psychic mechanisms.

ARGUMENTS FAVORING HYPNOSIS–DISSOCIATION LINKAGE

Before we can meaningfully explore how clinical theorists have struggled with the relationship between hypnosis and dissociation, we must understand what moved them to do so. The answer is straightforward. Four fundamental observations concerning hypnosis and dissociation have been noted by researchers and clinicians from Puysegur, Braid, Charcot, and Bernheim to Freud, Pavlov, E. R. Hilgard, and Fromm. Together, these four observations pose an intriguing possibility, one that was not lost on the earliest investigators of abnormal psychology

---

Jonathan E. Whalen and Michael R. Nash • Department of Psychology, University of Tennessee at Knoxville, Knoxville, Tennessee 37996.

Handbook of Dissociation: Theoretical, Empirical, and Clinical Perspectives, edited by Larry K. Michelson and William J. Ray. Plenum Press, New York, 1996.

(e.g., Charcot, Janet, Prince, Freud, and Sidis)—that by understanding hypnosis we may better understand dissociative pathology.

1. *Phenotypic similarities*. During hypnotic trance, behavioral and experiential phenomena characteristic of dissociation can be elicited in nonsymptomatic subjects. When otherwise nonsymptomatic subjects are hypnotized, they can elicit a host of behavioral and experiential phenomena characteristic of dissociative pathology. Hypnotic alterations in perception and sensation (hallucinations, time sense distortion, anesthesia, deafness, blindness, anosmia), cognition (amnesia, depersonalization, derealization), emotion (rage, lability, depression, anxiety), and behavior (compulsions, automatic writing, impulsivity) are quite common, even in the relatively neutral context of the experimental laboratory. These functional aberrations associated with a dissociative disorder and those associated with hypnosis are indeed alike in that they generally do not conform to patterns of organic illness that might otherwise explain the shift in function or experience (head injury, damage to peripheral nervous system, intoxication states) (see Blum, Porter, & Geiwitz, 1978; Grosz & Zimmerman, 1965; Loomis, Harvey, & Hobart, 1936; Pattie, 1935; Theodor & Mandelcorn, 1973). In addition, there is some reason to believe that, at least in the case of generalized sensory-based symptoms, hypnotically induced functional aberrations are behaviorally and cognitively similar to their dissociative disorder counterparts, and dissimilar to organically based disease (Malmo, Boag, & Raginsky, 1954; Sackheim, Nordlie, & Gur, 1979).

2. *Hypnosis as an effective treatment*. Another argument for a shared underlying process linking hypnosis and psychopathology has been the long and well-documented record of hypnosis as an agent of cure for many types of mental disorders over two centuries of clinical practice, especially dissociative disorders. Claims have sometimes been exaggerated, but there remains a solid and respectable research literature that supports the general clinical efficacy of hypnosis (Beutler, 1979; Deabler, Fidel, Dillenkoffer, & Elder, 1973; DePiano & Salzberg, 1979; Friedman & Taub, 1978; Scagnelli-Jobsis, 1982; Wadden & Anderton, 1982). It seems reasonable that if an intervention can alter or even cure debilitating symptoms, then it probably affects whatever process underlies the symptoms. Though reasonable, the logic of this argument is not without flaw. Even if it can be shown that hypnosis is indeed an especially efficacious therapeutic modality in cases of dissociative disorder, there are many ameliorative interventions in general medicine that may have only obscure and very limited relevance to the essential features of the disease process (e.g., aspirin for headaches). Still, the clinical efficacy of hypnosis in treating dissociative disorders is highly touted among many practitioners who contend that hypnosis itself is an essential underlying feature of the dissociative disorder.

3. *Subjective similarities*. "Time stood still," "I felt dazed," "Everything happened automatically," "Sometimes I did not know where I was," "Things seemed unreal," "Parts of my body moved without my conscious assistance," "I felt uninhibited": statements like these (taken form Field's Scale of Hypnotic Depth; Field, 1965) indicate a striking similarity between normal hypnotic subjective experiences and dissociative subjective experiences. Many theorists have noted these similarities and hypothesized that spontaneously occurring self-hypnosis episodes

are the root source of various pathological states such as anxiety, conversions, and so forth (Breuer & Freud, 1893-1895/1955; Frankel, 1974; Janet, 1919/1925; Spiegel & Spiegel, 1978).

4. *Common traumagenic etiology for hypnotizability and dissociation*. An association between early sexual trauma and dissociative states has been posited since the nineteenth century. Freud (1893/1959, 1900/1953), Janet (1889), and Prince (1906) believed that dissociative states resulted from defensive processes arrayed against the experiences of sexual trauma.

Modern researchers contend that early trauma engenders the repeated use of dissociative techniques, resulting in dramatic alterations in experiences of self and environment; experiences highly similar to hypnotic experiences (Frischholz, 1985a; Kluft, 1987; Putnam, 1985; Spiegel, Hunt, & Dondershine, 1988). Indeed, Bliss (1984), Frischholz (1985b), and Spiegel (1986), among others, argue that hypnotizability levels are sensitive indices of dissociation, and thus reliable markers of pathology presumably rooted in trauma.

Early Theoretical Formulations of the Hypnosis–Dissociation Link

Taken together, these four observations are as difficult to ignore now as they were 100 years ago at La Salpetriere. The similarities between hypnosis and certain forms of psychopathology, along with the clinical efficacy of hypnosis, seem to be valid and highly suggestive of shared processes. Many explanations of these four key observations have been offered by clinical theorists since Charcot began his work on hysteria in the 1870s.

First, Janet (1919/1925) understood most psychopathology and all genuine hypnosis to be manifestations of a common process—dissociation; under special circumstances, certain ideas, motives, sensations, and memories operate outside of conscious awareness. These fixed ideas can function quite automatically via amnesic barriers separating clusters of perceptual-cognitive activity from one another. Janet's ideas lost currency for several reasons most thoroughly reviewed by Ellenberger (1970). Experiments failed to support the idea that dissociated tasks could be so completely separated that they would not, and could not, interfere with one another (White & Shevach, 1942). Furthermore, in the first quarter of the twentieth century, the mushrooming of interest in psychoanalysis obscured Janet's important work.

Second, Freud was acutely interested in hypnosis and its relationship to psychopathology, especially hysteria. In an early work coauthored with his mentor, Josef Breuer (Breuer & Freud, 1893-1895/1955), Freud theorized that symptoms of hysteria were actually manifestations of self-induced "hypnoid states" brought about by the threatened eruption of early traumatic memories into awareness and the subsequent conversion (expression) of these memories in the somatic or functional sphere. In this very early Freudian formulation, the underlying process shared by hypnosis and hysteria was a "splitting off" of certain mental contents from the mainstream of awareness. Therapy then was curative to the extent that the therapist could exploit the ability of hypnosis to isolate and focus on the somatically expressed yet profoundly repressed affect-laden memories. Hypnotherapy sessions with these patients were often very dramatic, with violent explosions of emotion when the original memories surfaced; these were then followed by symptom relief. Later, Freud came to view both hypnosis and psychopathology from a more developmental perspective, with psychopathology and hypnosis representing a return to earlier modes of psychological functioning and relating (Freud 1917/1957).

CONTEMPORARY FORMULATIONS

There are two contemporary theoretical traditions that attempt to explain a link between hypnosis and dissociation: one evolving from the early clinical work with dissociative disordered patients and one evolving from cognitive psychology. Most contemporary clinical theorists studying multiple personality disorder (MPD), and other dissociative disorders, focus on the etiologic role of early trauma. They have adopted models similar to that of Breuer and Freud (Breuer & Freud, 1893-1895/1955), contending that early childhood trauma leads to repeated overuse of dissociation until it becomes the individual's primary psychological defense, manifesting itself in dramatic alterations in the experience of self and world (Frischholtz, 1985b; Kluft, 1987; Putnam, 1985; Spiegel et al., 1988). Based on a wealth of clinical observation, these models define a causal continuity between trauma in childhood and subsequent adult symptoms. What is so appealing about these traumagenic models of psychopathology is that they also chart a sure course for treatment, involving a therapeutic regression to the developmental stage in question, reemergence of long repressed (or dissociated) memories, and gradual resumption of development from that point.

The second theoretical tradition positing an underlying shared process in hypnosis and dissociation is the neodissociation theory of Ernest Hilgard's (1992). By bringing the study of consciousness back into the mainstream of scientific inquiry, Hilgard has revitalized the concept of dissociation and spawned vigorous experimental and clinical interest in the related phenomena of absorption, imaginative involvement, fantasy proneness, and dissociative disorders (Hilgard, 1979a; Tellegen & Atkinson, 1974; Lynn & Rhue, 1986; Bliss, 1984). Hilgard notes that both hypnotic and dissociative pathological states are characterized by intense absorption, amnesias, cognitive inconsistencies, and experience of involuntariness. He postulates a hierarchical system of cognitive control such that the relationship between the higher executive levels and actual behavior become transiently disconnected. Thus behaviors are experienced as involuntary by the hypnotic subject (e.g., "My arm got quite heavy and began to move down by itself").

From this theoretical perspective, the logic of a hypnosis-dissociation link is as follows: Dissociative psychopathology is characterized by intense absorption, amnesias, fantasy proneness, automatism, depersonalization, and cognitive inconsistencies. Since these same phenomena figure so prominently in hypnosis, a propensity for spontaneous self-hypnosis may underlie dissociative disorders. If true, then patients suffering from these disorders should test as more hypnotizable than control individuals.

THE RESEARCH EVIDENCE

Clinical observation and theoretical formulations strongly suggest some kind of relationship between hypnosis and dissociation. We now examine the empirical evidence for such a link. If hypnosis and dissociative disorders do indeed share important underlying psychic mechanisms, three core findings should obtain across clinical and nonclinical samples. First, if the trait of dissociativity captures something essential about the trait of hypnotizability, then these two abilities should be positively correlated, with highly hypnotizables also being highly dissociative (overlapping traits). Second, if hypnosis and dissociativity share common developmental pathways involving trauma, then a history of trauma should be associated with increased hypnotizability and increased dissociativity (common etiology). Third, if hypnosis captures some essential pathological feature of dissociative disorders, it may be especially effective in the treatment of these disorders (clinical efficacy). Below we examine the empirical evidence regarding each of these questions.

Hypnotizability and Dissociativity as Overlapping Traits

If measures of hypnotizability and dissociativity can be shown to positively correlate, we have then demonstrated that the two traits share some important feature(s). Other chapters in the present volume adequately describe the various self-report scales used to index an individual's dissociativity. However, measurement of hypnotic susceptibility involves a radically different procedure. Before we examine the empirical findings on the question of covariation between hypnotizability and dissociativity, we first must describe how hypnosis is measured and the nature of hypnotic susceptibility in general.

Observations that people differ in their general level of responsiveness to hypnotic procedures date back to the eighteenth century. Attempts to measure hypnotic susceptibility began in the early nineteenth century, with Braid and Bernheim (Zangwill, 1987) leading the way. But it was not until the late 1950s that a rigorously normed and standardized procedure for measuring hypnotizability emerged from the programmatic research of Ernest Hilgard at Stanford University: The Stanford Hypnotic Susceptibility Scales, Forms A, B, and C. While the Stanford Scales (especially Form C) remain somewhat of a "gold standard" in hypnosis research, many other standardized protocols have been developed in the ensuing years. But all operate from the basic premise that hypnotic responsiveness is best measured by hypnotizing a subject, administering a series of suggestions that are either passed or failed, and adding the number of "passed" items to obtain a score. For example, the Stanford Scales involve administration of an induction along with 12 suggestions, including ideomotor suggestions (e.g., an extended arm becomes unbearably heavy and moves down by itself), cognitive suggestions (e.g., amnesia), and perceptual suggestions (e.g., positive visual or auditory hallucination). Specific behavioral criteria are established for obtaining a "pass" score on each of these 12 items. The total number of suggestions *is* the subject's score. The range of possible scores is thus 0 to 12, with individuals scoring on the lower end of the spectrum being less hypnotizable and those at the upper end being more hypnotizable.

This methodological breakthrough enabled researchers and clinicians to more confidently examine the nature of hypnotizability, especially its relative stability. Four important discoveries emerged from this work. First, hypnotic susceptibility is for the most part normally distributed across the population, with almost everyone able to experience hypnosis to some extent. Second, a person's responsiveness to hypnosis is relatively unaffected by the technique used, environmental surroundings, and the hypnotist. In other words, the person's ability to be hypnotized accounts for his/her responsiveness, not the specific techniques used, not the expertise of the hypnotist, not the situational variables surrounding the test administration. Third, hypnotic susceptibility is a personality trait that changes little, if any, across time. Test-retest reliabilities for hypnotizability scales compare favorably with those of IQ tests. In fact, Piccione, Hilgard, and Zimbardo (1989) reported a 15-year follow-up study that revealed an impressive correlation of .82 between the scores subjects obtained in 1970 and the ones these same subjects obtained in 1985. Fourth, children as young as 4 years of age can be hypnotized. Hypnotizability appears to increase with age into early adolescence, when it plateaus, perhaps decreasing slightly among the elderly.

Thus the mode of measurement for dissociativity and hypnosis are quite distinct, with dissociativity usually indexed via self-report scales and hypnotizability indexed via behavioral responses. At first flush this might seem to bode ill for obtaining statistically and clinically meaningful results. But in fact just the opposite is true. Cook and Cambell (1979) recommend precisely this type of arrangement where related constructs are indexed across modes of measurement, such as behavioral, physiological, and self-report, so as to minimize what they term "method variance" (which can lead to spurious correlations attributable to the similarity in method of measurement rather than commonality in construct).

We have then an opportunity to rigorously assess the extent to which dissociativity and hypnosis overlap. Table 1 summarizes the 11 studies to date that have

Table 1. Correlations between Measures of Hypnotizability and Dissociation

Study	Measures	N	Pearson r, p value
Clinical samples			
Segal & Lynn (1992-93)	HGSHS/DES	85	.17, p = NS
Green & Lynn (1990)	HGSHS/DES	218	.09, p = NS
Nadon et al. (1991)	HGSHS/DES	475	.08, p = NS
Frischholz et al. (1992)	HGSHS/DES	309	.12, $p < .05$
Putnam et al. (unpublished)	SCHCS:C CDC	105	.11, p = NS
Nash et al. (1992)	SHSS:A/IDS	98	.16, p = NS
Nonclinical samples			
Spanos et al. (1993)	CURSS:O/DES	75	.11, p = NS
DiTomasso & Routh (1993)	HGSHS/DES	312	.16, $p < .01$
Silva & Kirch (1992)	CURSS:O/DES	190	.15, p = NS
Johnson et al. (1992)	SHSS:A/DES	148	.20, $p < .05$
Tanabe & Kasai (1993)	HGSHS/DES	107	.15, p = NS

correlated measures of dissociativity with measures of hypnotizability. In general, scores on standard hypnosis scales are not significantly corelated with scores of dissociativity across clinical and nonclinical samples (Faith & Ray, 1994; Green & Lynn, 1990; Nash, Hulsey, Sexton, Harralson, & Lambert, 1993; Putnam, Helmers, & Trickett, submitted; Segal & Lynn, 1992, 1993; Silva & Kirch, 1992; Spanos, Arango, & de Groot, 1993; Tanabe & Kasai, 1993). In the few cases where correlations reach statistical significance, the magnitude of correlation is small (.15 to .20), accounting for only 2-4% of the variance (DiTomasso & Routh, 1993; Frischholtz, Lipman, Braun, & Sachs, 1992; Johnson & Kirsch, 1990).

Some researchers have investigated the degree of correlation between fantasy proneness, absorption, hypnotizability, and dissociativity (Barrett, 1992; Glisky, Tataryn, Tobais, Kihlstrom, & McConkey, 1991; Lynn & Rhue, 1986). Absorption is thought to be trait-like and is defined as the ability to absorb self-altering experiences. Fantasy proneness is the tendency to live in a self-created world of imagination and fantasy. Fantasy proneness is thought to be a personality type.

Basically, these studies find moderate-to-strong correlations between absorption and fantasy proneness, absorption and hypnotizability, and absorption and dissociation. Fantasy proneness is moderately correlated with both hypnotizability and dissociativity. Overall, hypnotizability and dissociativity are correlated more strongly to absorption and fantasy proneness than to each other.

In sum, there is no compelling evidence to support the proposition that hypnotizability and dissociativity are overlapping traits. Even for samples including trauma victims, correlations either failed to reach significance or were so weak that they are conceptually unimportant. Sharing little variance, hypnotizability and dissociativity, in fact, seem to exist fairly independently of one another. They are probably not overlapping, and are certainly not synonymous, personality constructs.

Common Traumagenic Etiologies for Hypnotizability and Dissociativity

If hypnosis and dissociativity share common developmental pathways involving trauma, then a history of trauma should be associated with increased hypnotizability and increased dissociativity. There are of course two components to this issue: Is a history of trauma associated with high hypnotizabilty and is a history of trauma associated with high dissociativity?

Hypnosis and Trauma. There was some early support for the contention that hypnotizability may be very modestly related to extent of physical punishment during childhood. The research of Hilgard and others (Hilgard, 1974; London, 1962; Nowlis, 1969) suggests that childhood experiences of severe punishment and discipline are positively correlated with hypnotizability (correlations of around .30). Nash and his colleagues (Nash & Lynn, 1985; Nash, Lynn, & Givens, 1984) found that subjects who reported physical and sexual abuse in childhood were more hypnotizable than subjects not reporting such a history (the effect size was in the range of .30). The authors of the latter two studies came to understand these findings as artifactual, attributable to contextual features of the testing situation (testing for hypnotizability immediately following the questioning about early trauma) (see Council, Kirsch, & Hafner, 1986). In fact, six subsequent studies examining the relationship between sexual abuse and hypnotizability found no significant relationship (see Table 2).

Two of these studies were large-scale and particularly instructive; one examined children, the other adults. Putnam et al. (submitted) compared abused and nonabused girls (6-15 years of age) on the Stanford Hypnotic Scale for Children and the Child Dissociative Checklist. Abused and nonabused children did not differ significantly on measures of hypnotizability. Nash et al. (1993) compared clinical abused and nonclinical abused adult women on measures of dissociation (Indiana Dissociative Symptom Scale, Dissociation Content Scale) and hypnotizability (Stanford Hypnotic Susceptibility Scale: A [SHSS:A]). No significant relationship between hypnotic susceptibility and abuse was detected, nor was the severity of abuse or age of onset of abuse significantly correlated with hypnotizability.

There is, however, a second body of research that seems to suggest a traumagenic path to high hypnotizability. First, 85-97% of clinical MPD patients report early life trauma (Coons, Bowman, & Milstein, 1988; Kluft, 1984; Putnam, Guroff, Silberman, Barban, & Post, 1986; Ross, Heber, Norton, & Anderson, 1989). Second, MPD patients are reported to be highly hypnotizable as a group (Bliss, 1984; Frischholz, 1985b; Frischholz, Spiegel, Spiegel, Lipman, & Bark, 1988; Frischholz et al., 1992). Taken together, these two sets of findings would seem to confirm some etiologic link between hypnosis and dissociation.

However, there is now some reason to question the generalizability of these findings. Ross et al. (1991) have studied dissociative phenomena, MPD, and self-report histories of childhood trauma in clinical as well as nonclinical populations using the Dissociative Experiences Scale (DES). They estimated that between 5 and 10% of the general population is affected by a dissociated disorder. Ross et al. (1991) also found incidents of MPD in the general population at a rate of 3.1% based on a 450-person sample administered the Dissociative Disorder Interview Schedule (DDIS) (Ross, Heber, Norton & Anderson, 1989). Ross et al. (1991) state that the data of individuals with MPD in the general population were radically different from the clinical MPD patient data. In the clinical MPD population, 85-97% of patients report a history of severe sexual and physical abuse (Coons & Milstein, 1986; Kluft, 1987; Putnam et al., 1986). In the Ross et al. (1991) study, MPD subjects in the

Table 2. Correlation Effect Sizes For Hypnotizability and Trauma

Study	Measure	*N*	Effect size	Comparison
Nonclinical samples				
DiTomasso & Routh (1993)	HGSHS	312	.005	Nonabused undergraduates
Putnam et al. (unpublished)	SHSS:C	116	.23	Matched, nonabused girls
Johnson & Kirsch (1992)	SHSS:A	148	.025	Nonabused undergraduates
Rhue et al. (1990)	HGSHS	100	.610	Nonabused undergraduates
Clinical samples				
Johnson & Kirsch (1992)	SHSS:A	40	.025	Nonabused outpatients
Clinical and nonclinical samples				
Nash et al. (1993)	SHSS:A	105	.12	Nonabused adults

general population rarely reported histories of abuse and reported experiencing little distress. This is an interesting report of a supposedly extremely pathological condition heretofore always associated with severe childhood abuse, but now found in the general population relatively unassociated with a history of abuse and profound distress. Earlier studies claiming to find evidence of a trauma-hypnotizability link (Bliss, 1984; Coons & Milstein, 1986; Kluft, 1987; Putnam et al., 1986) may need to be reexamined in light of the Ross et al. (1991) findings.

Finally, there is one study that unambiguously demonstrates a relationship between trauma and hypnotizability among Vietnam combat veterans. Veterans suffering posttraumatic stress disorder (PTSD) are found to be more hypnotizable than are non-PTSD veterans (Spiegel et al., 1988). Spiegel (1986) contends that measures of hypnotizability may be a useful diagnostic tool in suspected cases of MPD/PTSD among this population. However, it must be noted that the concept of the developmental genesis of hypnotizability is strained in this study in large part because these traumas were not in childhood.

In sum, there is little evidence for a broadband relationship between early trauma and hypnotizability. Researchers do not find differences in hypnotizability between individuals who have been traumatized and those who have not. Among individuals with MPD, there is reason to suspect that trauma may not be the certain comorbid sign that it was once assumed to be. Thus, reports of high hypnotizability among MPD patients may not be so easily linked with early trauma in these cases. The Spiegel study does suggest that among certain narrowly selected clinical populations systematic covariance between hypnotizability and trauma may obtain. But this is far from establishing a broad association between trauma and hypnotizability.

Trauma and Dissociation. One can make a stronger case for a relationship between dissociativity and trauma, though there are methodological and definitional problems that plague the literature. First, of the 14 studies examining trauma and dissociativity, all have found higher levels of dissociativity among individuals who have been traumatized. Five of these studies were with nonclinical samples (Briere & Runtz, 1988; DiTomasso & Routh, 1993; Johnson & Kirsch, 1990; Putnam et al., submitted; Sanberg & Lynn, 1992), eight were with clinical samples (Bremner et al., 1992; Briere & Runtz, 1989; Chu & Dill, 1990; Goff et al., 1991; Pribor & Dinwiddie, 1992; Sanders & Giolas, 1991; Strick & Wilcoxon, 1991; Warshaw et al., 1993); and one was with both clinical and nonclinical samples (Nash et al., 1993). The magnitude of the relationship between trauma and dissociation appears to be in the $r = .20$ to $.45$ range. Second, the severity of trauma was positively correlated with dissociation scores in four studies (Branscomb, 1991; Cardeña & Spiegel, 1993; Carlson & Rosser-Hogan, 1991; Kirby, Chu, & Dill, 1992), but not in a fifth (Nash et al., 1993). In sum, there does seem to be some empirical support for the contention that trauma and dissociation are associated.

It is important to consider some methodological difficulties with this literature in general. First, the problem of defining trauma plagues the literature. For instance, many theorists have assumed that childhood sexual abuse is by definition traumatic. Yet, a more recent review questions whether all cases of sexual abuse necessarily involve overwhelming affect, fear for safety, and helplessness (Kendall-Tackett,

Williams, & Finkelhor, 1993). Second, there are also some problems in defining and operationalizing dissociation. The DES (Bernstein & Putnam, 1986) is widely employed in this area, and it does demonstrate satisfactory split-half and test-retest reliability. But there is some evidence that a large component of an individual's DES score may be attributable not to dissociative pathology specifically, but to gross psychopathology in general. Nash et al. (1993), Norton, Ross, and Novotny (1990), and Sanberg and Lynn (in press) detected a confound between general psychological impairment and DES scores, with high DES scores being associated with greater general psychopathology. In the Nash et al. (1993) study, the DES correlated .70 with the F-scale of the Minnesota Multiphasic Personality Inventory. Similar findings were obtained for two other scales: the Dissociation Content Scale (Boswell, Sanders, & Hernandez, 1985) and the Indiana Dissociative Symptom Scale (Levitt, 1989). Thus, when the DES scores of traumatized patients exceed those of non-traumatized patients, it is possible that the difference has less to do with dissociation per se and more to do with gross pathology.

Third, and perhaps most importantly, all but one of the above cited studies linking trauma and dissociation neglected to consider other pathogenic factors in the child's environment that might explain subsequent pathology. Families in which abuse occurs are more pathological than nonabusing families, with higher levels of role or boundary confusion, more rigid behavioral control, and less cohesiveness and adaptability (Alexander & Lupfer, 1987; Harter, Alexander, & Neimeyer, 1988; Hoagwood & Stewart, 1988). Thus, differences between abused and nonabused samples on measures of psychopathology in general (and dissociation in particular) may be due, not to the effects of trauma necessarily, but to the nonspecific effect of a pathogenic home environment. Indeed, recent empirical work seems to suggest that some adult pathology associated with childhood sexual trauma may reflect the effects of a broadly pathogenic family environment rather than the effects of sexual abuse per se (Harter et al., 1988; Fromuth, 1986; Wyatt & Newcomb, 1990). In the only dissociation study controlling for pathogenic factors other than trauma, Nash et al. (1993) found that subjects who were sexually traumatized in childhood were significantly more dissociative than nonabused subjects. However, when family environment was used as a covariate, the effect for early trauma receded into nonsignificance.

Evidence for the common etiology hypothesis—that early trauma exaggerates an individual's hypnotizability and dissociativity—is scant. First, trauma does not appear to be an important feature in the development of high hypnotizability. The overwhelming preponderance of high hypnotizables have not been traumatized; and those subjects who have been traumatized are no more hypnotizable than nontraumatized controls. Though there may be some possibility for an association between trauma and hypnotizability within narrow diagnostic categories, there is no convincing evidence that a history of early trauma is associated with high hypnotizability. Second, there is a fairly extensive research literature that finds an association between trauma and dissociation. Though serious methodological and definitional issues compromise our certainty, at this time it appears that trauma and dissociation may be linked. At the same time, however, it seems probable that this link is not a linear cause-effect relationship. Indeed, given the confounding of dissociation measures with measures of gross pathology and the neglect of other pathogenic factors, what dissociation researchers may be finding is simply that people who have had horribly troubling and chaotic home environments are more grossly pathological than those who had reasonably stable childhood home environments. But even if we accept the premise that dissociativity is directly associated with trauma, hypnosis is not. Therefore, experiences of early trauma do not exaggerate both an individual's dissociativity *and* hypnotizability. In this sense, then, hypnotizability and dissociativity are not "fellow travelers," following parallel trajectories in response to early trauma. Here again we find reason to reject the conclusion that these phenomena involve shared psychic mechanisms.

Hypnosis as an Effective Treatment. As stated earlier, there has been an interest in using hypnosis as treatment for mental disorders for over two centuries. Charcot, Janet, and Freud all employed hypnotic techniques to treat hysterical symptoms. Large-scale use of hypnosis in the treatment of trauma occurred during and after World War I where hypnotherapy was used to treat debilitating trauma or, as it was then called, shell shock. Typical treatment involved the modification of the traumatic memory, such that the soldier in question might return to normal levels of functioning.

Such examples illustrate how therapeutic hypnosis can provide controlled access to painful memories. This modulated access allows patients to experience a sense of mastery over previously overwhelming affect-laden memories. Once accomplished, the patient begins to reframe those memories such that he or she understands the memories to be a part of, but not all of, themselves (Spiegel, 1987).

Of note are two studies that found psychotherapy with hypnosis to be no more effective than psychotherapy without hypnosis in the treatment of MPD patients (Putnam et al., 1986; Ross & Norton, 1989). These are the only extant outcome studies examining whether hypnosis is particularly effective in the treatment of dissociative disorders; they provide no evidence to support a link between hypnosis and dissociation, however.

SUMMARY

If there is any relationship between the constructs of dissociation and hypnosis, it is complex and indirect. The three propositions, rooted in the assumption of a hypnosis-dissociation link, are not supported empirically. The overlapping trait proposition has been thoroughly tested: hypnotizability and dissociativity do not covary—positive correlations between these measures are rare and nonreplicable. Neither has the common traumagenic etiology proposition been confirmed empirically. No definitive developmental pathway conjoining trauma, dissociativity, and hypnotizability has emerged from the data. The specific and seemingly more secure link between trauma and dissociation is still uncertain, owing to numerous methodological and definitional problems (pathological family confounds, etc.).

Finally, the question of a special role for hypnosis in the treatment of dissociative disorders has not really been addressed adequately by the research literature. Empirically demonstrated unique effects for *any* psychological intervention are few and far between in psychotherapy outcome literature. A definitive test of the importance of hypnosis in the treatment of dissociative disorders has not been attempted and is sorely needed.

Given this state of affairs, we make the following recommendations for future investigations. First, the time for unrefined examination of correlations between hypnotizability and dissociativity scales has passed. Perhaps within specific diagnostic categories there is some nonrandom covariation between hypnosis and dissociation, but for normal populations the bulk of the evidence speaks against correlations between the two phenomenon.

Second, research examining the proposed traumagenic etiology of hypnotizability and dissociativity needs to be far more sophisticated. For instance, investigators must take care to disentangle the effects of sexual abuse from the effects of other sources of pathology in which the abuse may be embedded. In addition, there is a clear and pressing need for longitudinal studies with child victims of trauma. Only longitudinal studies can provide definitive data on proposed causal pathways linking trauma with dissociation and hypnosis. Likewise, following the lead of Ross et al. (1991), research should be undertaken to examine dissociative pathology among nontreatment populations. Specifically, why do dissociative and hypnotizability scores correlate for clinical MPD-PTSD populations but not for nonclinical MPD-PTSD populations. A final methodological point is related to extent of trauma. Specifically, among trauma victims, is the extent of trauma associated with the extent of dissociativity?

Our third recommendation addresses the clear need for empirically driven assessments of the clinical efficacy of hypnotic interventions with dissociative-disordered patients. Anecdotal evidence supportive of the efficacy of hypnosis abounds. Yet, there are too few adequately designed studies in this area to allow confident and satisfactory assessment of hypnotherapy efficacy. Methodologically, time series designs are well suited for this type of research, as are the more traditional control group approaches.

REFERENCES

Alexander, P., & Lupfer, S. (1987). Family characteristics and long term consequences associated with sexual abuse. *Archives of Sexual Behavior, 16*, 235-245.

Barrett, D. (1992). Fantasizers and dissociaters: Data on two distinct subgroups of deep trance subjects. *Psychological Reports, 71*, 1011-1014.

Bernstein, E. M., & Putnam, F. W. (1986). Development, reliability, and validity of a dissociation scale. *Journal of Nervous and Mental Disease, 174*, 727-735.

Beutler, L. E. (1979). Toward specific psychological therapies for specific conditions. *Journal of Consulting and Clinical Psychology, 47*, 882-897.

Bliss, E. L. (1984). Spontaneous self-hypnosis in multiple personality disorder. *Psychiatric Clinics of North America, 7*, 135-148.

Blum, G. S., Porter, M. L., & Geiwitz, P. J. (1978). Temporal parameters of negative visual hallucination. *International Journal of Clinical and Experimental Hypnosis, 26*, 30-44.

Branscomb, L. (1991). Dissociation in combat-related posttraumatic stress disorder. *Dissociation, 4*, 13-20.

Bremner, J. D., Southwick, S., Brett, D., Fontana, A., Rosenheck, R., & Charney, D. S. (1992). Dissociation and posttraumatic stress disorder in Vietnam combat veterans. *American Journal of Psychiatry, 149*, 328-332.

Breuer, J., & Freud, S. (1955). Studies on hysteria: I. On physical mechanisms of hysterical phenomena: Preliminary communication. In J. Strachey (Ed. and Trans.), *The standard edition of the complete psychological works of Sigmund Freud* (Vol. 2, pp. 1-181). London: Hogarth Press. (Original work published in 1893-1895.)

Briere, J., & Runtz, M. (1988). Post sexual abuse trauma. *Journal of International Violence, 2*, 367-379.

Briere, J., & Runtz, M. (1989). The trauma symptom checklist (TSC-33): Early data on a new scale. *Journal of Interpersonal Violence, 4*, 151-163.

Cardeña, E., & Spiegel, D. (1993). Dissociative reactions to the San Francisco Bay area earthquake of 1989. *American Journal of Psychiatry, 150*, 474-478.

Carlson, E. B., & Rosser-Hogan, R. (1991). Trauma experiences, posttraumatic stress, dissociation, and depression on Cambodian refugees *American Journal of Psychiatry, 149*, 1548-1551.

Chu, J. A., & Dill, D. L. (1990). Dissociative symptoms in relation to childhood physical and sexual abuse. *American Journal of Psychiatry, 147*, 887-892.

Cook, T. D., & Campbell, D. T. (1979). *Quasi-experimentation: Design and analysis issues for field settings*. Boston: Houghton Mifflin.

Coons, P. M., Bowman, E. S., & Milstein, V. (1988). Multiple personality disorder: A clinical investigation of 50 cases. *Journal of Nervous and Mental Disorders, 176*, 519-527.

Coons, P. M., & Milstein, V. (1986). Psychosexual disturbances in multiple personality: Characteristics, etiology, and treatment. *Journal of Clinical Psychiatry, 47*, 106-110.

Council, J. R., Kirsch, I., & Hafner, L. P. (1986). Expectancy versus absorption in the prediction of hypnotic responding. *Journal of Personality and Social Psychology, 50*, 182-189.

Deabler, H. L., Fidel, E., Dillenkoffer, R. L., & Elder, S. T. (1973). The use of relaxation and hypnosis in lowering blood pressure. *American Journal of Clinical Hypnosis, 16*, 75-83.

DePiano, F. A., & Salzberg, H. C. (1979). Clinical applications of hypnosis to three psychosomatic disorders. *Psychological Bulletin, 86*, 1223-1235.

DiTomasso, M. J., & Routh, D. K. (1993). Recall of abuse in childhood and three measures of dissociation. *Child Abuse and Neglect, 17*, 477-485.

Ellenberger, H. F. (1970). *The discovery of the unconscious: The history and evolution of dynamic psychiatry*. New York: Basic Books.

Faith, M., & Ray, W. J. (1994). Hypnotizability and dissociation in a college age population: Orthogonal individual differences. *Journal Of Personality and Individual Differences.*

Field, P. B. (1965). An inventory scale of hypnotic depth. *International Journal of Clinical and Experimental Hypnosis, 13*, 238-249.

Frankel, F. H. (1974). Trance capacity and the genesis of phobic behavior. *Archives of General Psychiatry, 31*, 261-262.

Freud, S. (1953). The interpretation of dreams. In J. Strachey (Ed. and Trans.), *The standard edition of the complete psychological works of Sigmund Freud* (Vol. 4, pp. 1-338; Vol. 5, pp. 229-621). London: Hogarth Press. (Original work published 1900.)

Freud, S. (1957). A metapsychological supplement to the theory of dreams. In J. Strachey (Ed. and Trans.), *The standard edition of the complete psychological works of Sigmund Freud* (Vol. 14, pp. 222-235). London: Hogarth Press. (Original work published in 1917.)

Freud, S. (1959). Charcot. In E. Jones (Ed.), J. Riviere (Trans.), *Sigmund Freud: Collected papers* (Vol. 1, pp. 9-23). New York: Basic Books. (Original work published 1893.)

Friedman, H., & Taub, H. A. (1978). A six-month follow-up of the use of hypnosis and biofeedback procedures in essential hypertension. *American Journal of Clinical Hypnosis, 20*, 184-188.

Frischholz, E. M. (1985a). The relationship among dissociation, hypnosis, and child abuse in the development of multiple personality. In R. P. Kluft (Ed.), *Childhood antecedents of multiple personality* (pp. 99-120). Washington, DC: American Psychiatric Press.

Frischholz, E. J. (1985b). Hypnotizability and psychosis: A meta-analytic review. In J. Fawcett (Chair), *Psychopathology and hypnotizability symposium*. Symposium conducted at the meeting of the American Psychiatric Association, Dallas, TX.

Frischholz, E. J., Lipman, L. S., Braun, B. G., & Sachs, R. G. (1992). Psychopathology, hypnotizability, and dissociation. *American Journal of Psychiatry, 149*, 1521-1525.

Frischholz, E. J., Spiegel, D., Spiegel, H., Lipman, L. S., & Bark, N. (1988). *Psychopathology and hypnotizability*. Unpublished manuscript.

Fromuth, M. E. (1986). The relationship of childhood sexual abuse with later psychological and sexual adjustment in a sample of college women. *Child Abuse and Neglect, 10*, 5-15.

Glisky, M. L., Tataryn, D. J., Tobais, B. A., Kihlstrom, J. F., & McConkey, K. M. (1991). Absorption, openness to experience, and hypnotizability. *Journal of Personality and Social Psychology, 60*, 263-272.

Goff, D. C., Brotman, A. W., Kindlon, D., & Waites, M. (1991). The delusion of possession in chronically psychotic patients. *Journal of Nervous and Mental Disease, 179*(9), 567-571.

Grosz, H. J., & Zimmerman, J. (1965). Experimental analysis of hysterical blindness: A follow-up report and new experimental data. *Archives of General Psychiatry, 13*, 255-260.

Harter, S., Alexander, P., & Neimeyer, R. A. (1988). Long-term effects of incestuous child abuse in college women: Social adjustment, social cognition, and family characteristics. *Journal of Consulting and Clinical Psychology, 56*, 5-8.

Hilgard, E. R. (1979a). Divided consciousness in hypnosis: The implications of the hidden observer. In E. Fromm & R. E. Shor (Eds.), *Hypnosis: developments in research and new perspectives*. (2nd ed., pp. 45-79). New York: Aldine.

Hilgard, E. R. (1979b), Consciousness and control: Lessons from hypnosis. *Australian Journal of Clinical and Experimental Hypnosis, 7*, 107-115.

Hilgard, E. R. (1992). Dissociation and theories of hypnosis. In E. Fromm & M. R. Nash (Eds.), *Contemporary hypnosis research* (pp. 69-100). New York: The Guilford Press.

Hilgard, J. R. (1974). Sequelae to hypnosis. *International Journal of Clinical and Experimental Hypnosis, 22*, 281-298.

Hoagwood, K., & Stewart, J. M. (1988, August). Family structural factors in cases of child sexual abuse. Paper presented at the Annual Meeting of the American Psychological Association, Atlanta, GA.

Janet, P. (1889). *L'automatisme psychologique*. Paris: Felix Alcan.

Janet, P. (1925). *Psychological healing: A historical and clinical study* (E. Paul & C. Paul, Trans.). New York: Macmillan. (Original work published in 1919)

Johnson, G., & Kirsch, I. (1990). Dissociation, hypnotizability, and fantasy proneness in a clinical sample of survivors of abuse. Annual meeting of the American Psychological Association, Washington, DC.

Kendall-Tackett, K. A., Williams, L. M., & Finkelhor, D. (1993). Impact of sexual abuse on children: A review and synthesis of recent empirical studies. *Psychological Bulletin, 113*, 164-180.

Kirby, J. S., Chu, J. A., & Dill, K. L. (1992). Correlates of dissociative symptomatology in patients with physical and sexual abuse histories. *Comprehensive Psychiatry, 34*, 258-263.

Kluft, R. P. (1982). Varieties of hypnotic interventions in multiple personality. *American Journal of Clinical Hypnosis, 24*, 230-240.

Kluft, R. P. (1984). Multiple personality disorder in childhood. *Psychiatric Clinics of North America, 7*, 1121-134.

Kluft, R. P. (1987). An update on multiple personality disorder. *Hospital and Community Psychiatry, 38*, 363-373.

London, P. (1962). Hypnosis in children: An experimental approach. *International Journal of Clinical and Experimental Hypnosis, 10*, 79-91.

Loomis, A. L., Harvey, E. N., & Hobart, G. A. (1936). Electrical potentials during hypnosis. *Science, 83*, 239-241.

Lynn, S., Green, J. P., Weekes, J. R., & Carlson, B. W. (1990, October). Literalism and hypnosis: hypnotic versus task motivated subjects. *American Journal of Clinical Hypnosis, 33*(2), 113-119.

Lynn, S. J., & Rhue, J. W. (1986). The fantasy-prone person: Hypnosis, imagination, and creativity. *Journal of Personality and Social Psychology, 51*, 404-408.

Malmo, R. B., Boag, T. J., & Raginsky, B. B. (1954). Electromyography study of hypnotic deafness. *International Journal of Clinical and Experimental Hypnosis, 2*, 305-317.

Nadon, R., Hoyt, I. P., Register, P. A., & Kihlstrom, J. F. (1991). Absorption and hypnotizability: Context effects re-examined. *Journal of Personality and Social Psychology, 60*(1), 144-153.

Nash, M. R., Hulsey, T. L., Sexton, M. C., Harralson, T. L., & Lambert, W. (1993). Long-term sequelae of childhood sexual abuse: Perceived family environment, psychopathology, and dissociation. *Journal of Consulting and Clinical Psychology, 61*, 276-283.

Nash, M. R., & Lynn, S. J. (1985). Child abuse and hypnotic ability. *Imagination, Cognition, and Personality 5*, 211-218.

Nash, M. R., Lynn, S. J., & Givens, D. L. (1984). Adult hypnotic susceptibility, childhood punishment, and child abuse: A brief communication. *International Journal of Clinical and Experimental Hypnosis 32*, 6-11.

Nash, M. R., Lynn, S. J., Stanley, S., & Carlson, V. (1987). Subjectively complete hypnotic deafness and auditory priming. *International Journal of Clinical and Experimental Hypnosis, 35*, 32-40.

Norton, G. R., Ross, C. A., & Novotny, M. F. (1990). Factors that predict scores on the Dissociative Experiences Scale. *Journal of Clinical Psychology, 46*(3), 273-277.

Nowlis, D. P. (1969). The child-rearing antecedents of hypnotic susceptibility and of naturally occurring hypnotic-like experience. *International Journal of Clinical and Experimental Hypnosis, 17*, 109-120.

Pattie, F. A. (1935). A report of attempts to produce uniocular blindness by hypnotic suggestion. *British Journal of Medical Psychology, 15*, 230-241.

Piccione, C., Hilgard, E. R., & Zimbardo, P. G. (1989). On the degree of stability of measured hypnotizability over a 25 year period. *Journal of Personality and Social Psychology, 56*, 289-295.

Pribor, E. F., & Dinwiddie, S. H. (1992). Psychiatric correlates of incest in childhood. *American Journal of Psychiatry, 149*, 52-56.

Prince, M. (1906). *The dissociation of a personality*. New York: Longmans, Green.

Putnam, F. W. (1985). Dissociation as a response to extreme trauma. In R. P. Kluft (Ed.), *Childhood antecedents of multiple personality* (pp. 65-98). Washington, DC: American Psychiatric Press.

Putnam, F. W., Guroff, J. J., Silberman, E. K., Barban, L., & Post, R. M. (1986). The clinical phenomenology of multiple personality disorder: Review of 100 recent cases. *Journal of Clinical Psychiatry, 47*(6), 285-293.

Putnam, F. W., Helmers, K., & Trickett, P. K. (submitted). *Hypnotizability and dissociativity in sexually abused girls.*

Rhue, J. W., Lynn, S. J., Henry, S., Buhk, K., & Boyd, P. (1990). Child abuse, imagination, and hypnotizability. *Imagination, Cognition, and Personality, 10*, 53-63.

Ross, C. A., Heber, S., Norton, G. R., & Anderson, G. (1989). Differences between multiple personality disorder and other diagnostic groups on structured interview. *The Journal of Nervous and Mental Disease, 177*(8), 487-491.

Ross, C. A., Miller, S. D., Bjornson, L., Reagor, P., Fraser, G. A., & Anderson, G. (1991). Abuse histories in 102 cases of multiple personality disorder. *Canadian Journal of Psychiatry, 36*, 97-101.

Ross, C. A., & Norton, G. R. (1989). Effects of hypnosis on the features of multiple personality disorder. *American Journal of Clinical Hypnosis, 32*(2), 99-105.

Sackheim, H. A., Nordlie, J. W., & Gur, R. C. (1979). A model of hysterical and hypnotic blindness: Cognition, motivation, and awareness. *Journal of Abnormal Psychology, 88*, 474-489.

Sandberg, P. A., & Lynn, S. J. (1992). Dissociative experiences, psychopathology and adjustment, and child and adolescent maltreatment in female college students. *Journal of Abnormal Psychology 101*(4), 717-723.

Sanders, B., & Giolas, M. H. (1991). Dissociation and childhood trauma in psychologically disturbed adolescents. *American Journal of Psychiatry 148*, 50-54.

Scagnelli-Jobsis, J. (1982). Hypnosis with psychotic patients: A review of the literature and presentation of theoretical framework. *American Journal of Clinical Hypnosis, 25*, 33-45.

Segal, D., & Lynn, S. J. (1992-93). Predicting dissociative experiences: Imagination, hypnotizability, psychopathology, and alcohol use. *Imagination, Cognition and Personality, 12*, 287-300.

Silva, C. E., & Kirsch, I. (1992). Interpretative sets, expectancy, fantasy proneness, and dissociation as predictors of hypnotic response. *Journal of Personality and Social Psychology, 63*, 847-856.

Skinner, B. F. (1953). *Science and human behavior*. New York: Macmillan.

Spanos, N. P., Arango, M., & de Groot, H. P. (1993). Context as a moderator in relationships between attribute variables and hypnotizability. *Personality and Social Psychology Bulletin, 19*, 71-77.

Spiegel, D. (1986). Dissociating damage. *American Journal of Clinical Hypnosis, 29*, 123-131.

Spiegel, D. (1987). Dissociation and hypnosis in posttraumatic stress disorders. *Journal of Traumatic Stress, 1*, 17-33.

Spiegel, D., Hunt, T., & Dondershine, H. E. (1988)., Dissociation and hypnotizability in posttraumatic stress disorder. *American Journal of Psychiatry, 145*(3), 301-305.

Spiegel, H., & Spiegel, D. (1978). *Trance and treatment: Clinical uses of hypnosis*. New York: Basic Books.

Strick, F. C., & Wilcoxon, S. A. (1991). A comparison of dissociative experiences in adult female outpatients with and without histories of early incestuous abuse. *Dissociation Progress in the Dissociative Disorders*, *4*(4), 193-199.

Tanabe, H.,. & Kasai, H. (1993). Dissociative experiences and hypnotic susceptibility. *Japanese Journal of Hypnosis*, *38*(1), 12-19.

Tellegen, A., & Atkinson, G. (1974). Openness to absorbing and self-altering experiences ("absorption"), a trait related to hypnotic susceptibility. *Journal of Abnormal Psychology*, *83*, 268-277.

Theodore, L. H., & Mandelcorn, M. S. (1973). Hysterical blindness: A case report and study using a modern psychophysical technique. *Journal of Abnormal Psychology*, *82*, 552-553.

Wadden, T. A., & Anderton, C. H. (1982). The clinical use of hypnosis. *Psychological Bulletin*, *91*, 215-243.

Watson, J. B. (1930). *Behaviorism*. New York: Norton.

West, L. (1967). Dissociative reactions. In *Comprehensive Testbook of Psychiatry* (pp. 885-899). Baltimore: Williams and Wilkins.

White, R. W., & Shevach, B. M. (1942). Hypnosis and the concept of dissociation. *Journal of Abnormal and Social Psychology*, *7*, 309-328.

Wyatt, G. E., & Newcomb, M. (1990). Internal and external mediators of women's sexual abuse in childhood. *Journal of Consulting and Clinical Psychology*, *59*, 758-767.

Zangwill, O. L. (1987). Experimental hypnosis. In R. L. Gregory (Ed.), *Oxford companion to the mind* (pp. 328-330). Oxford: Oxford University Press.

10

Emotional Dissociation in Response to Trauma

An Information-Processing Approach

Edna B. Foa and Diana Hearst-Ikeda

Pathological reactions to trauma and extreme stress have been noted in the psychological literature for over a century. These reactions were codified in the psychiatric literature as posttraumatic stress disorder (PTSD) (American Psychiatric Association, 1980). The diagnosis of PTSD is made when posttrauma symptoms occur in three domains: emotional, cognitive, and visual reexperiencing of the trauma; avoidance of trauma-relevant stimuli; and general arousal. Since the inception of PTSD as a diagnostic entity, experts have focused on the fear and anxiety components of the disorder (Foa, Steketee, & Rothbaum, 1989; Keane, Zimering, & Caddell, 1985). More recently, trauma researchers have become interested in the phenomenon of affective and cognitive avoidance that is commonly observed following a trauma and has been referred to as dissociation (e.g., Spiegel, Hunt, & Dondershine, 1988), denial (Horowitz, 1986; van der Kolk, 1987), or numbing (e.g., Foa, Riggs, & Gershuny, 1995; Horowitz, Wilner, Kaltreider, & Alvarez, 1980; Litz, 1993; van der Kolk & Ducey, 1989). Common to these constructs is a diminished awareness of one's emotions or thoughts, which is hypothesized to be motivated by self-preservation.

In this chapter we will discuss the construct of emotional dissociation, de-

Edna B. Foa • Center for the Treatment and Study of Anxiety, Medical College of Pennsylvania, Eastern Pennsylvania Psychiatric Institute, Philadelphia, Pennsylvania 19129. **Diana Hearst-Ikeda** • National Center for Posttraumatic Stress Disorder, Women's Health and Sciences Division, Boston Department of Veterans Affairs Medical Center, Boston, Massachusetts 02130.

Handbook of Dissociation: Theoretical, Empirical, and Clinical Perspectives, edited by Larry K. Michelson and William J. Ray. Plenum Press, New York, 1996.

scribe the measures that have been used to evaluate it, and review the relevant literature. Finally we will discuss mechanisms that are hypothesized to underlie dissociation and will propose that the presence of dissociation is an indicator of incomplete emotional processing of the trauma.

DISSOCIATION, DENIAL, AVOIDANCE, AND NUMBING: CONCEPTUAL ISSUES

The phenomenon of emotional detachment has gained considerable attention in the late nineteenth century and was conceptualized as a defense against overwhelming emotions (e.g., Breuer & Freud, 1985; Janet 1907, 1989). But it was Janet (1907) who coined the term *dissociation* to describe the lack of connection between aspects of memory or conscious awareness observed during and after extreme stress.

Since these early writings, many experts have noted that dissociation occurs in nonpathological as well as in pathological states (e.g., Bliss, 1984; Braun & Sachs, 1985; Hilgard, 1977; Spiegel, 1963). Nemiah (1981) has proposed two characteristics of pathological dissociation. The first is an alteration in one's sense of identity, as in multiple personality disorder, and the second is a disturbance in the memory of the specific experiences during a dissociative period (usually traumatically induced). The *Diagnostic and Statistical Manual of Mental Disorders*, Fourth Edition (DSM-IV) has endorsed this dual view, stating "The essential feature of the dissociative disorders is a disruption in the usually integrated functions of consciousness, memory, identity, or perception of the environment" (American Psychiatric Association, 1994, p. 477).

A third characteristic of dissociation that has been proposed by several experts (e.g., Coons & Milstein, 1986; Putnam, 1989; Spiegel, 1986) is its association with traumatic experience. Accordingly, Spiegel and Cardena (1990) proposed that "posttraumatic phenomenology frequently involves alterations in the relationship to the self (e.g., depersonalization and multiple personality disorder), to the world (e.g., derealization and hallucinatory phenomena), and to memory processes (e.g., psychogenic amnesia, fugue, and multiple personality disorder)" (p. 368). Support for the view that dissociation is etiologically connected to traumatic experiences also comes from clinical observations of children who have suffered repeated exposure to extreme stress such as sexual, physical, or psychological abuse (Terr, 1991). Terr reported that children often use dissociation and numbing to escape the trauma-related memories and the arousal they trigger.

It seems that the construct of dissociation is largely defined by a set of symptoms that have been observed in persons who experienced trauma. These include amnesia, emotional detachment, feelings of depersonalization, out-of-body experiences, dreamlike recall of events, feelings of estrangement, flashbacks, and abreaction. In a review of psychological reactions that ensue from a traumatic experience, Cardena and Spiegel (1993) have suggested that posttrauma dissociative symptoms can be classified into three types of responses: (1) detachment from others and the physical environment, (2) alterations in perceptions, and (3) impairments in memory.

A second construct, denial, was proposed by Horowitz (1986), who noted that a common reaction to trauma is "the massive ideational denial of the event" (p. 16). An examination of the items contained in the scale that Horowitz and his colleagues developed to measure denial (i.e., the Impact of Events Scale; Horowitz, Wilner, & Alvarez, 1979) indicates that denial denotes attempts at cognitive and emotional avoidance (e.g., "I avoid letting myself get upset when I thought about it [the trauma] or was reminded of it," and "I tried to remove it from memory") but not alteration in perception and memory impairment.

A third term that had been introduced into the DSM-III (American Psychiatric Association, 1980) is "emotional numbing." This term is sometimes used interchangeably with denial and avoidance to describe the lack of affective expression in trauma victims (American Psychiatric Association, 1980; Horowitz, 1986). Seven symptoms comprise the avoidance-numbing symptom cluster of DSM-III-R (American Psychiatric Association, 1987) and DSM-IV (American Psychiatric Association, 1994). These include effortful cognitive and behavioral avoidance of trauma reminders, memory loss, and emotional numbing (e.g., loss of interest in activities, detachment from others, restricted affect, sense of a foreshortened future). Thus, the effortful avoidance symptoms are grouped together with those of emotional numbing in the diagnostic nomenclature.

The grouping of avoidance and numbing symptoms into one cluster suggests that the DSM-IV authors had conceptualized emotional numbing and effortful avoidance as an equivalent concept. However, a review of literature on experimental paradigms that elicit PTSD-like symptoms in animals suggests that effortful avoidance and numbing involve separate mechanisms (Foa, Zinbarg, & Rothbaum, 1992). Foa and Riggs (1993) suggested that effortful avoidance may be regulated by strategic psychological processes, whereas numbing may be mediated by biological mechanisms resembling those underlying the freezing behavior in frightened animals. They further proposed that on exposure to trauma-related information, victims first mobilize effortful strategies to avoid the arousal associated with the traumatic memories. When such strategies fails, a "shutting-down" of the affective system occurs; this process is expressed as numbing symptoms. Consistent with the view that effortful avoidance and numbing reflect separate phenomena are findings from a factor analytical study of PTSD symptoms in female assault victims. The numbing symptoms loaded on one factor that also included symptoms of irritability and concentration problems; the effortful avoidance symptoms loaded on a separate factor that included intrusive thoughts, emotional reactivity, hypervigilance, and excessive startle (Foa et al., 1995).

MEASURES OF DISSOCIATION, DENIAL, AVOIDANCE, AND NUMBING

As we noted earlier, many experts agree that dissociation, denial, avoidance, and numbing are common responses to extreme stress. The first accounts of dissociation relied on clinical observations of trauma victims. More recently, information about this phenomenon has been based on measures that have been constructed to serve as operational definitions of dissociation. It is therefore important to describe measures of dissociation before discussing the empirical data that have employed these measures.

1. *Dissociative Events Scale* (DES) (Bernstein & Putnam, 1986). This is a 28-item scale to assess the frequency and intensity of a range of experiences commonly conceptualized as dissociation and depersonalization in a psychiatric population in general and in traumatized individuals in particular. The DES items pertain to disturbances of memory, attention, identity, and perception. According to Bernstein and Putnam, the DES is a trait measure, although this has not been empirically validated. There are no items about numbing or cognitive avoidance in this scale.

2. *Stanford Acute Stress Reaction Questionnaire* (SASRQ) (Cardena, Classen, & Spiegel, 1991). The long version of this scale has 73 items that tap dissociation and anxiety experiences during and immediately after a trauma. Thirty-three items comprise the dissociation scale that assesses five features: psychic numbing, depersonalization, derealization, amnesia, and stupor. Forty items comprise the anxiety scale that also assesses five features: intrusive thinking, somatic anxiety, hyperarousal, attention disturbance, and sleep disturbance.

3. *Perceptual Alterations Scale* (PAS) (Sanders, 1986). This is a 25-item scale designed to measure normal and pathological dissociation. Like the DES, it conceptualizes dissociation as a trait rather than a state or a pathological feature of a disorder. The scale items were selected from the Minnesota Multiphasic Personality Inventory. A factor analysis yielded three factors: affect and depersonalization, depersonalization and loss of body control, and memory impairment.

4. *Peritraumatic Dissociation Experiences Questionnaire* (PDEQ-RV) (Marmar & Weiss, 1990). This scale is available in two versions: (1) interview (nine items) and (2) self-report (eight items). Similar to the SASRQ, it is designed to obtain information about dissociative reactions and experiences during and immediately after a trauma. The content of the items involve memory loss specific to the trauma, depersonalization, and derealization.

5. *Impact of Events Scale* (IES) (Horowitz et al., 1979). This is a 15-item scale that assesses intrusive reexperiencing and cognitive and affective avoidance. The eight avoidance items assess effortful attempts to avoid emotional reactions to trauma-related stimuli and thoughts about the trauma, but not depersonalization, derealization, and emotional numbness.

6. *PTSD Symptom Scale* (PSS) (Foa, Riggs, Dancu, & Rothbaum, 1993b). Both interview (PSS-I) and self-administered (PSS-SR) versions of this 17-item scale have been validated with female victims of sexual and nonsexual assault. The items correspond to the PTSD symptoms listed in the DSM-IV. Paralleling the DSM-IV, the items are divided into three clusters: reexperiencing (four items), avoidance-numbing (seven items), and arousal (six items). A factor analysis of this scale yielded a numbing factor that combined the following symptoms: detachment from others, irritability, sense of foreshortened future, and emotional numbness (Foa et al., 1995).

7. *The Dissociative Disorders Interview Schedule* (DDIS) (Ross, Heber, Norton, Anderson, Anderson, & Barchet, 1989). The DDIS is a 131-item structured interview developed to make diagnoses of dissociation somatization, major depression, and borderline personality disorder. Ross and colleagues (1989) recommend

the use of this scale with the DES to provide a complete picture of the range and type of dissociation experiences and severity of psychopathology.

Examination of the measures here described suggests that the constructs of dissociation, numbing, and avoidance primarily involve three features. The first pertains to derealization, depersonalization, and memory loss; the second denotes the absence of affect in emotional contexts; and the third relates to effortful cognitive avoidance. Most measures focus on one or two of these features, with the exception of the SASRQ, which includes all three. With these distinctions in mind, we will now proceed to review the empirical literature on dissociation, numbing, and avoidance.

STUDIES OF DISSOCIATION, NUMBING, AND AVOIDANCE

Researchers have documented the presence of dissociative features following a variety of traumatic experiences. The results of these empirical investigations are summarized below, according to the type of trauma.

War Exposure

Using the DES with Vietnam War veterans, several studies have demonstrated that PTSD is associated with increased use of dissociative strategies (Bernstein & Putnam, 1986; Branscombe, 1991; Bremner et al., 1992; Coons, Bowman, Pellow & Schneider, 1989; Huska & Weathers, 1991; Orr et al., 1990). The degree of dissociation, as measured by the DES, was higher in male veterans with PTSD than in alcoholics, agoraphobics, and normals (Bernstein & Putnam, 1986). DES scores were also positively related to the severity of PTSD in combat veterans (Bremner et al., 1992; Waid & Urbanczyk, 1989). However, DES scores were also highly correlated with depression and anxiety, suggesting that the relationship of dissociation to PTSD is not specific but rather reflects the relationship between dissociation and psychopathology.

Several factor analytical studies of posttrauma symptoms in war veterans have identified dissociation as a core feature of PTSD. Silver and Iacono (1984) have conducted a factor analysis on psychiatric symptoms reported by Vietnam combat veterans and have identified four factors: depression, grief-guilt, reexperiencing, and detachment-anger. The latter factor was characterized by emotional detachment and difficulty experiencing emotions. Since PTSD diagnosis was not determined, the relationship of these symptoms to traumatic experiences was not determined. Davidson, Smith, and Kudler (1989) also factor analyzed the DSM-III-R symptoms of PTSD reported by 116 veterans of World War II, Korea, and Vietnam. Three factors were identified: reexperiencing and arousal, avoidance and detachment, and constricted affect and memory impairment. In a third study, Solomon, Mikulincer, and Benbenishty (1989) interviewed soldiers 1 year after the combat and submitted their reported symptoms to a factor analysis. A psychic numbing factor emerged that accounted for 20% of the variance (Solomon et al., 1989). The symptoms that loaded on this factor were: detachment from others and from one's surroundings, numbing of responses, mental escape, and distraction. The second factor, anxiety reactions, accounted for 11% of the variance. These results point to the prominent position of dissociation in posttrauma sequela.

Several studies have demonstrated that the use of dissociative strategies during combat were associated with chronic posttrauma reactions. Using the IES, Solomon and Mikulincer (1992) evaluated symptoms of intrusion and avoidance in two groups of soldiers: those who suffered combat stress response (CSR), or "battle shock," and those who did not. Soldiers with CSR reported more intrusion and avoidance symptoms 3 years after combat than those without CSR. However, in both groups, intrusion and avoidance symptoms decreased as a function of the time that had elapsed since combat exposure.

In a retrospective study, Bremner et al. (1992) compared the reported dissociation at the time of specific traumatic events in Vietnam veterans with and without PTSD. Dissociation during combat was evaluated using a modified version of the DES. PTSD patients reported more dissociative symptoms during combat traumas than did those without PTSD. A similar study was conducted by Marmar and coworkers (1992). These researchers also examined retrospectively the emotional experiences during combat of female and male Vietnam theatre veterans using the DES and the PDEQ-interviewer version. Consistent with the findings of Solomon et al. (1989) and Bremner et al. (1992), dissociative experiences reported during combat were highly associated with chronic posttrauma reactions.

Taken together, the above studies seem to indicate a common tendency to dissociate during a combat experience, and that such dissociation results in prolonged pathological reactions. However, it is important to note that all three studies used retrospective methodology, and therefore the results should be interpreted with caution. It is possible that individuals with more severe posttrauma pathology are more likely to report the dissociative experiences during the traumatic event than do individuals who have successfully recovered, irrespective of the degree of dissociation they had actually experienced during the traumatic event itself. If the reported dissociation during trauma accurately reflects the degree of dissociation during the trauma, then the argument can be made that although dissociation may provide short-term relief during a stressful event, the use of this coping style hinders recovery later on.

Several laboratory studies have explored dissociative phenomena in combat veterans. Spiegel et al. (1988) found that combat veterans with PTSD were more hypnotizable than their non-PTSD cohorts. Conceptualizing hypnotizability as a measure of dissociation, they concluded that individuals with PTSD dissociate more than those without PTSD. To study emotional numbing, veterans with and without PTSD were given an affective recognition task. As expected, veterans with PTSD had more difficulty evaluating and identifying emotions than those without PTSD (Zimering, Caddell, Fairbank, & Keane, 1993). A different method to examine numbing was employed by Orr (1991). Veterans with and without PTSD were asked to imagine a pleasant scene. No differences emerged between the PTSD and non-PTSD subjects on psychophysiology, self-report of emotional reactions, and facial expression of emotions. Influenced by results from animal experiments demonstrating opiate-mediated analgesia following uncontrollable electrical shocks, Pitman, van der Kolk, Orr, and Greenberg (1990) hypothesized that numbing symptoms in PTSD sufferers is mediated by endogenous opiates. To test this hypothesis, veterans with and without PTSD were exposed to combat movies. Pain tolerance was used as a measure of numbing. Veterans with PTSD showed decreased pain sensitivity in response to an ice-cold water test after watching the movies. No such decrease occurred when naloxone, an opiate antagonist, was administered, suggesting an opiate-mediated stress-induced analgesia in PTSD. The non-PTSD veterans showed no decrease in pain following the movies.

Abuse in Childhood

Several studies have investigated the relationship between dissociation and PTSD in individuals who were sexually abused in childhood. Using the DES, Coons et al. (1989) evaluated dissociation in psychiatric patients with a variety of diagnoses, including PTSD. A significantly higher incidence of childhood abuse was found among female patients who were referred to a counseling center than among female bulimics attending an eating disorders clinic. Further, the incidence of dissociation and PTSD was significantly higher in the former group.

Using the DES, Sanders and Giolas (1991) examined dissociation and childhood abuse in a group of emotionally disturbed adolescents. Modest correlations between history of childhood abuse and DES score were obtained in this sample, replicating the findings that have been obtained in college students (Sanders, McRoberts, & Tollefson, 1989). Chu and Dill (1990) also found that female psychiatric inpatients with childhood physical or sexual abuse scored significantly higher on the DES than did women without such a history. However, unlike the results of Coons et al. (1989), the severity of the DES scores was not related to diagnoses of PTSD or to dissociative disorders.

Several authors have postulated a relationship between symptoms of borderline personality and childhood abuse (Gelinas, 1983; Herman, Perry, & van der Kolk, 1989). In a retrospective study, Herman et al. (1989) examined the relationship between childhood trauma histories of patients with borderline personality disorder, PTSD symptoms (measured by IES), and the DES. They found a significant relationship between severity of trauma history, severity of PTSD symptoms, and the presence of borderline personality disorder. Also, patients with this disorder generally reported higher DES scores than those without this diagnosis, suggesting a link between sexual abuse, borderline personality, dissociation, and PTSD.

Similar results were reported in a study evaluating the sexual and physical abuse experiences in female and male adults diagnosed with borderline personality disorder using the Diagnostic Interview for Borderline Patients (DIB) (Gunderson, Kolb, & Austin, 1982). Although the DIB is not specifically designed to evaluate a wide range of dissociative experiences, a few items about derealization and depersonalization are included. The results of the study confirmed the hypothesized relationship among childhood sexual abuse, borderline personality, and dissociative symptoms (Ogata, Silk, Goodrich, Lohr, Westen, & Hill, 1990). Finally, Boon and Draijer (1991) reported a high prevalence of child abuse among patients who met criteria for dissociative and personality disorders using the Structured Clinical Interview for DSM-III-R Dissociative Disorders (SCID-D).

The studies described above converge to suggest a relationship among childhood abuse, psychopathology (including PTSD, dissociative disorders, and personality disorders), and tendency to employ dissociative strategies. However, this tendency is associated with general psychopathology and is not specific to PTSD.

Adult Victims of Assault

Symptoms of anxiety and dissociation have also been observed in adult victims of assault (Burgess & Holmstrom, 1976). Moderate dissociation (measured by the DES) in female victims of sexual and nonsexual assault was observed immediately after the assault, which declined over time, reaching a normal range 3 months later (Dancu, Riggs, Hearst-Ikeda, Shoyer, & Foa, in press). As with victims of childhood abuse, dissociation was related to posttrauma psychopathology (e.g., RIES, Beck Depression Inventory, State Trait Anxiety Inventory) in both rape and nonsexual assault victims. Dissociation was also related to PTSD diagnosis in nonsexual victims but not in rape victims. Thus, these results support the view that dissociation is related to general psychopathology rather than PTSD. Riggs, Dancu, Gershuny, Greenberg, and Foa (1992) also found that victims with a history of childhood sexual abuse reported more dissociation than victims without such a history. These findings are consistent with those of Chu and Dill (1990), and together they suggest that trauma in childhood may predispose victims to dissociate after a subsequent trauma in adulthood.

In the factor analytical study mentioned earlier that used the DSM-III-R symptoms of PTSD in recent female assault victims, Foa et al. (1993a) identified three factors: arousal-avoidance, numbing, and intrusion. The items that loaded on the numbing factor were: numbing of feelings, detachment from others, loss of interest, and a sense of foreshortened future. The numbing symptoms best distinguished assault victims with PTSD from those without PTSD 3 months after the assault. These findings concur with those of Solomon and colleagues using the DES with Israeli war veterans (Solomon et al., 1989; Solomon & Mikulincer, 1992). Although the symptoms that comprised the numbing factor differ from those of the DES, both studies reveal association between dissociation and the experience of trauma.

Abduction and Incarceration

In two studies, Kinzie and colleagues (Kinzie, Sack, Angell, Manson, & Rath, 1986; Kinzie, Sack, Angell, Clarke, & Rath, 1989) evaluated the posttrauma reactions of Cambodian adolescents 4 years after being incarcerated in the Pol Pot concentration camps. The victims reported a variety of traumas including separation from family members, starvation, being beaten, and witnessing the deaths of their companions. Four years after incarceration, half of these youths met DSM-III-R criteria for PTSD, 58% avoided memories of the camp, and 43% avoided discussing their traumas. Seven years after incarceration, 48% of the participants had PTSD and 41% exhibited moderate to severe depression. Thus, avoidance of trauma reminders was most common in victims of incarceration years after their traumatic experiences. While no other dissociation symptoms were reported in this study, the high prevalence of PTSD suggests that many victims experienced numbing symptoms. More direct evidence for the presence of dissociative symptoms following incarceration comes from a review of anecdotal accounts of prisoners of war about their emotional experiences during the trauma (Siegel, 1984). Twenty-six percent of the prisoners evidenced emotional numbing and depersonalization, and 13% experienced out of body experiences.

Accidents

Two studies by Noyes and colleagues examined dissociation in survivors of life-threatening situations (e.g., an automobile accident, a drowning, a fall, a serious illness). The first study consisted of interviewing accident survivors and administering a questionnaire inquiring about dissociative experiences during the trauma. The questionnaire revealed a wide range of dissociative symptoms including detachment, depersonalization, absence of affect, perceptual distortions, and feelings of unreality (Noyes & Kletti, 1977). In the second study, the dissociative symptoms of hospitalized automobile accident survivors and psychiatric patients were examined (Noyes, Hoenk, Kuperman, & Slymen, 1977). Accident victims were asked about their dissociative experiences during the trauma, and psychiatric patients were asked about dissociative experiences during the most recent episode of their illness. A 56-item questionnaire administered in this study was submitted to factor analysis. Three factors emerged for both populations: detachment, mental clouding, and alertness. Both victims and psychiatric patients reported experiences of depersonalization and dissociation; "mental clouding" was prevalent in psychiatric patients, whereas perceptual and time distortions were the predominant symptoms in accident victims. High prevalence of avoidance and numbing symptoms (about 25 to 40%) was also found among adult survivors of severe flame, chemical, electrical, or scald burns (Roca, Spence, & Munster, 1992) and among survivors of the Hyatt Regency Hotel skywalk collapse (Wilkinson, 1983) 4 to 5 months after the trauma.

Natural Disasters

Dissociation and avoidance symptoms have also been reported in victims of natural disasters and appear to be associated with persistent posttrauma psychopathology. Using an expanded version of the Hopkins Symptom Checklist to include PTSD items, Madakasira and O'Brien (1987) evaluated the posttrauma reactions of disaster victims after a tornado in North Carolina. Five months after the trauma, 82% of the victims were bothered by intrusive thoughts, 61% suffered memory loss of the trauma, 57% experienced feelings of estrangement, and 31% avoided trauma reminders.

Two studies used the SASRQ to examine dissociation after a natural disaster. In the first study, two groups of earthquake survivors were compared. One group was evaluated 1 week after the earthquake and the other 4 months later. As expected, more symptoms of dissociation and anxiety were reported by the former than the latter group (Cardena & Spiegel, 1993). In the second study, firestorm survivors were evaluated on two occasions: within the first month after the fire and 7 to 9 months later. Dissociation and anxiety were highly correlated within the first month posttrauma and both symptom clusters followed similar recovery courses. Interestingly, dissociative symptoms were stronger predictors of chronic posttrauma reactions than symptoms of anxiety (Koopman, Cardeña, Classen, & Spiegel, Ch. 17, this volume). Similarly, McFarlane (1986) reported that DSM-III-R symptoms of avoidance predicted persistent PTSD in survivors of the Ash Wednesday brush fires. These findings, like those of Foa et al. (1995a), point to the cardinal role of dissociation in PTSD.

Witnessing Trauma

Using a short version of the SASRQ, Freinkel, Koopman, and Spiegel (1994) studied anxiety and dissociation symptoms of journalists during and immediately after witnessing an execution. Symptoms of emotional numbing, cognitive avoidance, and derealization were more prevalent than anxiety symptoms. The frequency of the dissociation symptoms reported by this sample was as high as that of survivors of natural disasters (Koopman, Classen, & Spiegel, 1994) but did not persist as long.

In summary, the studies reviewed above indicate that dissociative experiences during and immediately after a trauma are frequent and are strongly associated with persistent posttrauma reactions. Moreover, dissociative symptoms during or shortly after a trauma may be a stronger predictor of PTSD than anxiety symptoms. It is unclear, however, whether the tendency to dissociate has a causal relationship to the development of chronic PTSD. It is possible that both the tendency to dissociate and the vulnerability to develop chronic PTSD are mediated by other factors such as childhood experiences. The strong relationship between childhood abuse and dissociation strongly supports this proposition. Most studies also indicate that dissociative symptoms are not unique to trauma victims; rather, they seem to reflect general psychopathology. How can we explain the relationship between traumatic experiences, dissociation, and psychopathology?

INFORMATION-PROCESSING PERSPECTIVE OF EMOTIONAL DISSOCIATION IN RESPONSE TO TRAUMA

Many authors have noted that emotional experiences are often relived long after the original emotional events have occurred (e.g., Freud, 1920; Lindemann, 1944; Rachman, 1980; Foa & Kozak, 1991). As is apparent from the studies reviewed above, this phenomenon is clearly exemplified in individuals who have experienced traumatic events. Usually, the frequency and intensity of this emotional reexperiencing of the trauma gradually diminishes over time. Thus, shortly after the attack, a rape victim may experience intense fear when reminded of the assault, and with time this fear lessens, although perhaps it never completely disappears.

Rachman (1980) discussed the significance of the processes that underlie the decline of emotional reexperiencing and suggested that when these processes are impaired, psychopathology surfaces. He further proposed that the persistence of neurotic symptoms such as intrusive thoughts, nightmares, excessive fears, and sleep disturbances are signs of unsatisfactory "absorption" of the emotional experience. The overlap between these signs and the symptom criteria for PTSD is striking, and it has lead Foa (1993) to propose that the presence of PTSD reflects impairment in emotional processing of a traumatic experience. If this is true, Foa (1993) suggested, the identification of factors that differentiate trauma victims with chronic PTSD from victims without PTSD would shed light on the mechanisms that facilitate or hinder emotional processing. Moreover, successful treatment of PTSD can be viewed as assisting in emotional processing, and thus, factors that distinguish individuals who improved with treatment from those who failed to show improvement may further our knowledge of the pathology underlying PTSD.

To explain the mechanism by which cognitive-behavioral therapy reduced pathological anxiety (i.e., signs of impaired processing), Foa and Kozak (1986) extended Lang's (1977, 1979) bioinformation model of pathological fear. Using this framework, we will provide an information-processing analysis of how dissociation impairs the normal processing of a traumatic event, thereby contributing to the development and maintenance of chronic PTSD. We will also provide an explanation of how exposure treatment prevents or negates the deleterious effects of dissociation.

The Cognitive Structure of Fear

Lang (1977, 1979) proposed that fear is represented in memory as a structure that comprises information about: (1) feared stimuli, (2) physiological and motor responses, and (3) interpretive information about their meaning. Lang further suggested that a fear structure constitutes a "program" for escape from threat. If a fear structure is a program for escaping danger, then it must involve information that trauma-related stimuli and/or responses are dangerous. And it is this meaning information, Foa and Kozak (1986) contended, that distinguishes a fear structure from other cognitive structures.

Most people experience fear in some circumstances, which implies the "running" of a fear program. "Normal" fear occurs when an individual perceives actual threat, and it subsides when the danger is removed. When does a fear become pathological? Foa and Kozak (1986) noted that several characteristics distinguish pathological fear. First, fear becomes pathological when it is extremely intense and when it persists, despite information that it is unrealistic. In other words, a pathological fear structure involves excessive response elements, such as representations of avoidance and physiological activity, that are resistant to modification. Second, a pathological fear structure includes unrealistic elements. This implies that stimulus-stimulus associations do not accurately represent the world. For example, for the rape victim who was raped at gunpoint by a tall, bearded man, the elements "tall, bearded man" may become erroneously associated with the stimulus "gun." Third, mistaken associations between nondangerous stimuli and escape or avoidance responses are also characteristic of a pathological fear structure. Indeed, running away from a "tall, bearded man" is not likely to enhance the safety of the victim.

In addition to erroneous association among elements, victims with pathological fear make several evaluative mistakes. First, they commonly believe that anxiety, once experienced, will persist unless they escape the feared situation. Second, they overestimate the probability that the feared stimuli or responses will cause physical or psychological harm. And third, their feared consequences have an extremely high negative valence.

According to Foa and Kozak (1986), different anxiety disorders represent different pathological fear structures. For example, there is evidence to suggest that erroneous interpretations of fear responses distinguish the structure of agoraphobia from that of simple phobia. Agoraphobics commonly interpret anxiety responses, themselves, as threatening, since they expect these responses to result in physical or psychological harm. For an agoraphobic, stimulus elements such as "tunnels" are not perceived as inherently dangerous; rather, the danger is perceived to exist in the anxiety that these elements engender. In contrast, for simple phobics, the danger lies in the stimulus situation itself, such as "snakes," "airplanes," or "insects."

Foa (1993) suggested that PTSD, like the other anxiety disorders, can be construed as reflecting a pathological fear structure that contains faulty associations and erroneous evaluations. She further proposed that a trauma memory can be viewed as a fear structure. It includes information about stimuli and responses related to the trauma, as well as information about their meaning. The trauma structure of a woman who was raped at gunpoint at her home in the suburbs will include the stimulus elements of "gun," "man," his physical characteristics such as "tall," and "beard," and environmental stimuli such as "home" and suburbs." The response elements will include physiological responses such as "tachycardia" and behavioral responses such as "struggling" and "screaming."

In a trauma memory of a non-PTSD victim, "rape" and "pointed gun" are associated with a "danger" meaning but neutral stimuli such as "man," "home," and "suburbs" are not. In a pathological trauma structure that underlies PTSD, stimuli that are inherently neutral such as "tall, bearded man," "home," and "suburbs" are associated with the meaning "danger." Because many stimuli become associated with danger meaning, the world as a whole is perceived as threatening by the victim with PTSD. Foa and Riggs (1993) have suggested that a pathological trauma structure includes not only erroneous interpretations of stimulus elements but also mistaken interpretations of response elements. In particular, they proposed that responses during the trauma such as "struggling" and "screaming" become associated with the meaning "self-incompetence." A pathological trauma structure also includes particularly intense response elements that are reflected in PTSD symptoms such as excessive avoidance and arousal. In summary, a pathological trauma structure is distinguished by excessive response elements, as well as erroneous interpretations of intrinsically neutral stimuli as dangerous and normal responses to trauma as reflecting self-incompetence.

Modification of the Trauma Structure

Studies have revealed that 95% of female rape victims and 75% of female nonsexual assault victims met symptom criteria for PTSD within the first 2 weeks after the trauma (Rothbaum, Foa, Riggs, Murdock, & Walsh, 1992). It follows that, for most people, immediately after a traumatic experience the trauma memory includes pathological elements such as excessive responses and faulty interpretations. Rothbaum et al. (1992) further noted that over time, only 50% of rape victims and 25% of nonsexual assault victims met criteria for the disorder. This finding suggests that, in the course of time, the trauma structure of many victims undergoes modification.

Foa and Kozak (1986) have suggested that the modification of a pathological fear structure is the essence of emotional processing, and that successful therapy promotes emotional processing. How does emotional processing occur in the natural progression of recovery from a trauma? We argue that the understanding of how cognitive behavioral therapy reduces pathological fear will help us conceptualize natural recovery from a trauma.

Foa and Kozak (1986) proposed that two conditions are necessary for emotional processing to occur. First, therapists must activate the fear structure by providing information that matches the information represented in the structure. For if the fear structure remains unaccused, it will not be available for correction. Second, information provided during therapy must also be incompatible with the pathological elements in the structure. Extending this model, we propose that in order to acquire a spontaneous decline of posttrauma emotional disturbances, the trauma memory, including its emotional elements, must be repeatedly activated by contact with trauma-related stimuli. Further, this contact should include corrective information about the world (e.g., "not all tall, bearded men carry guns and rape") and about oneself (e.g., "screaming during the rape does not mean that I am incompetent").

Dissociation Impedes Emotional Processing

The view that repeated engagement with the trauma memory is important for a successful resolution of the traumatic experience has been shared by many theorists (e.g., Freud, 1920; Horowitz, 1986). In fact, Horowitz (1986) invented the term *completion principle* to denote the natural tendency to process new information until it is "brought up to date" with inner schemas of the self and of the world. A stressful life event, he suggested, includes by definition information that is incompatible with a person's inner cognitive models, and thus requires more processing activity than nonstressful experiences. But the completion principle conflicts with the tendency to avoid trauma reminders in order to protect oneself from emotional pain, the pain that is associated with the trauma. Dissociation or numbing, like avoidance, is a strategy to avert trauma-related distressing emotions (Davidson & Foa, 1991; Spiegel et al., 1988). If recovery (i.e., emotional processing) requires repeated engagement with the trauma memory, then dissociation is expected to impede this process.

Indirect evidence supporting the hypothesis that dissociation impairs emotional processing and hence impedes recovery comes from the repeated finding that dissociation during or immediately after the traumatic experience is associated with later psychopathology. More direct evidence comes from a study examining the facial fear expression of assault victims during therapy that involved reliving of the trauma (Foa, Riggs, Massie, & Yarczower, in press). Assault victims who displayed more intense facial fear expressions and reported greater subjective distress during the first reliving session benefited more from treatment than those who displayed less intense fear. These findings converge with those of other studies that measured fear activation via increase in heart rate. With simple phobics, Lang, Melamed, and Hart (1970) found that clients who evidenced higher heart rate response during the first imaginal exposure to feared stimuli manifested greater improvement in their phobias. Similar results were reported with obsessive-compulsives: a strong positive correlation was found between heart rate increase during the first in vivo exposure to the patients' most feared situations and change in measures of obsessional fear (Kozak, Foa, Steketee, & Grayson, 1988). In all of these studies, emotional engagement with the feared memory enhanced emotional processing. Conversely, emotional disengagement (i.e., dissociation) hampered emotional processing. Interestingly, in the Foa and co-workers' (in press) study described above, victims who reported more anger prior to treatment displayed less fear during reliving of the trauma and benefited less from treatment. These results correspond with the finding that intense anger shortly after an assault predicts PTSD severity 1 month later in female victims (Riggs et al., 1992). If, as we suggested, PTSD reflects a failure to emotionally process the traumatic event, then anger appears to impede the mechanisms underlying both the "natural" emotional processing and emotional processing during treatment. The negative association between anger and facial fear expression implies that anger impedes processing of the trauma by inhibiting the activation of fear. It is possible that anger, like effortful avoidance and dissociation, is a means by which victims with PTSD regulate their arousal and emotional distress.

FURTHER CONSIDERATIONS

In this chapter we have adopted the view that dissociation or numbing may represent a strategy for reducing or avoiding trauma-related emotional distress. We have proposed that excessive use of dissociation prevents the activation of the traumatic memory, and that repeated activation is a necessary condition for emotional processing to occur. It follows that dissociation is one factor underlying the persistence of posttrauma disturbances, and thus, it is implicated in the development of chronic PTSD and related psychopathology.

The conceptualization of dissociation that we have offered here carries implications for the treatment of trauma-related psychopathology. If recovery from a trauma requires emotional engagement with the traumatic memory, then treatment of chronic PTSD should involve the promotion of such engagement. Indeed, successful treatments for PTSD consist of the reliving of the trauma in imagination (Boudewyns & Wilson, 1972; Boudewyns, 1975; Foa, Rothbaum, Riggs, & Murdock, 1991; Keane, Fairbank, Caddell, & Zimering, 1989; Keane & Kaloupek, 1985).

The use of exposure therapy to promote emotional processing assumes that the tendency to dissociate will be conquered by therapeutic instructions to engage in the emotional reliving of the trauma. The results of treatment studies that employed exposure support this presumption.

For the most part, successful reduction of trauma-related distress via treatment should eliminate the function of dissociation, and thus reduce dissociative responses. However, clinical observations reveal that some traumatized individuals continue to dissociate during the reliving of the trauma, rendering exposure therapy ineffective. For such individuals, therapeutic techniques directly aimed at reducing dissociation must be implemented. Such interventions are reported in the literature (for a summary of treatment for multiple personality disorder, see Putnam, 1989), but studies of their efficacy are awaiting controlled investigation.

ACKNOWLEDGMENTS. This research was supported by NIMH grant #MH42178-07 to the first author.

REFERENCES

American Psychiatric Association. (1980). *Diagnostic and statistical manual of mental disorders* (3rd ed.) Washington, DC: Author.

American Psychiatric Association. (1987). *Diagnostic and statistical manual of mental disorders* (3rd ed., rev.) Washington, DC: Author.

American Psychiatric Association. (1994). *Diagnostic and statistical manual of mental disorders* (4th ed.). Washington, DC: Author.

Bernstein, E. M., & Putnam, F. W. (1986). Development, reliability and validity of a dissociation scale. *Journal of Nervous and Mental Disease, 174,* 727-734.

Bliss, E. L. (1984). Multiple personalities: A report of 14 cases with implications for schizophrenia and hysteria. *Archives of General Psychiatry, 37,* 1388-1397.

Boon, S., & Draijer, N. (1991). Diagnosing dissociative disorders in the Netherlands: A pilot study with the structured clinical interview for D-III-R dissociative disorders. *American Journal of Psychiatry, 148,* 458-462.

Boudewyns, P. (1975). Implosive therapy and desensitization therapy with inpatients: A five-year follow-up. *Journal of Abnormal Psychology, 84,* 159-160.

Boudewyns, P. A., & Wilson, A. E. (1972). Implosive therapy and desensitization therapy using free association in the treatment of inpatients. *Journal of Abnormal Psychology, 79,* 259-268.

Branscombe, L. B. (1991). Dissociation in combat-related post-traumatic stress disorder. *Dissociation, 4,* 13-20.

Braun, B. G. & Sachs, R. G. (1985). The development of multiple personality disorder: Predisposing, precipitating, and perpetuating factors. In R. P. Kluft (Ed.), *Childhood Antecedents of Multiple Personality* (pp. 37-64). Washington, DC: American Psychiatric Press.

Bremner, J. D., Southwick, S., Brett, E., Fontana, A., Rosenheck, R., & Charney, D. (1992). Dissociation and posttraumatic stress disorder in Vietnam combat veterans. *American Journal of Psychiatry, 149,* 328-332.

Breuer, J., & Freud, S. (1985). *Studies on hysteria.* New York: Basic Books.

Burgess, A. W., & Holmstrom, L. L. (1976). Coping behavior of the rape victim. *American Journal of Psychiatry, 133,* 413-418.

Cardena, E., & Spiegel, D. (1993). Dissociative reactions to the Bay Area earthquake. *American Journal of Psychiatry, 150,* 474-478.

Cardena, E., Classen, K., & Spiegel, D. (1991). *Stanford acute stress reaction questionnaire.* Stanford, CA: Stanford University Medical School.

Chu, J. A., & Dill, D. L. (1990). Dissociative symptoms in relation to childhood physical and sexual abuse. *American Journal of Psychiatry, 147,* 887-892.

Coons, P., & Milstein, V. (1986). Rape and post-traumatic stress in multiple personality. *Psychological Reports, 55,* 839-845.

Coons, P. M., Bowman, E. S., Pellow, T. A., & Schneider, P. (1989). Post-traumatic aspects of the treatment of victims of sexual abuse and incest. *Treatment of Victims of Sexual Abuse, 12,* 325-335.

Dancu, C. V., Riggs, D. S., Hearst-Ikeda, D., Shoyer, B., & Foa, E. B. (in press). *Dissociative experiences and post-traumatic stress disorder among female victims of criminal assault and rape. Journal of Traumatic Stress.*

Davidson, J., & Foa, E. B. (1991). Diagnostic issues in post-traumatic stress disorder: Consideration for the DSM-IV. *Journal of Abnormal Psychology, 100,* 346-355.

Davidson, J., Smith, R., & Kudler, H. (1989). Validity and reliability of the DSM-III criteria for posttraumatic stress disorder: Experience with a structured interview. *Journal of Nervous and Mental Disease, 177,* 336-341.

Foa, E. B. (1993, August). *Psychopathology and treatment of PTSD in rape victims*. Paper presented at the 101st American Psychological Association Annual Convention, Toronto, Canada.

Foa, E. B., & Kozak, M. J. (1986). Emotional processing of fear: Exposure to corrective information. *Psychological Bulletin, 99*, 20-35.

Foa, E. B., & Kozak, M. J. (1991). Emotional processing: Theory, research and clinical implications for anxiety disorder. In J. Safran & L. S. Greenberg (Eds.), *Emotion psychotherapy and change* (pp. 21-49). New York: Guilford Press.

Foa, E. B., & Riggs, D. S. (1993). Post-traumatic stress disorder in rape victims. In J. Oldham, M. B. Riba, & A. Tasman (Eds.), *American psychiatric press review of psychiatry* (Vol. 12, pp. 273-303). Washington, DC: American Psychiatric Press.

Foa, E. B., Riggs, D. S., Dancu, C. V., & Rothbaum, B. O. (1993). Reliability and validity of a brief instrument for assessing post-traumatic stress disorder. *Journal of Traumatic Stress, 6*, 459-473.

Foa, E. B., Riggs, D. S., & Gershuny, B. (1995). Arousal, numbing, and intrusion: Symptom structure of posttraumatic stress disorder following assault. *American Journal of Psychiatry, 152*, 116-120.

Foa, E. B., Riggs, D. S., Massie, E. D., & Yarczower, M. (in press). *The impact of fear activation and anger on the efficacy of exposure treatment for PTSD. Behavior Therapy.*

Foa, E. B., Rothbaum, B. O., Riggs, D. S., & Murdock, T. (1991). A prospective examination of post-traumatic stress disorder in rape victims. *Journal of Traumatic Stress, 5*, 455-475.

Foa, E. B., Steketee, G., & Rothbaum, B. O. (1989). Behavioral/cognitive conceptualization of post-traumatic stress disorder. *Behavior Therapy, 20*, 155-176.

Foa, E. B., Zinbarg, R., & Rothbaum, B. O. (1992). Uncontrollability and unpredictability in posttraumatic stress disorder. *Psychological Bulletin, 112*, 218-238.

Freinkel, A., Koopman, C., & Spiegel, D. (1994). *Dissociative symptoms in media eyewitnesses of an execution. American Journal of Psychiatry, 157*, 1335-1339.

Freud, S. (1950). Beyond the pleasure principle. In J. Strachey (Ed. and Trans.), *Complete psychological works, standard edition.* (Vol. 3, pp. 9-11). London: Hogarth Press. (Originally published in 1920.)

Gelinas, D. (1983). The persisting negative effects of incest. *Psychiatry, 46*, 312-332.

Gunderson, J. G., Kolb, J. E., & Austin, V. (1982). The diagnostic interview for borderline patients. *American Journal of Psychiatry, 138*, 896-903.

Herman, J., Perry, J. C., & van der Kolk, J. B. (1989). Childhood trauma in borderline personality disorder. *American Journal of Psychiatry, 146*, 490-495.

Hilgard, E. R. (1977). *Divided consciousness: Multiple controls in human thoughts and action*. New York: Wiley.

Horowitz, M., Wilner, N., Kaltreider, N., & Alvarez, W. (1980). Signs and symptoms of posttraumatic stress disorders. *Archives of General Psychiatry, 37*, 85-92.

Horowitz, M. J. (1986). *Stress-response syndromes* (2nd ed.). Northvale, NJ: Jason Aronson.

Horowitz, M. J., Wilner, N., & Alvarez, W. (1979). Impact of event scale: A measure of subjective distress. *Psychosomatic Medicine, 41*, 207-218.

Huska, J. A., & Weathers, F. W. (1991). *Reliability and validity of the dissociative experiences scale in combat-related PTSD*. Unpublished manuscript. Boston, MA: Behavioral Sciences Division, National Center for PTSD, Boston DVAMC.

Janet, P. (1989). *L'Automisme psychologique*. Paris: Felix Alcan.

Janet, P. (1907). *The major symptoms of hysteria*. New York: Macmillian.

Keane, T. M., & Kaloupek, D. G. (1985). Imaginal flooding in the treatment of post-traumatic stress disorder. *Journal of Consulting and Clinical Psychology, 50*, 138-140.

Keane, T. M., Zimering, R. T., & Caddell, J. M. (1985). A behavioral formulation of post-traumatic stress disorder in Vietnam veterans. *Behavior Therapist, 8*, 9-12.

Keane, T. M., Fairbank, J. A., Caddell, J. M., & Zimering, R. T. (1989). Implosive (flooding) therapy reduces symptoms of PTSD in Vietnam combat veterans. *Behavior Therapy, 20*, 245-260.

Kinzie, J. D., Sack, W. H., Angell, R. H., Manson, S., & Rath, B. (1986). The psychiatric effects of massive trauma on Cambodian children: I. The children. *Journal of the American Academy of Child Psychiatry, 25*, 370-376.

Kinzie, J. D., Sack, W. H., Angell, R. H., Clarke, G., & Rath, B. (1989). A three-year follow-up of Cambodian young people traumatized as children. *Journal of the American Academy of Child and Adolescent Psychiatry, 28*, 501-504.

Koopman, C., Classen, C., & Spiegel, D. (1994). *Predictors of post-traumatic stress symptoms among Oakland/Berkeley firestorm survivors. American Journal of Psychiatry, 151,* 888-894.

Kozak, M. J., Foa, E. B., Steketee, G., & Grayson, (1988). Process and outcome of exposure treatment with obsessive-compulsives: Psychophysiological indicators of emotional processing. *Behavior Therapy, 19,* 157-169.

Lang, P. J. (1977). Imagery in therapy: An information processing analysis of fear. *Behavior Therapy, 8,* 862-886.

Lang, P. (1979). A bio-informational theory of emotional imagery. *Psychophysiology, 16,* 495-512.

Lang, P., Melamed, B., & Hart, J. D. (1970). A psychophysiological analysis of fear modification using automated desensitization. *Journal of Abnormal Psychology, 31,* 220-234.

Lindemann, E. (1944). Symptomatology and management of acute grief. *American Journal of Psychiatry, 101,* 141-148.

Litz, B. T. (1993). Emotional numbing in combat-related post-traumatic stress disorder: A critical review and reformulation. *Clinical Psychology Review, 12,* 417-432.

Madakasira, S., & O'Brien, K. (1987). Acute posttraumatic stress disorder in victims of natural disaster. *Journal of Nervous and Mental Disorders, 175,* 286-290.

Marmar, C. R., & Weiss, D. S. (1990). *Peritraumatic dissociative experiences questionnaire-subject version.* Unpublished scale. San Francisco, CA: San Francisco Medical School.

Marmar, C. R., Weiss, D. S., Schlenger, W. E., Fairbank, J. A., Jordan, B. K., Kulka, R,. A., & Hough, R. L. (1994). Peritraumatic dissociation and post-traumatic stress in male Vietnam theatre veterans. *American Journal of Psychiatry, 151,* 902-907.

McFarlane, A. C. (1986). Posttraumatic morbidity of a disaster: A study of cases presenting for psychiatric treatment. *Journal of Nervous and Mental Disease, 174,* 4-14.

Nemiah, J. (1981). Dissociation disorders. In A. M. Freeman & H. I. Kaplan (Eds.), *Comprehensive textbook of psychiatry.* (3rd ed., pp. 1554-1561). Baltimore: Williams & Wilkins.

Noyes, Jr., R., & Kletti, R. (1977). Depersonalization in the face of life-threatening danger: A description. *Psychiatry, 39,* 19-27.

Noyes, Jr., R., Hoenk, P. R., Kuperman, S., & Slymen, D. J. (1977). Depersonalization in accident victims and psychiatric patients. *Journal of Nervous Disorder and Mental Disease, 164,* 401-407.

Ogata, S. N., Silk, K. R., Goodrich, S., Lohr, N., Westen, D., & Hill, E. M. (1990). Childhood sexual and physical abuse in adult patients with borderline personality disorder. *American Journal of Psychiatry, 147,* 1008-1013.

Orr, W. (1991). Psychophysiological studies of posttraumatic stress disorder. In E. L. Giller, Jr. (Ed.), *Biological assessment and treatment of posttraumatic stress disorder* (pp. 135-157). Washington, DC: American Psychiatric Press.

Orr, S. P., Claiborn, J. M., Altman, B., Forgue, D. F., De Jong, J. B., Pitman, R. K., & Herz, L. R. (1990). Psychometric profile of posttraumatic stress disorder, anxiety, and healthy Vietnam veterans: Correlations with psychophysiologic responses. *Journal of Consulting and Clinical Psychology, 58,* 329-335.

Pitman, R., van der Kolk, B., Orr, S., & Greenberg, L. (1990). Nalaxone-reversible analgesic response to combat-related stimuli in posttraumatic stress disorder: A pilot study. *Archives of General Psychiatry, 47,* 541-544.

Putnam, F. W. (1989). *Diagnosis and treatment of multiple personality disorder.* New York: Guilford Press.

Rachman, S. (1980). Emotional processing. *Behaviour Research and Therapy, 18,* 51-60.

Riggs, D. S., Dancu, C. V., Gershuny, B. S., Greenberg, D., & Foa, E. B. (1992). Anger and post-traumatic stress disorder in female crime victims. *Journal of Traumatic Stress, 5,* 613-625.

Roca, R. P., Spence, R. J., & Munster, A. (1992). Posttraumatic adaptation and distress among adult burn survivors. *American Journal of Psychiatry, 149,* 1234-1238.

Ross, C. A., Heber, S., Norton, G. R., Anderson, D., Anderson, G., & Barchet, (1989). The dissociative disorders interview schedule: A structured interview. *Dissociation: Progress in the Dissociative Disorders, 2(3),* 169-189.

Rothbaum, B. O., Foa, E. B., Riggs, D. S., Murdock, T., & Walsh, W. (1992). A prospective examination of post-traumatic stress disorder in rape victims. *Journal of Traumatic Stress, 5,* 455-475.

Sanders, B. (1986). The perceptual alterations scale: A scale measuring dissociation. *American Journal of Clinical Hypnosis, 29,* 95-102.

Sanders, B., & Giolas, M. H. (1991). Dissociation and childhood trauma in psychological disturbed adolescents. *American Journal of Psychiatry, 148*, 50-54.

Sanders, B., McRoberts, G., & Tollefson, C. (1989). Childhood stress and dissociative in a college population. *Dissociation, 2*, 17-23.

Silver, S., & Iacano, C. (1984). Factor analytic support for DSM-III post traumatic stress disorder for Vietnam veterans. *Journal of Clinical Psychology, 40*, 5-14.

Solomon, Z., & Mikulincer, M. (1992). Aftermaths of combat stress reactions: A three year study. *British Journal of Clinical Psychology, 31*, 21-32.

Solomon, Z., Mikulincer, M., & Benbenishty, B. (1989). Combat stress reaction: Clinical manifestations and correlates. *Military Psychology, 1*, 35-47.

Siegel, R. K. (1984). Hostage hallucinations. *Journal of Nervous and Mental Disorders, 172*, 264-272.

Spiegel, D. (1986). Dissociating damage. *American Journal of Clinical Hypnosis, 29*, 123-131.

Spiegel, D., & Cardena, E. (1990). dissociative mechanisms in posttraumatic stress disorder. In M. E. Wolf & A. D. Mosnian (Eds.), *Posttraumatic stress disorder: Etiology, phenomenology, and treatment* (pp. 23-34). Washington, DC: American Psychiatric Press.

Spiegel, D., Hunt, T., & Dondershine, H. E. (1988). Dissociation and hypnotizability in posttraumatic stress disorder. *American Journal of Psychiatry, 145*, 310-305.

Spiegel, H. (1963). The dissociation-association continuum. *Journal of Nervous and Mental Disorders, 136*, 374-378.

Terr, L. C. (1991). Childhood trauma: An outline and overview. *American Journal of Psychiatry, 148*, 10-16.

van der Kolk, B. (1987). *Psychological trauma*. Washington, DC: American Psychiatric Press.

van der Kolk, B., & Ducey, C. P. (1989). The psychological processing of traumatic experiences and Rorschach patterns in PTSD. *Journal of Traumatic Stress, 2*, 259-274.

Waid, L. R., & Urbanczyk, S. A. (1989, August). A comparison of high versus low dissociative Vietnam veterans with PTSD. Poster presented at the Annual Meeting of the American Psychological Association, New Orleans.

Wilkinson, C. B. (1983). Aftermath of a disaster: The collapse of the Hyatt Regency Hotel skywalk. *American Journal of Psychiatry, 140*, 1134-1139.

Zimering, R. T., Caddell, J. M., Fairbank, J. A., & Keane, T. M. (1993). Posttraumatic stress disorder in Vietnam veterans: An experimental validation of the DSM-III diagnostic criteria. *Journal of Traumatic Stress, 6*, 327-342.

IV
ASSESSMENT

Janet suggested that dissociation lies at the basis of almost all psychopathology. This idea has been supported in previous chapters with the many comments describing the manner in which dissociative experiences co-occur with a variety of affect psychopathologies. However, if dissociation is related to everything, then it becomes problematic to differentiate dissociative processes from other forms of psychopathology. This section approaches this important question and begins to ask how to assess dissociative processes. In Chapter 11, Cardeña and Spiegel begin to address the broad questions related to diagnostic issues including comorbidity of dissociative disorders. In Chapter 12, the focus becomes more specific in terms of DSM-IV criteria and the development of the SCID-D by Steinberg. Finally, Chapter 13, by Zahn, Moraga, and Ray, focuses on concomitant psychophysiological processes and hints at some physiological mechanisms involved in dissociative disorders.

Historically, some authors have identified dissociative disorders with hysteria. By doing so, they have included conversion reactions as well as somatizations along with severe shifts in identity, memory, and consciousness within the rubric of dissociation. To aid in our clarification of the boundaries of the term dissociation, Cardeña and Spiegel consider the speculations and formulations that informed DSM-IV by examining the five DSM-IV dissociative disorders: dissociative amnesia, dissociative fugue, dissociative identity disorder, depersonalization disorders, and dissociative disorders not otherwise specified. The chapter also raises the question of whether acute stress disorder, which is seen as an anxiety disorder in DSM-IV, should be considered to be a dissociative disorder. This, of course, raises a larger question as to the relationship of dissociation to other types of affective disorders such as anxiety and depression. In Chapter 12, Steinberg describes a variety of measures for diagnosing dissociative experiences and disorders. She also describes the development of the SCID-D with its structured and semistructured formats and its ability to assess the presence and severity of dissociative symptoms. In the final chapter of this section, Zahn, Moraga, and Ray examine psychophysiological indicants of dissociative processing. One intriguing finding within the folklore of dissociative identity disorder is the possibility that each identity can be organized differently in terms of physiology. This would mean that one identity, for example, could be allergic to one substance and another not show any signs of allergy. The initial part of this chapter examines the question as to whether different identities show differential physiological patterns, especially in terms of autonomic nervous system measures, and begins with the earliest psychophysiological study of DID, which was published by Morton Prince in 1908. The second part of the chapter focuses on central nervous system measures of dissociative processes. Since temporal lobe epilepsy patients may display dissociative symptoms, an important question asks if epilepsy lies at the heart of dissociative disorders. This chapter suggests that although epilepsy may produce dissociative symptoms, it is not logical to conclude that dissociation implies epilepsy.

11

Diagnostic Issues, Criteria, and Comorbidity of Dissociative Disorders

Etzel Cardeña and David Spiegel

> The fear of being nothing but an empty body that anybody—I or anyone else—could occupy, and the wretchedness of watching yourself, alive, and the doubt that it is—it is not—real.
>
> XAVIER VILLAURRUTIA, *Nocturno Miedo* (translated by Eliot Weinberger)

INTRODUCTION

While the interest in and concern with the dissociative disorders have grown exponentially in the last decade, with annual conventions, a journal exclusively devoted to dissociation, monographs, and so forth, this state of affairs represents more a rediscovery of concepts and phenomena than a brand new area of inquiry (cf. Spiegel & Cardeña, 1991; van der Kolk & van der Hart, 1989). Hysteria, a concept closely connected with the dissociative disorders, can be traced back at least to Pharaonic Egypt (cf. Kihlstrom, 1994). Closer to our times, just about every one of the forebears of modern psychopathology studied disorders involving a "disruption in the usually integrated functions of consciousness, memory, identity, or perception of the environment" (American Psychiatric Association, 1994, p. 477). For

Etzel Cardeña • Department of Psychiatry, Uniformed Services University of the Health Sciences, Bethesda, Maryland 20814. **David Spiegel** • Department of Psychiatry and Behavioral Sciences, Stanford University School of Medicine, Stanford, California 94305.

Handbook of Dissociation: Theoretical, Empirical, and Clinical Perspectives, edited by Larry K. Michelson and William J. Ray. Plenum Press, New York, 1996.

example, Breuer and Freud, Pierre Janet, William James, and Morton Prince, among a longer list of distinguished psychologists at the turn of the century, all described fascinating cases of pronounced shifts in identity, memory, somatic reactivity, and consciousness.

Still more recently, the drive to create a reliable psychiatric nosology gave rise to the first edition of a project that is now in its fourth decade and edition, namely the *Diagnostic and Statistical Manual of Mental Disorders* (DSM) of the American Psychiatric Association. The first edition of the DSM (American Psychiatric Association, 1952), under the subheading of psychoneurotic disorders, included "dissociative reaction" and "conversion reaction." The second edition of the DSM (DSM-II, American Psychiatric Association, 1968)) was a more elaborate taxonomy that, for the purposes of this chapter, classified what are currently regarded as dissociative disorders in the categories of "depersonalization neurosis" and "hysterical neurosis;" the latter either of a "conversion type" or a "dissociative type" (the latter including amnesia, fugue, and multiple personality). A shift toward a more descriptive and less theoretically laden taxonomy (e.g., note the deletion of the term "neurosis") is evident in the third edition of the DSM (DSM-III, American Psychiatric Association, 1980), which included a specific category for the dissociative disorders (i.e., psychogenic amnesia, psychogenic fugue, depersonalization disorder, multiple personality disorder, and atypical dissociative disorder) as a major diagnosis. A new term, "somatoform disorders," was devised for what used to be called "conversion type neurosis." Although there were some important changes in the criteria for the various diagnoses, the revised 3rd edition of the DSM (DSM-III-R, American Psychiatric Association, 1987) maintained the same general categories for the dissociative disorders. (For a more thorough review of the conceptual transformation of the concept of "dissociative disorders," consult Kihlstrom, 1994).

FROM DSM-III-R TO DSM-IV

A great wealth of information and theory has accumulated since the DSM-III-R, particularly with respect to the most severe form of the dissociative disorders, "dissociative identity disorder [or DID, previously known as multiple personality disorder (MPD)]. Nonetheless, some basic conceptual issues are controversial and far from solved, among them the uncertainty of whether dissociation is a descriptive or a theoretical term and what its boundaries are (cf. Cardeña, 1994). Another important issue is whether what are now called the somatization disorders (previously known as conversion) should be included under the rubric of the dissociative disorders. There are at least four arguments that can be adduced for subsuming somatization under the dissociative disorder: (1) historically, what used to be called hysteria typically included somatization phenomena such as hysterical paralysis and blindness, along with other dissociative phenomena; (2) even within the province of the current categorization of the dissociative disorder, somatization symptoms are frequently found among individuals with dissociative disorders (see comorbidity section); (3) most, if not all, of the somatization disorders can be conceptualized as a dissociation between the patient's anatomical or functional status and his/her conscious awareness of that status; and (4) The International Classification of

Diseases, 10th edition (ICD-10) includes a dissociative (conversion) disorder; a parallel development in the DSM would thus increase the compatibility between the two systems (cf. Garcia, 1990). While this is not the place to fully develop this argument, the interested reader can consult Nemiah (1991) and Kihlstrom (1994) for cogent discussions of this issue.

The bulk of this chapter provides the data and rationale for the changes made to the dissociative disorders in the DSM-IV. The appendix shows a comparison between the diagnostic criteria of the DSM-IV and those of its predecessor, the DSM-III-R along with the proposed criteria for a diagnosis that, by virtue of being placed in the appendix of the DSM-IV is under consideration for the 5th edition of the DSM, namely dissociative trance disorder. The criteria and rationale for a diagnosis that was not accepted, secondary dissociative disorder due to a non-psychiatric medical condition, will also be briefly reviewed.

The appendix also contains the criteria for a new diagnosis, acute stress disorder, that includes dissociative symptoms. This diagnosis, while added to the DSM-IV under the anxiety stress disorders, was initially proposed by the Working Group on Dissociative Disorders of the Task Force on DSM-IV under the term "brief reactive dissociative disorder" (Spiegel & Cardeña, 1991).

Dissociative Amnesia

Amnesia can be considered to be a disorder in its own right, and a building block for other disorders such as fugue and DID. Indeed, personal identity requires the sense of temporal continuity that personal, or episodic memory, provides. In contrast with many forms of organic amnesia in which typically there is anterograde loss (i.e., impairment with learning new material), dissociative amnesia is typically retrograde (i.e., loss of memory for events preceding the episode) and is organized according to affective rather than temporal dimensions (e.g., Schacter, Wang, Tulving, & Freedman, 1982). A patient with dissociative amnesia may not be able to remember a specific episode or personal information dealing with a stressful event (e.g., forgetting a marriage and a family in the midst of a divorce) while preserving "islets" of other information. In a recent study of dissociative amnesia, Coons and Milstein (1992) found that out of 25 patients (23 women), 76% had amnesia for selective information, 8% had a more generalized amnesia, while the remaining 16% had both types of amnesia; most patients had chronic cases of amnesia not of sudden onset.

Dissociative amnesia is typically associated with stressful situations such as early abuse, war or financial disaster, depression, and suicide attempts (Kopelman, 1987; Loewenstein, 1991). Coons and Milstein (1992) found the following precipitants for amnesic episodes: child abuse (60%), severe marital troubles (24%), disavowed sexual or illegal behavior (16%), and suicide attempts (16%).

Differential diagnoses for amnesia include malingering (particularly for patients with legal problems) and various organic disorders. Among the latter are transient global amnesia, which is a transient, single amnestic episode involving confusion and probably caused by transient vascular insufficiency (Rollinson, 1978), drug toxicity, Korsakoff's psychosis, head injury, epilepsy, dementia, amnesic stroke, posttraumatic amnesia, postoperative amnesia, postinfectious amnesia, alcoholic "blackout," and anoxic amnesia (Benson, 1978; Keller & Shaywitz, 1986; Kopelman, 1987). Generally, dissociative amnesia seems to differ from organic amnesia in the lack of temporal arrangement, the fast resolution, the preponderance of personal memory loss, a stressful precipitant, and a discernible motivation. Specific cases, however, might differ from this profile.

The changes in the diagnostic criteria for DSM-IV are:

1. The name of the condition itself became dissociative amnesia, instead of psychogenic amnesia, to achieve compatibility with the nomenclature of the International Classification of Diseases and to further link other dissociative disorders that have amnesia as a constituent component (dissociative fugue, dissociative identity disorder).
2. Criterion A was modified in the following ways: The term "sudden" to qualify the onset of the condition was removed because it is unduly restrictive. The course of dissociative amnesia may be gradual and insidious rather than abrupt; amnesia may present as a discrete episode or as a chronic series of episodes of varying intensity and duration. Based on the literature reviewed above, phrasing was added in the DSM-IV to indicate that trauma and stress are the typical precipitants of amnesia, and that dissociative amnesia should be distinguished from the common amnesia for early years.
3. The list for differential diagnoses is more specific than that for the DSM-III-R.

Dissociative Fugue

Fugue states have been documented at least since the late 1800s. The most famous case may be that of the Reverend Ansel Bourne, who reported leaving his home and adopting a new identity after he had become amnestic for his previous life (James, 1890/1923). Since World War II, when fugue states were frequently observed, there have been very few systematic studies of pure dissociative fugue other than DID-involving episodes of fugue. This may be because of the lack of the widespread stressful effect of war in the United States, but also because of a "nonclassic" presentation of fugue in which patients may not present with amnesia and dissociative symptoms unless queried about it. This group includes individuals who are unlikely to come under the care of clinicians, including adolescent runaways from abusive homes, homeless individuals, and so forth (cf. Loewenstein, 1991).

A recent review of the literature concluded that the definition of dissociative fugue as a condition in which there is an adoption of a new identity is unduly restrictive. Cases of fugue may involve only the loss of a personal identity or other alterations in consciousness of personal identity without the assumption of a new identity (Riether & Stoudemire, 1988). A case study by Keller and Shaywitz (1986) of a 16-year-old male found entangled in a shrubbery along a state highway, who had amnesia for personal identity, is a good example of fugue without the adoption of a new identity. As with amnesia, fugue is typically associated with traumatic or very stressful circumstances.

Differential diagnosis for fugue includes complex partial seizure episodes involving postictal episodes of aimless wandering, followed by retrograde amnesia and disorientation, or "poriomania" (Gross, 1979; Mayeux, Alexander, Benson, Brandt, & Rosen, 1979). The clinician should also take into consideration other organic conditions that could give rise to "fuguelike" states, including organic, nonepileptic factors (e.g., migraine, brain tumors), schizophrenia, alcohol- and drug-related fugues, and so on (Akhtar & Brenner, 1979).

Changes in criteria for the DSM-IV include:

1. The change of name from "psychogenic" to "dissociative" fugue, for the reasons explained above.
2. A change in criterion B from the requirement of the assumption of a new identity to the more general "confusion about personal identity or assumption of a new identity."
3. A more specific list of exclusion diagnoses.

Dissociative Identity Disorder

The central feature of this condition is the presence within the individual of two or more distinct identities. Without question, DID has been the most controversial and researched of the dissociative disorders. DID is the most extreme disorder within a spectrum of dissociation and it typically involves dissociative amnesia, fugue, and depersonalization, along with other symptoms (e.g., Braun, 1993; Putnam, 1989). For instance, DID patients have been found to have more elevated Minnesota Multiphase Personality Inventory (MMPI) F and SC scales than amnestic patients (Coons & Milstein, 1992) and a higher incidence of other diagnoses such as borderline personality and somatization than patients with dissociative disorders not otherwise specified (Ross et al., 1992).

Opinions on DID range from considering it a fiction cocreated by patient and clinician, to accepting its validity. Within the latter position, a cogent case can be made that DID should be included on Axis II (personality disorders) rather than on Axis I, considering that it is a chronic, pervasive condition that represents a failure in development rather than a regression from a previously higher level of functioning. Nonetheless, the eminently dissociative nature of DID argues strongly for its continued presence within the dissociative disorders category.

DID has also been considered a subtype or variant of borderline personality disorder (cf. Buck, 1983; Clary, Burstin, & Carpenter, 1984). There is considerable diagnostic overlap between both conditions. For instance, Ross and colleagues (1992) reported that 61% of DID patients could also be diagnosed as borderline. The general view, however, is that they are separate categories (cf. Horevitz & Braun, 1984; Kemp, Gilbertson, & Torem, 1988). The conclusion by Ross, Norton, and Wozney (1989c) that "the reciprocal relationship between the two disorders is complex, and awaits further elucidation" is worth heeding.

Of the preexisting dissociative entities, DID shows the most changes in the new edition of the DSM. The first and most obvious change is its name from multiple personality disorder to dissociative identity disorder. The original name has a long and controversial history. This fact was reflected in the divided opinion among members of the Working Group on Dissociative Disorders for the DSM-IV on whether to adopt the new name. The prevailing view advanced the idea that the classical definition of "personality" denotes a stable individual pattern. The fact that, in the case of DID patients, individual consistency is formed by abrupt changes in mood and identity does not alter this concept.

The new name also emphasizes the fact that the fundamental problem is a failure of integration of various aspects of identity, memory, and consciousness rather than a proliferation of "personalities." In addition, it brings the name into line with others in the category and "preempts" the disorder from some of its metaphysical connotations. The name and description of the condition now refer to changes in "identity" rather than "personality." In a similar vein, DSM-IV defines DID as the "presence of two or more distinct identities" rather than "the existence ... of two or more distinct personalities," to avoid the ontological suggestion that two or more personalities may reside within the individual.

The most critical change in diagnostic criteria, however, is the readoption of the criterion of amnesia, which could be considered essential to the construct of DID itself. DSM-III contained this criterion, which was deleted because of the risk that DID patients may not be aware of this symptom, or even deny it, so that keeping the amnesia criterion would give rise to false-negative diagnoses (Kluft, Steinberg, & Spitzer, 1988). Conversely, an argument could be made that not requiring amnesia for a DID diagnosis may give rise to false-positive diagnoses, such as not distinguishing ego states from actual DID. While at the time of the DSM-III revision there was little systematic research investigating the possibility of false positive- versus false-negative diagnoses in DID, we now have a number of studies directly relevant to this issue.

In a study with 236 DID cases from various sources, Ross et al. (1989c) found that 95% reported some form of amnesia at least among some alter identities. In a survey of 100 cases, Putnam, Guroff, Silberman, Barban, & Post, (1986) reported that 98% of DID patients had amnesia, while Bliss's (1984) figure was 85% of his DID sample.

While these figures are very high, use of structured instruments shows an even higher incidence of amnesia among DIDs. In one study, all 102 DID patients given the Dissociative Disorders Interview Schedule (DDIS) endorsed at least one of six amnesia criteria (Ross et al., 1990). Complete endorsement by other samples of DID patients was also found with the use of the Dissociative Experiences Scale (DES) (Putnam, 1989), and the Structured Clinical Interview for the Dissociative Disorders (SCID-D) (Steinberg, Rounsaville, & Ciccheti, 1990; Steinberg, 1991; Boon & Draijer, 1991). The data unequivocally show that the risk of false-negative diagnoses is negligible when a systematic form of inquiry is used.

Finally, the single word "full" in criterion B, which addresses the intermittent control of the person's behavior by different identities or personality states was deleted based on the clinical observation of members of the Work Force, whose experience shows that control of the individual's behavior may be at times divided among two or more identities, or one identity may have a subtle influence on the presenting one.

The diagnosis of DID is particularly difficult, since the disorder typically presents with multiple symptoms and may also coexist with other psychiatric disorders. In his review of differential diagnoses, Coons (1984) pointed out that DID may be difficult to differentiate from the other dissociative disorders, psychotic states, some personality disorders, drug and alcohol abuse, epilepsy, nonpsychotic dissociative states, malingering, conversion and somatization disorders, depression, and psychosexual disorders.

Along these lines, Putnam et al. (1986) found in their review that 95% of DID patients had received one or more psychiatric and/or neurological diagnoses (a mean of 3.6 diagnoses) before being recognized as DIDs. The most common previous diagnoses included depression (in about 70% of cases), neurotic disorders (about 55%), personality disorder (about 50%), and schizophrenia (about 50%). There was an average length of 6.8 years between the first diagnosis and the eventual diagnosis of MPD. Coons, Bowman, and Milstein (1988), in their study of 50 cases of DID, showed that there was a mean of 3.8 diagnoses per patient. Besides DID, the diagnoses included personality disorders, alcohol abuse, conversion disorders, drug abuse, and affective disorders. Finally, Ross et al. (1989c) found that the 236 patients they studied had received an average of 2.74 diagnoses, including affective disorder, personality disorder, anxiety disorder, and schizophrenia.

Patients with DID or other dissociative disorders may be misdiagnosed as schizophrenics on account of their auditory hallucinations, distrust, feelings of depersonalization, and performance on the MMPI (Kluft, 1987; Spiegel & Fink, 1979; Steingard & Frankel, 1985). Coons (1984), however, concluded that the resemblance between the two disorders is merely superficial, and suggested that the best way to differentiate schizophrenia from DID is on the basis of Bleuler's primary symptoms.

In summary, criteria changes for DID include:

1. Changing of the name of the condition multiple personality disorder to dissociative identity disorder.
2. Introducing language that does not objectify the individual's experience (e.g., "existence of ... distinct personalities" to "presence ... of distinct identities").
3. The reintroduction of the criterion of amnesia.
4. A more specific differential diagnosis list than before.

Depersonalization Disorder

Depersonalization disorder has been mentioned in the literature for more than a century, although there has been little systematic research on it. It is defined as an alteration in the perception or experience of the self in which the usual sense of one's own reality is temporarily lost or altered. The self may be experienced as being unreal, "dead," not having any emotions, or the person may observe him- or herself from an external perspective. Our review (Kubin, Pakianathan, Cardeña & Spiegel, 1989) of the symptomatology of depersonalization in 17 case reports on 41 patients indicated that the four most common features were: (1) an altered sense of self (e.g., "no sense of self," "my body doesn't belong to me"); (2) a precipitating event (e.g., an accident, marijuana use); (3) a sense of unreality or a dreamlike state (e.g., "nothing seems real," "I'm not real"); and (4) sensory alterations (e.g., "colors are less vibrant," "voices sound strange").

A distinction must be made between depersonalization *symptoms* and depersonalization *syndrome*. The former are very prevalent among psychiatric conditions, but also are not uncommon as transient and not necessarily distressing symptoms among young adults, or in the context of traumatic events and risk of death, or even during some forms of meditation and hypnosis. In contrast, depersonalization syndrome is chronic, severe, distressing, and impairing and not associated with diminished reality testing. Steinberg (1991) has also made a distinction between depersonalization as a predominant disturbance (but which may co-occur with other dissociative symptoms or other disorders such as depression, panic, or anxiety) or as a transient or secondary event.

The differential diagnosis of depersonalization should include other dissociative disorders, anxiety disorders (frequently co-occurring with depersonalization), depression, obsessions and hypochondriacal symptoms, schizophrenia, borderline personality disorder, substance abuse disorders, seizure disorders, organic illness, and medication side effects (Steinberg, 1991).

Changes in the criteria of depersonalization for the DSM-IV consisted of minor wording changes:

1. Criterion A was rephrased for greater clarity.
2. On criterion C, phrasing was added to indicate that the diagnosis would require distress *or* impairment in social or occupational functioning, to further distinguish transient and benign depersonalization from depersonalization syndrome.
3. The differential diagnosis criterion was further clarified.

Acute Stress Disorder

Acute stress disorder (ASD) is defined by peritraumatic, short-term dissociative and anxiety symptomatology that brings pronounced distress and/or maladjustment. This new diagnosis is placed in the anxiety disorders section of the DSM-IV, although in its earlier forms it was conceived of as a dissociative disorder since it consists of prominent dissociative symptoms (cf. Spiegel & Cardeña, 1991). Although posttraumatic stress disorder (PTSD) also involves a reaction to trauma, it differs from this diagnosis in that it cannot be diagnosed for 1 month after the traumatic event and its criteria do not contain as explicit a list of dissociative symptoms as ASD. Because the rationale for the adoption of this new diagnosis is included in this handbook (see Chapter 17) and has been developed elsewhere (e.g., Cardeña et al., 1995), it will not be presented here. Suffice it to say that the literature contains by now a number of studies that show that dissociative reactions to disasters and traumatic events are not only common but, in their more extreme form, bring distress and maladjustment and are significant predictors of long-term PTSD (Cardeña, 1995).

Some of the issues that arose during the consideration of this diagnosis included the following: (1) whether dissociative reactions following a disaster or trauma are prevalent enough to warrant a new diagnosis; or (2) even if they are present, whether a new diagnosis would not pathologize a normal reaction to an abnormal situation. The reviews cited above show that dissociative and anxiety symptomatology are indeed quite prevalent during or following disaster or trauma, and that individuals showing extreme dissociative reactions may not only endanger themselves but are prone to develop a long-standing PTSD syndrome. The new diagnosis of ASD should foster investigation of the type of interventions that will alleviate ongoing symptoms and prevent long-term negative sequelae. The criteria for ASD are included in the appendix.

Dissociative Disorders Not Otherwise Specified

As with other catchall diagnoses in DSM-IV, DDNOS refers to disorders that are clearly dissociative in nature but do not fit any of the previously described categories. Coons (1992) listed the following as DDNOS variants: Ganser's syndrome (the use of approximate answers usually accompanied by other dissociative phenomena), ego state disorders (in which changes in personality do not have the amnesia and profound identity disturbance of DIDs), trance states, simple derealization, dissociative states following coercive persuasion, different personality states associated with gender identity disorder, secondary dissociative disorder due to a nonpsychiatric medical condition, dissociation associated with culture-bound syndromes, and so on. One of the greatest challenges for editors of future editions of the DSM will be to obtain greater taxonomical clarity, considering that the majority of diagnosed dissociative disorders do not fit the established criteria.

In India, Saxena and Prasad (1989) found that 90% of clinic outpatients receiving a DSM-III dissociative diagnosis were "atypical dissociative disorder," or DDNOS. In a very extensive study ($N = 11{,}292$) in the U.S. with general psychiatric patients, Mezzich, Fabrega, Coffman, and Haley (1989) reported that the majority (57%) of dissociative diagnoses were "atypical." Finally, Saxe et al. (1993) found that within the subgroup of general psychiatric patients reporting clinical levels of dissociation, 60% warranted a diagnosis of DDNOS.

The DSM-III-R contained some examples of DDNOS and the following changes have been made, as shown in Appendix 1:

1. A previous example that described identity confusion following purposeful behavior and amnesia was deleted since it is now covered by the definition for "dissociative fugue."
2. A description of DID in which a second identity does not assume full control was also deleted because of the change of criteria for DID.
3. The definition of derealization was expanded to exclude these episodes among children, since fantasy life at that age may be very prevalent and nonpathological.
4. A thorough description of various forms of dissociative or possession phenomena was included to account for the fact that these may be the most prevalent forms of dissociation in non-Western cultures.
5. An example of loss of consciousness, stupor, or coma not attributable to a general medical condition was added.
6. Dissociative amnesia or fugue were made superordinate to Ganser's syndrome (giving approximate answers to questions).

Dissociative Trance Disorder

This proposed diagnosis would include distressing or impairing alterations in consciousness (i.e., narrowing of consciousness and stereotyped movements) or identity (experience of possession by an external agent). In our proposal we have been careful to distinguish between alterations of consciousness or identity that are prevalent in other cultures and are part of a cultural or religious practice (cf. Bourguignon, 1976) and those forms of trance or possession that are not culturally accepted and are distressing or impairing to the individual. Subsuming culture-bound syndromes within a Western form of psychiatric nosology is not bereft of problems (cf. Lewis-Fernández, 1992). Conversely, the lack of a specific diagnosis for one of the most common forms of dissociative disorder in other cultures (cf. Saxena & Prasad, 1989) and ours (Cardeña, 1992) may prevent development in treatment, research, and conceptualization. We describe the rationale for and against this proposal elsewhere (Cardeña et al., 1995).

Discussions of earlier revisions of the DSM have also remarked on the need for a diagnosis similar to the one we have proposed. We hope that the inclusion of this proposal in the appendix of DSM-IV will foster research and cross-cultural collaboration so that a much larger data base may be considered in future revisions of the DSM. Appendix 1 describes the criteria for this diagnosis.

Secondary Dissociative Disorder due to a Nonpsychiatric Medical Condition

This proposal includes dissociative symptomatology associated with a medical condition (typically a complex partial seizure), not whether DID patients show abnormal electroencephalograms. This new category was introduced into the ICD-10 based on a number of studies suggesting a high number of dissociative symptoms or disorders among complex seizure patients (e.g., Devinsky, Putnam, Grafman, Bromfield, & Theodore, 1989; Litwin & Cardeña, 1993; Ross, Heber, Norton, & Anderson, 1989a; Schenk & Bear, 1981). In a review of this literature, we concluded that, whereas seizure patients do not have the extent of dissociation that DID or PTSD have, they nonetheless show a higher incidence of amnesia and depersonalization symptoms than the nonclinical population (Cardeña et al., 1995).

While this proposal was not accepted, the diagnostician should be aware of the possibility of dissociative symptomatology in seizure patients. The differential diagnosis between psychologically based and neurologically based conditions is an important area currently being developed (cf. Sivec & Lynn, 1995). Good (1993) has developed the concept of an organic dissociative syndrome produced by various drugs and medical conditions. Appendix 1 includes the proposed criteria for this diagnosis.

COMORBIDITY

As a separate major category, the dissociative disorders can be traced back only to the third edition of the DSM (American Psychiatric Association, 1980); reliable and valid diagnostic instruments are even younger still. This may help explain why few studies have evaluated the comorbidity of the dissociative disorders, particularly in conditions other than DID. Dissociative disorders are typically polysymptomatic, and major surveys of DID (e.g., Putnam et al., 1986; Ross et al., 1990) have found that these patients usually receive a number of psychiatric and/or neurological diagnoses before being classified as DID. Previous diagnoses frequently included affective disorder, personality disorder, anxiety disorder, schizophrenia, substance abuse, and others. We will concentrate on the conditions most commonly associated with the dissociative disorders in general, namely depression, anxiety, somatization, and first-rank symptoms, with the assumption that superordinate diagnoses such as DID include other dissociative symptoms (amnesia and not uncommonly fugue, depersonalization, "going into trances," etc.). In the DID section, we have already alluded to the conceptual and empirical overlap between borderline personality disorder and DID, so we will not revisit the topic.

Depression and Affective Lability

Depression is the most common comorbid symptom of DID patients. Bliss (1980) reported that 100% of his 14 DID cases reported depression, whereas in their study with 50 DID patients, Coons et al. (1988) found that 88% were depressed, similar to the percentage found by Putnam et al. (1986) in their review of 100 cases treated by different clinicians. In a study using a structured interview with 102 DID patients in four centers, Ross et al. (1990) reported that 91% had a concurrent diagnosis of major depressive disorder; Martínez-Taboas (1991), in a sample of 15 Puerto Rican DID patients, found depressive symptomatology in 93%, the same percentage that Saxe et al. (1993) found among their highly dissociative psychiatric inpatients. These studies explain why the most common previous diagnosis of a DID patient is depression (about 70% for Putnam et al., 1986) or affective disorder (64% for Ross et al., 1989c; see also Bliss, 1984; Kluft, 1985). A cross-cultural comparison of DID showed a 36% concurrent diagnosis of depression and 87% incidence of depressive symptomatology (Coons, Bowman, Kluft, & Milstein, 1991).

Other studies have compared the rate of depression of dissociative patients to that of other clinical groups. While Ross et al. (1989) did not find that a major depressive episode differentiated a group of 20 DID patients from an equal number of patients with schizophrenia, panic disorder, or eating disorders, Saxe et al. (1993) reported that major depression was significantly more prevalent among 15 patients with confirmed dissociative diagnoses than among a comparison group of 15 clinical patients who reported few episodes of dissociation. In a study with 15 women treated for incestuous abuse and 15 women treated for depression, Vohra (1991) found that the abuse patients reported levels of depression similar to the depressive patients, and that depression and dissociative experiences were highly correlated.

In their study with 25 amnestic patients, Coons and Milstein (1992) found that 28% had a secondary diagnosis of dysthymia and 21% of major depression. These percentages are substantially lower than those for DID, which could be explained by the greater prevalence of abuse among DID than among amnesia patients. Substantially higher rates were found among patients with DDNOS: 88% with depression in the study by Ross et al. (1992) and 84% in the study by Coons (1992), suggesting that DDNOS is a more severe group of syndromes than dissociative amnesia. A recent study (Coons, 1994) gathered independent corroboration for reports of child abuse.

Labile moods, or mood swings, are also very prevalent among DID: 87%, 70%, and 64% in the surveys conducted by Martínez-Taboas (1991), Putnam et al. (1986), and Coons et al. (1988), respectively.

Suicidal ideation and actual suicidal attempts or self-injurious behaviors are related to depressive episodes and are very prevalent among patients with dissociative disorders (Ross & Norton, 1989). Suicidal ideation was found among 100% of 71 Dutch DID patients (Boon & Draijer, 1991) and 92% of the patients studied by Ross et al. (1990). Dissociative patients frequently engage in self-destructive behavior (e.g., overdoses, wrist slashing, cigarette burning) frequently associated with episodes of depersonalization or of self-injury by a sadistic alter identity. Self-mutilation has ranged between 33 and 56% across various DID samples (Coons et al., 1988, 1991; Martínez-Taboas, 1991; Putnam et al., 1986). Among patients with DDNOS, 34% presented with self-mutilation (Coons, 1992). Actual suicide attempts were reported by 80%, 72%, and 71% of the samples of Martínez-Taboas (1991), Ross and Norton (1989), and Putnam et al. (1986), respectively.

Although depression may very well be the most common psychiatric complaint, the almost universal presence of depression among the most severe dissociative disorders and the very high incidence of suicidal and parasuicidal behavior suggest that these symptoms are sensitive markers of dissociative pathology. A likely explanation of this pattern is the extraordinarily high incidence of various forms of early abuse and familial chaos, particularly in the more severe syndromes, which have effects not only on the prevalence of dissociation but on fundamental issues of identity, trust, and self-worth (cf. Putnam et al., 1986; Ross & Norton, 1989; Saxe et al., 1993).

Anxiety

Even though they are indexed as different categories, it is clear that some anxiety disorders, particularly PTSD, include both anxiety and dissociative symptomatology (cf. Hyer, Albrecht, Poudewyns, Woods, & Brandsma, 1993; Spiegel & Cardeña, 1990). We have briefly alluded to this conceptual and empirical relationship when discussing the new diagnosis, acute stress disorder, whose criteria include dissociative and anxiety reactions to traumatic events. A recent study with a nonclinical population exposed to the 1989 San Francisco earthquake found that somewhere between 36 and 57% of the sample shortly after the event experienced some types of anxiety, whereas about 40% experienced some forms of derealization or depersonalization (Cardeña & Spiegel, 1993). Another study with survivors of the Oakland/Berkeley firestorm of 1991 shows that dissociative symptoms related to the disaster were significantly correlated with measures related to PTSD symptomatology, namely the Civilian Mississippi Scale and the Impact of Event Scale (r = .59 and .53, respectively) and significantly predicted PTSD at a 7-month follow-up (Koopman, Classen, & Spiegel, 1994).

With respect to DID, Bliss (1980) found that 100% of his sample had reported anxiety symptoms, including acute anxiety attacks and palpitations. Forty-four percent of the 236 DID patients in the study by Ross et al. (1989c) had a previous diagnosis of anxiety disorder, whereas 81% of Boon and Draijer's (1991) sample presented with PTSD symptomatology and 30% with anxiety disorder. Panic attacks were present in about 55% of Putnam and colleagues' (1986) sample. These consistent results show that anxiety is prevalent among the dissociative disorders, although unfortunately few studies have provided specific data for the various forms of anxiety symptomatology. Despite the current separation of the anxiety and dissociative disorders, the fact is that traumatic and severely stressful events typically produce both short- and long-term anxiety and dissociative symptoms. The phenomenology of the symptoms and the relationship between anxiety and dissociation require a more thorough investigation than has been the case so far. This relationship is probably not a simple casual one. For instance, dissociation in the sense of detaching from an event could be a way to reduce the distress produced by a dangerous situation, as in the so-called near-death experiences. Alternately, dissociation in the sense of the emergence of isolated distressing memory units could be the trigger for distress and anxiety (cf. Cardeña, 1994).

Conversion

The relatively recent separation of conversion from the dissociative disorders represents more a classification fashion than an absolute distinction between the disorders. Both have similar underlying dissociative mechanisms and they frequently co-occur. Patients with dissociative disorders frequently complain of headaches, unexplained pain, various forms of paresthesias and analgesias, sexual dysfunctions, and so forth (cf. Ross, Heber, Norton, & Anderson, 1989b). In fact, the association between somatization disorder, dissociative symptoms, and history of abuse which Janet, among others, had postulated, has been confirmed recently in a study with 79 female psychiatric patients (Priber, Yutzi, Dean, & Wetzel, 1993).

The authors reviewed below do not always make a distinction between conversion and somatization, making further clarification of this overlapping symptomatology difficult. In a well-controlled study by Saxe and collaborators (1994), 64% of dissociative disorder patients also met criteria for somatization disorder as compared with none from a matched group of psychiatric patients with few reported dissociative symptoms.

Ross et al. (1990) found that 92% of their 102 DID patients had reported five or more somatic symptoms. In a smaller sample of 20 DID patients compared with the same number of eating disorder, panic disorder, and schizophrenia patients, Ross et al. (1989b) found that the DID patients reported more somatic symptoms (sometimes significantly so) than the other patients. Somatization in DID ranged between 73 and 36% across other studies (Coons et al., 1988, 1991; Martínez-Taboas, 1991; Putnam et al., 1986). Rates of diagnoses for somatization disorder, rather than symptomatology, were 16, 21, and 61% in the studies of Boon and Draijer (1991), Coons et al. (1991), and Ross et al. (1990), respectively. Coons et al. (1988) also reported a 40% incidence of conversion in their sample. Headache is the most common somatic symptom among DID, ranging from 55 to 100% across various studies (Bliss, 1980; Coons et al., 1988, 1991; by Martínez-Taboas, 1991; Putnam et al, 1986; Ross et al., 1989c).

In the case of dissociative amnesia, conversion disorder was a secondary diagnosis among 24% of patients (Coons & Milstein, 1992). Among DDNOS patients, Ross et al. (1992) reported 25% of somatization disorder, whereas Coons (1992) found 26% of somatization, 14% of conversion symptoms, and 32% incidence of headaches.

Sexual dysfunction is also common among dissociative patients, ranging from 50 to 84% across various samples (Coons et al., 1988; Martínez-Taboas, 1991; Putnam et al., 1986; Ross et al., 1989). Coons et al. (1991) reported a secondary diagnosis of sexual dysfunction in 50% and of symptomatology in 73% of their patients. For DDNOS patients, Coons (1992) reported 48% of sexual dysfunction.

Bliss (1984) has suggested that the preponderance of somatic symptoms found among dissociative patients may be the result of an abuse of self-hypnotic techniques, since hypnotic techniques can produce a number of physiological changes among highly hypnotizable individuals (Spiegel & Vermutten, 1994). In this context it is of interest that DID patients, who as a group, are very hypnotizable, almost universally complain of headaches and that the outcome of a few hypnosis inductions is a headache (e.g., Hilgard, 1974). Indeed, the intensity of migraine symptoms is positively correlated with measured hypnotizability (Andreychuk & Skriver, 1975). Clearly there is a strong link between dissociation and somatization that requires far more attention than it has received so far.

First-Rank Symptoms

Even though Schneiderian first-rank symptoms are sometimes assumed to be pathognomic of schizophrenia, that is clearly not the case since they are also found in a number of other conditions (Kluft, 1987). The phenomenology of DID, involving the influence and presence of different identities, is similar to some first-rank symptoms, and, of course, dissociative symptoms may underlie some acute psychosis (Spiegel & Fink, 1979; Steingard & Frankel, 1985). However, unlike schizophrenics, individuals with dissociative disorders are typically found to have an adequate sense of reality outside of specific events such as a fugue, they typically lack the "negative" symptoms of chronic schizophrenics, and do not respond to neuroleptics but do respond to psychotherapy employing hypnosis (Hollender & Hirsch, 1964; Mallet & Gold, 1964; Spiegel & Fink, 1979).

In the first systematic study of this topic, Kluft (1987) found that all 30 DID patients presented at least one first-rank symptom (mean of 3.6 symptoms, but excluding audible thoughts, thought diffusion or broadcasting, and delusional perception), Boon and Draijer (1991) observed in their study that "most of the subjects" had these symptoms, and Ross et al. (1990) reported that 90% of their sample presented with Schneiderian symptoms. Some specific examples of first-rank symptoms include the experience of "someone trying to influence the patient," present in 73% of Bliss's sample (1980), and reports of "voices" ranging from 30 to 72% across various studies (Coons et al., 1988; Martínez-Taboas, 1991; Putnam et al., 1986; Ross et al., 1989c).

The lack of this information for dissociative disorders other than DID may be the result of a lack of inquiry into this area, or of the absence of these symptoms among patients who have a more integrated identity than do DID patients. Nonetheless, more research is needed on failures of reality testing in the various dissociative syndromes and on, conversely, the presence of dissociative symptomatology in psychotic populations.

Substance Abuse and Eating Disorders

These disorders, although sometimes present, have been less frequently associated with dissociative pathology than other disorders reviewed here. For the DID population, rates for drug and alcohol abuse range from 31 to 64% across various samples (Boon & Draijer, 1991; Coons et al., 1988; Martínez-Taboas, 1991; Putnam et al., 1986; Ross et al., 1989c; Saxe et al., 1993). Coons et al. (1988) report a 42% incidence of alcohol abuse. In their cross-cultural study of DID, Coons et al. (1991) found the same percentage (13%) for a secondary diagnosis of alcohol or substance abuse (13%), and symptoms of alcohol abuse in 53% and of drug abuse in 27% of their sample. Although substance abuse is present in many other conditions, the specific function that it plays in the dissociative disorders has not been systematically studied.

Alcohol abuse/dependence was present in 24% and drug abuse in 20% of the sample of 50 amnestic patients studied by Coons and Milstein (1992). For DDNOS patients, substance abuse was present in 42% of Ross and co-workers' sample (1992), and in 46% for alcohol and 16% for drug abuse in Coons' sample (1992).

Some researchers have also pointed to previous or concurrent diagnoses of eating disorders among dissociative disorder patients. Demitrack, Putnam, Brewerton, Brandt, and Gold (1990) describe various links between dissociation and eating disorders: reports of increased hypnotizability, particularly among bulimics (e.g. Pettinati, Horne, & Staats, 1985; Barabasz, 1990); the usefulness of hypnosis in the treatment of these disorders; the frequent incidence of early abuse among eating-disorder patients; the early historical association of "hysteria" and a number of gastrointestinal and eating disturbances; the presence of dissociative states in eating disorders patients; and, conversely, the incidence of eating disorders in dissociative disorders patients. For instance, McCallum, Lock, Kulla, Rorty, and Wetzel (1992) report that 29% of their patients with eating disorders also fulfilled criteria for dissociative disorders (18% of depersonalization, 10% of DID), and that dissociation was associated with binging-purging or severe restrictions, sexual behavior, and self-harm.

Reported percentages of eating disorders among DID patients include 27% of anorexia and about 15% of bulimia in Putnam and co-workers' (1986) study and a 76% history of eating problems in the sample of Boon and Draijer (1991). Sixteen percent of the patients in Ross and colleagues' (1989c) sample had received a previous diagnosis of eating disorder (23% for Boon & Draijer). Finally, 20% of the amnestic patients in Coons and Milstein's (1992) sample presented with bulimia.

Nonetheless, these relationships are probably more complex than originally thought. For instance, Greenes, Fava, Cioffi, and Herzog (1993) found in a clinical sample that the relationship between bulimia and dissociation is confounded by the relationship between dissociation and depression. Also, in a recent review of the literature, Pope, Mangweth, Negrao, Hudson, and Cordas (1994) found no consistent evidence for a link between abuse and bulimia. Thus, reported correlations between eating disorders and dissociation may be mediated by other factors.

CONCLUSION

The various changes in criteria for previous dissociative disorders and the proposal for new diagnostic entities represent a developing view of dissociative psychopathology. The rather recent history of these disorders as an independent category and the various changes and reconceptualizations made so far show an evolving and far from complete perspective on dissociation. Many basic questions remain, among them: What differentiates normal from dysfunctional dissociation? Why do some traumatized individuals develop dissociative pathology while others develop different or no pathology? Why do some pathologies co-occur with the dissociative disorders while others are rarely encountered?

Some major tasks to be accomplished in the following years include developing a more precise phenomenology and neurophysiology of these disorders, elucidating the cultural variants of normal and pathological dissociation, and establishing a clear theoretical and empirical basis to study the relationship between dissociative phenomena and other related disorders such as depression, anxiety, conversion, substance abuse, and eating disorders.

APPENDIX

DSM-IV	DSM-III-R
Dissociative amnesia	*Psychogenic amnesia*
A. The predominant disturbance is one or more episodes of inability to recall important personal information, usually of a traumatic or stressful nature, that is too extensive to be explained by ordinary forgetfulness. B. The disturbance does not occur exclusively during the course of Dissociative Identity Disorder, Dissociative Fugue, Posttraumatic Stress Disorder, Acute Stress Disorder, or Somatization Disorder and is not due to the direct physiological effects of a substance (e.g., a drug of abuse, medication) or a neurological or other general medical condition (e.g., Amnestic Disorder due to Head Trauma). C. The symptoms cause clincally significant distress or impairment in social, occupational, or other important areas of functioning.	A. The predominant disturbance is an episode of sudden inability to recall important personal information that is too extensive to be explained by ordinary forgetfulness B. The disturbance is not due to Multiple Personality Disorder or to an Organic Mental Disorder (e.g., blackouts during Alcohol Intoxication).
Dissociative fugue	*Psychogenic fugue*
A. The predominant disturbance is sudden, unexpected travel away from home or one's customary place of work, with inability to recall one's past. B. Confusion about personal identity or assumption of a new identity (partial or complete).	A. The predominant disturbance is sudden, unexpected travel away from home or one's customary place of work, with inability to recall one's past B. Assumption of a new identity (partial or complete).

C. The disturbance does not occur exclusively during the course of Dissociative Identity Disorder, and is not due to the direct physiological effects of a substance (e.g., a drug of abuse, a medication) or a general medical condition (e.g., temporal lobe epilepsy).
D. The symptoms cause clincally significant distress or impairment in social, occupational, or other important areas of functioning.

C. The disturbance is not due to Multiple Personality Disorder or to an Organic Mental Disorder (e.g., partial complex seizures in temporal lobe epilepsy).

Dissociative identity disorder

A. The presence of two or more distinct identities or personality states (each with its own relatively enduring pattern of perceiving, relating to, and thinking about the environment and self).
B. At least two of these identities or personality states recurrently take control of the person's behavior.
C. Inability to recall important personal information that is too extensive to be explained by ordinary forgetfulness
D. The disturbance is not due to the direct physiological effects of a substance (e.g., blackouts or chaotic behavior during Alcohol Intoxication) or a general medical condition (e.g., complex partial seizures). NOTE: In children, the symptoms are not attributable to imaginary playmates or other fantasy play.

Multiple personality disorder

A. The existence within the person of two or more distinct personalities or personality states (each with its own relatively enduring pattern of perceiving, relating to, and thinking about the environment and self).
B. At least two of these personalities or personality states recurrently take full control of the person's behavior.

Depersonalization disorder

A. Persistent or rcurrent experiences of feeling detached from, and as if one is an outside observer of, one's mental processes or body (e.g., feeling like one is in a dream).
B. During the depersonalization experience, reality testing remains intact.
C. The depersonalization causes significant impairment in social, occupational, or other important areas of functioning.
D. The depersonalization experience does not occur exclusively during the course of another mental disorder, such as Schizophrenia, Panic Disorder, Acute Stress Disorder, or another Dissociative Disorder, and is not due to the direct

Depersonalization disorder

A. Persistent or recurrent experiences of depersonalization as indicated by either (1) or (2):
   (1) an experience of feeling detached from, and as if one is an outside obsever of, one's mental processes or body
   (2) an experience of feeling like an automaton or as if in a dream
B. During the depersonalization experience, reality testing remains intact.
C. The depersonalization is sufficiently severe and persistent to cause marked distress.
D. The depersonalization experience is the predominant disturbance and is not

physiological effects of a substance (e.g., a drug of abuse, a medication) or a general medical condition (e.g., temporal lobe epilepsy).

Dissociative disorders not otherwise specified

This category is included for disorders in which the predominant feature is a dissociative symptom (i.e., a disruption in the usually integrated functions of consciousness, memory, identity, or perception of the environment) that does not meet the criteria for a specific Dissociative Disorder. Examples include:

(1) Clinical presentations similar to Dissociative Identity Disorder that fail to meet full criteria for this disorder. Examples include presentations in which:
 (a) there are not two or more distinct personality states, or
 (b) amnesia for important personal information does not occur.
(2) Derealization unaccompanied by depersonalization in adults.
(3) States of dissociation that occur in individuals who have been subjected to periods of prolonged and intense coercive persuasion (e.g., brainwashing, thought reform, or indoctrination while captive).
(4) Dissociative trance disorder: single or episodic disturbances in the state of consciousness, identity or memory that are indigenous to particular locations and cultures. Dissociative trance involves narrowing of awareness of immediate surroundings or stereotyped behaviors or movements that are experienced as being beyond one's control. Possession trance involves replacement of the customary sense of personal identity by a new identity, attributed to the influence of a spirit, power, deity, or other person, and associated with stereotyped "involuntary" movements or amnesia. Examples include ***amok***

a symptom of another disorder, such as Schizophrenia, Panic Disorder, or Agoraphobia without History of Panic Disorder but with limited symptom attacks of depersonalization, or temporal lobe epilepsy.

Dissociative disorders not otherwise specified

Disorders in which the predominant feature is a dissociative symptom (i.e., a disturbance or alteration in the normally integrative functions of identity, memory, or consciousness) that does not meet the criteria for a specific Dissociative Disorder. Examples:

(1) Ganser's syndrome: the giving of "approximate answers" to question, commonly associated with other symptoms such as amnesia, disorientation, perceptual disturbance, fugue, and conversion symptoms
(2) Cases in which there is more than one personality state capable of assuming executive control of the individual, but not more than one personality state is sufficiently distinct to meet the full criteria for Multiple Personality Disorder, or cases in which a second personality never assumes complete executive control
(3) Trance states, i.e., altered states of consciousness with markedly diminished or selectively focused responsiveness to environmental stimuli. In children this may occur following physical abuse or trauma
(4) Derealization unaccompanied by depersonalization
(5) Dissociated states that may occur in people who have been subjected to periods of prolonged and intense coercive persuasion (e.g., brainwashing, thought reform, or indoctrination while the captive of terrorists or cultists)
(6) Cases in which sudden, unexpected travel and organized, purposeful behavior with inability to recall one's past are not accompanied by the assumption of a new identity, partial or complete.

(Indonesia), *bebainan* (Indonesia), latah (Malaysia), pibloktoq (Artic), ataque de nervios (Latin America), and possession (India). The dissociative or trance disorder is not a normal part of a broadly accepted collective cultural or religious practice.

(5) Loss of consciousness, stupor, or coma not attributable to a general medical condition.

(6) Ganser's syndrome: the giving of approximate answers to questions (e.g., "2 plus 2 equals 5") when not associated with Dissociative Amnesia or Dissociative Fugue.

Dissociative Trance Disorder

Possession and trance states are common and normal components of religious and other ceremonies in many cultures. However, Dissociative Trance Disorder (leading to distress and dysfunction) is also the most common dissociative disorder reported in non-Western culture. DSM-III mentioned trancelike states as an example of Atypical Dissociative Disorder. DSM-III-R expanded the example and provided a definition of trance. ICD-10 has included a new category, Dissociative Trance Disorders, within the Dissociative Disorders.

A. Either (1) or (2):
   (1) trance, i.e., temporary marked alteration in the state of consciousness or loss of customary sense of personal identity, without replacement by an alternate identity, associated with at least one of the following:
      (a) narrowing of awareness of immediate surroundings, or unusually narrow and selective focusing on environmental stimuli
      (b) stereotyped behaviors or movements that are experienced as being beyond one's control
   (2) possession trance, i.e., a single or episodic alteration in the state of consciousness, characterized by the replacement of (the) customary sense of personal identity by a new identity. This is attributed to the influence of a spirit, power, deity or other person, as evidenced by one (or more) of the following:
      (a) stereotyped and culturally determined behaviors or movements that are experienced as being controlled by the possessing agent
      (b) full or partial amnesia for the event
B. The trance or possession state is not a normal part of a clinically collective cultural or religious practice.
C. The trance or possession state causes clinically significant distress or impairment in social, occupational, or other important areas of functioning.
D. The trance or possession state does not occur exclusively during the course of a Psychotic Disorder (including Mood Disorder with Psychotic Features and Brief Reactive Psychosis) or Dissociative Identity Disorder, and is not

due to the direct physiological effects of a substance or general medical condition.

Secondary Dissociative Disorder due to a Nonpsychiatric Medical Condition

This category has been proposed but not accepted for DSM-IV and is included in ICD-10. It is supported by studies that suggest an elevated prevalence of dissociative symptoms in individuals with complex partial seizures and that dissociative symptoms accompanying complex partial seizures are not associated with a history of physical and sexual trauma.

A. Amnesia, fugue, depersonalization, derealization, or other dissociative symptoms.
B. There is evidence from the history, physical examination, or laboratory findings that a general medical condition (e.g., complex partial seizure or drug toxicity) is etiologically related to the dissociative symptoms.
C. The dissociative symptoms cause significant impairment in social or occupational functioning, or cause marked distress.
D. Does not meet criteria for a secondary Cognitive Impairment Disorder (i.e., due to a general medical condition).

Acute Stress Disorder

This is a proposed new diagnosis, parallel to one included in ICD-10 (as "Acute Stress Reaction"), which may help to describe cases that do not meet the criteria for Posttraumatic Stress Disorder (because of differences in onset, duration, and symptom presentation) and are more specific and severe than Adjustment Disorder.

A. The person has been exposed to a traumatic event in which both of the following have been present:
   (1) the person has experienced, witnessed, or been confronted with an event or events that involve actual or threatened death or serious injury, or a threat to the physical integrity of oneself or others.
   (2) the person's response involved intense fear, helplessness, or horror.
B. Either while experiencing, or immediately after experiencing, the distressing event, the individual has at least three of the following dissociative symptoms:
   (1) subjective sense of numbing, detachment, or absence of emotional responsiveness
   (2) a reduction in awareness of one's surroundings (e.g., "being in a daze")
   (3) derealization
   (4) depersonalization
   (5) dissociative amnesia, ie., inability to recall an important aspect of the trauma
C. The traumatic event is persistently reexperienced in at least one of the following ways: recurrent images, thoughts, dreams, illusions, flashback

episodes, or a sense of reliving the experience; or distress upon exposure to reminders of the traumatic event.

D. Marked avoidance of stimuli that arouse recollections of the trauma (e.g., thoughts, feelings, conversations, activities, places or people)
E. Marked symptoms of anxiety or increased arousal (e.g., difficulty sleeping, irritability, poor concentration, hypervigilance, exaggerated startle response, and motor restlessness.
F. The disturbance causes clinically significant distress or impairment in social, occupational, or other important areas of functioning, or the individual is prevented from pursuing some necessary task, such as obtaining necessary medical or legal assistance or mobilizing personal resources by telling family members about the traumatic experience.
G. The symptoms last for a minimum of two days and a maximum of four weeks and occur within four weeks of the traumatic event.
H. Not due to the direct effects of a substance (e.g., drugs of abuse, medication) or a general medical condition, and is not merely an exacerbation of a preexisting Axis I or Axis II disorder.

REFERENCES

Akhtar, S., & Brenner, I. (1979). Differential diagnosis of fugue-like states. *Journal of Clinical Psychiatry*, *9*, 381-385.

American Psychiatric Association. (1952). *Diagnostic and statistical manual: Mental disorders*. Washington, DC: Author.

American Psychiatric Association. (1968). *Diagnostic and statistical manual of mental disorders* (2nd ed.). Washington, DC: Author.

American Psychiatric Association. (1980). *Diagnostic and statistical manual of mental disorders* (3rd ed.). Washington, DC: Author.

American Psychiatric Association. (1987). *Diagnostic and statistical manual of mental disorders* (3rd ed., rev.). Washington, DC: Author.

American Psychiatric Association. (1994). *Diagnostic and statistical manual of mental disorders* (4th ed.). Washington, DC: Author.

Andreychuk, Y., & Skriver, C. (1975). Hypnosis and biofeedback in the treatment of migraine headache. *International Journal of Clinical and Experimental Hypnosis*, *23*, 172-183.

Barabasz, M. (1990). Bulimia, hypnotizability and dissociative capacity. In R. Van Dyck, Ph. Spinhoven, A. J. W. Van der Does, Y. R. Van Rood, and W. De Moor (Eds.), *Hypnosis. Current theory, research and practice* (pp. 207-213). Amsterdam: VU University Press.

Benson, D. F. (1978). Amnesia. *Southern Medical Journal*, *71*, 1221-1227.

Bliss, E. L. (1980). Multiple personalities: A report of 14 cases with implications for schizophrenia and hysteria. *Archives of General Psychiatry*, *37*, 1388-1397.

Bliss, E. L. (1984). A symptom profile of patients with multiple personalities, including MMPI results. *Journal of Nervous and Mental Disease*, *172*, 197-202.

Boon, S., & Draijer, N. (1991). Diagnosing dissociative disorders in the Netherlands: A pilot study with the Structured Clinical Interview for the DSM-III-R Dissociative Disorders. *American Journal of Psychiatry*, *148*, 458-462.

Bourguignon, E. (1976). *Possession*. San Francisco: Chandler.

Braun, B. G. (1993). Multiple personality disorder and posttraumatic stress disorder. In J. P. Wilson & B. Raphael (Eds.), *International handbook of traumatic stress syndromes* (pp. 35-47). New York: Plenum Press.

Buck, O. D. (1983). Multiple personality as a borderline state. *Journal of Nervous and Mental Diseases*, *171*, 62-65.

Cardeña, E. (1992). Trance and possession as dissociative disorders. *Transcultural Psychiatric Research Review, 29*, 287-300.

Cardeña, E. (1994). The domain of dissociation. In S. J. Lynn & R. W. Rhue (Eds.), *Dissociation: Theoretical, clinical, and research perspectives* (pp. 15-31). New York: Guilford Press.

Cardeña, E. (1995, August). Hypnosis and dissociation: New research findings. Paper presented at the 103rd Annual Meeting of the American Psychological Association, New York.

Cardeña, E., & Spiegel, D. (1993). Dissociative reactions to the San Francisco Bay Area earthquake of 1989. *American Journal of Psychiatry, 150*, 474-478.

Cardeña, E., Lewis-Fernández, R., Bear, D., Pakianathan, I., & Spiegel, D. (1995). Dissociative disorders. In *DSM-IV sourcebook* (Vol. 2, pp. 973-1005). Washington, DC: American Psychiatric Press.

Clary, W. F., Burstin, K. J., & Carpenter, J. S. (1984). Multiple personality and borderline personality disorder. *Psychiatric Clinics of North America, 7*, 89-99.

Coons, P. M., (1984). The differential diagnosis of multiple personality. *Psychiatric Clinics of North America, 7*, 51-67.

Coons, P. M. (1992). Dissociative disorders not otherwise specified: A clinical investigation of 50 cases with suggestions for typology and treatment. *Dissociation, 5*, 187-195.

Coons, P. M. (1994). Confirmation of childhood abuse in child and adolescent cases of multiple personality disorder and dissociative disorder not otherwise specified. *Journal of Nervous and Mental Disease, 182*, 461-464.

Coons, P. M., & Milstein, V. (1992). Psychogenic amnesia: A clinical investigation of 25 cases. *Dissociation, 5*, 73-79.

Coons, P. M., Bowman, E. S., & Milstein, V. (1988). Multiple personality disorder: A clinical investigation of 50 cases. *Journal of Nervous and Mental Diseases, 176*, 519-527.

Coons, P. M., Bowman, E. S., Kluft, R. P., & Milstein, V. (1991). The cross-cultural occurrence of MPD: Additional cases from a recent survey. *Dissociation, 4*, 124-128.

Demitrack, M. A., Putnam, F. W., Brewerton, T. D., Brandt, H. A., & Gold, P. W. (1990). Relation of clinical variables to dissociative phenomena in eating disorders. *American Journal of Psychiatry, 147*, 1184-1188.

Devinsky, O., Putnam, F., Grafman, J., Bromfield E., & Theodore, W. H. (1989). Dissociative states and epilepsy *Neurology, 39*, 835-840.

Garcia, F. O. (1990). The concept of dissociation and conversion in the new edition of the International Classification of Diseases (ICD-10). *Dissociation, 3*, 204-208.

Good, M. I. (1993). The concept of an organic dissociative syndrome: What is the evidence? *Harvard Review of Psychiatry, 1*, 145-157.

Greenes, D., Fava, M., Cioffi, J., & Herzog, D. (1993). The relationship of depression to dissociation in patients with bulimia nervosa. *Journal of Psychiatric Research, 27*, 133-137.

Gross, M. (1979). Pseudoepilepsy: A study in adolescent hysteria. *American Journal of Psychiatry, 136*, 213-213.

Hilgard, J. (1974). Sequelae to hypnosis. *International Journal of Clinical and Experimental Hypnosis, 22*, 281-296.

Hollender, M. H., & Hirsch, S. J. (1964). Histerical psychosis. *American Journal of Psychiatry, 120*, 1066-1074.

Horevitz, R. P., & Braun, B. G. (1984). Are multiple personalities borderline? *Psychiatric Clinics of North America, 7*, 69-87.

Hyer, L. A., Albrecht, W., Poudewyns, P. A., Woods, M. G., & Brandsma, J. (1993). Dissociative experiences of Vietnam veterans with chronic post-traumatic stress disorder. *Psychological Reports, 73*, 519-530.

James, W. (1890/1923). *Principles of psychology*. New York: Holt.

Keller, R., & Shaywitz, B. A. (1986). Amnesia or fugue state: A diagnostic dilemma. *Developmental and Behavioral Pediatrics, 7*, 131-132.

Kemp, K., Gilbertson, A. D., & Torem, M. (1988). The differential diagnosis of multiple personality disorder from borderline personality disorder. *Dissociation, 1*, 41-46.

Kihlstrom, J. F. (1994). One hundred years of hysteria. In S. J. Lynn & R. W. Rhue (Eds.) *Dissociation: Theoretical, clinical, and research perspectives* (pp. 365-394). New York: Guilford Press.

Kluft, R. P. (1985). The natural history of multiple personality disorder. In R. Kluft (Ed.), *Childhood antecedents of multiple personality* (pp. 197-238). Washington DC: American Psychiatric Press.

Kluft, R. (1987). First-rank symptoms as a diagnostic clue to multiple personality disorder. *American Journal of Psychiatry, 144*, 293-298

Kluft, R. P., Steinberg, M., & Spitzer, R. L. (1988). DSM-III-R revisions in the dissociative disorders: An exploration of their derivation and rationale. *Dissociation, 1*, 39-46.

Koopman, C., Classen, C., & Spiegel, D. (1994). Predictors of post-traumatic stress symptoms among Oakland/Berkeley firestorm survivors. *American Journal of Psychiatry, 151*, 888-894.

Kopelman, M. D. (1987). Amnesia: Organic and psychogenic. *British Journal of Psychiatry, 150*, 428-442.

Kubin, M., Pakianathan, I., Cardeña, E., & Spiegel, D. (1989). Depersonalization disorder. *Unpublished manuscript*. Stanford University.

Lewis-Fernández, R. (1992). The proposed DSM-IV trance and possession disorder category: Potential benefits and risks. *Transcultural Psychiatric Research Review, 29*, 301-317.

Litwin, R. G., & Cardeña, E. (1993). Dissociation and reported trauma in organic and psychogenic seizure patients. Paper presented at the 101st Annual Convention of the American Psychological Association, Toronto.

Loewenstein, R. J. (1991). Psychogenic amnesia and psychogenic fugue: A comprehensive review. In A. Tasman & S. M. Goldfinger (Eds.), *American Psychiatric Press Review of Psychiatry* (Vol. 10, pp. 189-222). Washington, DC: American Psychiatric Press.

Mallet, B., & Gold, S. (1964). A pseudo-schizophrenic hysterical syndrome. *British Journal of Medical Psychology, 37*, 59-70.

Martínez-Taboas, A. (1991). Multiple personality in Puerto Rico: Analysis of fifteen cases. *Dissociation, 4*, 189-192.

Mayeux, R., Alexander, M. P., Benson, F., Brandt, J., & Rosen, J. (1979). Poriomania. *Neurology, 29*, 1616-1619.

Mezzich, J. E., Fabrega, H., Coffman, G. A., & Haley, R. (1989). DSM-III disorders in a large sample of psychiatric patients: Frequency and specificity of diagnoses. *American Journal of Psychiatry, 146*, 212-219.

McCallum, K., Lock, J., Kulla, M., Rorty, M., & Wetzel, R. D. (1992). Dissociative symptoms and disorders in patients with eating disorders. *Dissociation, 5*, 227-235.

Nemiah, J. (1991). Dissociation, conversion, and somatization. In A. Tasman & S. M. Goldfinger (Eds.), *American Psychiatric Press Review of Psychiatry* (Vol. 10, pp. 248-260). Washington, DC: American Psychiatric Press.

Petinatti, H. M., Horne, R. L., & Staats, J. M. (1985). Hypnotizability in patients with anorexia nervosa and bulimia. *Archives of General Psychiatry, 42*, 1014-1016.

Pope, H. G., Mangweth, M. A., Negrao, A. B., Hudson, J. I., & Cordas, T. A. (1994). Childhood sexual abuse and bulimia nervosa: A comparison of American, Austrian, and Brazilian Women. *American Journal of Psychiatry, 151*, 732-737.

Pribor, E. F., Yutzy, S. H., Dean, J. T., & Wetzel, R. D. (1993). Briquet's syndrome, dissociation, and abuse. *American Journal of Psychiatry, 150*, 1507-1511.

Putnam, F. W. (1989). *Diagnosis and treatment of multiple personality disorder*. New York: Guilford Press.

Putnam, F. W., Guroff, J. J., Silberman, E. K., Barban, L., & Post, R. M. (1986). The clinical phenomenology of multiple personality disorder: Review of 100 recent cases. *Journal of Clinical Psychiatry, 47*, 285-293.

Riether, A. M., & Stoudemire, A. (1988). Psychogenic fugue states: A review. *Southern Medical Journal, 81*, 568-571.

Rollinson, R. D. (1978). Transient global amnesia—A review of 213 cases from the literature. *Australian and New Zealand Journal of Medicine, 8*, 547-549.

Ross, C. A., & Norton, G. R. (1989). Suicide and parasuicide in multiple personality disorder. *Psychiatry, 52*, 365-371.

Ross, C. A., Heber, S., Norton, G. R., & Anderson, G. (1989a). Differences between multiple personality disorder and other diagnostic groups on structured interview. *Journal of Nervous and Mental Disease, 177*, 487-491.

Ross, C. A., Heber, S., Norton, G. R., & Anderson, G. (1989b). Somatic symptoms in multiple personality disorder. *Psychosomatics, 30*, 154-160.

Ross, C. A., Norton, G. R., & Wozney, K. (1989c). Multiple personality disorder: An analysis of 236 cases. *Canadian Journal of Psychiatry, 34*, 413-418.

Ross, C. A., Miller, S. D., Reagor, P., Bjornson, L., Fraser, G. A., & Anderson, G. (1990). Structured interview data on 102 cases of multiple personality disorder from four centers. *American Journal of Psychiatry, 147*, 596-601.

Ross, C. A., Anderson, G., Fraser, G. A., Reagor, P., Bjornson, L., & Miller, S. D. (1992). Differentiating multiple personality disorder and dissociative disorder not otherwise specified. *Dissociation, 5*, 87-90.

Saxe, G. N., Chinman, G., Berkowitz, R., Hall, K., Lieberg, G., Schwartz, J., & van der Kolk, B., (1994). Somatization in patients with dissociative disorders. *American Journal of Psychiatry, 151*, 1329-1334.

Saxe, G. N., van der Kolk, B. A., Berkowitz, R., Chinman, G., Hall, K., Lieberg, G., & Schwartz, J. (1993). Dissociative disorders in psychiatric patients. *American Journal of Psychiatry, 150*, 1037-1042.

Saxena, S., & Prasad, K. V. (1989). DSM-III subclassification of dissociative disorders applied to psychiatric outpatients in India. *American Journal of Psychiatry, 146*, 261-262.

Schacter, D. L., Wang, P. L., Tulving, E., & Freedman, M. (1982). Functional retrograde amnesia: A quantitative case study. *Neuropsychologia, 20*, 523-532.

Schenk, L., & Bear, D. (1981). Multiple personality and related dissociative phenomena in patients with temporal lobe epilepsy. *American Journal of Psychiatry, 138*, 1311-1316.

Sivec, H. J., & Lynn, S. J. (1995). Dissociative and neuropsychological symptoms: The question of differential diagnosis. *Clinical Psychology Review, 15*, 297-316.

Spiegel, D., & Cardeña, E. (1990). New uses of hypnosis in the treatment of posttraumatic stress disorder. *Journal of Clinical Psychiatry, 51*(Suppl.), 39-43.

Spiegel, D., & Cardeña, E. (1991). Disintegrated experience: The dissociative disorders revisited. *Journal of Abnormal Psychology, 100*, 366-378.

Spiegel, D., & Fink, R. (1979). Hysterical psychosis and hypnotizability. *American Journal of Psychiatry, 136*, 777-781.

Spiegel, D., & Vermutten, E. (1994). Physiological efects of hypnosis and dissociation. In D. Spiegel (Ed.), *Dissociation: Culture, mind, and body* (pp. 185-209). Washington, DC: American Psychiatric Press.

Steinberg, M. (1991). The spectrum of depersonalization: Assessment and treatment. In A. Tasman & S. M. Goldfinger (Eds.), *American Psychiatric Press review of psychiatry* (Vol. 10, pp. 223-247). Washington, DC: American Psychiatric Press.

Steinberg, M., Rounsaville, B., & Ciccheti, D. (1990). The Structured Clinical Interview for DSM-III-R Dissociative Disorders. *American Journal of Psychiatry, 147*, 76-82.

Steingard, S., & Frankel, F. H. (1985). Dissociation and psychotic symptoms. *American Journal of Psychiatry, 142*, 953-955.

van der Kolk, B. A., & van der Hart, O. (1989). Pierre Janet and the breakdown of adaptation in psychological trauma. *American Journal of Psychiatry, 146*, 1530-1540.

Vohra, S. (1991). Dissociative experiences and their relationship with depression in women with a history of incestuous abuse in childhood. *Dissertation Abstracts International, 52*(2-B), 1086.

12

The Psychological Assessment of Dissociation

Marlene Steinberg

INTRODUCTION

The five dissociative disorders included in the *Diagnostic and Statistical Manual of Mental Disorders*, 4th Edition (DSM-IV) [dissociative amnesia, dissociative fugue, depersonalization disorder, dissociative identity disorder (multiple personality disorder), and dissociative disorder not otherwise specified (DDNOS)] are characterized by disturbances in the integrative functions of memory, consciousness, and/or identity (American Psychiatric Association, 1994). In recent years, mental health professionals and researchers have found that dissociative disorders occur frequently in psychiatric patients, and comprise as much as 10% of inpatient psychiatric populations (Bliss & Jeppsen, 1985). Moderate-to-severe dissociative symptoms are also common in patients with other psychiatric disorders, particularly the anxiety disorders (including posttraumatic stress disorder), mood disorders, eating disorders, and borderline personality disorder (Coons, 1984; Fink, 1991; Horevitz & Braun, 1984; Kluft, 1987c; Putnam, Guroff, Silberman, Barban, & Post, 1986; Schultz, Braun, & Kluft, 1989; Torem, 1986; Steinberg, 1995).

Despite growing recognition of the prevalence of dissociative symptoms, they are often overlooked because of their intrinsic complexity and multiform presentation. Severe dissociation is recognized as being a posttraumatic defense mechanism (Chu & Dill, 1990; Coons, Cole, Pellow, & Milstein, 1990; Kluft, 1987a; Wilbur, 1984); a patient may be unaware of his or her dissociative symptoms as well as of the

Marlene Steinberg • Department of Psychiatry, Yale University School of Medicine, New Haven, Connecticut 06510.

Handbook of Dissociation: Theoretical, Empirical, and Clinical Perspectives, edited by Larry K. Michelson and William J. Ray. Plenum Press, New York, 1996.

memories of the traumatic event(s) (Coons, 1984; Edwards & Angus, 1972; Kluft, 1984a, 1991; Steinberg, 1991, 1995). In addition, the occurrence of hallucinations and affective lability in patients with undetected dissociative disorders has led to misdiagnoses of schizophrenia, affective disorder, and borderline personality disorder (Bliss, 1986; Clary, Burstin, & Carpenter, 1984; Coons, 1984; Horevitz & Braun, 1984; Kluft, 1984a, 1987c; Marcum, Wright, & Bissell, 1985; Putnam et al., 1984; Putnam et al., 1986; Rosenbaum, 1980). Patients with undetected dissociative symptoms often remain misdiagnosed and improperly treated (Coons, Bowman, & Milstein, 1988; Kluft, 1984b, 1991). Conversely, such patients who are properly diagnosed usually respond well to appropriate treatment (Coons, 1986; Kluft, 1984b, 1991). In fact, the dissociative disorders are one of the few categories of psychiatric illness for which a record of success with appropriate therapy is developing (Spiegel, 1993). The recent development of reliable diagnostic instruments, such as the Structured Clinical Interview for DSM-IV Dissociative Disorders (SCID-D) (Steinberg, 1993b), allows for effective early identification and proper treatment of patients with dissociative disorders.

This chapter offers an overview of testing methods available for the assessment and diagnosis of dissociative symptoms and disorders. It will summarize the results of both screening and diagnostic measures of dissociation and discuss the characteristic profiles of patients with dissociative disorders on standard psychological measurements such as the Minnesota Multiphasic Personality Inventory (MMPI). The use of standard measurement techniques allows for reliable diagnoses of dissociative symptoms and disorders. Moreover, specialized interviews such as the SCID-D (Steinberg, 1993b) can facilitate the training of clinicians in the accurate assessment of dissociative symptomatology.

DIAGNOSTIC INSTRUMENTS AND SYSTEMATIC ASSESSMENT OF GENERAL PSYCHOPATHOLOGY

The introduction of standardized criteria and structured assessment tools has raised the level of diagnostic accuracy for major disorders, in both clinical and research settings (Endicott & Spitzer, 1978; Endicott et al., 1976; Helzer et al., 1977; Maier, Phillipp, & Buller, 1988; Robins, Helzer, Croughan, & Ratcliff, 1981; Spitzer, Williams, Gibbon, & First, 1990). Both structured diagnostic instruments and symptom screeners enhance the validity of diagnostic procedures by limiting variability between interviews, focusing inquiry on diagnostically discriminating features, and insuring the analysis of a broader range of psychiatric issues (MacKinnon & Yudofsky, 1986; Spitzer, 1983).

A variety of instruments are currently used in general psychiatric assessment. These tools are based on criteria derived from several sources, including DSM (American Psychiatric Association, 1987; Spitzer et al., 1990), Research Diagnostic Criteria (Spitzer, Endicott, & Robins, 1978; Endicott & Spitzer, 1978; Robins et al., 1981), and the International Classification of Diseases (ICD) (Garcia, 1990; Spitzer, Williams, Gibbon, & First, 1992). The Present State Examination (PSE) (Wing, Birley, Cooper, Graham, & Isaacs, 1967), and the National Institutes of Mental Health Diagnostic Interview Schedule (DIS) (Robins et al., 1981) are structured interviews with rating scales that make computerized diagnoses. The DIS was the first instrument to incorporate DSM-III's comprehensive nosology (American Psychiatric Association, 1980). It is highly structured, allowing for use by nonclinician interviewers. The Structured Clinical Interview for DSM-III-R Dissociative Disorders (SCID) (Spitzer et al., 1990) is an open-ended structured clinical interview based on DSM-III-R criteria, requiring the interviewer to draw on clinical judgment throughout. The SCID was designed to be administered by experienced clinicians trained to ask appropriate probing questions (Spitzer et al., 1992).

Although these instruments have increased the reliability of general psychiatric diagnosis, none of them are specifically designed for the diagnosis of dissociative symptoms or disorders. As a result, patients with dissociative disorders may be diagnosed as suffering from schizophrenia or mood disorder, particularly when questions for the dissociative disorders are omitted and/or questions worded to include dissociative symptoms are included in subscales that score for nondissociative disorders.

ASSESSMENT OF DISSOCIATIVE DISORDERS

Self-Administered Screening Tools for Dissociative Symptoms

Self-administered instruments are time-efficient screening tools; they are therefore useful in studies involving large patient samples or several questionnaires. Patients suspected of having dissociative disorders may then be followed up with a confirmatory diagnostic interview. The disadvantages of self-administered instruments include their limited scope, their tendency to result in false negatives in patients unaware of their symptoms or unmotivated/aversive to symptom disclosure (MacKinnon & Yudofsky, 1986), and their high susceptibility to malingering of dissociative symptoms (Gilbertson et al., 1992).

Depersonalization Questionnaires. Prior to the last decade, a variety of questionnaires were designed exclusively for the measurement of depersonalization. These questionnaires provided the basis for descriptive papers on the incidence of depersonalization in college populations (Dixon, 1963; Myers & Grant, 1972; Roberts, 1960), psychiatric patients (Brauer, Harrow, & Tucker, 1970), and survivors of life-threatening trauma (Noyes & Kletti, 1977; Noyes et al., 1977). These instruments are highly structured, have not been tested on different clinical populations, and have not been evaluated in terms of their psychometric properties. Nonetheless these questionnaires have provided important descriptive information regarding the symptom of depersonalization.

The Dissociative Experiences Scale. The Dissociative Experiences Scale (DES) (Bernstein & Putnam, 1986) is a self-administered dissociative experience screener, consisting of 28 items rated with a visual analogue scale. The subject marks a point on a line between two extremes (0 and 100%), according to the frequency of the experience, yielding a total DES score between 0 and 100, which represents an average of the scores for all 28 items. A second version of the DES asks the subject to circle a frequency percentage from 0 to 100%, spaced at 10% intervals. Subjects are instructed to report only those experiences that occur without the use of drugs or alcohol.

Factor analysis yielded five categories of dissociation: amnestic dissociation, depersonalization, derealization, absorption (preoccupation with a particular activity), and imaginative involvement (Carlson et al., 1991). Good test–retest and internal reliability have been shown for the DES (Bernstein & Putnam, 1986; Frischholz, 1985; Frischholz et al., 1990; Strick & Wilcoxon, 1991). Good convergent and discriminant validity with respect to other measures were also found in a number of other studies (Bernstein & Putnam, 1986; Branscomb, 1991; Frischholz et al., 1991; Nadon, Hoyt, Register, & Kihlstrom, 1991). Steinberg, Rounsaville, and Cicchetti (1991) recommend the use of a DES cutoff of 15 to 20 when screening for individuals suspected of having a dissociative disorder. Subjects with scores of greater than 15 should then be followed up with a confirmatory diagnostic tool such as the Structured Clinical Interview for DSM-IV Dissociative Disorders (SCID-D) (Steinberg 1994a).

A number of researchers have pinpointed several limitations of the DES. In a study of 100 substance abusers (Ross et al., 1992), the DES failed to discriminate between patients with comorbid dissociative disorders and patients without dissociative disorders. A factor analytic study of 507 undergraduates given the DES and Perceptual Alteration Scale (PAS) (Fischer & Elnitsky, 1990) found different principal factors for each scale (PAS: disturbance in affect control; DES: disturbance in cognition control), indicating that neither tool assesses dissociation in its entirety. Last, studies by Antens et al. (1991) and Gilbertson et al. (1992) indicate that the DES, as well as the PAS and the Questionnaire of Experiences of Dissociation, is susceptible to malingerers: "all of these scales are very transparent to individuals taking the test and thus are easily faked in either direction" (North et al., 1993, p. 104).

The Perceptual Alteration Scale. The Perceptual Alteration Scale (PAS) (Sanders, 1986) assesses dissociative symptoms using items adapted from the MMPI (Hathaway & McKinley, 1970), selected on the basis of Hilgard's (1984) conceptualization of neo-dissociation. This self-administered, 60-item questionnaire contains Likert scale ratings ranging from 1 to 4. The PAS was used to discriminate between a sample of binge eaters and control subjects (N = 114, t = 5.12), finding higher severity and frequency of PAS items in binge eaters than in normal subjects. The PAS has reported limited data on reliability and validity, and its clinical usefulness requires further exploration.

The Questionnaire of Experiences of Dissociation. The Questionnaire of Experiences of Dissociation (QED) (Riley, 1988) contains 26 true–false items related to a variety of dissociative phenomena. The items on the QED are simply worded for ease of understanding. With a sample of over 1200 subjects, the QED reported a reliability of .77, and discriminated between control subjects and patients with somatization disorder (N = 21) and multiple personality disorder (MPD) (N = 3). Eleven items indicate dissociative psychopathology when marked true, and half indicate the presence of dissociation when marked false. The QED's simple one-page format allows for rapid screening for dissociative symptoms. Further research is recommended using the QED on a variety of patient populations.

OTHER TOOLS NOT SPECIFIC TO DISSOCIATIVE DISORDERS

The Dissociative Disorders Interview Schedule

The Dissociative Disorders Interview Schedule (DDIS) (Ross et al., 1989a) is a highly structured interview developed to diagnose the presence of dissociative disorders, as well as major depression, borderline personality, and somatization disorder. Though some studies have suggested that the DDIS has shown good interrater reliability and sensitivity (Ross, Heber, Norton, & Anderson, 1989b), others indicate poorer results (Ross et al., 1989a). The limitations of the DDIS include its highly structured format, which incorporates only one item for each DSM criterion, resulting in diagnoses that hinge on a "yes" response to only a few items. Furthermore, many items in the DDIS are not diagnostic of the dissociative disorders (e.g., items related to somatization disorder, major depression, and borderline personality), and can be reliably evaluated by existing tools such as the Structured Clinical Interview for DSM-III-R (Spitzer et al., 1990). Clinicians and researchers should also note the limited utility of the DDIS in identifying dissociative disorders in the chemically dependent population.

Nonspecific Tests Used in Psychological Assessment (Not Diagnostic for Dissociative Disorders)

Administration of standard psychological tests to patients with dissociative and nondissociative disorders has proved to be inadequate in detecting the presence of MPD or other dissociative disorders (North et al., 1993). Such tests may be useful in providing relevant information about the subject's personalities once the MPD diagnosis has otherwise been made, and may be helpful to the clinician in determining the presence and nature of other forms of psychopathology that may coexist with dissociative disorders (Armstrong, 1991). But dependence on standard psychological tests (i.e., MMPI, Rorschach) to diagnose dissociative disorders has often led to tragic cases of misdiagnosis (Hall, 1989).

Patients with DID have been frequently misdiagnosed as schizophrenics on the basis of their MMPI responses (Bliss, 1984; Coons & Sterne, 1986; Solomon, 1983). These misdiagnoses occur because the MMPI includes dissociative symptoms such as amnesia on the schizophrenia scale. North et al. (1993) likewise conclude that administration of the MMPI may be useful to clinicians in evaluating the severity and nature of the co-ordinate or subordinate diagnoses of patients with polysymptomatic/polysyndromic disorders, but not in diagnosing the presence of DID as such.

Conflicting results have also emerged from the use of the Rorschach on patients with dissociative identity disorder. North et al. (1993) assert that "the Rorschach is unlikely to be a good screening instrument for detecting currently undiagnosed cases of MPD" (p. 106).

Finally, intelligence testing of patients with DID has yielded mixed results. While some researchers have reported similar IQs across personalities (Berman, 1973; Ludwig, Brandsma, Wilbur, Benfeldt, & Jameson, 1972), others have observed differences in scores (Ohberg, 1984). North et al. (1993) report that nonstandard intelligence examinations may be required in order to obtain the best estimate of a dissociative patient's true abilities, but, "as a group, patients with DID do not appear to have significant cognitive or neuropsychological deficits on the tests described to this point" (p. 74).

Diagnostic Tools Specific to Dissociative Disorders: The Structured Clinical Interview for DSM-IV Dissociative Disorders (SCID-D) Interview

In order to fill the gap left by general diagnostic instruments, the SCID-D (Steinberg, 1993b, 1994b) was developed to assess dissociative symptoms and disorders. This instrument has proven useful in studying the phenomenology, of dissociative symptoms, and comorbidity with nondissociative symptoms and disorders, and is widely recognized as a standard in the field of diagnosis and assessment of dissociative symptoms and disorders. The use of the SCID-D, which has undergone rigorous field-testing for reliability and validity has improved diagnostic accuracy with regard to dissociative disturbances, and has allowed for clinical investigations of the phenomenology and prevalence of dissociative symptoms and disorders. This semistructured clinical interview comprehensively assesses five specific dissociative symptoms and makes diagnoses of the dissociative disorders based on DSM-IV criteria. The SCID-D's structure is based on the format of the Structured Clinical Interview for DSM-III-R (SCID; Spitzer et al., 1990); it uses open-ended questions and embeds DSM-IV criteria throughout the interview. Guidelines for the administration, scoring, and interpretation of the SCID-D are described in the *Interviewer's Guide to the SCID-D* (Steinberg, 1993a, 1994a).

The SCID-D systematically evaluates the presence and severity of five core dissociative symptoms (amnesia, depersonalization, derealization, identity confusion, and identity alteration) (Steinberg, 1994b, 1994c); and allows the interviewer to make DSM-IV diagnoses of dissociative amnesia, dissociative fugue, depersonalization disorder, dissociative identity disorder (multiple personality disorder), and dissociative disorder not otherwise specified (DDNOS). Disorders newly proposed in DSM-IV consisting of predominantly dissociative symptoms, including acute dissociative (stress) disorder and possession trance disorder (in the DSM-IV appendix) can also be assessed with the SCID-D (see Spiegel & Cardeña, 1991; Steinberg, 1994a).

Development and Field Trials of the SCID-D. Good-to-excellent reliability and discriminant validity were reported for the SCID-D with respect to the five dissociative symptoms and the dissociative disorders, on the basis of over 400 administrations of the instrument (Steinberg, Rounsaville, & Cicchetti, 1990; Steinberg, Cicchetti, Buchanan, Hall, & Rounsaville, 1989–1992). These results were replicated by researchers at Harvard (Goff, Olin, Jenike, Baer, & Buttolph, 1992) and in the Netherlands (Boon & Draijer, 1991). Preliminary results regarding SCID-D psychometrics led to the award of an National Institute of Mental Health grant to field-test the instrument (Steinberg et al., 1989–1992). The SCID-D was field-tested on 140 patients with a variety of psychiatric disorders, including the affective, psychotic, anxiety, substance abuse, and personality disorders. SCID-D interviews were rated by two of five interviewers blind to the referring clinician's diagnosis. Each subject was given two interviews with 1-week interval, and 50 were given a third interview at 6-month follow-up. Analysis of the results of this field testing has indicated good-to-excellent reliability and validity for dissociative symptoms and disorders (Steinberg et al., 1989–1992). In addition, multicenter field trials of the SCID-D have been completed with expert researchers at four sites: in Philadelphia (Drs. Kluft, Fine, and Fink); Indianapolis (Drs. Coons and Bowman); Summit, New Jersey (Dr. Pamela Hall); and New Haven (Drs. Steinberg, Rounsaville, and Cicchetti) (Steinberg et al., 1989–1993). SCID-D interviews were performed at each of the four sites and then corated by experts at the other sites. Preliminary analysis (based on results from three of the four sites) continues to indicate good-to-excellent interrater reliability for each of the five dissociative symptoms as well as the diagnosis of the dissociative disorders. In addition, the SCID-D interview was able to distinguish between patients with dissociative disorders, patients with substance abuse disorders, and those with substance abuse disorder and a coexisting dissociative disorder.

Format of the SCID-D. The SCID-D's semistructured format and use of diagnostically discriminating questions allows for a clinically rich interview in which interviewers are encouraged to add unscripted follow-up questions that clarify or elaborate the subject's response.

The SCID-D is divided into five major sections, one for each of the five dissociative symptoms. In addition, the instrument includes questions related to associated features of identity disturbance, follow-up sections on identity confusion and alteration, and intrainterview dissociative cues. DSM-IV criteria are embedded throughout the interview. Each DSM-IV criterion is assessed with a series of questions that follow a preliminary screening question. Exclusionary factors for these disorders (for medical illness, alcohol and drug use) are assessed within each dissociative symptom section.

Due to the complexity and subtlety of dissociative identity disturbances, they are further assessed in follow-up sections on identity confusion and alteration. Follow-up sections are administered at the interviewer's discretion to subjects who have endorsed significant dissociative symptoms. One or two of these modules may be administered. A series of questions assess the degree of volition and distinctness of personality states, drawing on patients' own terminology for their altered state(s) of identity. The completion of this section allows the rater to determine whether the subject's symptoms meet DSM-IV criteria for multiple personality disorder and DDNOS. After the interview, the rater records the five symptom severities and dissociative disorder diagnosis on the summary score sheet, which records this summary information in a visually concise form.

Throughout the SCID-D interview, responses to each item are recorded with the following codes: ? = unclear, 1 = absent, 3 = present, 4 = inconsistent information. A rating of 4 is given when a subject provides contradictory responses to a question, which may occur in patients with significant identity confusion. A rating of "?" is often given when patients are amnestic for information that is being assessed (which frequently occurs in patients with dissociative disorders). Descriptive responses to open-ended inquiries are recorded in the space provided.

Severity rating definitions are provided in the *Interviewer's Guide* (Steinberg, 1993a) and allow the interviewer to determine symptom severity based on the subject's responses to each section of the SCID-D. The severity of each dissociative symptom is assessed through questions concerning the frequency, duration, distress, and dysfunction associated with each dissociative experience. Severity rating codes are 1 = none, 2 = mild, 4 = moderate, and 5 = severe. A subject receives a score from 1 to 5 for each of the five dissociative symptoms and also receives a total score for all the symptoms ranging from 5 to 20.

All scores are recorded on a summary score sheet, which is intended to be filed with the patient's records. The score sheet (together with the patient's responses as recorded by the examiner in the SCID-D booklet) can be admitted as courtroom evidence in forensic contexts. These records, when accurately scored and interpreted, offer the clinician documentary protection against potential allegations of iatrogenic symptom production. In addition, these symptom profiles can be represented iconically on a SCID-D symptom profile graph, as demonstrated by the characteristic profiles of patients with dissociative and nondissociative disorders (see Figures 12.1 and 12.2).

Features of the SCID-D's Semistructured Interview Format. Numerous authors have remarked on the benefits of semistructured interviews in improving the reliability, validity, and richness of a psychiatric assessment (Cicchetti & Tyler, 1988; Endicott & Spitzer, 1978; Endicott et al., 1976; Helzer et al., 1977; MacKinnon & Yudofsky, 1986; Maier et al., 1988; Robins et al., 1981; Saghir, 1971; Spitzer, 1983; Spitzer et al., 1990). Semistructured interviews "enhance both the reliability and validity of a respondent's information about a given subject ... [providing] more accurate descriptions than might be possible with other modes of test administration" (Cicchetti & Tyler, 1988). This is accomplished by balancing unstructured features, such as open-ended responses and rapport, with structured features, such as operationalized rating scales and interview instructions. According to Anastasi (1976), such a design can "provide a rich harvest of leads for further exploration ... permit[ting] more flexibility of search and more effective utilization of cues than would be possible with a test, questionnaire, or other standardized procedure" (pp. 464, 484). The advantages of structured or semistructured interviews over highly structured checklists have been described by a number of authors (Anastasi, 1976; Maier et al., 1988; Robins et al., 1981; Saghir, 1971). Whereas highly structured interviews require the clinician to take a yes–no response at face value, SCID-D interviewers can evaluate the descriptions offered by patients for each endorsed symptom. This flexibility also permits clinicians to consider the intent of a response rather than merely its face value conformity to a question (Spitzer, 1983). The SCID-D's format also allows for exploration of the complexities and interconnections of dissociative symptomatology. For example, patients may volunteer material suggestive of the presence of identity confusion or identity alteration during earlier portions of the interview. The SCID-D allows the interviewer to follow up on specific descriptions of symptoms in order to clarify the existence of identity confusion or alteration.

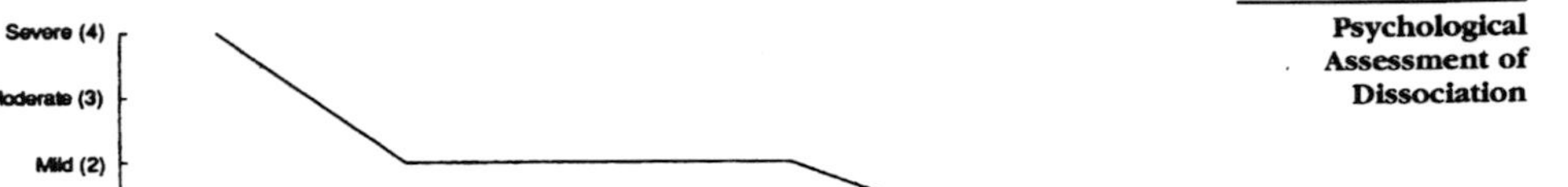

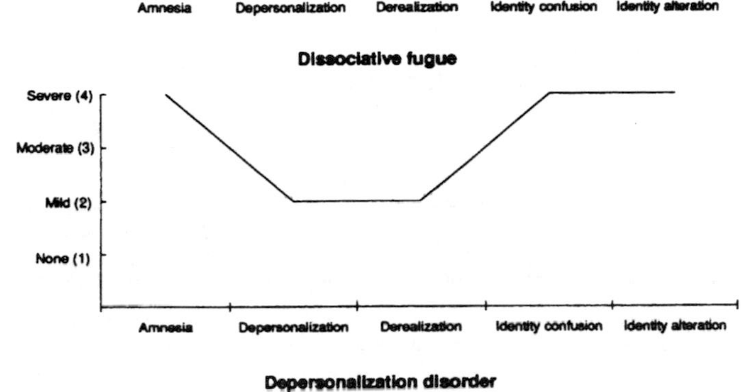

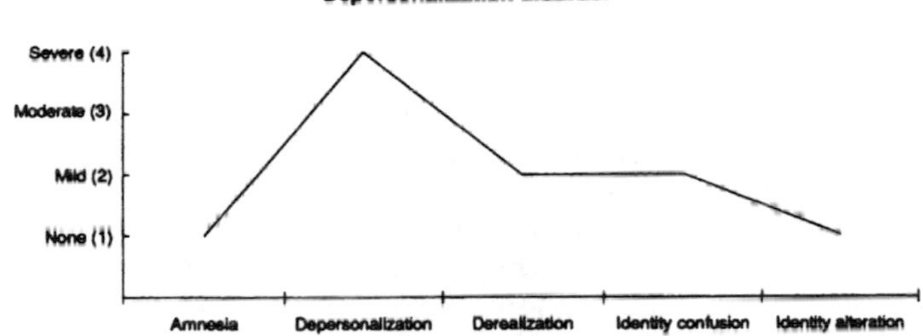

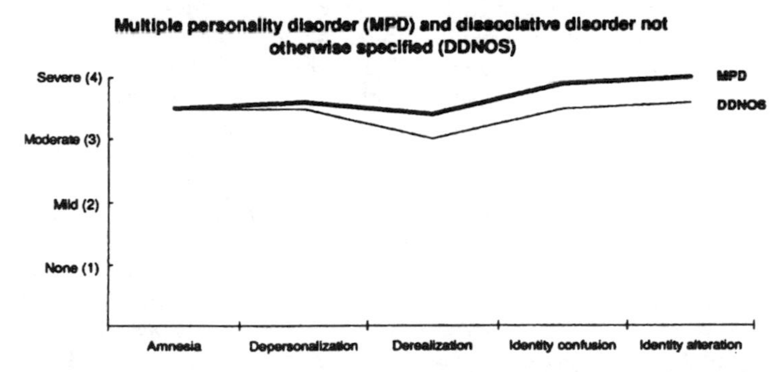

Figure 1 SCID-D symptom profiles of the dissociative disorders. ***Interviewer's Guide to the Structured Clinical Interview for DSM-IV Dissociative Disorders***. Reprinted with permission from M. Steinberg (SCID-D, Revised).

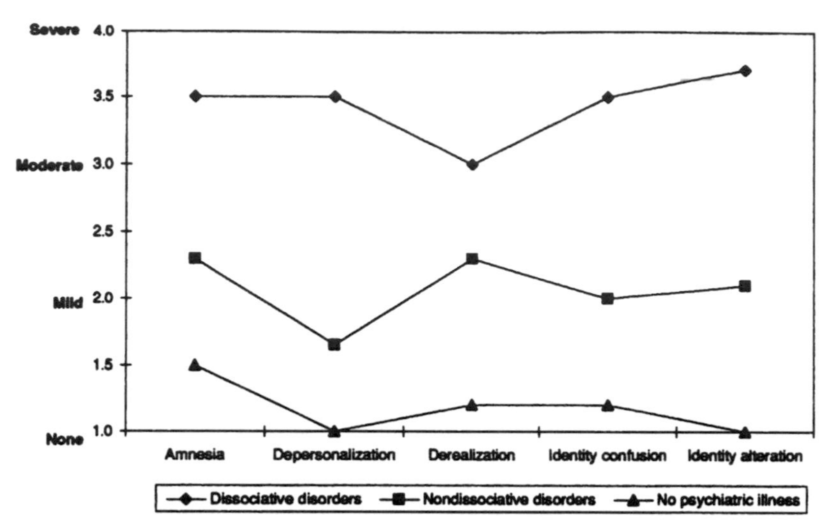

Figure 2 SCID-D dissociative symptom profiles for patients with dissociative disorders, patients with nondissociative disorders, and subjects without psychiatric illness. *Interviewer's Guide to the Structured Clinical Interview for DSM-IV Dissociative Disorders*. Reprinted with permission from M. Steinberg (SCID-D, Revised). Copyright 1994 American Psychiatric Press.

Moreover, semistructured interviews such as the SCID and SCID-D allow the clinician to skip questions that are not pertinent to the subject. This pattern of questioning resembles a seasoned clinician's diagnostic decision tree and focuses the interview on diagnostically discriminating issues (Spitzer, 1983).

In addition, the open-ended responses elicited by a semistructured format contribute to the interviewer's access to nonverbal, behavioral cues that would not be available in a self-administered or highly structured format. Kluft (1987b) notes the importance of intrainterview amnesia, as well as fluctuations in voice, speech, and movement characteristics, which can be essential clues to the presence of a dissociative disorder. He adds that extended interviews (lasting over 4 hours) may elicit observable symptoms in a patient with a dissociative disturbance; however, the clinician must be informed and attuned to the possibility of their manifestation. The SCID-D interview booklet includes a section for the clinician's notation and description of intrainterview cues.

Structured Features. The incorporation of structure in a clinical interview offers several advantages. The primary advantage is the exclusion of uncontrolled variables. Systematic interviews reduce variability in the symptom areas assessed, interpretations made from test results, and the types of questions asked of each patient (Spitzer, 1983). This uniformity allows for the comparison of clinical data from different sources, particularly in research settings (Saghir, 1971). The unreliability, skepticism, and omissions of dissociative disorder diagnoses were major factors motivating the development of the SCID-D.

For example, structured rating scales developed for the SCID-D allow the interviewer to quantify the severity of individual dissociative symptoms, rather than merely record their presence or absence. The SCID-D operationalized definitions of severity according to multiple factors, which include: frequency, duration, and onset of symptoms; degree of distress; and dysfunction. These detailed and standardized criteria allow researchers to compare SCID-D results reliably across different patient populations.

Finally, because dissociative symptoms are posttraumatic, they are often difficult to detect. In order to obtain indications of these more elusive symptoms, clinicians must routinely ask questions that can directly or indirectly retrieve information essential to a correct diagnosis. The SCID-D was designed to assess signs of dissociation whose significance may not be apparent to the subjects themselves. For example, blank spells or time loss are indications of amnesia, and being told by others that the subject acted in an uncharacteristic way is a sign of identity alteration. As Kluft writes, "The Structured Clinical Interview for the DSM-III-R Dissociative Disorders (Steinberg et al., 1990) is extremely comprehensive and sensitive and has shown the capacity to pick up previously unsuspected cases of dissociative disorders" (Kluft, 1991, p. 173). Thus, use of the SCID-D should become an integral part of the diagnostic evolution process.

Clinical Applications of the SCID-D. The SCID-D is a time- and cost-effective instrument with a variety of clinical applications. Indeed, given the high costs of misdiagnosis of dissociative symptoms, health insurers would be wise to cover the minimal expense of the use of the SCID-D interview. Its uses include diagnosis for treatment, identification of symptoms for treatment planning, estimating the prevalence and comorbidity of dissociative symptoms and disorders, and investigation of symptom phenomenology. Because the SCID-D's format facilitates long-term follow-up of patients' symptoms, a clinician can administer the instrument at 6-month or yearly intervals in order to monitor changes in symptomatology and reassess treatment strategy accordingly. This feature makes the instrument particularly useful to practitioners of hypnosis, in that it can be administered to patients prior to the induction of formal hypnotic trance, in order to establish the patient's symptomatic baseline. Moreover, the SCID-D is a tool that can be used for patient education (during a follow-up session with the subject) regarding the nature and significance of the patient's dissociative symptoms. Many patients have reported immediate therapeutic benefits from the opportunity to discuss their symptoms with the interviewer. Last, since the instrument is designed to be filled with patients' charts, it secures easily accessible documentation of symptoms, for recordkeeping and psychological reports. This feature is particularly beneficial to clinicians involved as expert witnesses in forensic cases, in that SCID-D results can be submitted as evidentiary material that is less controversial than amytal interviews, hypnosis, or the results of psychological tests such as the MMPI. As North et al. (1993) have remarked with regard to the MMPI:

> [MMPI] validity scale patterns present a clear problem in forensic settings. Because many patients with MPD, borderline personality disorder, and/or Briquet's syndrome present invalid test results, one cannot confidently attribute the production of invalid profiles to malingering alone.... In forensics, one must simply conclude that one's test data are equivocal to some extent and that the scientific conclusions that can be drawn from them are quite limited. (p. 81)

For a comprehensive overview of the dissociative symptoms and disorders, as well as an explanatory guide to the clinical applications of the SCID-D, the reader is referred to the *Handbook for the Assessment of Dissociation: A Clinical Guide* (Steinberg, 1995).

A Sample SCID-D Evaluation Report. As an illustration of the SCID-D's specific applications in symptom documentation, psychological reports, and treatment planning, a sample patient report follows:

(For the sake of conciseness, the past psychiatric history of this patient is abbreviated and this sample protocol will focus primarily on the SCID-D evaluation.)

> Jane Smith is a 35-year-old single woman. She has experienced intermittent panic attacks, depression, auditory hallucinations, "trances," "blackouts," and self-mutilating behaviors, since she was 12 years old. Jane reports a family history of emotional and physical abuse at the hands of both parents. She has been treated in outpatient psychotherapy four times since age 14, for periods of up to 2 years; past diagnoses include bipolar disorder, schizophrenia, atypical psychosis, and depression. She was referred for a diagnostic consultation by her present therapist.
>
> *Dates of Evaluation*
>
> On 5/24/94, I administered the *Structured Clinical Interview for DSM-IV Dissociative Disorders* (Steinberg, 1993b). Scoring and interpretation of the SCID-D were performed according to the guidelines described in the *Interviewer's Guide to the SCID-D* (Steinberg, 1993a). On 5/31/94, I met with Jane Smith to review the findings of the SCID-D interview and discussed recommendations for treatment.
>
> *SCID-D Evaluation and Diagnostic Assessment*
>
> A review of the significant findings from the SCID-D interview is as follows: Jane suffers from bimonthly episodes of severe amnesia since age 9, which are the "blackouts" she describes. She also experiences recurrent episodes of depersonalization, which include her "trances," during which she feels she leaves her body and is sitting on her own shoulder. She reports that she occasionally cuts herself with a razor in order to alleviate the feelings of depersonalization. She endorses symptoms of recurrent derealization and identity confusion. In addition, Jane reports evidence of identity alteration: she receives mail addressed to "Samantha" and "Freddie," from two other students at different undergraduate institutions; she has also reported that people had greeted her on the street as "Samantha." During administration of the follow-up sections, Jane endorsed having recurrent feelings that different people existed inside her, including a child of toddler age, a "Biker" in her late teens, a rageful person called "Son-of-a-Bitch" of uncertain age, and a person named "Idiot." She reported that she experiences these people as separate from her "normal self" and that they assume control of her behavior. As examples, she mentioned that "Idiot" was talking to me during part of the interview; and that her boyfriend broke up with her because the "Biker" came out several times during their dates and displayed inappropriate behavior. During the SCID-D interview, I observed changes in Jane's affect, speech, and physical posture consistent with her child alter, such as curling up in the chair and sucking her thumb.
>
> Jane's SCID-D symptom profile and past history of traumatic experiences are consistent with a primary diagnosis of a dissociative disorder. Based on the

SCID-D evaluation, Jane's symptoms of amnesia, depersonalization, derealization, identity confusion, and identity alteration are all present at a severe level. She has suffered from chronic dissociative symptoms that interfere with her schoolwork and relationships and that appear to be related to her self-cutting. She has also described the presence of other personalities within her that take control of her behavior to the extent of forming alternate sets of relationships and behaviors. The constellation of Jane's symptoms meets DSM-IV criteria for a diagnosis of dissociative identity disorder. Her depression appears to be secondary to the disruptions in her life caused by the alter personalities.

Recommendation

I recommended weekly individual therapy focused on the reduction of Jane's dissociative symptoms. Patient education regarding these symptoms and their triggers is recommended during the initial treatment phase. A subsequent goal should be increased cooperation among the alternate personalities in order to reduce the severity of Jane's amnesia, identity confusion, and identity alteration. Finally, the use of an antidepressant may relieve some of the immediate symptoms of depression.

SCID-D Research and the Differential Diagnosis of Dissociation. The SCID-D can be useful to clinicians in detecting and assessing the severity of dissociative symptomatology in patients diagnosed with a nondissociative disorder, as well as in patients with a high index of suspicion for a dissociative disturbance. Clinicians should note that dissociative symptoms may manifest in any of the disorders classified under Axes I and II and DSM-IV. Research indicates that the relationship between dissociative symptoms and nondissociative disorders will fall into one of two basic patterns: (1) the primary disorder is nondissociative, but coexists with some dissociative symptoms; and (2) the nondissociative disorder has been masking the presence of an underlying, previously undetected dissociative disorder. Since accurate diagnosis is essential to the planning and implementation of appropriate treatment, selective administration of the SCID-D is helpful in preventing misinterpretation of a patient's dissociative symptoms. Research findings indicate that the SCID-D is effective in detecting previously undiagnosed dissociative disorders and in distinguishing between patients with dissociative disorders and other psychiatric disorders (including the anxiety disorders, personality disorders, substance abuse and eating disorders, and the psychotic disorders) (see Goff et al., 1992; Steinberg, Cicchetti, Buchanan, Raakfeldt, & Rounsaville, 1994). In addition, the SCID-D can be used to discriminate between dissociative disorders and seizure disorders (E. Bowman, 1994, personal communication). The reader is referred to the *Handbook for the Assessment of Dissociation* (Steinberg, 1995) for a more detailed discussion of the use of the SCID-D in differential diagnosis of dissociative symptomatology in nondissociative as well as in dissociative disorders.

CONCLUSION

In summary, the last decade has witnessed the development of diagnostic instruments which are specific for the dissociative disorders. Clinicians and researchers can now choose from a variety of self-administered screeners, in order to screen patients for dissociative symptomatology rapidly, as well as effective and time-efficient clinician-administered tools for the diagnosis of the dissociative disorders. Among these clinician-administered instruments, the SCID-D offers the advantage of assessing the severity as well as the presence of dissociative symptoms and disorders. Although IQ tests and projective and psychological tests such as the Rorschach and MMPI respectively are not diagnostic of the presence of dissociation and should not be used for that purpose, they may provide evidence of coexisting psychopathology in some subjects, necessitating follow-up with instruments specific for the dissociative disorders.

ACKNOWLEDGMENTS. This research was supported by NIMH Grant R01-43352.

REFERENCES

American Psychiatric Association. (1980). *Diagnostic and statistical manual of mental disorders* (3rd ed.). Washington, DC: Author.

American Psychiatric Association. (1987). *Diagnostic and statistical manual of mental disorders* (3rd ed., rev.). Washington, DC: Author.

American Psychiatric Association. (1994). *Diagnostic and statistical manual of mental disorders* (4th ed.). Washington, DC: Author.

Anastasi, A. (1976). *Psychological testing* (4th ed.). New York: Macmillan.

Antens, E., Frischholz, E. J., Braun, B. G., et al. (1991). The simulation of dissociative disorders on the Dissociative Experiences Scale. Paper presented to the 8th annual meeting of the International Society for the Study of Multiple Personality Disorder and Dissociation, Chicago, November 15-17.

Armstrong, J. (1991). The psychological organization of multiple personality disordered patients as revealed in psychological testing. *Psychiatric Clinics of North America*, *14*(3), 533-546.

Berman, E. (1973). *The development and dynamics of multiple personality*. Ann Arbor, MI: University Microfilms International.

Bernstein, E., & Putnam, F. W. (1986). Development, reliability and validity of a dissociation scale. *Journal of Nervous and Mental Disease*, *174*, 727-735.

Bliss, E. (1986). *Multiple personality, allied disorders and hypnosis*. New York: Oxford University Press.

Bliss, E. L. (1984). A symptom profile of patients with multiple personalities, including MMPI results. *Journal of Nervous and Mental Disease*, *172*, 197-202.

Bliss, E. L., & Jeppsen, E. A. (1985). Prevalence of multiple personality among inpatients and outpatients. *American Journal of Psychiatry*, *142*(2), 250-251.

Boon, S., & Draijer, N. (1991). Diagnosing dissociative disorders in the Netherlands: A pilot study with the Structured Clinical Interview for DSM-III-R Dissociative Disorders. *American Journal of Psychiatry*, *148*(4), 458-462.

Branscomb, L. (1991). Dissociation in combat-related post-traumatic stress disorder. *Dissociation*, *4*(1), 13- 20.

Brauer, R., Harrow, M., & Tucker, G. (1970). Depersonalization phenomena in psychiatric patients. *British Journal of Psychiatry*, *117*, 509-515.

Carlson, E. B., Putnam, F. W., Ross, C. A., Anderson, G., Clark, P., Torem, M., Coons, P. M., Bowman, E. S., Chu, J. A., & Dill, D. (1991). Factor analysis of the Dissociative Experiences Scale: A multicenter study. In B. G. Braun & E. B. Carlson (Eds.), *Proceedings of the eighth international conference on multiple personality and dissociative states* (pp.). Chicago: Rush Presbyterian.

Chu, J. A., & Dill, D. L. (1990). Dissociative symptoms in relation to childhood physical and sexual abuse. *American Journal of Psychiatry*, *147*(7), 887-892.

Cicchetti, D. V., & Tyler, P. (1988). Reliability and validity of personality assessment. In P. Tyler (Eds.), *Personality disorders: Diagnosis, management, and course* (pp. 63-73). London: Wright.

Clary, W. F., Burstin, K. J., & Carpenter, J. S. (1984). Multiple personality and borderline personality disorder. *Psychiatric Clinics of North America*, *7*, 89-100.

Coons, P. M. (1984). The differential diagnosis of multiple personality: A comprehensive review. *Psychiatric Clinics of North America*, *12*, 51-67.

Coons, P. M. (1986). Treatment progress in 20 patients with multiple personality. *Journal of Nervous and Mental Disease, 174*, 715-721.

Coons, P. M., & Sterne, A. L. (1986). Initial and follow-up psychological testing on a group of patients with multiple personality disorder. *Psychological Reports, 58*, 43-49.

Coons, P. M., Bowman, E. S., & Milstein, V. (1988). Multiple personality disorder: A clinical investigation of 50 cases. *Journal of Nervous and Mental Disease, 176*(5), 519-527.

Coons, P. M., Cole, C., Pellow, T., & Milstein, V. (1990). Symptoms of posttraumatic stress and dissociation in women victims of abuse. In R. P. Kluft (Eds.), *Incest-related syndromes of adult psychopathology* (pp. 205-226). Washington, DC: American Psychiatric Press.

Dixon, J. C. (1963). Depersonalization phenomena in a sample population of college students. *British Journal of Psychiatry, 109*, 371-375.

Edwards, G., & Angus, J. (1972). Depersonalization. *British Journal of Psychiatry, 120*, 242-244.

Endicott, J., & Spitzer, R. L. (1978). A diagnostic interview: The Schedule for Affective Disorders and Schizophrenia. *Archives of General Psychiatry, 35*, 837-844.

Endicott, J., Spitzer, R. L., Fleiss, J. L., et al. (1976). The Global Assessment Scale: A procedure for measuring overall severity of psychiatric disturbance. *Archives of General Psychiatry, 33*, 766-771.

Erickson, M. H., & Rappaport, D. (1980). Findings on the nature of the personality structures in two different dual personalities by means of projective and psychometric tests. In E. L. Rossi (Eds.), *The collected papers of Milton Erickson: Vol 3. Investigations of psychodynamic processes* (pp.). New York: Irvington.

Fink, D. (1991). The comorbidity of multiple personality disorder and DSM-III-R Axis II disorders. *Psychiatric Clinics of North America, 14*(3), 547-566.

Fischer, D., & Elnitsky, S. (1990). A factor analytic study of two scales measuring dissociation. *American Journal of Clinical Hypnosis, 32*(3), 201-207.

Frischholz, E. (1985). The relationship among dissociation, hypnosis, and child abuse in the development of multiple personality disorder. In R. P. Kluft (Eds.), *Childhood antecedents of multiple personality* (pp. 99-126). Washington, DC: American Psychiatric Press.

Frischholz, E. J., Braun, B. G., Sachs, R. G., Hopkins, L., Schaeffer, D. M., Lewis, J., Leavitt, F., Pasquotto, M. A., & Schwartz, D. R. (1990). The Dissociative Experiences Scale: Further replication and validation. *Dissociation, 3*(3), 151-153.

Frischholz, E. J., Braun, B. G., Sachs, R. G., Schwartz, D. R., Lewis, J., Schaeffer, D., Westergaard, C., & Pasquotto, J. (1991). Construct validity of the Dissociative Experiences Scale (DES): The relationship between the DES and other self-report measures of DES. *Dissociation, 4*(4), 185-188.

Garcia, F. O. (1990). The concept of dissociation and conversion in the new edition of the International Classification of diseases (ICD-10). *Dissociation, 3*(4), 204-208.

Gilbertson, A., Torem, M., Cohen, R., et al. (1992). Susceptibility of common self-report measures of dissociation to malingering. *Dissociation, 5*(4), 216-220.

Goff, D. C., Olin, J. A., Jenike, M. A., Baer, L., & Buttolph, M. L. (1992). Dissociative symptoms in patients with obsessive-compulsive disorder. *Journal of Nervous and Mental Disease, 180*(5), 332-337.

Hall, P. (1989). Multiple personality disorder and homicide: Professional and legal issues. *Dissociation, 2*, 110-115.

Hathaway, S. R., & McKinley, J. C. (1970). *Minnesota multiphasic personality inventory, revised*. Minneapolis: University of Minnesota.

Helzer, J., Clayton, P., Pambakian, R., et al. (1977). Reliability of psychiatric diagnosis, II: The test-retest reliability of diagnostic classification. *Archives of General Psychiatry, 34*, 136-141.

Hilgard, E. R. (1984). The hidden observer and multiple personality. *International Journal of Clinical and Experimental Hypnosis, 32*(2), 248-253.

Horevitz, R. P., & Braun, B. G. (1984). Are multiple personalities borderline? *Psychiatric Clinics of North America, 7*, 69-87.

Kluft, R. P. (1984a). An introduction to multiple personality disorder. *Psychiatric Annals, 14*, 19-24.

Kluft, R. P. (1984b). Treatment of multiple personality: A study of 33 cases. *Psychiatric Clinics of North America, 7*, 9-29.

Kluft, R. P. (1987a). First rank symptoms as a diagnostic clue to multiple personality disorder. *American Journal of Psychiatry, 144*, 293-298.

Kluft, R. P. (1987b). Making the diagnosis of multiple personality disorder. In F. F. Flach (Eds.), *Diagnostics and psychopathology* (pp. 207-225). New York: Norton.

Kluft, R. P. (1987c). An update on multiple personality disorder. *Hospital and Community Psychiatry*, *38*, 363-373.

Kluft, R. P. (1991). Multiple personality disorder. In A. Tasman & S. Goldfinger (Eds.), *Psychiatric update* (pp.). Washington, DC: American Psychiatric Press.

Lovitt, R., & Lefkof, G. (1985). Understanding multiple personality with the comprehensive Rorschach system. *Journal of Personality Assessment*, *49*, 289-294.

Ludwig, A. M., Brandsma, J. M., Wilbur, C. B., Benfeldt, F., & Jameson, D. H. (1972). The objective study of a multiple personality. *Archives of General Psychiatry*, *26*, 298-310.

MacKinnon, R. A., & Yudofsky, S. C. (1986). *The psychiatric evaluation in clinical practice*. Philadelphia: Lippincott.

Maier, W., Phillipp, M., & Buller, R. (1988). The value of structured clinical interviews. *Archives of General Psychiatry*, *45*, 963-964.

Marcum, J. M., Wright, K., & Bissell, W. G. (1985). Chance discovery of multiple personality disorder in a depressed patient by amobarbital interview. *Journal of Nervous and Mental Disease*, *174*, 489-492.

Myers, D., & Grant, G. (1972). A study of depersonalization in students. *British Journal of Psychiatry*, *121*, 59-65.

Nadon, R., Hoyt, I. P., Register, P. A., & Kihlstrom, J. F. (1991). Absorption and hypnotizability: Context effects reexamined. *Journal of Personality and Social Psychology*, *60*, 144-153.

North, C. S., Ryall, J.-E. M., Ricci, D. A., & Wetzel, R. D. (1993). *Multiple personalities, multiple disorders, psychiatric classification and media influence*. New York and Oxford: Oxford University Press.

Noyes, R., Jr., & Kletti, R. (1977). Depersonalization in response to life-threatening danger. *Comprehensive Psychiatry*, *18*, 375-384.

Noyes, R. J., Hoenk, P., Kuperman, S., et al. (1977). Depersonalization in accident victims and psychiatric patients. *Journal of Nervous and Mental Disease*, *164*, 401-407.

Ohberg, H. G. (1984). Test results for a blind multiple. Paper presented at the First International Conference on Multiple Personality/Dissociative States, Chicago, IL, September.

Putnam, F. W., Loewenstein, R. J., Silberman, E. K., et al. (1984). Multiple personality disorder in a hospital setting. *Journal of Clinical Psychiatry*, *45*, 172-175.

Putnam, F. W., Guroff, J. J., Silberman, E. K., Barban, L., & Post, R. M. (1986). The clinical phenomenology of multiple personality disorder: 100 recent cases. *Journal of Clinical Psychiatry*, *47*, 285-293.

Riley, K. (1988). Measurement of dissociation. *Journal of Nervous and Mental Disease*, *176*, 449-450.

Roberts, W. (1960). Normal and abnormal depersonalization. *Journal of Mental Science*, *106*, 478-493.

Robins, L. N., Helzer, J. E., Croughan, J., & Ratcliff, K. (1981). National Institute of Mental Health Diagnostic Interview Schedule: Its history, characteristics, and validity. *Archives of General Psychiatry*, *38*, 381-389.

Rosenbaum, M. (1980). The role of the term schizophrenia in the decline of the diagnoses of multiple personality. *Archives of General Psychiatry*, *37*, 1383-1385.

Ross, C. A., Heber, S., Norton, G. R., Anderson, D., Anderson, G., & Barchet, P. (1989a). The Dissociative Disorders Interview Schedule: A structured interview. *Dissociation*, *2*(3), 169-189.

Ross, C. A., Heber, S., Norton, G. R., & Anderson, G. (1989b). Differences between multiple personality disorder and other diagnostic groups on structured interview. *The Journal of Nervous and Mental Disease*, *177*(8), 487-491.

Ross, C. A., Kronson, J., Koensgen, S., Barkman, K., Clark, P., & Rockman, G. (1992). Dissociative comorbidity in 100 chemically dependent patients. *Hospital and Community Psychiatry*, *43*(8), 840-842.

Saghir, M. T. (1971). A comparison of some aspects of structured and unstructured psychiatric interviews. *American Journal of Psychiatry*, *128*(2), 180-184.

Sanders, S. (1986). The Perceptual Alteration Scale: A scale measuring dissociation. *American Journal of Clinical Hypnosis*, *29*, 95-102.

Schultz, R., Braun, B. G., & Kluft, R. P. (1989). Multiple personality disorder: Phenomenology of selected variables in comparison to major depression. *Dissociation*, *2*(1), 45-51.

Spiegel, D. (1993). Multiple posttraumatic personality disorder. In R. P. Kluft & C. G. Fine (Eds.), *Clinical Perspectives on Multiple Personality Disorder* (pp. 87-99). Washington, DC: American Psychiatric Press.

Spiegel, D., & Cardeña, E. (1991). Disintegrated experience: The dissociative disorders revisited. *Journal of Abnormal Psychology*, *100*(3), 366-378.

Spitzer, R. L. (1983). Psychiatric diagnosis: Are clinicians still necessary? *Comprehensive Psychiatry, 24*(5), 399-411.

Spitzer, R. L., Endicott, J., & Robins, E. (1978). Research Diagnostic Criteria. *Archives of General Psychiatry, 35*, 773-782.

Spitzer, R. L., Williams, J. B. W., Gibbon, M., & First, M. B. (1990). *The Structured Clinical Interview for DSM-III-R (SCID)*. Washington, DC: American Psychiatric Press.

Spitzer, R. L., Williams, J. B., Gibbon, M., & First, M. B. (1992). The Structured Clinical Interview for DSM-III-R (SCID) I. History, rationale and description. *Archives of General Psychiatry, 49*, 624-629.

Steinberg, M. (1991). The spectrum of depersonalization: Assessment and treatment. In A. Tasman & S. Goldfinger (Eds.), *American psychiatric press review of psychiatry* (Vol 10, pp. 223-247). Washington, DC: American Psychiatric Press.

Steinberg, M. (1993a). *Interviewer's guide to the structured clinical interview for DSM-IV dissociative disorders (SCID-D)*. Washington, DC: American Psychiatric Press.

Steinberg, M. (1993b). *Structured clinical interview for DSM-IV dissociative disorders (SCID-D)*. Washington, DC: American Psychiatric Press.

Steinberg, M. (1994a). Structured Clinical Interview for DSM-IV Dissociative Disorders-Revised (SCID-D-R). Washington, DC: American Psychiatric Press.

Steinberg, M. (1994b). *Interviewer's guide to the structured clinical interview for DSM-IV dissociative disorders-revised (SCID-D-R)*. Washington, DC: American Psychiatric Press.

Steinberg, M. (1994c). Systematizing dissociation: Symptomatology and diagnostic assessment. In D. Spiegel (Ed.), *Dissociation: Culture, mind and body* (pp. 59-88). Washington, DC: American Psychiatric Press.

Steinberg, M. (1995). *Handbook for the assessment of dissociation: A clinical guide*. Washington, DC: American Psychiatric Press.

Steinberg, M., Cicchetti, D. V., Buchanan, J., Hall, P. E., & Rounsaville, B. J. (1989-1992). NIMH field trials of the Structured Clinical Interview for DSM-IV Dissociative Disorders (SCID-D). Yale University School of Medicine, New Haven, CT.

Steinberg, M., Kluft, R. P., Coons, P. M., Bowman, E. S., Buchanan, J., Fine, C. G., Fink, D. L., Hall, P. E., Rounsaville, B. J., & Cicchetti, D. V. (1989-1993). Multicenter field trials of the Structural Clinical Interview for DSM-IV Dissociative Disorders (SCID-D). New Haven, CT, Yale University School of Medicine.

Steinberg, M., Rounsaville, B. J., & Cicchetti, D. V. (1990). The Structured Clinical Interview for DSM-III-R Dissociative Disorders: Preliminary report on a new diagnostic instrument. *American Journal of Psychiatry, 147*(1), 76-82.

Steinberg, M., Rounsaville, B. J., & Cicchetti, D. V. (1991). Detection of dissociative disorders in psychiatric patients by a screening instrument and a structured diagnostic interview. *American Journal of Psychiatry, 148*(8), 1050-1054.

Steinberg, M., Cicchetti, D. V., Buchanan, J., Raakfeldt, J., & Rounsaville, B. J. (1994). Distinguishing between schizophrenia and multiple personality disorder: Systematic evaluation of overlapping symptoms using a structured interview. *Journal of Nervous and Mental Disease, 182*, 495-502.

Strick, F. L., & Wilcoxon, A. (1991). A comparison of dissociative experiences in adult female outpatients with and without histories of early incestuous abuse. *Dissociation, 4*(4), 193-199.

Torem, M. (1986). Dissociative states presenting as eating disorders. *American Journal of Clinical Hypnosis, 29*, 137-142.

Walters, S. B. (1981). *A delineation and study of the nature of multiple personality: Toward earlier diagnosis of the multiple personality syndrome*. Ann Arbor, MI: University Microfilms International.

Wilbur, C. B. (1984). Multiple personality and child abuse. *Psychiatric Clinics of North America, 7*, 3-8.

Wing, J. K., Birley, J. L. T., Cooper, J. E., Graham, P., & Isaacs, A. (1967). Reliability of a procedure for measuring and classifying "present psychiatric state." *British Journal of Psychiatry, 113*, 499-515.

13

Psychophysiological Assessment of Dissociative Disorders

Theodore P. Zahn, Richard Moraga, and William J. Ray

The study of dissociative disorders by experimental methods such as those used in psychophysiological experiments presents special challenges not encountered in most other forms of psychopathology. In most disorders, patients are considered relatively stable for some period of time, lasting for days to years, and data gathered at any time is assumed to be representative of data gathered at any other time. In the typical study, a group of patients is tested (usually when symptomatic with the disorder) and compared with groups of patients with other disorders and/or normal controls. In the few instances where repeated testing in different symptomatic states is done at all, it is done for some extended period of time such as weeks or months. In major psychoses, for example, the periods of interest would be essentially when ill and in remission; or to take another example, manic, depressed, and euthymic could be the periods of interest. Likewise, the effects of a specific type of treatment such as behavior therapy or pharmacotherapy are investigated.

Most of the relatively few psychophysiological studies on dissociative disorders have been done on dissociative identity disorder (DID) (previously referred to as multiple personality disorder), and here the interest has been in the differences in psychophysiology and behavior occurring in different states, which may change on a time scale of minutes, hours, or days, rather than whether such patients are

Theodore P. Zahn • Laboratory of Psychology and Psychopathology, National Institute of Mental Health, Bethesda, Maryland 20892. **Richard Moraga and William J. Ray** • Department of Psychology, Pennsylvania State University, University Park, Pennsylvania 16802.

Handbook of Dissociation: Theoretical, Empirical, and Clinical Perspectives, edited by Larry K. Michelson and William J. Ray. Plenum Press, New York, 1996.

psychophysiologically different from normal controls or from patients with depression or anxiety disorders. Indeed, since the states (alternate identities) are so different from each other behaviorally, this question, as applied to the individual patient, may be thought to be essentially meaningless. The other difficulty is that the "states" appear to be idiosyncratic or specific for each individual patient. Therefore, this area has lent itself to the case study method to an extent not seen in other disorders, even when objective measures of behavior or psychophysiology have been used. In this chapter, those psychophysiological measures that focus on the autonomic nervous system (ANS) and musculoskeletal system will be discussed first, and research using electrocortical measures—electroencephalography and event-related potentials—will then be covered.

One of the major objectives of psychophysiological studies of DID has been simply to see if these variables can distinguish between different identities. Sometimes this has been done with the motivation of providing objective evidence that the different identity manifestations are "real" rather than some kind of pretense. Whatever the motivation for the study, it would seem that exhibiting consistent psychophysiological differences between alternate identities would be a valuable and necessary first step in determining how these measures might help to understand the phenomenology of this disorder.

That real physiological differences may exist between different alter identities is suggested by clinical anecdotal evidence. A survey of a large series of cases (Putnam, Guroff, Silberman, Barban, & Post, 1986) reported that one or more alternates (but not all) had headaches in 74% of the cases. Differential responses to drugs, alcohol, and food and the presence of allergies in different alters were observed in substantial proportions of cases. Handedness was different among alters in 37% of the cases. These observations are suggestive of differences in biological functioning among alters in many cases, but do not allow us to make predictions about psychophysiological activity.

AUTONOMIC NERVOUS SYSTEM STUDIES

The potential of ANS studies to contribute to an understanding of DID has been only minimally explored. Before getting to the very sparse literature on this topic, it may be worthwhile to present brief reviews of the non-DID literature on ANS activity in relation to normal personality, psychopathology, and emotion to give the reader a feel for the advantages and limitations of such measures for studying this disorder.

Psychophysiology and Normal Personality

Anyone who has done psychophysiological recording from a large series of normal subjects using a variety of ANS measures cannot help but be impressed by the wide range of individual differences that one observes, not only for each measure separately but particularly in the patterning of different measures. It is compelling to believe that such individual differences must have some relationship to the personality of the subjects. Research has shown that these variables are both state- and trait-related. They can be altered predictably by life situations and by laboratory procedures such as task- or threat-induced stressors or long vigilance procedures. There are marked individual differences in both the extent and the patterning of such reactions. Under reasonably similar conditions, they appear to have adequate stability over time. The test-retest reliability of electrodermal activity (EDA), probably the most widely studied of such measures, varies with the parameter measured, the conditions of the study (resting vs. stressed), and the time period, but satisfactory reliabilities (.65 to .9) for major parameters such as skin conductance level (SCL), skin conductance response (SCR) amplitude, and the frequency of spontaneous SCRs for periods of a few weeks to a year have been reported (Boucsein, 1992).

Despite this, finding consistent correlations with personality traits has been difficult. For example, although ANS indices of activation and arousal increase reliably under conditions under which subjects rate themselves as more anxious, subjects within the normal population who rate themselves high on trait-anxiety do not necessarily show greater activation than low trait-anxious persons under either resting or stressful conditions (Myrtek, 1984; Zahn, Nurnberger, Berrettini, & Robinson, 1991). Even when rather consistent and statistically significant relationships have been found between personality and psychophysiology, they typically account for a fairly small (10-20%) proportion of the variance (Gale & Edwards, 1986; Stelmack, 1990) and may be quite specific to a small set of conditions or variables. Thus it is not clear from this literature how much variation in ANS activity one might expect from different alternate personalities.

Psychophysiology and Psychopathology

DID is not a normal condition, so perhaps a more relevant data base is the literature concerning ANS markers of psychopathology. This is particularly so because DID patients frequently present in clinical settings as some other form of serious psychopathology—various major psychoses, obsessive-compulsive disorder, panic disorder, and so on (Putnam, 1989). This is usually attributed to one of the alternate identities who is "out" at the time of these diagnoses. In such cases, where it is possible to elicit an alter with a diagnosable form of psychopathology, it might be possible to test whether this personality resembles non-DID subjects with that diagnosis. This literature (for reviews, see Turpin, 1989; Zahn, 1986) shows, for example, that subjects with major psychoses have been found generally to have absent or attenuated psychophysiological reactions to environmental stimuli. Indices of arousal such as heart rate (HR), SCL, or spontaneous SCR rate may be either higher or lower than normal but only infrequently are at moderate levels. Patients with chronic schizophrenia and retarded depression tend to be unusually low on EDA, while schizophrenics undergoing an acute episode and agitated or anxious depressed subjects may be very high on these indices. Subjects with anxiety disorders, on the other hand, as might be expected, generally show high baseline arousal and frequently exaggerated reactions and slow habituation of ANS responses to innocuous stimuli. Obsessive-compulsive disorder patients tend to be higher than controls on both arousal and reactivity, but not extremely so.

In the present context, it is relevant that some investigators have found extremely high arousal indices and slow habituation in patients with conversion disorder. Lader and Sartorius (1968) reported that patients who had conversion symptoms had even higher indices of arousal than patients with anxiety states. This was replicated by Meares and Horvath (1972) in a subgroup of conversion disorder patients with long-standing difficulties and poor prognosis, but not in patients with a good premorbid adjustment and short-lived conversion symptoms, who were at normal levels. An interesting facet of the Lader and Sartorius (1968) study was that the ANS data correlated with self-rated anxiety, but not with an observer's rating of anxiety in the patient. Thus the patients may have been manifesting classical *la belle indifference*, thought to be characteristic of conversion disorder, behaviorally but not subjectively or autonomically. This illustrates the general point that patients may not always be subjectively and autonomically what they appear to be, which is a good argument for the use of ANS measures in a disorder like DID where intentional and/or unintentional disguising of feelings may be an issue. The data from these studies suggest, contrary to the usual theory of this disorder, that conversion symptoms do not necessarily protect against high anxiety-arousal.

Somewhat in contrast, Lader (1975) reported several instances in which depersonalization and derealization spontaneously occurred in very anxious patients, and this was accompanied by profound decreases in EDA and HR. Lader suggests that the reduction in sensory input occurring in these conditions may be linked to an emergency physiological mechanism that protects the individual from excessive arousal by blocking sensory input.

An implication of this section for DID is that in cases where one or more personalities appear to have a diagnosable disorder, ANS recording may be useful in determining whether the outward appearance of psychopathology is consistent with what is known about psychophysiological activity in similar types of psychopathology occurring in non-DIDs. To the authors' knowledge, no study of DID has used this approach.

Psychophysiology and Emotion

When one reads the literature on DID written by clinicians who have had much experience with this disorder (e.g., Putnam, 1989), it is clear that most patients have alter identities whose function is to express certain emotions that the "main" or "host" identity finds impossible to feel or express. The specific emotions characterized by alters may be fairly similar from one patient to another. Hostile and aggressive alters are quite frequent, as are anxious and fearful ones. Frequently the host, or one or more alters, is withdrawn and/or sad and depressed, while others may be lively, extroverted, and seductive. Therefore, the literature on the psychology of emotion may be highly relevant in deriving hypotheses about specific cases of DID.

There has been considerable controversy about the specificity of psychophysiological patterns in relation to different emotions. From the standpoint of studying DID, it is probably sufficient that there is general agreement that many emotional states can be differentiated from nonemotional states by an arousal dimension. Therefore, in studying the psychophysiology of alter identities, any theory would predict more arousal in those alters who are expressing an active emotion. A relevant question here is whether such patterns can be faked. Ekman and his colleagues (cf., Levenson, Ekman, & Friesen, 1990), who were able to teach subjects to produce facial expressions characteristic of different emotions, found that this tended to produce the appropriate subjective judgments and also to lead to distinctive psychophysiological patterns. Although the efficacy of biofeedback in producing therapeutically meaningful changes in cardiovascular and other systems is controversial, there is no doubt that measurable changes can be produced by these methods (Ray, Raczynski, Rogers, & Kimball, 1979; Hatch, Fisher, & Rugh, 1987). Increases in arousal can also be produced by hypnosis in highly hypnotizable subjects (Maslach, 1979; Zimbardo, La Berge, & Butler, 1993), and patients with DID are thought to be generally easily hypnotized (Putnam, 1989). Although in the above lines of research subjects are taught to change their ANS activity by others, some voluntary control over ANS activity would seem to be possible through self-teaching and self-hypnosis.

ANS Studies of DID

The preceding sections suggest that there are good reasons for expecting at least some alter identities to exhibit distinct psychophysiological patterns compared to others. Most of the few studies that have been done in this area have been single case studies. In an abstract, Bahnson and Smith (1975) reported that they found "consistent differences" between four different identities in EDA, HR, and respiration reactions recorded in a therapeutic setting. They also observed dramatic pauses in respiration of up to 2 minutes with accompanying bradycardia and decreases in skin potential during the switch from one personality to another.

Larmore, Ludwig, and Cain (1977) reported another single session on a single case in which EDA, muscle activity, HR, blood pressure, EEG, and ERPs were recorded from four different alter identities. Possible differences in EDA were obscured by marked habituation effects. HR was very high (98 to 110 beats per minute) for all identities. Rather marked muscle activity and blood pressure elevations were seen in an alter whose function was to "absorb all physical and emotional pain." This identity was also a marked "reducer" on a stimulus-intensity ERP paradigm. Otherwise, the differences were unremarkable. Definite conclusions cannot be drawn without replication in the same subject, but there is an interesting parallel to the case to be reported next.

Brende (1984) recorded bilateral electrodermal responses (EDRs) in three alter identities of a patient in several therapy sessions over the course of more than a year. A protective identity demonstrated reduced EDRs and a victim identity exhibited increased EDRs in each of the four sessions in which they both "appeared," but only in left hand recordings. This replicated finding is conceptually similar to the elevated electromyogram and blood pressure in the victim personality reported by Larmore et al. (1977). In the experience of the senior author of this chapter (T.P.Z.), it is highly unusual to see the marked lateral differences in EDA reported by Brende (1984), even in brain-injured subjects with unilateral damage or in a study of DID to be described below (Putnam, Zahn, & Post, 1990). Unfortunately, Brende's (1984) data were collected using techniques that did not permit evaluation of commonly used EDA variables and seemingly did not permit control over sources of artifacts.

However, the unilateral nature of the changes find a parallel in a clinical report of two cases of DID studied neurologically (Ischlondsky, 1955) in which unilateral changes in sensory function, pupil size, salivation, palmar sweating, and abdominal reflexes occurred in an aggressive hypomanic identity and the opposite laterality was shown by a timid dependent personality. A second case also showed different laterality patterns in two alters, but the relationships between active and passive identity and the specific lateral patterns were opposite of those shown by the first case. This is explained by differences in handedness in the two patients.

The only study of ANS activity on more than one patient (Putnam et al., 1990) was designed to provide a rigorous test of the hypothesis of consistent ANS differences between alternate identities. Nine DID patients and five controls had bilateral EDA, HR, and respiration recorded during a short protocol consisting of a rest period, a series of innocuous tones, and a reaction time task. For the DID subjects, the same three identities were tested during each of four to five sessions, each time in different order. Controls produced "alter" states by simulation and by hypnosis or deep relaxation. Thus each subject constituted a separate experiment for which the data for each individual variable were subjected to an identity × sessions analysis of variance (ANOVA). The number of significant F ratios for identity for each subject was the basic measure of psychophysiological consistency.

Eight of the nine DID subjects showed more significant results at the .01 level than would be expected by chance and all nine showed more results than chance at the .05 level. This demonstrates that alter identities do show reliable differences in ANS activity, interpreted by Putnam et al. (1990) to suggest that "the alter personalities of MPD subjects are highly organized, discrete states of consciousness" (p. 256). Some caution in interpreting the data is indicated by the fact that both hypnotized controls and one of the three nonhypnotized controls showed more psychophysiological differences than expected by chance. However, it was noted that the deviant state for the hypnotized controls was very deep relaxation—low arousal—during the hypnotic trance, whereas the deviant states of the DID subjects were increases in arousal in one or more alters compared to the host personality. It was not attempted to produce increases in arousal hypnotically, but this might be a worthy control in future studies. A separate set of tests of the hypothesis that there were consistent differences among personalities in the laterality of EDA showed that none of the subjects had appreciably more of these than would be expected by chance.

The reliable differences shown among identities in ANS activity do not *prove* that subjects were not voluntarily producing these patterns, since as shown above such processes can be brought under voluntary control. However, only one of three controls who adopted an alternate identity and relaxed without the benefit of hypnosis was able to produce reliable changes in psychophysiology. Therefore, the results seem highly suggestive that the distinctive psychophysiological states reliably accompanying different alter identities are natural accompaniments, or possibly determinants, of the state of consciousness represented by that identity.

Despite the positive results, this study has inherent limitations in design that might have attenuated the differences among identities. Chief among these is the rather artificial nature of the timing; the alter identities were called up for 10- to 15-minute periods for the same, rather boring, testing sequence, a procedure that figures to dampen the emotional responsivity of the alters compared to the natural life situation in which a given alter spontaneously appears to cope with a life event. The short periods during which each alter was out precludes measuring the influences of changes in slow-acting endocrine processes. Some limitations might be overcome by the use of longer periods of recording, possibly using telemetering of psychophysiological data, although here the control over environmental factors would be less than optimal. In addition, Putnam et al. (1990) did not attempt to relate any of the ANS data to particular clinical data on the patients. From the data on personality, psychopathology, and emotion on normal subjects, it should be possible in many patients to make definite predictions about the psychophysiology from clinical knowledge of the alters.

Within-Identity Differences on Other Measures

Visual functions by means of a battery of optical tests were studied in 9 DID patients and 9 controls by Miller (1989) and in 20 patients and 20 controls by Miller, Blackburn, Scholes, White, and Mamalis (1991). In each study, three alter identities were tested in the DID group and three play-acted personalities were tested in the controls on visual acuity, visual field, manifest refraction, and eye muscle balance, and the groups were compared on the pooled within-subject variance. Both studies found that the variability among the alter identities was larger than that for the controls on visual acuity and visual field. Miller (1989), but not Miller et al. (1991), also found a similar difference for eye muscle balance. Pupil size, which is under autonomic control, was assessed only by qualitative ratings, and showed no group difference in variability. The same critical comments could be applied to this study as were applied above to Putnam et al. (1990). It would appear that visual acuity and field could be even more under voluntary control and subject to differences in attention and motivation than ANS activity.

In a case study, Mathew, Jack, and West (1985) measured regional cerebral blood flow (CBF) with the ^{133}Xe inhalation technique in one patient on four occasions. The major finding was that a fearful 7-year-old identity showed a marked elevation in right temporal lobe CBF compared to the host identity, to the integrated identities after therapy, and to normal controls. In contrast, Saxe, Vasile, Hill, Bloomingdale, and van der Kolk (1992), using the higher-resolution single-photon emission method of measuring regional CBF, reported elevated CBF in the left temporal area of all four alter identities of a DID patient relative to whole brain activity and to a control site. Although these studies conflict greatly in their findings, both show changes specific to the temporal lobe. This brings to mind the association between temporal lobe epilepsy and dissociative symptoms, which have been reported in some patients (Mesulam, 1981; Schenk & Bear, 1981) and will be discussed later in this chapter.

Studies of the Amnestic Relationships between Alter Identities

Another use of psychophysiological methods has been to test the claim that certain identities are unaware of the experiences of certain other identities, frequently to convince skeptics of the reality of DID as presented by the patients. We will first review the few studies on this topic and then critique the methodology from the standpoint of what is known about ANS activity and consciousness, with a view to determining what can and cannot be learned from such studies.

The first psychophysiological study of DID was done by the eminent neurologist-psychologist Morton Prince and a psychiatrist colleague (Prince & Peterson, 1908). The objective was not to study DID per se, but to determine if the psychogalvanic reaction (SCR) could be useful to corroborate the existence of coconscious (sometimes called subconscious) ideas. The DID patient was "made use of" as particularly suitable for this purpose. The patient had a "normal" identity and two alters, one of which claimed amnesia for both other identities. The identities could all be hypnotized, and only one of these hypnotic states was coconscious with the other hypnotic states as well as the unhypnotized identities. A number of studies were performed on this patient using electrodermal reactions to words that on the basis of bad dreams or past experiences had conscious emotional significance to some identities (and/or hypnotic states) and not to others.

The data show unequivocally that SCRs occurred to emotionally significant words *even when the personality or state being tested claimed to be unaware of the experience that produced the emotional valence for that word*. The studies seem adequately controlled; the target words were presented unpredictably in a series of control words; the authors were aware of habituation effects and attempted to take them into account when comparing the magnitudes of the responses. However, comparative magnitudes are not critical in interpreting the data; most of the data simply show that obvious SCRs were obtained to significant words whether consciously perceived as significant or not and not to neutral words. One possible problem is that presumably the words were presented verbally by one of the investigators who would be familiar with the details of the case, so that an unintentional change in intonation for the target words could have occurred. However, in another experiment each of the identities was given a "strong tactile stimulus" when in a hypnotic state. In two of these three states the subject was "absolutely anesthetic" (Prince & Peterson, 1908, p. 124) yet marked SCRs were obtained during all three of these hypnotic states, confirming the word studies that SCRs occurred to stimuli whose emotional significance was out of conscious awareness.

Prince and Peterson (1908) interpret the data as supporting their theory of psychical subconscious processes that preserve memories that cannot be recalled consciously but can influence electrodermal activity. It is difficult to know how general the conclusions can be from data obtained on a single case of DID. This patient had one alter identity that, in both her normal and hypnotized state, claimed coconsciousness of the experiences of all other identities when they were out. The authors suggest that the memories from all identities and states were preserved in this alter and that she reacted to them electrodermally even when an amnestic identity or state was being tested. This suggests that different results might be obtained in cases in which there was no completely aware identity to remember everything. An alternative hypothesis, of course, is that this patient was confabulating about her amnesia and also her anesthesia. It is not mentioned how the latter condition was confirmed objectively. It does not seem possible to verify the amnesia independently, so the confabulation hypothesis in this case seems untestable on the basis of the data presented.

There seem to have been no subsequent studies of this kind until the comprehensive case study reported by Ludwig, Brandsma, Wilber, Bendfeldt, and Jameson (1972). This subject had a primary identity who was unaware of the three alters. Each of the alters had "intimate" knowledge of the primary but only "peripheral" knowledge of each other. Like Prince and Peterson (1908), these investigators recorded SCRs to words that had emotional significance to one of the four identities tested but not to the others. Each of the identities, which were elicited by means of hypnosis, was given the same word list consisting of his own emotional words, those of the other identities, and neutral words. The results showed clearly that each of the alters gave large SCRs to their own significant words and to those of the primary personality but much smaller SCRs to each other's significant words. The primary identity was only moderately responsive to his own emotional words, despite being tested first, but much less responsive to the significant words of the alters. Thus, unlike the case reported by Prince and Peterson (1908), the electrodermal responsivity to the emotionally significant words covaried with the reported amnestic relationships among the personalities, even when amnesia was not absolute. In this case none of the identities claimed coconsciousness with all of the others. There does not seem to be a reasonable explanation of these results based on a confabulation hypothesis.

In contrast to these neat results, equivocal results were obtained with an SCR classical conditioning procedure. Here, a different conditioned stimulus (CAS) was used for each identity, the unconditioned stimulus (UCS) being an electric shock. Following the establishment of conditioning for one identity, each of the other identities was called forth in turn via hypnosis and exposed to two CS-only (test) trials. After all the other identities had been tested, the original (conditioned) identity was brought back and given two CS-only trials to index extinction. Cross-conditioning between identities was said to occur when the mean SCR magnitude to the test stimuli was greater than that obtained for that identity on his own extinction trials. The results showed that of the 12 possible instances of cross-conditioning, 9 were positive, and these did not bear any systematic relationship to the amnestic relationships between identities. This leads to a different conclusion than the word study. Although order of testing is an uncontrolled variable here, it is difficult to imagine how this could artifactually produce the results obtained.

Another interesting result of this study was that, unlike the case of Prince and Peterson (1908), one of the alter identities, who was found to be hyperalgesic on a neurological exam, was very difficult to condition and even then gave small conditioned SCRs. This alter did not show generally attenuated EDA, since he was quite responsive on the words procedure.

In another approach to testing carryover effects between different identities, a cross-habituation paradigm was used by Putnam et al. (1990). In this study, it will be recalled, in nine DID cases and five controls the same three identities or states were tested on four or five separate days in a different order in a protocol that included a series of ten tones. In the DID group, since most alter identities claimed to be unaware of the experiences of the others and since novel stimuli elicit larger SCRs, which habituate over trials, it was expected that the DID group would show less carryover of habituation across segments within a session than controls. The results showed that, on the contrary, for both the number and amplitudes of SCRs significant carryover of habituation was shown by the DID group, and this did not differ significantly from the controls. This result leads to the same conclusion of "communication" between identities, at some level, as the conditioning results of Ludwig et al. (1972) but not those of their word-stimulation procedure.

ANS Activity and Awareness

The emotional word, conditioning, and habituation protocols were used in the above studies in part to provide objective tests of the purported amnesia of one identity for another. The implicit assumption is that EDA reflects or is congruent with the conscious experience of the eliciting stimulus or situation. Under this assumption the evidence of cross-communication of EDA between identities who profess to be unaware of each other would be grounds for seriously questioning this claim. We thus need to ask what the evidence is for the assumption of congruence between EDA and cognition.

A strict congruence was questioned in Öhman's (1979) influential model of the orienting response in which the novelty of the stimulus, and thus its probability of eliciting an orienting response, was determined by preattentive processing of the stimulus. This question was addressed in the context of differential electrodermal conditioning by Dawson and Furedy (1976), who concluded from a review of a number of studies that awareness of the stimulus contingencies (i.e., which of two potential CSs may be followed by an aversive UCS) is a necessary but not a sufficient condition for obtaining conditioning. They hypothesized, without presenting data, that awareness of the termination of the CS-UCS relationship is a necessary but ***not a sufficient condition*** for extinction to occur. Evidence for this latter point was provided by Bridger and Mandel's (1965) finding that instructions that shock would no longer be delivered and removal of the shock electrodes was not sufficient to eliminate conditioned SCRs. It has also been shown that conditioned SCRs can be elicited by stimuli that are out of awareness by virtue of being presented in the unattended ear while subjects are attending to the other ear continuously in order to perform a task (Dawson & Schell, 1982). Although this seems to occur unambiguously when the unattended ear is the left ear but not when it is the right ear (Dawson & Schell, 1982), it is a demonstration of a dissociation between awareness and psychophysiological responding nevertheless. Similarly, Öhman and Soares (1993) reported that phobic subjects who had been differentially conditioned using fearful stimuli maintained the conditioning when a backward masking procedure prevented conscious recognition of the stimuli. These lines of research all show that conditioned responses may be "remembered" in a part of the nervous system that is not available to conscious awareness.

Other evidence on this point may be cited. Tranel and Damasio (1985), making use of a finding that pictures of faces of famous persons elicit larger SCRs than pictures of unknown persons (Tranel, Fowles, & Damasio, 1985), found that this was true also in prosopagnosic patients despite a complete lack of conscious recognition of the faces. In a quite different type of study of unexplained arousal (Maslach, 1979; Zimbardo et al., 1993), subjects are hypnotized and given a posthypnotic suggestion that they will feel aroused and that their EDA, HR, and respiration rate will increase. They are further told that they will not be aware of the source of their arousal. Large posthypnotic increases in the physiological variables and in ratings of subjective arousal have been demonstrated under these conditions in highly hypnotizable subjects who profess to be unaware of the source of their arousal. These increases were larger than those shown by low hypnotizable subjects and even larger than those of both groups when they remained aware that the source of their arousal was a hypnotic suggestion. These studies show that increases in autonomic responsivity and base levels may occur without conscious awareness of the conditions producing these phenomena.

An implication of these studies for the investigation of DID is that they suggest that a test of the amnestic relationships between identities based on conditioning one identity and testing others will not necessarily be definitive. One might say that a transfer of conditioning from identity A to identity B is a necessary but not a sufficient condition for disproving the reality of the amnesia of B for A. If A is conditioned to respond to circles and not to squares, and B subsequently shows CRs to circles and not to squares, then a definite conclusion as to whether B's purported amnesia for A's experiences is valid cannot be made. However, if there is no transfer, then the claim of amnesia is strengthened considerably.

In the case study of Ludwig et al. (1972), it will be recalled that whereas there was transfer of conditioning between mutually amnestic identities, there was no transfer of responsivity to stimuli that were uniquely emotional for the separate identities, findings that at face value seem conflicting. The evidence presented above, however, suggests that the amnesia implied by the emotional word results is not necessarily refuted by the conditioning results since the latter are not definitive. But this raises the further question of why the affective reactions to the emotional stimuli were not transferred. The answer here might lie in the complexity of the stimuli. In a review of information processing without awareness, Greenwald (1992) concludes that "unconscious cognition [is] severely limited in its analytic capability" and that it might be limited to the "analysis of partial meanings of single words" (p. 775), although this particular limitation may be dependent on the method of investigation (Kihlstrom, Barnhardt, & Tataryn, 1992). Therefore, it is possible to hypothesize that there may be information transmitted between amnestic identities that is similarly limited in complexity, and that tests using simple sensory stimuli, such as the CSs used by Ludwig et al. (1972) and simple tones used by Putnam et al. (1990) in their habituation paradigm will not be definitive, whereas paradigms using more complex stimuli might actually provide a more conclusive test of amnesia. It will be recalled, however, that Prince and Peterson's (1908) patient did show transfer of electrodermal reactions to emotional word stimuli between her identities, attributed to a coconscious identity who was always present. The methods discussed here would not seem to be able to test this assertion.

CENTRAL NERVOUS SYSTEM MEASURES OF DISSOCIATIVE DISORDERS

Psychophysiological assessment of dissociative disorders offers one way to address the complex relationship between the brain, consciousness, and behavior. However, the scope and limitations of explicit and implicit views on mind-brain relationships have constrained progress in understanding dissociative disorders.

Early models of the brain suggesting telephone switchboardlike processing or even Freud's somewhat linear models involving repression make a physiological understanding of dissociation difficult. Jung with his parallel model of cortical processes offered a more compatible model. More recently, speculation from the neurosciences has emphasized modular processes within the cortex. Neuropsychology has demonstrated such modular relationships for vision, pain, and speech, but these relationships have yet to be articulated in relation to dissociative states and the brain. To this end current models of the mind suggest a promising approach to psychophysiological assessment of dissociation. Neural networks propose parallel information processing by neural control systems (coordinating brain and behavior) with processing distributed among localized and broad brain areas and overlapping control systems. Such models can enhance CNS research on the relationship between the brain and dissociative phenomena. As was true of the ANS studies reported earlier, DID has also been the most widely studied dissociative disorder in terms of the central nervous system.

DID Studies

Electroencephalography (EEG) and evoked potentials (ERP) have been the most widely used CNS measures in the study of dissociation. To date, much of this research has consisted of single-case studies with only a few controlled group studies. Among the first studies to examine EEG differences in different identity states were reports of differences between identities (Thigpen & Cleckley, 1954; Ludwig et al., 1972; Larmore et al., 1977). Larmore et al. (1977) describe a DID patient who presented with suicidal ideation, memory gaps, medical problems, and conversion symptoms. The neurological examination and the EEG were normal. In terms of history, there was possible sexual abuse. Visual evoked response recorded from the vertex (C_z to A_1) revealed significantly larger differences in latency and amplitude of three components (P_1, N_1, and P_2) across identities. The average evoked response types were so distinct for each identity that the authors likened them to having been elicited from four different individuals. The possibility of faking the alternate identities was deemed unlikely based on clinical interviews and psychological testing.

However, Coons, Milstein, and Marley (1982) investigated EEG differences among the alters of two DID patients and a control with less clear-cut findings. The control was a subject's therapist who simulated the client's alters. Significant right central-temporal (C4-T4) amplitude differences were found among the identities of one subject in delta, theta, and beta frequencies. Significant right temporal (T4-T6) differences were found in the second patient in theta and beta bands. The control, however, exhibited the greatest differences, predominantly in the right hemisphere. Although the assessment procedure differed for the subjects, the authors concluded that subject and control EEG differences merely reflected emotional changes not related to dissociation.

Despite these contradictory findings, recent researchers report that there are indeed significant EEG differences among alter identities. Ongoing work reported by Putnam (1991b) obtained significant spontaneous and evoked EEG differences among identities of DID subjects not duplicated by the controls. Braun (1983) hypothesizes that conflicting findings may be accounted for by some "common denominator" responsible for the suppression or expression of the physiological response. He suggests that emotionally cued autohypnotic or state-dependent learning mechanisms may determine the physiological expression of dissociative states.

Of course there exists a number of possible factors that may influence EEG studies. For example, in the study by Coons et al. (1982) the greatest differential EEG responding among alters was by a patient familiar with the clinical laboratory from prior studies. Likewise, differential responding may also be due to relationship variables between the patients and therapists who elicited the alters. Another possibility is the type of EEG measure used, since it has been observed that visual evoked potentials appear to best elicit differences (Putnam, 1991). Lowenstein (1993) also reports that visual evoked potentials "show more significant differences between bona fide DID alters than between simulator controls switching between sham alters" (pp. 598-599). Given the current state of EEG research with dissociative disorders, it is not surprising that this work has been critically described as both "varied and conflicting" (Putnam, 1991a, p. 155) and with "little systematic effort to study the neurophysiologic basis of dissociation" (Spiegel, 1991, p. 442). Further, few of the researchers explain what type of EEG differences should be found. For example, it is unclear if one would expect to find continuous EEG differences during baseline conditions, whereas differences might be possible in response to specific stimuli, e.g., emotional situations, by the different identities of a DID individual.

DID, Epilepsy, and Seizure Disorder

An important neurological question is the relationship between dissociative processes and temporal lobe epilepsy. There are actually two questions being asked. First, can individuals with temporal lobe epilepsy show dissociative symptoms. And second, does the presence of dissociative symptoms suggest temporal lobe epilepsy. The answer to the first question appears to be yes. The appearance of dissociative phenomena among individuals with temporal lobe epilepsy has been well documented (Devinsky, Putnam, Grafman, Bromfield, & Theodore, 1989; Mesulam, 1981; Schenk & Bear, 1981). Schenk and Bear (1981) reported EEG and neuropsychological data for three patients who developed DID "years after the onset of complex partial seizures" (p. 1311). They also summarized data for 40 patients with temporal lobe epilepsy. Repeated EEGs in one subject "... revealed theta slowing over the left temporal region and from the left nasopharyngeal lead" in the first and "... sharp activity from the left nasopharyngeal lead" in the second (p. 1311). Neuropsychological testing indicated left temporal dysfunction in this patient. EEG in two other patients revealed bilateral temporal lobe abnormalities, prominent in the right. Recurrent dissociative episodes were reported for one third of the 40 patients with complex partial seizures and EEG confirmed temporal lobe epilepsy.

Schenk and Bear (1981) described these findings as "highly distinctive" and "... suggestive of a causal relationship between temporal lobe epilepsy and dissociative experiences, including multiple personality disorder" (p. 1314). They hypothesized that the effect of seizure activity on the limbic system resulted in heightened affective associations between the limbic system and sensory association cortex. Patients with temporal lobe epilepsy would be predisposed to dissociate as a response to this intensified affect.

Mesulam (1981) also proposed a similar mechanism for dissociative phenomena in patients with a temporal lobe focus of complex partial seizures. Clearly abnormal EEG with a temporal lobe focus was found in 10 of 12 cases consistent with psychomotor epilepsy. Dissociative experiences consisted of DID-like symptoms in seven patients and the illusion of possession in the others. The dissociative phenomena were hypothesized to be a manifestation of the abnormal temporal lobe activity based on the rich interconnections between the association cortex, temporal lobes, and limbic structures. Such manifestations due to excitation, or kindling, could be interictal as well as ictal in nature.

An interesting ancillary finding was that asymmetrical EEG abnormalities were predominant in the nondominant temporal lobe in five of seven cases. Mesulam (1981) conjectured that dominant (language) hemispheric mental phenomena are less likely to be dissociative, or ego alien, relative to the nondominant hemisphere. Both the limbic system and right hemisphere are central to emotional processing and memory and involved in mental activity outside conscious awareness (Joseph, 1990). The questions raised in these studies regarding the possible roles of the limbic system and the temporal lobes in dissociative phenomena have generated much research.

The answer to the second question—does the presence of dissociative symptoms suggest temporal lobe epilepsy—appears less certain. The idea of a neurological model of DID has been coined the "temporal lobe/complex partial seizure/kindling model" (Putnam, 1991b, p. 498). Kindling is a process studied in animals by which repeated stimuli lead to behavioral sensitization and convulsive responses. A kindling theory of dissociation would suggest that brain structures can be altered with repeated electrical stimulation, which could result from severe stress and trauma (van der Kolk & Greenberg, 1987; Shearer, Peters, Quaytman, & Ogden, 1990; Teicher, Glod, Surrey, & Swett, 1993). However, EEG studies using subjects with diagnosed dissociative disorders have not supported this model in the etiology of dissociative disorders (Putnam, 1991a,b; Spiegel, 1991). One such study reported intensive video-EEG monitoring of patients diagnosed with DID and dissociative screening of 71 patients with generalized seizures (Devinsky et al., 1989). The referring diagnosis of seizure disorder was not confirmed by the EEG for the DID patients. The prevalence of nonepileptiform abnormal EEGs suggested that seizures and neurophysiological abnormalities might contribute to dissociative states. However, the data did not support a seizure disorder model as a primary mechanism for dissociation.

Likewise, Coons, Bowman, and Milstein (1988) conducted an extensive assessment, including EEG and the Dissociative Experiences Scale (DES) (Bernstein and Putnam, 1986) of 50 patients diagnosed with DID. EEGs were collected for 30 patients of which 7 showed abnormalities. Psychogenic seizures were found in 6 patients and organic seizures in 5 subjects. The DES was administered to 13 patients with a group mean score of 41. The authors concluded that the etiology of DID in this sample was not due to temporal lobe or chronic limbic epilepsy. Overall, these studies indicate that neurologically diagnosable epileptic or complex partial seizures do not account for DID.

Spiegel's (1991) assessment of this literature supports the idea of temporal lobe activity in the production of dissociative symptoms, especially since this relationship is found during the interictal period. The work by Mesulam (1981) and Schenk and Bear (1981) did not so much attribute DID per se to limbic and temporal lobe seizure activity, but rather identified the contribution of these areas to the development of dissociative phenomena in certain individuals. Devinsky et al. (1989) found that seizure-disordered patients' DES scores fell between those of normals and DID and suggested the role of seizures in dissociative states for selected individuals (p. 840). Mesulam (1981) also raised the possibility of differential susceptibility to drastic changes in affective, perceptual, and cognitive balance leading to impaired personality integration and dissociative states. Precisely what factors constitute "selected" or "susceptible" is unclear, but trauma is clearly implicated as a factor in dissociation (Chu & Dill, 1990; Loewenstein, 1993; Ludwig, 1983; Teicher et al., 1993; Putnam et al., 1986).

Psychogenic seizures, concomitant dissociative symptoms, and EEG abnormalities are suspected to be related to physical or psychological trauma. However, research in this area is often complicated by the difficulty in distinguishing between organic and psychogenic seizures. Briefly stated, psychogenic seizures are diagnosed when a patient presents clinical seizure disorder activity in the absence of change in preictal, ictal, or postictal EEG (Rachmandi & Schindler, 1993). Chu (1991) further suggests that dissociative symptoms in patients with temporal lobe epilepsy are less severe and that DES scores of patients with organic seizure are generally lower than those with psychogenic seizures.

Rachmandi and Schindler (1993) were able to distinguish two groups of pseudoseizure patients: those that mimic complex partial type seizures and those that mimic grand mal type seizures. Dissociative symptoms were more prominent among pseudoseizure patients with the pseudo-complex partial type. These patients also showed recognizable psychological conflict in their histories before the onset of the symptoms. For example, one pseudoseizure patient reported dissociative experiences following the death of her homosexual son from AIDS, which she was unable to explain to co-workers.

In terms of trauma, studies have reported a high incidence of dissociative symptoms and/or pseudoseizures in individuals with histories of early abuse. In one study, complex partial seizures were frequently found in women with a history of childhood abuse (Shearer et al., 1990). Bowman (1993) assessed 27 diagnosed pseudoseizure patients, 5 with concomitant epilepsy, using video-EEG monitoring. Most of these patients received an unstructured DSM-III-R-based interview and the DES. Trauma was reported by 88% of the subjects (sexual = 77%; physical = 70%). The mean DES score (26.7) was below that typical of DID but comparable to posttraumatic stress disorder subjects. Affective, dissociative, and posttraumatic stress disorders were the most prevalent Axis I disorders. In this study, all abused subjects had a dissociative disorder. Twenty-five percent of the subjects had abnormal EEGs possibly related to physical abuse. Bowman (1993) states, "it appears that abuse experiences operate to produce both dissociative disorders and pseudoseizures" (p. 339).

Overall, current attempts to identify neurophysiological factors in dissociative disorders have not been successful. The convergence of developing psychological models of dissociation, neurological models of trauma, and EEG technology may help clarify this issue. Recently a developmental model proposed repetitive trauma, especially in childhood, as an etiologic factor in dissociative disorders (Loewenstein, 1993). Teicher et al. (1993) developed a self-report measure of symptoms related to temporal lobe epilepsy and limbic system dysfunction, the Limbic System Checklist-33 (LSCL). Based on self-report data of 253 psychiatric outpatients, strong statistical relationships were found between the LSCL-33 and both the DES and self-reports of childhood abuse via the Life Experiences Questionnaire. Although exploratory in nature, this study supported a relationship between EEG abnormalities and trauma, in particular early childhood sexual and physical abuse.

FUTURE DIRECTIONS

In conclusion, this review of the DID literature and related literature in the field of psychophysiology suggests that the phenomena reported in DID patients can, in principle, be accounted for by what is known about the relationships between psychophysiological variables and psychopathology and emotion and awareness of eliciting conditions. However, techniques used for studying this unique disorder have not generally been appropriate and the research has generally not progressed beyond the laboratory curiosity stage. Some variant of the case study method to investigate the relationships between different personalities and psychophysiological patterns would still seem valuable because of the clinical complexity of individual cases, but this should involve repeated testing on individual cases in order to assess the reliability of the differences obtained. Similarly, studies of more than single cases will be necessary in order to determine if any consistencies exist between frequently occurring types of alter personalities and psychophysiological patterns.

Since there is still skepticism about the "reality" of this disorder, it is particularly critical to develop valid techniques to test the limits of communication across identities in relation to their purported degree of awareness of one another. Likewise, the issue of what sorts of information are communicated across amnestic states in DID is an important one, and psychophysiological methods may be very useful tools in addressing the problem. It may be observed that the conditions for the use of the emotional word paradigm—namely, that different personalities have uniquely emotional words—might not be able to be met in every case. However, this paradigm can be seen as a variant of what is known as the Guilty Knowledge Test (Lykken, 1981) used in the detection of deception in criminal cases. In this method, a suspect, while hooked up to a polygraph, is queried about details of the crime that only the criminal could know (i.e., was the victim wearing a red dress?), so that larger reactions to questions about these details compared to equally plausible but untrue alternatives (was the victim wearing slacks?) indicate familiarity and thus guilt. This technique, of course, does not detect lying per se, but simply reflects the obvious and well-established finding that psychophysiological reactions to more significant stimuli are larger than those to less significant ones. This technique might be used to test the psychophysiological "recognition" of the life experiences of one personality by an amnestic alternate personality. Laboratory tests using this approach have been well developed (see Ben-Shakhar & Furedy,

1990) and could be adapted for use with DID patients. In both of these approaches, and also if transfer of conditioning is the method of choice, it would seem important to study the level of complexity of the information whose transmission is to be tested for. In this way one might learn something useful about a given patient, about DID patients in general, and even be informed about unconscious cognition in normal subjects. Much more work along these lines needs to be done before a definitive two-way test of the validity of the existence of mutually amnestic identities on a case-by-case basis can be devised. Similarly, there is much current interest and development in the general problem of unconscious information processing, and as this field develops, a deeper understanding of the processes involved in dissociative disorders will be possible.

REFERENCES

Bahnson, C. B., & Smith, K. (1975). Autonomic changes in a multiple personality patient. *Psychosomatic Medicine, 37*, 85-86.

Ben-Shakhar, G., & Furedy, J. J. (1990). *Theories and applications in the detection of deception*. New York: Springer-Verlag.

Bernstein, E., & Putnam, F. W. (1986). Development, reliability, and validity of a dissociation scale. *Journal of Nervous and Mental Disease, 174*, 727-735.

Bowman, E. (1993). Etiology and clinical course of pseudoseizures: Relationship to trauma, depression, and dissociation. *Psychosomatics, 34*, 333-342.

Boucsein, W. (1992). *Electrodermal activity*. New York: Plenum Press.

Braun, B. G. (1983). Psychophysiologic phenomena in multiple personality and hypnosis. *American Journal of Clinical Hypnosis, 26*, 124-137.

Brende, J. O. (1984). The psychophysiologic manifestations of dissociation. *Psychiatric Clinics of North America, 7*, 41-50.

Bridger, W. H., & Mandel, I. J. (1965). Abolition of the PRE by instruction in GSR conditioning. *Journal of Experimental Psychology, 69*, 476-482.

Chu, J. A. (1991). Letters to the editor. *American Journal of Psychiatry, 148*, 1106-1107.

Chu, J. A., & Dill, D. L. (1990). Dissociative symptoms in relation to childhood physical and sexual abuse. *American Journal of Psychiatry, 147*, 887-892.

Coons, P. M., & Milstein, V. (1992). Psychogenic amnesia: A clinical investigation of 25 cases. *Dissociation, 5*, 73-78.

Coons, P. M., Milstein, V., & Marley, C. (1982). EEG studies of two multiple personalities and a control. *Archives of General Psychiatry, 39*, 823-825.

Coons, P. M., Bowman, E. S., & Milstein, V. (1988). Multiple personality disorder: A clinical investigation of 50 cases. *The Journal of Nervous and Mental Disease, 176*, 519-527.

Dawson, M. E., & Furedy, J. J. (1976). The role of awareness in human differential autonomic classical conditioning: The necessary gate hypothesis. *Psychophysiology, 13*, 50-53.

Dawson, M. E., & Schell, A. M. (1982). Electrodermal responses to attended and nonattended significant stimuli during dichotic listening. *Journal of Experimental Psychology: Human Perception and Performance, 8*, 315-324.

Devinsky, O., Putnam, F., Grofman, J., Bromfield, E., and Theodore, W. H. (1989). Dissociative states and epilepsy. *Neurology, 39*, 835-840.

Gale, A., & Edwards, J. A. (1986). Individual differences. In M. G. H. Coles, E. Donchin, & S. W. Porges (Eds.), *Psychophysiology: Systems, processes, and applications* (pp. 431-507). Amsterdam: Elsevier (North-Holland).

Greenwald, A. G. (1992). New Look 3: Unconscious cognition reclaimed. *American Psychologist, 47*, 766-779.

Hatch, J., Fisher, J., & Rugh, J. (1987). *Biofeedback, studies in clinical efficacy*. New York: Plenum Press.

Ischlondsky, N. D. (1955). The inhibitory process in the cerebro-physiological laboratory and in the clinic. *Journal of Nervous and Mental Disease*, *121*, 5-18.

Joseph, R. (1990). *Neuropsychology, neuropsychiatry, and behavioral neurology*. New York: Plenum Press.

Kihlstrom, J. F., Barnhardt, T. M., & Tataryn, D. J. (1992). The psychological unconscious: Found, lost, and regained. *American Psychologist*, *47*, 788-791.

Lader, M. (1975). *The psychophysiology of mental illness*. London: Routledge & Kegan Paul.

Lader, M. H., & Sartorius, N. (1968). Anxiety in patients with hysterical conversion symptoms. *Journal of Neurology, Neurosurgery and Psychiatry*, *31*, 490-497.

Larmore, A. M. (1983). The psychobiological functions of dissociation. *American Journal of Clinical Hypnosis*, *26*, 93-99.

Larmore, K., Ludwig, A. M., & Cain, R. L. (1977). Multiple personality: An objective case study. *British Journal of Psychiatry*, *131*, 35-40.

Levenson, R. W., Ekman, P., & Friesen, W. V. (1990). Voluntary facial action generates emotion-specific autonomic nervous system activity. *Psychophysiology*, *27*, 363-384.

Loewenstein, R. J. (1993). Dissociation, development, and the psychobiology of trauma. *Journal of the American Academy of Psychoanalysis*, *21*, 581-603.

Ludwig, A. M. (1983). The psychobiological functions of dissociation. *American Journal of Clinical Hypnosis*, *26*, 93-99.

Ludwig, A. M., Brandsma, J. M., Wilbur, C. R., Bendfeldt, F., & Jameson, D. (1972). The objective study of a multiple personality: Or are four heads better than one? *Archives of General Psychiatry*, *26*, 298-310.

Lykken, D. T. (1981). *A tremor in the blood: Uses and abuses of the lie detector*. New York: McGraw-Hill.

Maslach, C. (1979). Negative emotional biasing of unexplained arousal. *Journal of Personality and Social Psychology*, *37*, 953-969.

Mathew, R. J., Jack, R. A., & West, W. S. (1985). Regional cerebral blood flow in a patient with multiple personality. *American Journal of Psychiatry*, *142*, 504-505.

Meares, R., & Horvath, T. (1972). "Acute" and "chronic" hysteria. *British Journal of Psychiatry*, *121*, 653-657.

Mesulam, M. M. (1981). Dissociative states with abnormal temporal lobe EEG: Multiple personality and the illusion of possession. *Archives of Neurology*, *38*, 176-181.

Miller, S. D. (1989). Optical differences in cases of multiple personality disorder. *Journal of Nervous and Mental Disease*, *177*, 480-486.

Miller, S. D., Blackburn, T., Scholes, G., White, G., & Mamalis, N. (1991). Optical differences in cases of multiple personality disorder: A second look. *Journal of Nervous and Mental Disease*, *179*, 132-135.

Myrtek, M. (1984). *Constitutional psychophysiology*. New York: Academic Press.

Öhman, A. (1979). The orienting response, attention, and learning: An information processing perspective. In H. D. Kimmel, E. H. van Olst, & J. F. Orlebeke (Eds.), *The orienting reflex in humans* (pp. 443-472). Hillsdale, NJ: Erlbaum.

Öhman, A., & Soares, J. J. F. (1993). On the autonomic nature of phobic fear: Conditioned electrodermal responses to masked fear-relevant stimuli. *Journal of Abnormal Psychology*, *102*, 121-132.

Prince, M., & Peterson, F. (1908). Experiments in psycho-galvanic reactions from co-conscious (subconscious) ideas in a case of multiple personality. *Journal of Abnormal Psychology*, *3*, 114-131.

Putnam, F. W. (1989). *Diagnosis and treatment of multiple personality disorder*. New York: Guilford Press.

Putnam, F. W. (1991a). Dissociative phenomena. In A. Tasman and S. Goldfinger (Eds.), *Annual Review of Psychiatry* (pp. 145-160). Washington, DC: American Psychiatric Press.

Putnam, F. W. (1991b). Recent research on multiple personality disorder. *Psychiatric Clinics of North America*, *14*(3), 489-502.

Putnam, F. W., Guroff, J. J., Silberman, E. K., Barban, L., & Post, R. M. (1986). The clinical phenomenology of multiple personality disorder: Review of 100 recent cases. *Journal of Clinical Psychiatry*, *47*, 285-293.

Putnam, F. W., Zahn, T. P., & Post, R. M. (1990). Differential autonomic nervous system activity in multiple personality disorder. *Psychiatric Research*, *31*, 251-260.

Rachmandi, D., & Schindler, B. (1993). Evaluation of pseudoseizures: A psychiatric perspective. *Psychomatics, 34*, 70-79.

Ray, W. J., Raczynski, J. M., Rogers, T., & Kimball, W. H. (1979). *Evaluation of clinical biofeedback*. New York: Plenum Press.

Saxe, G. N., Vasile, R. G., Hill, T. C., Bloomingdale, K., & van der Kolk, B. A. (1992). Brief reports: SPECT imaging and multiple personality disorder. *The Journal of Nervous and Mental Disease, 180*, 662-663.

Schenk, L., & Bear, D. (1981). Multiple personality and related dissociative phenomena in patients with temporal lobe epilepsy. *American Journal of Psychiatry, 60*, 1311-1316.

Shearer, S. L., Peters, C. P., Quaytman, S. S., & Ogden, R. L. (1990). Frequency and correlates of childhood sexual and physical abuse histories in adult female borderline inpatients. *American Journal of Psychiatry, 147*, 214-216.

Spiegel, D. (1991). Neurophysiological correlates of hypnosis and dissociation. *The Journal of Neuropsychiatry and Clinical Neurosciences, 3*, 440-445.

Stelmack, R. (1990). Biological bases of extraversion: Psychophysiological evidence. *Journal of Personality, 58*, 293-311.

Teicher, M. H., Glod, C. A., Surrey, J. S., & Swett, C. (1993). Early childhood abuse and limbic system ratings in adult psychiatric outpatients. *Journal of Neuropsychiatry and Clinical Neurosciences, 5*, 301-306.

Thigpen, C. H., & Cleckly, H. (1954). A case of multiple personality. *Journal of Abnormal and Social Psychology, 49*, 135-151.

Tranel, D., & Damasio, A. R. (1985). Knowledge without awareness: An autonomic index of facial recognition by prosopagnosics. *Science, 228*, 1453-1454.

Tranel, D. T., Fowles, D. C., & Damasio, A. R. (1985). Electrodermal discrimination of familiar and unfamiliar faces: A methodology. *Psychophysiology, 22*, 403-408.

Turpin, G. (1989). *Handbook of clinical psychophysiology*. New York: Wiley.

van der Kolk, B. A., & Greenberg, M. S. (1987). The psychobiology of trauma response: Hyperarousal, constriction, and addiction to traumatic reexposure. In B. A. van der Kolk (Ed.), *Psychological trauma* (pp. 63-87). Washington, DC: American Psychiatric Press.

Zahn, T. P. (1986). Psychophysiological approaches to psychopathology. In M. G. H. Coles, E. Donchin, & S. W. Porges (Eds.), *Psychophysiology: Systems, processes, and applications* (pp. 508-610). New York: Guilford Press.

Zahn, T. P., Nurnberger, Jr., J. I., Berrettini, W. H., & Robinson, Jr., T. N. (1991). Concordance between anxiety and autonomic nervous system activity in subjects at genetic risk for affective disorder. *Psychiatry Research, 36*, 99-110.

Zimbardo, P. G., LaBerge, S., & Butler, L. D. (1993). Psychophysiological consequences of unexplained arousal: A posthypnotic suggestion paradigm. *Journal of Abnormal Psychology, 102*, 466-473.

V
DIAGNOSTIC CLASSIFICATIONS

This section is the most formal part of the handbook. The first three chapters describe the specified dissociative disorders of DSM-IV. These include depersonalization and derealization, amnesia, fugue, and dissociative identity disorders. DSM-III included depersonalization and derealization without depersonalization as a separate disorder, whereas in DSM-IV, only depersonalization is listed as a dissociative disorder.

In Chapter 14, Coons point out that although the term was coined in the 1890s, little is known about the epidemiology of depersonalization. What we do know suggests that depersonalization is experienced by 80 percent of the general population at some time and in some form and is the third most common psychiatric symptom after depression and anxiety.

In Chapter 15, a discussion of amnesia and fugue is presented by Loewenstein. This chapter updates earlier reviews by Loewenstein, demonstrating the strong connection between trauma and amnesia. In terms of this discussion, three other issues are raised: (1) the historical relationship and differentiation between the construct of repression and that of dissociation; (2) the nature of amnesia described by each; and (3) the influence the legal system has had on the question of trauma, amnesia, and one's ability to remember past events. Finally, the question of treatment is considered.

Dissociative identity disorder is the focus of Chapter 16. In this chapter, Kluft traces the history of the disorder, including the first modern description of it in 1787. Although until recently considered a North American disorder, Kluft reports its existence throughout the world. As can be seen from this chapter, great debate has been associated with the disorder even within the DSM-IV committee itself. The question of what exactly is an "identity" is one of the core issues of this chapter. Phenomenologically, DID patients display approximately two to four identities at the time of diagnosis, although more identities may become apparent within treatment. An important discussion in this chapter describes the course of the disorder as well as the models that have been presented to understand DID.

During the past few years there has been a proposal to consider a new DSM diagnosis, that of acute stress disorder. Chapter 17, by Koopman and her colleagues, raises this possibility and begins to forge the links between dissociative disorders and stress and trauma situations such as PTSD. Using the 1991 Oakland/Berkeley fire, these researchers present empirical support to suggest that a combination of dissociative and anxiety symptoms is able to define a diagnosis of acute stress disorder.

The final chapter of the section continues the discussion of posttraumatic response and describes the final dissociative disorder—dissociative disorder, not otherwise specified. How to treat dissociation and abuse is a question that has been discussed throughout the book and will continue in great detail in the next section. In this chapter, Chu revisits the complex question of how to treat abuse and describes the early, middle, and later stages of treatment.

14

Depersonalization and Derealization

Philip M. Coons

> How did I know that someday—at college, in Europe, somewhere, anywhere—the bell jar, with its stifling distortions, wouldn't descend again?
>
> Sylvia Plath,
> *The Bell Jar* (1971)

INTRODUCTION

Depersonalization and derealization consist of altered perceptions about the self and the environment. Both of these phenomena may be symptoms of a wide variety of psychiatric disorders with exceedingly diverse etiologies. Both depersonalization and derealization without depersonalization are listed as dissociative disorders in the *Diagnostic and Statistical Manual of Mental Disorders*, 4th Edition (DSM-IV) (American Psychiatric Association, 1994).

The scientific literature on both depersonalization and derealization is sparse. Only 150 references are listed for both in an extensive bibliography on the dissociative disorders (Goettman, Greaves, & Coons, 1990); of these, only eight refer to derealization, and only two of these refer to derealization unaccompanied by depersonalization.

Philip M. Coons • Department of Psychiatry, Indiana University School of Medicine, Indianapolis, Indiana 46202.

Handbook of Dissociation: Theoretical, Empirical, and Clinical Perspectives, edited by Larry K. Michelson and William J. Ray. Plenum Press, New York, 1996.

Very little is known about the epidemiology of either depersonalization disorder or derealization without depersonalization. In fact, the existence of the psychiatric syndrome of derealization without depersonalization has recently been challenged (Coons, 1992). Until the recent introduction of selective serotonin reuptake inhibitors, the treatment of depersonalization disorder was problematic.

The remainder of this chapter will outline what is known about depersonalization and derealization. Sections include history, definition, diagnosis, differential diagnosis, epidemiology, etiology, a typical case example, treatment, and future directions in research.

HISTORY

Dugas (1898) coined the term "depersonalization" to describe what Krishaber had called "cerebro-cardiac neurosis" in 1872 (as quoted in Ackner, 1954a). Although numerous nineteenth- and early twentieth-century luminaries in psychology, such as Ribot, Oestrreich, Bleuler, Freud, Breuer, and Janet, briefly commented on the phenomenon or listed it as a symptom in numerous celebrated cases, scant attention was paid to it in textbooks until depersonalization was officially listed as a psychiatric diagnosis in the DSM-III (American Psychiatric Association, 1980).

There were about a dozen papers on depersonalization between 1930 and 1960. Mayer-Gross (1935) began the modern study of depersonalization with his classical paper in which he described 26 patients. Eleven years later, Shorvon (1946) described an additional 66 patients, and 8 years after that, Ackner (1954a,b) published a series with an additional 54 patients.

Since the 1960s, there has been a steady increase of papers on depersonalization to about 30–40 per decade. In the early 1960s, interest in depersonalization was ignited by Roth's (1959) description of the phobic anxiety-depersonalization syndrome. Interest in depersonalization was kept alive by Sedman's writings in the 1960s (Sedman, 1966; Sedman & Kenna, 1963; Sedman & Reed, 1963), studies by Noyes and his colleagues on trauma and depersonalization in the 1970s (Noyes, Hoenk, Kupperman, & Slymen, 1977; Noyes & Kletti, 1977), and Torch's (1987) writings on the psychotherapy of depersonalization in the 1980s. Most recently, Hollander and his colleagues (1990) have discussed the psychopharmacological treatment of depersonalization.

DEFINITIONS

Depersonalization

The DSM-IV (American Psychiatric Association, 1994, p. 488) defines the symptom of depersonalization as "a feeling of detachment or estrangement from one's self." Depersonalization can take many forms, but only two are listed in the DSM-IV: "a feeling of detachment from one's self" combined with "a sensation of being an outside observer of one's body" (i.e., an out-of-body experience) and "feeling like an automaton or as if he or she is living in a dream" (p. 488). Other examples of depersonalization include emotional numbing, feeling as if one were in a fog or a trance, not recognizing one's self in the mirror, feeling that behavior or emotions are not under the individual's control, or feeling like body parts are detached, absent, unreal, foreign, or changed in size (Simeon & Hollander, 1993; Steinberg, 1993a).

Jacobs and Bovasso (1992) described five subtypes of depersonalization. The first is inauthenticity, or the loss of genuineness in the experience of the self. The second, derealization will be described below. The third is self-objectification, wherein "the world is experienced as rapidly changing and basic distinctions between the self and objects are blurred" (p. 353). The fourth, or self-negation, "involves denial that one is performing certain actions or that one is witnessing certain events occurring in the environment" (pp. 353-354). In the fifth type of depersonalization, body detachment, there is the perception that the body is distorted or detached.

Derealization

The DSM-III-R (American Psychiatric Association, 1987, p. 269) defines derealization as "an alteration in the perception of one's surroundings so that a sense of the reality of the external world is lost." Examples of derealization include feeling that people or surroundings are fading away or disappearing or are unreal or foreign and the inability to recognize friends, relatives, or familiar surroundings (Steinberg, 1993a,b).

Derealization is distinct from depersonalization. It is not a subset of depersonalization as some investigators have asserted (American Psychiatric Association, 1984; Jacobs & Bovasso, 1992; Sedman, 1966). An easy way to make the distinction between depersonalization and derealization is to remember that depersonalization is a feeling of estrangement from or unreality about the self while derealization is a feeling of estrangement from or unreality about the environment (i.e., anything outside the self).

TRANSIENT DEPERSONALIZATION

Depersonalization may occur either as a transient symptom or a syndrome called depersonalization disorder in which the depersonalization is severe, prolonged, and causes marked distress. As symptoms, depersonalization and derealization may occur in a variety of psychiatric and medical disorders (American Psychiatric Association, 1987, 1994). These symptoms are usually transient, but occasionally prolonged depersonalization is seen with marijuana abuse.

Depersonalization and derealization are common symptoms in dissociative disorders (American Psychiatric Association, 1987, 1994; Steinberg, 1993a,b), including multiple personality disorder (MPD) (Coons, Bowman, & Milstein, 1988; Loewenstein, 1991; Putnam, Guroff, Silberman, Barban, & Post, 1986), psychogenic amnesia (Coons & Milstein, 1992), and dissociative disorder not otherwise specified

(DDNOS) (Coons, 1992). They also occur in schizophrenia (Bezzubova, 1991; Rosenfeld, 1947; Sedman & Kenna, 1963); severe affective disorders including major depression with psychosis and bipolar disorder (Blank, 1954; Sedman & Reed, 1963; Tucker, Harrow, & Quinlan, 1973); agoraphobia and panic disorder (Ambrosino, 1973; Cassano et al., 1989; Hollander, Fairbanks, Decaria, & Liebowitz, 1989; James, 1961; Roth, 1959; Shraberg, 1977); posttraumatic stress disorder; personality disorders including schizotypal personality disorder, borderline personality disorder (Hunter, 1966), and obsessive personality disorder (Sedman & Reed, 1963; Torch, 1978); substance abuse disorders involving marijuana (Mathew, Wilson, Humphreys, Lowe, & Weithe, 1993; Melges, Tinklenberg, Hollister, & Gillespie, 1970; Moran, 1986; Szymanski, 1981), and the hallucinogens LSD (Waltzer, 1972) and mescaline (Guttmann & Maclay, 1936). A wide range of conditions associated with medical or neurological illnesses (Pies, 1991) and the use of a wide variety of different medications can also result in depersonalization and derealization.

Medical or neurological conditions associated with depersonalization include hyperventilation, migraine headaches, temporal lobe epilepsy (Devinsky, Feldmann, Burrowes, & Bromfield, 1989; Harper & Roth, 1962; Kenna & Sedman, 1965), temporal lobe tumors, fever, delirium, cerebral trauma (Grigsby, 1986), cerebrovascular disease, encephalitis, Alzheimer's disease, Huntington's chorea, Menière's disease (Grigsby & Johnson, 1989), hypopituitarism, and hypothyroidism. Medications that cause depersonalization include fluoxetine (Black & Wojeieszek, 1991), fluphenazine (Musa & Wollcott, 1982) and other antipsychotics, anxiolytics, and indomethacin (Schwartz & Moura, 1983). Withdrawal from nitrazepam has also been implicated (Terao, Yoshimura, Terao, & Abe, 1992).

Other nonmedical causes of depersonalization include brainwashing, hypnosis (Wineberg & Straker, 1973), sleep deprivation, sensory deprivation (Horowitz, 1964; Reed & Sedman, 1964), exposure to trauma (Noyes et al., 1977; Noyes & Kletti, 1977; Rosen, 1955), and relaxation-meditation (Castillo, 1990; Edinger, 1985; Fewtrell, 1984; Kennedy, 1976; Signer, 1988).

DEPERSONALIZATION DISORDER

Diagnostic Criteria

The diagnostic criteria of depersonalization disorder from DSM-IV include the following:

> A. Persistent or recurrent experiences of feeling detached from, and as if one is an outside observer of, one's mental processes or body (i.e., feeling like one is in a dream).
> B. During the depersonalization experience reality testing remains intact.
> C. The depersonalization causes clinically significant distress or impairment in social, occupational, or other important areas of functioning.
> D. The depersonalization experience does not occur exclusively during the course of another mental disorder, such as Schizophrenia, Panic Disorder, Acute Stress Disorder, or another Dissociative Disorder, and is not due to the

physiological effects of a substance (e.g., a drug of abuse, a medication) or a general medical condition (e.g., temporal lobe epilepsy) (American Psychiatric Association, 1994, p. 490).

Epidemiology

Depersonalization disorder has been reported in adolescents (Meares & Grose, 1978; McKellar, 1978; Meyer, 1961; Munich, 1977; Shimizu & Sakamoto, 1986). Only two cases have been reported in children, one, a 10-year-old boy who felt "as if I were always dreaming, and I didn't realize whether I was there or not" (Shimizu & Sakamoto, 1986, p. 605), and the other, an 8-year-old boy, who felt "... a ghost feeling... like a machine ..." (Fast & Chethik, 1976, p. 484). Interestingly, a number of patients with depersonalization disorder retrospectively report the onset of their symptoms in childhood anywhere from age 5 to 10 years (Fast & Chethik, 1976). Transient depersonalization has been reported in both children (Elliott, Rosenberg, & Wagner, 1984) and adolescents (Dixon, 1963). The rarity of depersonalization and derealization in children may reflect the child's inability to abstract and adequately describe these phenomena.

In Mayer-Gross's (1936) pioneering study of 26 patients, there were six patients between the ages of 30-39 years, two under 20, and the rest in their 20s. Their mean age was 26.6 years. Not all of his patients may have had genuine depersonalization disorder since there were 12 with depression and 6 with schizophrenia. In Shorvon's (1946) series, the ages of onset ranged from 10 to 38 years with a mean age of onset of about 24 years. Chee and Wong (1990) found an age range of 25 to 47 years with a mean age of onset of 25 years.

Although depersonalization is an apparently uncommon psychiatric disorder whose precise incidence in the general population is unknown, the symptom of depersonalization is the third most common psychiatric symptom after depression and anxiety (Cattel, 1966). Depersonalization is experienced by 80% of the general population (Probst & Jansen, 1991), 12-56% of normal college students (Dixon, 1963; Myers & Grant, 1970; Trueman, 1984), and 40-80% of psychiatric inpatients (Brauer, Harrow, & Tucker, 1970; Noyes et al., 1977). Differences in reporting statistics on depersonalization probably are caused by the use of different phraseology in asking about depersonalization.

The sex ratio of those experiencing depersonalization and depersonalization disorder is unclear. Of supposedly genuine cases of depersonalization, Mayer-Gross (1935) reported a 4:1 female:male ratio, and Shorvon (1946) reported a 2:1 ratio. Of normal college students experiencing the symptom of depersonalization, Roberts (1960) reported a 3:1 ratio in favor of females, Myers and Grant (1970) reported a 2:1 preponderance of men over women, and Dixon (1963), Sedman (1966), and Chee and Wong (1990) found no sex differences. Of the available reports of depersonalization in adolescents, there is an approximately equal sex incidence. Unfortunately, no large studies of patients with depersonalization disorder have occurred since the introduction of the DSM-III, so the precise sex ratio of patients with genuine depersonalization disorder is unknown.

There is no known familial pattern of inheritance for those with depersonalization disorder.

Clinical Features

Depersonalization disorder is characterized by persistent or recurrent symptoms of depersonalization severe enough to cause marked distress. It may not be diagnosed in the presence of schizophrenia, panic disorder, multiple personality disorder, or temporal lobe epilepsy. Symptoms of depersonalization are egodystonic and reality testing remains intact. Although the onset of depersonalization disorder is described as usually rapid, Shorvon (1946) and Chee and Wong (1990) found that onset was gradual in 3 and 33% of cases, respectively.

Derealization symptoms are frequently present with depersonalization disorder. Depression and obsessionality also frequently accompany depersonalization disorder (Grinberg, 1966; Lower, 1972; Sedman & Reed, 1963; Torch, 1978). Suicide attempts are frequent with depersonalization, and occasionally the feelings of depersonalization may be so distressing that successful suicide results (Chee & Wong, 1990). Somatization, dizziness, time distortion, and a fear of becoming insane may also be present (American Psychiatric Association, 1987). The course of depersonalization disorder is chronic. Remissions and exacerbations are common.

Individual case reports reveal that predisposing factors may include military combat, severe auto accidents, or some other type of trauma. However, most of the older case reports do not list trauma as a precipitating factor.

Diagnostic Aids

Two recent diagnostic instruments, the Dissociative Experiences Scale (DES) (Bernstein & Putnam, 1986) and the Structured Clinical Interview for Dissociative Disorders (SCID-D) (Steinberg, 1993a,b), have been introduced for use in diagnosing dissociative disorders.

The DES is a self-administered screening instrument for dissociative symptoms. It consists of 28 questions about depersonalization, derealization, amnesia, fugue, absorption phenomena, identity confusion, and identity alteration. It requires about 10–15 minutes to complete. Scores range from 1–100. Scores above 20 are thought to be significant. Normals score in the 0–10 range, with adolescents somewhat higher. Scores are elevated for those with schizophrenia, borderline personality disorder, dissociative disorders, and posttraumatic stress disorder.

The SCID-D is a structured clinical interview used for assessing dissociative symptoms. There are sections on amnesia, depersonalization, derealization, identity confusion, and identity alteration as well as a number of follow-up sections if the examiner desires more information. The interview takes anywhere from 30–90 minutes to administer depending on the degree of dissociative psychopathology present. After the interview is complete, the examiner rates each of the five dissociative areas on a 1- to 4-point scale. A decision is then made on a dissociative disorder diagnosis based on DSM-IV criteria.

Differential Diagnosis

The differential diagnosis of depersonalization is vast. All of the transient causes of depersonalization must be considered. A thorough review of psychiatric, medical, family, and social histories is indicated in addition to a physical and neurological examination and mental status examination. Screening blood chemistries such as a complete blood count, thyroid function tests, chemical profiles, and drug screens may be indicated. Electroencephalogram (EEG), computerized tomography, or magnetic resonance imaging of the head may be indicated as well.

The diagnosis of depersonalization disorder may not be made if the depersonalization is not persistent and does not cause marked distress. Since depersonalization disorder is quite uncommon, perhaps even rare, the clinician will usually find that depersonalization symptoms are due to some other more common disorder such as schizophrenia, panic disorder, multiple personality disorder, dissociative disorder not otherwise specified, borderline personality disorder, temporal lobe epilepsy, or medication use.

Etiology

The etiology for depersonalization symptoms is as diverse as the differential diagnosis. It is likely that depersonalization symptoms are produced by a bewildering variety of biological and psychological agents acting through one final common pathway: the temporal lobe and its various cerebral connections. More specifically, serotonergic dysfunction has recently been suggested as the mechanism whereby depersonalization symptoms are produced (Hollander et al., 1989, 1990).

The psychological triggering of depersonalization is well known. Emotional stress caused by a variety of situations, including natural or human-made traumas, overwhelming anxiety, conflict over anger or sexuality, or painful depressive affect, causes patients with severe dissociative disorders such as multiple personality disorder and dissociative disorder not otherwise specified to depersonalize and even to dissociate into another ego state. Such a switch has been postulated to serve as a defensive function to protect the individual against overwhelming anxiety regarding conflicted impulses or painful affects (Feigenbaum, 1937; Kluft, 1987). Based on improvement of depersonalization in patients treated with clozapine and benzodiazepines, Nuller (1982) has postulated that depersonalization occurs as a result of anxiety.

Treatment

The treatment for dissociative symptoms caused by the various psychiatric and medical conditions listed previously should follow the treatment of the underlying psychiatric or medical condition. Fortunately, depersonalization symptoms due to these other conditions are usually transient, so no specific treatment is necessary other than education, support, and reassurance that the depersonalization will resolve.

The treatment of depersonalization disorder is more problematic. A wide variety of treatments have been attempted, including electroconvulsive therapy, anxiolytics, antipsychotics, stimulants, antidepressants, behavior therapy, and psychotherapy. Because depersonalization disorder is so rare and may spontaneously remit, no large controlled studies of therapeutic efficacy have been undertaken.

Behavior Therapy. Blue (1979) described a 50-year-old woman with depersonalization who successfully responded to a six-session behavioral approach consisting of establishing a baseline on dissociative symptoms through record keeping, then recording feelings and activities associated with the depersonalization, and finally involving behavioral prescriptions including paradoxical intention. Previous treatment with 16 different psychopharmacological agents had been unsuccessful.

Sookman and Solyom (1978) reported two cases. A 48-year-old woman experienced marked reduction of depersonalization through 20 1-hour flooding treatments using fantasy over a 10-week period. A 40-year-old man was treated with a combination of flooding through fantasy and paradoxical intention. His depersonalization symptoms diminished enough for him to return to work, but did not entirely disappear.

Psychopharmacotherapy. *Traditional Antipsychotics, Electroconvulsive Therapy, and Other Heroic Treatments.* Electroconvulsive therapy, traditional antipsychotic medication, and other heroic treatments including continuous narcosis, leucotomy, vasodilators, metrazol, and insulin therapy have all been tried for depersonalization disorder. None have shown much benefit, except in rare single cases (Shorvon, 1946).

Stimulants. Both Shorvon (1946) and Davison (1964) found that a one-time intravenous administration of amphetamines could abort an episode of depersonalization disorder. About half of the patients treated with amphetamines responded to such treatment, and, of these, about half quickly relapsed.

Antidepressants. Tricyclic antidepressants are sometimes useful in the treatment of depersonalization disorder (Walsh, 1975; Noyes, Kupperman, & Olson, 1987). More recently treatment with selective serotonin reuptake inhibitors has shown surprising success. Hollander et al. (1990) treated eight patients (five women and two men) with fluoxetine; six were very much improved and two were only minimally improved on dosages of fluoxetine that ranged from 5 to 80 mg/day.

Anxiolytics and Novel Antipsychotic Medication. Nuller (1982) reported on 57 patients with depersonalization, some of whom had an accompanying depression and some who had previously experienced acute psychosis. Forty-two were treated with phenazepam and 15 were treated with clozapine. Of those treated with clozapine, nine improved and six did not. Of those treated with phenazepam, 13 experienced complete remission, 21 experienced moderate to considerable improvement, and 8 experienced no improvement.

Recently Stein and Uhde (1989) reported a single patient, a 28-year-old woman, who responded in a single-blind study to the benzodiazepine anticonvulsant clonazepam, but not to carbamazepine. Symptoms worsened upon challenge with caffeine while on both study drugs but not while on placebo.

Psychotherapy. Torch (1987) is a strong advocate of the use of psychodynamic psychotherapy. Torch believes that depersonalization develops as a result of low self-esteem and a compensatory hypervigilance in which the self serves as an obsessional focus. The individual's low self-esteem is postulated to result from an inability to satisfy excessive parental demands. Successful treatment occurs by attending to self-esteem issues and transferring responsibility for feelings of worthlessness back to the parents.

Schilder (1939) perhaps best summarizes the effects of dynamic psychotherapy. He indicates that psychotherapy for depersonalization is difficult, time-consuming, does not always work, and does not prevent relapses. However, the positive results achieved in some patients make this a technique that should be considered when supportive and psychopharmacological measures fail.

Treatment Precautions. Numerous clinicians have observed that depersonalization disorder is frequently accompanied by depression and suicidal behavior. Chee and Wong (1990) found that almost half of the nine patients in their series had attempted suicide and one was eventually successful. Although the precise suicide rate in depersonalization disorder is unknown, the clinician should be aware that suicide attempts are extremely common and should take appropriate precautions.

Because depersonalization disorder has frequently been associated with affective disorders, the clinician should be especially cautious when treating with stimulants or antidepressants. Liebowitz, McGrath, and Bush (1980) described two young women, a 21-year-old and a 17-year-old, who became floridly psychotic after being treated with moderately large doses of dextroamphetamine (30 mg/day) and amitriptyline (300 mg/day), respectively. Therefore, the clinician should be careful to inquire about previous symptoms of mania and take a family history for recurrent affective disorder prior to instituting treatment with stimulants or antidepressants.

Case Example

Mrs. Brown (not her real name) was a 32-year-old married woman with a 10th grade education. She was born in the South of Catholic parentage. In her early 20s she had a 3- or 4-month period of depersonalization that was not severe enough to require treatment. She had been steadily employed as a factory worker since age 19. She married at age 20 a truck driver who was employed intermittently and abused alcohol. They had two children. The marital relationship was distant, partly due to Mrs. Brown's aloof, almost schizoid personality traits.

Her current psychiatric illness had no obvious precipitant and was characterized by a 6-month period of pervasive and unremitting depersonalization. Associated symptoms included headaches and dizziness. She described her symptoms as follows:

> I don't feel anything. It's like I'm on a bad, bad trip and everything feels like a shell with nothing inside. Only my mind is working. My face and arms feel numb. It's like being in a fog. I feel empty.

Although she denied feeling depressed, she experienced fatigue, guilt, low self-esteem, and had tried to kill herself in order to escape the extremely dysphoric feelings of depersonalization. Family history revealed that both her father and brother had suffered from depression and that her brother and both grandfathers were alcoholic.

Prior to her referral to a tertiary-care, psychiatric research hospital, her psychiatrists had tried a wide array of therapeutic doses of antipsychotics, anxiolytics, and antidepressants including haloperidol, thioridazine, nortriptyline, amitriptyline, doxepin, maprotiline, trazodone, lithium carbonate, carbamazepine, bupropion, diazepam, and lorazepam. A course of ten bilateral electroconvulsive treatments had also been unsuccessful.

Her referring psychiatrists were not really sure of her diagnosis; by the time she reached our hospital, she had been labeled with major depression, agoraphobia, bipolar disorder, dysthymic disorder, schizotypal personality, borderline personality, passive aggressive personality, and dependent personality. She had never shown any psychotic symptoms nor symptoms of panic disorder.

Further history revealed that she had been sexually abused by an uncle for about a year when she was 7 or 8. From age 16 to 18 she had abused alcohol and marijuana. During a move 5 years previously she had experienced a 2-day period of amnesia. However, she had never experienced fugues or symptoms characteristic of multiple personality.

Her physical and neurological examinations were normal, as were an EEG and computed tomography scan. Laboratory tests including a urinalysis, complete blood count, a chemistry-24 panel, thyroid function tests, and VDRL were all negative. Psychological testing revealed an IQ of 110, absence of a thought disorder and signs of organicity, but evidence of a mixed personality disorder.

She was placed on desipramine, involved in ward activities and occupational therapy, and treated with supportive psychotherapy. A brief try of marital therapy was ineffective due to her husband's refusal to return after three sessions. Her symptoms gradually remitted and she was discharged to return to her factory job. No follow-up information is available.

Comment. This case represents a classic case of depersonalization disorder. Her first episode began in her early 20s. Depersonalization symptoms were pervasive, unremitting, and caused marked distress and dysfunction. Associated symptoms included headaches, dizziness, and depression. Onset of her illness was rapid with a gradual remission. No evidence was present for the diagnoses of schizophrenia, panic disorder, multiple personality, epilepsy, or other forms of organic brain dysfunction. It is not known whether her remission was simply spontaneous or was brought about by treatment with desipramine.

DEREALIZATION UNACCOMPANIED BY DEPERSONALIZATION

In the seven available case reports or studies on derealization (Fast & Chethik, 1976; Fleiss, Gurland, & Goldberg, 1975; Krizek, 1989; Rosen, 1955; Sarlin, 1962; Selinsky, 1968; Trueman, 1984), six patients, three adults and three children, are mentioned. Analysis of these case reports reveals that five experienced both derealization and depersonalization and one experienced depersonalization only.

Trueman's study (1984) was a nonclinical sample of 221 undergraduate students: 30.1% reported depersonalization experiences, 28.3% reported derealization experiences, and 25.7% reported both types of experiences. Trueman reported that some students experienced derealization without depersonalization, but failed to indicate the exact number or percentage.

Shorvon (1946) and Chee and Wong (1990) reported on 61 and 9 cases of depersonalization disorder, respectively. Although both found that derealization could accompany depersonalization, neither found any cases of derealization unaccompanied by depersonalization. In the extensive review of the literature contained in this chapter, no cases of the disorder of derealization unaccompanied by depersonalization were found.

Neither the DSM-III-R nor the DSM-IV (American Psychiatric Association, 1987, 1994) contain a clinical description of derealization unaccompanied by depersonalization, although both list this disorder under dissociative disorder not otherwise specified. Because of the lack of a single case of derealization unaccompanied by depersonalization, it would be best to list this as a possible syndrome in an appendix (Coons, 1992).

FUTURE DIRECTIONS IN RESEARCH

Because of the rarity of depersonalization disorder, little is known about etiology, prevalence, predisposing factors, associated features, familial patterns, and treatment. No studies of depersonalization disorder have been published that have used either the DES as a screening instrument or the SCID-D as a study instrument. The question of whether derealization unaccompanied by depersonalization exists remains unanswered. Regarding treatment, there is one open study using serotonin reuptake blockers to treat depersonalization disorder in eight patients (Hollander et al., 1990) and one single-blind study using clonazepam in a single patient.

Because of the rarity of depersonalization disorder, the only conceivable way to study it is with a multicenter approach whereby patients with depersonalization are recruited from dissociative disorder programs throughout North America. Clear inclusion and exclusion criteria should be established, especially for derealization. Patients enrolled in such studies should have a thorough psychiatric evaluation including psychiatric, medical, family, and social histories, mental status examination, physical and neurological examinations, blood chemistries, EEGs, neuropsychological testing, administration of the DES, SCID-D, and other structured interviews such as the SCID. The treatment of these patients would then be followed prospectively in a double-blind fashion.

REFERENCES

Ackner, B. (1954a). Depersonalization: I. Aetiology and phenomenology. *Journal of Mental Science, 100*, 838–853.

Ackner, B. (1954b). Depersonalization: II. Clinical syndromes. *Journal of Mental Science, 100*, 854–872.

Ambrosino, S. V. (1973). Phobic anxiety-depersonalization syndrome. *New York State Journal of Medicine, 73*, 419–425.

American Psychiatric Association (1980). *Diagnostic and statistical manual of mental disorders* (3rd ed.). Washington, DC: Author.

American Psychiatric Association (1984). *The American Psychiatric Association's psychiatric glossary* (p. 28). Washington, DC: Author.

American Psychiatric Association (1987). *Diagnostic and statistical manual of mental disorders* (3rd ed., rev., pp. 269-277). Washington, DC: Author.

American Psychiatric Association (1994). *Diagnostic and statistical manual of mental disorders* (4th ed.). Washington, DC: Author.

Bernstein, E. M., & Putnam, F. W. (1986). Development, reliability, and validity of a dissociation scale. *Journal of Nervous and Mental Disease, 174*, 727-735.

Bezzubova, E. B. (1991). Clinical characteristics of vital depersonalization in schizophrenia. *Zh Nevropatol Psikhiatr, 91*(7), 83-86.

Black, D. W., & Wojeieszek, J. (1991). Depersonalization syndrome induced by fluoxetine. *Psychosomatics, 32*, 468-469.

Blank, H. R. (1954). Depression, hypomania, and depersonalization. *Psychoanalytic Quarterly, 23*, 20-37.

Blue, F. R. (1979). Use of directive therapy in the treatment of depersonalization neurosis. *Psychological Reports, 49*, 904-906.

Brauer, R., Harrow, M., & Tucker, G. J. (1970). Depersonalization phenomena in psychiatric patients. *British Journal of Psychiatry, 117*, 509-515.

Cassano, G. B., Petracca, A., Perugi, G., Toni, C., Tundo, A., & Roth, M. (1989). Derealization and panic attacks: A clinical evaluation on 150 patients with panic disorder/agoraphobia. *Comprehensive Psychiatry, 30*, 5-12.

Castillo, R. J. (1990). Depersonalization and meditation. *Psychiatry, 53*, 158-168.

Cattel, J. P. (1966). Depersonalization phenomena. In S. Arieti (Ed.), *American handbook of psychiatry* (pp. 766-799). New York: Basic Books.

Chee, K. T., & Wong, K. E. (1990). Depersonalization syndrome—A report of 9 cases. *Singapore Medical Journal, 31*, 331-334.

Coons, P. M. (1992). Dissociative disorder not otherwise specified: A clinical investigation of 50 cases with suggestions for typology and treatment. *Dissociation, 4*, 187-195.

Coons, P. M., & Milstein, V. (1992). Psychogenic amnesia: A clinical investigation of 25 cases. *Dissociation, 4*, 73-79.

Coons, P. M., Bowman, E. S., & Milstein, V. (1988). Multiple personality disorder: A clinical investigation of 50 cases. *Journal of Nervous and Mental Disease, 176*, 519-527.

Davison, K. (1964). Episodic depersonalization: Observations on 7 patients. *British Journal of Psychiatry, 110*, 505-513.

Devinsky, O., Feldmann, O., Burrowes, K., & Bromfield, E. (1989). Autoscopic phenomena with seizures. *Archives of Neurology, 46*, 1080-1088.

Dixon, J. C. (1963). Depersonalization phenomena in a sample population of college students. *British Journal of Psychiatry, 109*, 371-375.

Dugas, L. (1898). Un cas de depersonalization [A case of depersonalization]. *Revue Philosophique, 45*, 500-507.

Edinger, J. D. (1985). Relaxation and depersonalization. *British Journal of Psychiatry, 146*, 103.

Elliott, G. C., Rosenberg, M., & Wagner, M. (1984). Transient depersonalization in youth. *Social Psychology Quarterly, 47*, 115-129.

Fast, I., & Chethik, M. (1976). Aspects of depersonalization-derealization in the experience of children. *International Review of Psychoanalysis, 3*, 483-490.

Feigenbaum, D. (1937). Depersonalization as a defense mechanism. *Psychoanalytic Quarterly, 6*, 4-11.

Fewtrell, W. D. (1984). Relaxation and depersonalization (letter to the editor). *British Journal of Psychiatry, 145*, 217.

Fleiss, J. L., Gurland, B. L., & Goldberg, K. (1975). Independence of depersonalization-derealization. *Journal of Consulting and Clinical Psychology, 43*, 110-111.

Goettman, C., Greaves, G. B., & Coons, P. M. (1990). *Multiple personality and dissociation, 1791-1990; A complete bibliography*. Norcross, GA: Ken Burrow & Co.

Grigsby, J. P. (1986). Depersonalization following minor closed head injury. *International Journal of Neuropsychology, 8*, 65-68.

Grigsby, J. P., & Johnson, C. L. (1989). Depersonalization, vertigo, and Menière's disease *Psychological Reports, 64*, 527-534.

Grinberg, L. (1966). The relationship between obsessive mechanism and a state of self disturbance: Depersonalization. *International Journal of Psychoanalysis, 46,* 177-183.

Guttmann, E., & Maclay, W. S. (1936). Mescalin and depersonalization: Therapeutic experiments. *Journal of Neurology and Psychopathology, 41,* 193-212.

Harper, M., & Roth, M. (1962). Temporal lobe epilepsy and the phobic-anxiety-depersonalization syndrome: Part I: A comparative study. *Comprehensive Psychiatry, 3,* 129-151.

Hollander, E., Fairbanks, J., Decaria, C., & Liebowitz, M. R. (1989). Pharmacological dissection of panic and depersonalization (letter to the editor). *American Journal of Psychiatry, 146,* 402.

Hollander, E., Liebowitz, M. R., Decaria, C., Fairbanks, J., Fallon, B., & Klein, D. F. (1990). Treatment of depersonalization with serotonin reuptake blockers. *Journal of Clinical Psychopharmacology, 10,* 200-203.

Horowitz, M. J. (1964). Depersonalization in spacemen and submariners. *Military Medicine,* 1058-1060.

Hunter, R. C. A. (1966). The analysis of episodes of depersonalization in a borderline patient. *International Journal of Psychoanalysis, 47,* 32-41.

Jacobs, J. R., & Bovasso, G. B. (1992). Toward the clarification of the construct of depersonalization and its association with affective and cognitive symptoms. *Journal of Personality Assessment, 59,* 352-365.

James, I. P. (1961). The phobic-anxiety-depersonalization syndrome. *American Journal of Psychiatry, 118,* 163-164.

Kenna, J. C., & Sedman, G. (1965). Depersonalization in temporal lobe epilepsy and the organic psychoses. *British Journal of Psychiatry, 111,* 293-299.

Kennedy, R. B. (1976). Self-induced depersonalization syndrome. *American Journal of Psychiatry, 133,* 1321-1328.

Kluft, R. P. (1987). An update on multiple personality disorder. *Hospital and Community Psychiatry, 38,* 363-373.

Krizek, G. O. (1989). Derealization without depersonalization. *American Journal of Psychiatry, 146,* 1360-1361.

Liebowitz, M. R., McGrath, P. J., & Bush, S. C. (1980). Mania occurring during treatment for depersonalization: A report of two cases. *Journal of Clinical Psychiatry, 41,* 33-34.

Loewenstein, R. J. (1991). An office mental status examination for complex chronic dissociative symptoms and multiple personality disorder. *Psychiatric Clinics of North America, 14,* 567-604.

Lower, R. B. (1972). Affect changes in depersonalization. *Psychoanalytic Review, 59,* 565-577.

Mathew, R. J., Wilson, W. H., Humphreys, D., Lowe, J. V., & Weithe, K. E. (1993). Depersonalization after marijuana smoking. *Biological Psychiatry, 33,* 431-441.

Mayer-Gross, W. (1936). On depersonalization. *British Journal of Medical Psychology, 15,* 103-126.

McKellar, A. (1978). Depersonalization in a 16-year-old boy. *Southern Medical Journal, 71,* 1580-1581.

Meares, R., & Grose, D. (1978). On depersonalization in adolescence: A consideration from the viewpoints of habituation and "identity." *British Journal of Medical Psychology, 51,* 335-342.

Melges, F. T., Tinklenberg, J. R., Hollister, L. E., & Gillespie, H. K. (1970). Temporal disintegration and depersonalization during marijuana intoxication. *Archives of General Psychiatry, 23,* 204-210.

Meyer, J. E. (1961). Depersonalization in adolescence. *Psychiatry, 24,* 537-560.

Moran, C. (1986). Depersonalization and agoraphobia associated with marijuana use. *British Journal of Medical Psychology, 59,* 187-196.

Munich, R. L. (1977). Depersonalization in a female adolescent. *International Journal of Psychoanalytic Psychotherapy, 6,* 187-197.

Musa, M. N., & Wollcott, P. (1982). Depersonalization as a side effect of fluphenazine. *Research Communications in Psychology, Psychiatry, and Behavior, 7,* 477-480.

Myers, D. H., & Grant, G. (1970). A study of depersonalization in students. *British Journal of Psychiatry, 121,* 59-65.

Noyes, R., & Kletti, R. (1977). Depersonalization in response to life-threatening danger. *Comprehensive Psychiatry, 18,* 375-384.

Noyes, R., Hoenk, P. R., Kupperman, B. A., & Slymen, D. J. (1977). Depersonalization in accident victims and psychiatric patients. *Journal of Nervous and Mental Disease, 164,* 401-407.

Noyes, R., Kuperman, S., & Olson, S. B. (1987). Desipramine: A possible treatment for depersonalization disorder. *Canadian Journal of Psychiatry, 32,* 782-784.

Nuller, Y. L. (1982). Depersonalization—symptoms, meaning, therapy. *Acta Psychiatrica Scandinavica, 66*, 451-458.

Pies, R. (1991). Depersonalization's many faces. *Psychiatric Times, 8*(4), 27-28.

Plath, S. (1971). *The bell jar*. New York: Harper & Row.

Probst, P., & Jansen, J. (1991). [Depersonalization and deja vu experiences: Prevalences in nonclinical samples]. *Zeitschrift fur Klinische Psychologie, Psychopathologie, und Psychotherapie, 39*, 357-368.

Putnam, F. W., Guroff, J. J., Silberman, E. K., Barban, L., & Post, R. M. (1986). The clinical phenomenology of multiple personality disorder: A review of 100 recent cases. *Journal of Clinical Psychiatry, 45*, 172-175.

Reed, G. F., & Sedman, G. (1964). Personality and depersonalization under sensory deprivation conditions. *Perceptual and Motor Skills, 18*, 659-660.

Roberts, W. W. (1960). Normal and abnormal depersonalization. *Journal of Mental Science, 106*, 478-493.

Rosen, V. H. (1955). The reconstruction of a childhood event in a case of derealization. *Journal of the American Psychoanalytic Association, 3*, 211-221.

Rosenfeld, H. (1947). Analysis of a schizophrenic state with depersonalization. *International Journal of Psychoanalysis, 28*, 130-139.

Roth, M. (1959). The phobic anxiety-depersonalization syndrome. *Proceedings of the Royal Society of Medicine, 52*, 587-595.

Sarlin, C. N. (1962). Depersonalization and derealization. *Journal of the American Psychoanalytic Association, 10*, 784-804.

Schilder, P. (1939). The treatment of depersonalization. *Bulletin of the New York Academy of Medicine, 15*, 258-272.

Schwartz, J. I., & Moura, R. J. (1983). Severe depersonalization and anxiety associated with indomethacin. *Southern Medical Journal, 76*, 679-680.

Sedman, G. (1966). Depersonalization in a group of normal subjects. *British Journal of Psychiatry, 112*, 907-912.

Sedman, G., & Kenna, J. C. (1963). Depersonalization and mood changes in schizophrenia. *British Journal of Psychiatry, 109*, 669-673.

Sedman, G., & Reed, G. F. (1963). Depersonalization phenomena in obsessional personalities and in depression. *British Journal of Psychiatry, 109*, 376-379.

Selinsky, H. (1968). Depersonalization and derealization: Present day concepts. *Journal of the Hillside State Hospital, 17*, 306-316.

Shimizu, M., & Sakamoto, S. (1986). Depersonalization in early adolescence. *Japanese Journal of Psychiatry, 40*, 603-608.

Shorvon, H. J. (1946). The depersonalization syndrome. *Proceedings of the Royal Society of Medicine, 39*, 779-785.

Shraberg, D. (1977). The phobic anxiety-depersonalization syndrome. *Psychiatric Opinion, 14*(6), 35-40.

Signer, S. F. (1988). Mystical-ecstatic and trance states. *British Journal of Psychiatry, 152*, 296-297.

Simeon, D., & Hollander, E. (1993). Depersonalization disorder. *Psychiatric Annals, 23*, 382-388.

Sookman, D., & Solyom, L. (1978). Severe depersonalization treated by behavior therapy. *American Journal of Psychiatry, 135*, 1543-1545.

Stein, M. B., & Uhde, T. W. (1989). Depersonalization disorder: Effects of caffeine and response to pharmacotherapy. *Biological Psychiatry, 26*, 315-320.

Steinberg, M. (1993a). *Interviewer's guide to the Structured Clinical Interview for DSM-IV Dissociative Disorders*. Washington, DC: American Psychiatric Press.

Steinberg, M. (1993b). *Structured Clinical Interview for DSM-IV Dissociative Disorders*. Washington, DC: American Psychiatric Press.

Szymanski, H. V. (1981). Prolonged depersonalization after marijuana use. *American Journal of Psychiatry, 138*, 231-233.

Terao, T., Yoshimura, R., Terao, M., & Abe, K. (1992). Depersonalization following nitrazepam withdrawal. *Biological Psychiatry, 31*, 212-213.

Torch, E. M. (1978). Review of the relationship between obsession and depersonalization. *Acta Psychiatrica Scandinavica, 58*, 191-198.

Torch, E. M. (1987). The psychotherapeutic treatment of depersonalization disorder. *Hillside Journal of Clinical Psychiatry, 9,* 133–143.

Trueman, D. (1984). Anxiety and depersonalization and derealization experiences. *Psychological Reports, 54,* 91–96.

Tucker, G. J., Harrow, M., & Quinlan, D. (1973). Depersonalization, dysphoria, and thought disturbance. *American Journal of Psychiatry, 130,* 702–706.

Walsh, R. N. (1975). Depersonalization: Definition and treatment (letter to the editor). *American Journal of Psychiatry, 132,* 873.

Waltzer, H. (1972). Depersonalization and the use of LSD: A psychoanalytic study. *American Journal of Psychoanalysis, 32,* 45–52.

Wineberg, E. N., & Straker, N. (1973). An episode of acute, self-limiting depersonalization following a first session of hypnosis. *American Journal of Psychiatry, 130,* 98–100.

15

Dissociative Amnesia and Dissociative Fugue

Richard J. Loewenstein

INTRODUCTION

In 1991, I published a comprehensive review of dissociative (psychogenic) amnesia (DA) and dissociative (psychogenic) fugue (DF), emphasizing the relationship of these conditions to overwhelming psychological trauma (Loewenstein, 1991b). Since the publication of that work, several additional studies have been published that support the basic premises of that review. Also, I have recently published a review of treatment of dissociative amnesia and dissociative fugue (Loewenstein, 1995). In addition, however, there has arisen an intense public and academic controversy about the validity of delayed adult recollections of childhood traumatic events, particularly those for which the individual reports prior amnesia (Loftus, 1993). Further, critics of the dissociation-trauma model have questioned whether DA for traumatic events *ever* occurs (McHugh, 1992). This chapter will update the prior review. In addition, however, I will discuss issues in the current controversy over the delayed recollection of traumatic events.

DIAGNOSTIC CRITERIA

The diagnostic criteria for DA and DF are found in Table 1 (American Psychiatric Association, 1994). The *Diagnostic and Statistical Manual of Mental Dis-*

Richard J. Loewenstein • Dissociative Disorders Service Line, Sheppard Pratt Health Systems, Baltimore, Maryland 21285; and Department of Psychiatry and Behavioral Sciences, University of Maryland School of Medicine, Baltimore, Maryland 21201.

Handbook of Dissociation: Theoretical, Empirical, and Clinical Perspectives, edited by Larry K. Michelson and William J. Ray. Plenum Press, New York, 1996.

Table 1. DSM-IV Diagnostic Criteria for Dissociative Amnesia and Dissociative Fugue[a]

Diagnostic criteria for dissociative amnesia

1. The predominant disturbance is one or more episodes of inability to recall important personal information, usually of a traumatic or stressful nature, that is too extensive to be explained by ordinary forgetfulness.
2. The disturbance does not occur exclusively during the course of dissociative identity disorder, dissociative fugue, posttraumatic stress disorder, acute stress disorder, or somatization disorder and is not due to the direct physiological effects of a substance (e.g., a drug of abuse, a medication) or a neurological or other general medical condition (e.g., amnestic disorder due to head trauma).
3. The symptoms cause clinically significant distress or impairment in social, occupational, or other important areas of functioning.

Diagnostic criteria for dissociative fugue

1. The predominant disturbance is sudden, unexpected travel away from home or one's customary place of work, with inability to recall one's past.
2. Confusion about personal identity or assumption of a new identity (partial or complete).
3. The disturbance does not occur exclusively during the course of dissociative identity disorder and is not due to the direct physiological effects of a substance (e.g., a drug of abuse, a medication) or a general medical condition (e.g., temporal lobe epilepsy).
4. The symptoms cause clinically significant distress or impairment in social, occupational, or other important areas of functioning.

[a]Reprinted by permission from the *Diagnostic and Statistical Manual of Mental Disorders*, Fourth Edition. Copyright 1994 American Psychiatric Association.

orders, 4th edition (DSM-IV) criteria for DA differ from DSM-III-R version in that the relationship to traumatic events and the chronic, recurrent nature of this condition are emphasized. The DSM-IV criteria for DF have changed in that they no longer require the development of an alternate identity at the termination of a fugue. Both of these changes were supported by recent systematic data or by expert consensus (Coons & Millstein, 1992).

Types of Dissociative Amnesia

Following Janet (1901), the discussion of amnesia in DSM-IV describes several types of disturbance in the process of recall in this disorder. These are listed in Table 2. In addition, there are a variety of disturbances in the content of memory that characterize DA, most of which are forms of localized, selective, and systematized amnesias (Table 3). Many patients meeting diagnostic criteria for DA or DF will actually have a far more extensive history of amnesia, fugue states, and dissociation if closely questioned in the clinical interview or followed up longitudinally. Thus, they will ultimately meet diagnostic criteria for dissociative identity disorder (DID) or dissociative disorder not otherwise specified (DDNOS) (Kluft, 1985). For a full discussion of the clinical presentation of individuals with complex forms of dissociative amnesia, see Loewenstein (1991a,b).

Table 2. Types of Dissociative Amnesia[a]

Type
Localized amnesia: Inability to recall events related to a circumscribed period of time.
Selective amnesia: Ability to remember some, but not all, of the events during a circumscribed period of time.
Generalized amnesia: Failure to recall the whole life of the patient.
Continuous amnesia: Failure to recall successive events as they occur.
Systematized amnesia: Amnesia for certain categories of memory such as all memories relating to one's family or a particular person.

[a]From American Psychiatric Association (1994), Janet (1901), Loewenstein (1991b).

EPIDEMIOLOGY

Using the Dissociative Experiences Scale (DES) (Bernstein & Putnam, 1986) and the Dissociative Disorders Interview Schedule (DDIS) (Ross, Heber, Norton, & Anderson, 1989), Ross (Ross, 1991; Ross, Joshi, & Currie, 1990) examined 1005 randomly selected people from the general population of Winnipeg, Canada. In this study, the lifetime prevalence of a dissociative disorder was 11.2%. When over half the respondents were followed up with the DDIS, about 7.0% of the sample met criteria for DA. Less than 1% met criteria for DF. DA was the most prevalent dissociative disorder in this sample. DF may be more common in settings where war or other forms of extreme social dislocation and violence are common (Putnam, 1985).

These data need replication in studies using more rigorous methodology (e.g., clinical examination of respondents given the DDIS, etc.). However, the prevalence figure for all dissociative disorders is comparable to those reported in population studies of individuals with posttraumatic stress disorder (Breslau, Davis, Andreski, & Peterson, 1991; Davidson & Fairbank, 1993). Similarly, these prevalence figures are consistent with the known high rates of childhood abuse and trauma as well as adult traumatic experiences found in the general population (Breslau et al., 1991; Davidson & Fairbank, 1993; Russell, 1983; van der Kolk, 1993).

CONCEPTUAL ISSUES

Amnesia is a specific disorder and also a diagnostic criterion for other disorders. In DSM-IV (American Psychiatric Association, 1994), amnesia is one of the diagnostic criteria for DID (previously known as multiple personality disorder, or MPD). It is also among the DSM-IV diagnostic criteria for somatization disorder (SD), acute stress disorder (ASD), and posttraumatic stress disorder (PTSD). This reflects the repeatedly described correlation of dissociative symptoms with traumatic or overwhelmingly stressful life events. Also, somatization and somatoform disorders are common in individuals with a history of trauma and vice versa (Bowman, 1993; Loewenstein, 1990; Saxe et al., 1994; Walker, Katon, Harrop-Griffiths, Holm, & Russo, 1988; Walker, Katon, Neraas, Jemelka, & Massoth, 1992;

Table 3. The Experience of Dissociative Amnesia[a]

Blackouts or "time loss"
Reports of disremembered behavior
Appearance of unexplained possessions
Perplexing changes in relationships
Fragmentary recall of the life history
Evidence of unusual fluctuations in skills, habits, tastes, knowledge
Fuguelike episodes
Recurrent, unexplained mistaken identity experiences
Brief, trancelike amnesia episodes ("microamnesias")

[a]From Loewenstein (1991a,b), Steinberg (1993, 1994).

Walker, Katon, Roy-Byrne, Jemelka, & Russo, 1993). In fact, the DSM-IV work group for PTSD proposed a superordinate category of the Trauma Disorders to encompass dissociative disorders, PTSD, ASD, and possibly conversion disorder and somatization disorder, among others (Davidson & Foa, 1993). This recommendation was not followed in DSM-IV, however.

Finally, amnesia can be viewed not only from a descriptive and psychopathological perspective, but from an adaptational, process-oriented, psychodynamic one as well. Here amnesia can be understood as a concomittant of cognitive and/or intrapsychic defensive processes (Schacter & Kihlstrom, 1989; Spiegel, 1986). Discussions of amnesia and fugue in the literature often blur the distinction between these ways of understanding dissociative phenomena, leading to imprecision in conceptualization.

As discussed in my earlier writing (Loewenstein, 1991b, p. 47),

> [Dissociative] amnesia can be more broadly defined as a reversible memory impairment in which groups of memories for personal experience that would ordinarily be available for recall to the conscious mind cannot be retrieved or retained in a verbal form (or, if temporarily retrieved, cannot be wholly retained in consciousness). In addition, this disturbance is not primarily due to destruction or dysfunction of neurobiological systems and structures that subserve memory or language but rather to a potentially reversible form of psychological inhibition.
>
> The diagnosis of dissociative amnesia generally connotes four factors. First, relatively large groups of memories and associated affects have become unavailable, not just single memories, feelings, or thoughts (Rapaport, 1942). Second, the unavailable memories usually relate to day-to-day information that would ordinarily be a more-or-less routine part of conscious awareness: who I am, what I did, where I went, whom I spoke to, what was said, what I thought and felt at the time, etc. (Hilgard, 1986). Third, the ability to remember new factual information, general cognitive functioning, and language capacity are usually intact (Lishman, 1987). Finally, the dissociated memories frequently indirectly reveal their presence in more-or-less disguised form such as intrusive visual images, somatoform symptoms, nightmares, conversion symptoms, and behavioral reenactments.

There are different schools of thought within academic psychology that debate the existence of "repression" (Singer, 1990). In general, representatives of these schools do not differentiate dissociation from repression in a systematic fashion (e.g., Loftus, 1993). This leads to additional conceptual confusion in evaluating and comparing various theoretical and experimental works in the debate about the existence of amnesia for traumatic circumstances.

Several of the recent popular and academic critics of the notion of posttraumatic dissociative amnesia for traumatic experiences neglect almost entirely the extensive literature on dissociation and trauma, particularly that on combat veterans, and rely instead on their own caricature of the psychoanalytic notion of repression to support their views (see, for example, Ofshe & Watters, 1994). This is an odd circumstance indeed, since many trauma researchers, theorists, and clinicians have found most psychoanalytic writings problematic, if not frankly inhospitable, to trauma-based notions of human psychopathology (van der Kolk & Herman, 1986). Also, as is well known, since Freud's famed renunciation of the "seduction theory," with few exceptions (e.g., Niederland, 1968, and other writers on the Nazi Holocaust), until very recently psychoanalytic thinkers have mostly neglected and/or discounted the importance of extreme psychological trauma in the genesis of human psychopathology, particularly urging doubt on the veracity of claims of paternal incest during childhood (Freud, 1933; Herman, 1981).

Conversely, psychoanalytic writers have found it difficult to fit dissociative disorders into their theoretical system (Kluft, 1992). For example, Fisher (1945), writing about patients with dissociative fugues associated with wartime and civilian violence, stated that: "It does not seem ... that fugues are explicable in terms of the usual concepts of ego and superego; that ultimately other operational principles will have to be utilized when we know more about fugues" (p. 466).

The distinction between repression and dissociation made in this chapter follows Rapaport (1942). In repression, single or a few memories, perceptions, affects, thoughts, and/or images are thought to become relatively unavailable to full conscious awareness. These are usually thought to have important but conflictual meaning for the person. Repression can relate to many aspects of human experience and does not require extreme psychological trauma for its occurrence. Also, in repression, large blocks of ordinary experience do not become unavailable to consciousness along with the psychologically conflictual information. Repressed information does not manifest itself indirectly in nightmares, flashbacks, intrusive images, somatoform symptoms, and so forth, although psychoanalytic formulations note the importance of slips of the tongue, dreams, and somatoform symptoms in understanding material that has been subject to repression (Freud, 1910).

Individuals with DA are often subjectively aware of distinct gaps or deletions in their sense of continuous memory for life history and/or experience (Steinberg, 1994). This is unusual in individuals conceptualized as manifesting repression, since the material that is unavailable is so limited in scope.

Finally, animal research on stress and studies of combat veterans and former prisoners of war and childhood abuse survivors. suggest that DA due to trauma may have a distinct psychobiology involving alterations in the neuronal structure of the hippocampus, possibly due to excess glucocorticoid production (Bremner, Davis, Southwick, Krystal, & Charney, 1993a; Bremner et al., 1995; Stein et al., 1995). Recent studies using the MRI have found decreased size of hippocampus in brains of combat veterans with PTSD and survivors of childhood sexual abuse (Bremner et al., 1995; Stein et al., 1995). In the Stein et al. study, these alterations were significantly correlated with measures of dissociation and the numbing/avoidance symptom cluster of the DSM-IV diagnostic criteria for PTSD. The latter include dissociative amnesia as a criterion symptom (American Psychiatric Association, 1994). Since the hippocampus is a structure vital to encoding of memory, it has been suggested that these findings support a biological basis for memory difficulties in individuals who have experienced extreme psychological trauma (see, for example, Bremner et al., 1993c). Alterations in the amygdala and other neuronal systems such as the benzodiazepine-GABA system, the opiate system, the norepinephrine system, and the corticotropin-releasing factor-hypothalamic-pituitary-adrenal axis system due to extreme stress may all contribute to the manifold memory disturbances caused by trauma (Bremner et al., 1993a). In addition to DA, these include depersonalization and the various forms of posttraumatic hyperamnesia including reexperiencing (flashback) episodes, intrusive posttraumatic imagery, and eidetic engraving of the traumatic experience in memory (Terr, 1988, 1991; van der Kolk, 1986).

In this chapter, dissociation is conceptualized as a basic part of the psychobiology of the human trauma response: a protective activation of altered states of consciousness in reaction to overwhelming psychological trauma (Putnam, 1991). Memories and affects relating to the trauma are encoded during these altered states. When the person returns to the baseline state, there is relatively less access to the dissociated information, leading, in many cases, to DA for at least some part of the traumatic events. However, the dissociated memories and affects can manifest themselves in nonverbal forms: posttraumatic nightmares, reenactments, intrusive imagery, and somatoform symptoms. Not only is there amnesia for the trauma, but the person frequently has dissociated that certain basic assumptions about the self, relationships, other people, and the nature of the world have been altered by the trauma (Classen, Koopman, & Spiegel, 1993; Spiegel, 1988a, 1991a; Terr, 1991).

This view of dissociation is supported by virtually every systematic study and comprehensive review of dissociation and dissociative disorders in the literature: overtly traumatic circumstances such as wartime trauma, concentration camp experiences, subjection to torture or atrocities, natural disasters, family violence, child abuse, and other forms of civilian violence are extraordinarily prevalent in the histories of dissociating patients or in the immediate circumstances in which dissociative symptoms are manifested (Cardena & Spiegel, 1993; Jaffe, 1968; Loewenstein, 1991b; Niederland, 1968; Putnam, 1985; Spiegel, 1991a). The converse is true as well. Studies of traumatized populations consistently document the presence of amnesia and other dissociative symptoms in the clinical phenomenology of these individuals (Cardena & Spiegel, 1993; Carlson & Rosser-Hogan, 1991; Davidson & Fairbank, 1993; Grinker & Spiegel, 1945; Jaffe, 1968; Kardiner & Spiegel, 1947; Kuch & Cox, 1993; Niederland, 1968; Sargent & Slater, 1941; Spiegel, 1991). In addition, cross-cultural studies of European and Asian samples support the universality of dissociative symptoms in response to psychological trauma (Boon & Draijer, 1993b; Carlson & Rosser-Hogan, 1991; Ensink, 1992).

Dissociative Amnesia, Normal Memory, and Ordinary Forgetfulness

The DSM-IV diagnostic criteria for DA specify that the amnesic disturbance must be "too extensive to be explained by ordinary forgetfulness" (American Psychiatric Association, 1994, p. 481). This definition raises the question of what is meant by "ordinary forgetfulness" and how DA differs from it. In addition, nonpathological forms of amnesia have been described such as infantile and childhood amnesia, amnesia for sleep and dreaming, and posthypnotic amnesia (Schacter & Kihlstrom, 1989). Little systematic research has been performed differentiating and characterizing different forms of DA and their relation to "repression," nonpathological forms of amnesia, ordinary forgetfulness, or to cognitive disturbances found in dementia, delirium, and other "organic" amnestic and cognitive disorders.

Most forms of DA are thought to primarily involve difficulties with the functioning of episodic-autobiographical memory not implicit-semantic memory (Schacter & Kihlstrom, 1989). However, several studies have confirmed the clinical observation that subjects with dissociative amnesia for their life history can demonstrate "implicit" autobiographical memory while amnesic (Schacter & Kihlstrom, 1989). Similar phenomena have been described in posthypnotic amnesia with implicit demonstration that the memories for which amnesia has been suggested have been encoded and stored, but without their being accessible directly for retrieval (Orne, 1966; Schacter & Kihlstrom, 1989).

Amnesic patients may also have intense reactions to stimuli that are emotionally significant without knowing consciously the reason for the reaction or the significance of the stimuli (Kaszniak et al., 1988; Pitman, 1993; Schacter & Kihlstrom, 1989). Clinically, this is most vividly demonstrated when a patient with PTSD has a behavioral reexperiencing episode triggered by an apparently benign everyday stimulus that the patient does not consciously connect with a traumatic experience. There is experimental evidence that the cues for flashbacks and reexperiencing episodes in patients with PTSD are very specific to the traumatic experiences that generated the PTSD-amnesia syndrome and not to more generic stressful life events (Pitman, 1993).

Infantile and childhood amnesia can be experimentally documented in experimental paradigms for autobiographic memory (Rubin, 1986). Clinically and experimentally, patients with DA have been found to have exaggerated or extended forms of childhood amnesia (Schacter, Kihlstrom, & Kihlstrom, 1989; Schacter, Wang, & Tulving, 1982). Recall of autobiographical information while amnesic seemed to be related to life events with positive affects that were unconnected with the traumatic events precipitating the amnesia. Implicit autobiographical memory phenomena was documented as well in these studies (Schacter et al., 1982, 1989). Similar findings have been reported for Vietnam combat veterans with PTSD who show deficits in retrieval of specific autobiographical memories, particularly after viewing videotapes of combat (McNally, Litz, Prassas, Shin, & Weathers, 1994).

HISTORICAL REVIEW

Dissociative amnesia has been described in the world literature at least since classical European accounts of demonic possession and exorcism where the possessed person is frequently described as showing amnesia for the period of possession and the exorcism (Ellenberger, 1970; Laurence & Perry, 1988). In Europe in the late eighteenth and early nineteenth centuries, amnesia was recognized as a concomitant of "artificial somnambulism," considered to be the prototype of modern hypnosis, developed by devotees of Mesmer's animal magnetism theories (Ellenberger, 1970; Laurence & Perry, 1988). In various countries during the nineteenth century, there were periods of great interest in artificial somnambulism and in "magnetic diseases," i.e., spontaneously occurring disorders with symptoms similar to those that appeared in artificial somnambulism.

By the late nineteenth century, there was an interweaving of the notions of the somnambulistic magnetic disorders with the concept of hysteria. In their classic descriptions of hysteria, both Briquet (1859) and Charcot (quoted in Janet, 1901) underscored the frequent occurrence of amnesia, memory problems, and fugue in hysterical patients. Outside of Europe during this time, there was interest in similar phenomena as well. For example, in the United States, William James described one of the paradigmatic cases of fugue with change of personal identity, that of Ansel Bourne (see Hilgard, 1986).

The work of Janet has vast importance for the modern study of dissociation. His giant contributions to psychology and psychiatry have been largely ignored until the rediscovery of the importance of the dissociation concept in recent decades (Ellenberger, 1970; van der Kolk & van der Hart, 1989). Janet was influenced by the work of the early "magnetizers," as well by Charcot (Ellenberger, 1970; van der Hart & Friedman, 1989). His discussion of the etiology and phenomenology of amnesia, fugue, and other dissociative conditions remains one of the most comprehensive in the literature and is quite similar to more modern conceptualizations (van der Hart & Friedman, 1989; van der Kolk & van der Hart, 1989).

Janet viewed amnesia as a basic part of the dissociative process in which complex subsystems of memories, feelings, thoughts, and ideas became autonomous through disconnection from the overall executive control of the total personality with failure to recognize these as part of the patient's own consciousness (Janet, 1901, 1907). He hypothesized that fugue was based on dissociation of more complex groups of mental functions than occurred in amnesia and was usually organized around a powerful emotion or feeling state that linked many trains of associations accompanied by a wish to run away.

The description of complex dissociative amnesia symptoms also can be found in the original case descriptions of hysterical patients by Breuer and Freud (Freud, 1893–1895). For example, patients such as Anna O. and Emmy von N. were described as having blackouts, episodes of disremembered behavior, extensive amnesic gaps for the life history, fluctuations in handwriting, handedness, and language, and spontaneous age regression with amnesia (Loewenstein, 1993).

Since the beginning of the twentieth century, there have been a number of systematic studies and case reports about patients with amnesia and fugue. They make up the bulk of the literature on amnesia and fugue cited in psychiatric textbooks and they form the underpinnings of most of the received notions about these conditions in the literature (Abeles & Schilder, 1935; Akhtar & Brenner, 1979; Berrington, Liddell, & Foulds, 1956; Croft, Healthfield, & Swash, 1973; Fisher, 1943, 1945; Fisher & Joseph, 1949; Geleerd, Hacker, & Rapaport, 1945; Gill & Rapaport, 1942; Kiersch, 1962; Kirshner, 1973; Leavitt, 1935; Luparello, 1970; Menninger, 1919; Parfitt & Carlyle-Gall, 1944; Stengel, 1939, 1941, 1943; Wilson, Rupp, & Wilson, 1950).

These studies have a multitude of methodological weaknesses. For example, some patients diagnosed with DA in these studies actually had clear-cut fuguelike episodes and vice versa. Also, some of these cases more closely approximate modern diagnostic criteria for DID or DDNOS rather than amnesia or fugue. Other cases seem to have had other disorders such as epilepsy, a primary mood disorder, or a psychotic disorder that could account for the memory disturbances and/or pathological wandering (Stengel, 1939, 1941, 1943).

Despite the heterogeneity of these studies, most supported the view of Abeles and Schilder (1935) that the psychosocial environment out of which DA and DF develop are massively stressful, with the patient experiencing intolerable emotions of shame, guilt, despair, rage, desperation, frustration, and conflict experienced as unresolvable without suicide or flight.

A group of psychoanalytic clinicians and researchers became interested in dissociation in the early 1940s. For example, Fisher (1943, 1945), Fisher and Joseph (1949), Geleerd et al. (1945), Gill and Brenman (1959), Gill and Rapaport (1942), and Rapaport (1942) described a number of cases of patients with amnesia, fugue, and other dissociative disturbances. Bornstein (1946) reported a case of recurrent amnesia and fuguelike symptoms in an 8-year-old girl. Fisher (1943, 1945; Fisher & Joseph, 1949) and other psychodynamically oriented clinicians also produced an extensive literature on amnesia and related disturbances resulting from combat during World War II (see, for example, Grinker & Spiegel, 1945; Kardiner & Spiegel, 1947).

Traumatic circumstances surrounded the amnesia-fugue episodes in most of the civilian cases reported by these authors. These included past wartime combat, incest, other forms of childhood sexual assault, adult rape, threats of death or physical violence, and other similarly overwhelming events. In addition to external dangers or traumas, the patients were often struggling with extreme emotions or impulses such as overwhelming fear and/or intense incestuous, sexual, suicidal, or violent urges. Thus, the patients were also described as suffering from massive psychological conflict from which fight or flight was impossible or psychologically unacceptable without dissociation.

A few other psychoanalytic case reports have stressed that amnesia, altered states of consciousness, "hypnoid states," and other forms of dissociation can be conceptualized as defensive reactions to childhood trauma including childhood sexual abuse, physical abuse, witness to violence, and so forth (Bychowski, 1962; Dickes, 1965; Fleiss, 1953; Paley, 1988; Silber, 1979). More recent psychoanalytic writing has begun to address the issues of trauma and dissociation in a more systematic fashion (Armstrong, 1995; Marmer, 1980, 1991; Ross & Loewenstein, 1992; Schwartz, 1994).

Greenberg and van der Kolk (1986) state that: "Pathologies of memory are characteristic features of posttraumatic stress disorder" (p. 191). A variety of memory disturbances for trauma are codified in the DSM-IV diagnostic criteria for PTSD. These include intrusive recollections and reexperiencing symptoms, depersonalization and detachment, and amnesia.

Combat-Related and Other Wartime Trauma

Amnesia and fugue are frequent concomitants of acute stress disorder produced by wartime experiences and were frequently described in association with "shell shock" and "traumatic war neuroses" in case reports of soldiers in World War I and II, respectively (Brown, 1918, 1919, 1920–1921; Grinker & Spiegel, 1945; Henderson & Moore, 1944; Kardiner, 1941; Kardiner & Spiegel, 1947; Kubie, 1943; Myers, 1915, 1916; Rivers, 1918; Sargent & Slater, 1941; Southard, 1919; Thom & Fenton, 1920; Tureen & Stein, 1949). For example, Brown (1919), in discussing his experiences during World War I using hypnotherapy for soldiers with severe posttraumatic disorders, stated: "All the severe cases of 'shell shock' of the hysterical type (that is, showing functional disturbance or loss, of sensory or motor powers) which I saw near the firing line in France *suffered from loss of memory*" (p. 735, italics added).

Grinker and Spiegel (1945) reported that the extent of amnesia experienced by psychiatric battlefield casualties in World War II ranged from relatively brief periods of time to complete generalized amnesia as well as fugue episodes. Sargent and Slater (1941) reported a 14.4% prevalence of amnesia as a "prominent symptom" in a consecutive series of 1000 combat soldiers admitted to the Neurological Unit of Sutton Emergency Hospital during World War II. Thirty-five percent of the 87 soldiers subjected to the most severe combat stress had amnesia for war experiences, compared with 13% with "moderate" stress, and 6% with "trifling" stress. Only about 10% of the soldiers had had a severe head injury that was related to development of symptoms. In other studies from World War II, prevalence rates for amnesia during combat ranged from 5 to 8.6% (Fisher, 1945; Henderson & Moore, 1944).

Some of Sargent and Slater's (1941) other findings are also consistent with data acquired about veterans of the Vietnam War with PTSD (Bremner, Southwick, Yehuda, Johnson, & Charney, 1993b; Foy, Sipprelle, Rueger, & Carroll, 1984; Kulka et al., 1990). In these studies, intensity of combat exposure was the critical factor in the development of posttraumatic stress symptoms and DA. However, there was a group of individuals with a childhood history of trauma or of a dissociative disorder who appeared to have a lower threshold for the development of overt dissociative or PTSD symptoms when retraumatized during combat. These individuals also may have a more severe and chronic course with PTSD after return to civilian life (Bremner et al., 1993b).

Several studies have documented memory problems and amnesia for trauma in veterans with delayed-onset PTSD from World War II, the Korean conflict, and the Vietnam War (Archibald & Tuddenham, 1965; Bremner, Steinberg, Southwick,

Johnson, & Charney, 1993c; Futterman & Pumpian-Mindlin, 1951; Grinker & Spiegel, 1945; Hendin et al., 1984; Kardiner, 1941; Kardiner & Spiegel, 1947; Laufer, Brett, & Gallops, 1984)

In a recent systematic study using structured interviews and other standardized measures, Bremner et al. (1993c) compared 40 Vietnam combat veterans with PTSD to 15 Vietnam combat veterans without this condition. Subjects were studied with the Structured Clinical Interview for DSM-IV Dissociative Disorders (SCID) (American Psychiatric Association, 1994) and the SCID-D (for DSM-III-R dissociative disorders) (Steinberg, 1993) to make diagnoses of PTSD and of dissociative disorders, respectively. Veterans with PTSD scored significantly higher on all subscales of the SCID-D. The amnesia score in the PTSD group was significantly higher than that of controls at the $p < .0001$ level. An earlier study (Bremner et al., 1992) found significantly higher scores on the DES in combat veterans with PTSD compared with those without PTSD. PTSD patients reported more dissociative symptoms, specifically dissociative amnesia, at the time of trauma.

In another study, Bremner and his colleagues (Bremner, Scott, Delaney, et al., 1993) found significantly lower scores in individuals with combat-related PTSD as compared with normal controls on a number of subscales of the Wechsler Memory Scale, including total recall, immediate recall, long-term storage, long-term retrieval, and several other measures. IQ did not differ significantly between patients and controls. Abnormal neuropsychological findings in PTSD patients were comparable to those in other clinical populations with temporal lobe/hippocampal damage, consistent with the findings of hippocampal damage in patients with PTSD (Bremner et al., 1995).

Systematic Studies of Amnesia and Fugue in Other Traumatized Populations

Kuch and Cox (1992) studied 124 Jewish survivors of the Nazi Holocaust who were seeking compensation from the German government. All were documented to have undergone traumatic experiences including labor-camp placement, concentration camp incarceration for one month or more, and a group who were tattooed survivors of Auschwitz. Almost half of the total sample and over two-thirds of the Auschwitz group met DSM-III-R criteria for PTSD. About 3 percent of the total sample and 10 percent of the Auschwitz sample were found to have dissociative amnesia for at least some aspect of their Holocaust experiences.

Carlson and Rosser-Hogan (1991) studied 50 randomly selected Cambodian refugees to the United States who had escaped from the Cambodian holocaust. Subjects had experienced a variety of severe traumas and atrocities, including murder of relatives in front of them, rape, forced labor and repatriation, torture, and so forth. Eighty-six percent of subjects met full DSM-III-R PTSD criteria, and most of the remainder had posttraumatic stress symptoms (mean number of PTSD symptoms per subject = 8.6). Forty percent met *all* DSM-III-R PTSD criteria that include amnesia. Ninety-six percent of Cambodian refugees had high scores on the DES translated into Cambodian (mean = 37.1) compared to Western samples in which a DES score of 30 or higher predicts a diagnosis of a severe, clinically significant dissociative disorder such as dissociative identity disorder.

Terr (1988) described 20 children who had experienced documented trauma before the age of 5, including physical trauma, sexual abuse, ritualistic abuse, kidnapping, child pornography, and so forth. Children's reports of trauma were compared with the documentary evidence. Single brief traumas were better remembered verbally, although little verbal memory was available for traumas that occurred before 28 months of age. Virtually all children, especially those traumatized repetitively, "remembered," often uncannily accurately, in behavioral reenactments of the trauma. Preverbal traumas also were reenacted in this way. The author suggests that the data support the hypothesis that trauma may be preferentially encoded visually. This leads to a greater likelihood of remembering in imagery, dreams, and behavioral reenactments, not in verbal recall.

Coons and Millstein (1992) studied a consecutive series of 25 patients referred to a dissociative disorders clinic who met DSM-III criteria for dissociative amnesia. Most patients had more than one episode of amnesia. Seventy-two percent of patients had a history of child abuse: 52% reported a history of sexual abuse and 40% described a history of physical abuse. Abuse was reported to be the main precipitant of the amnesia in almost 60% of cases. However, distressing personal circumstances and behaviors that were being disavowed such as financial or sexual indiscretions were found to be precipitants in 30% of cases.

Herman and Schatzow (1987) reported on 53 women in a 12-week time-limited group therapy for the sequelae of reported childhood sexual abuse. Sixty-four percent reported some amnesia for the abuse. Twenty-eight percent were said to have "severe" memory deficits such as dense amnesia for many years of childhood. Earlier and more violent forms of reported abuse correlated with more severe memory deficits. Patients with later abuse (e.g., during latency) described more depersonalization and less amnesia. Almost three quarters of this sample of women reported corroboration of their reports of abuse by perpetrator admission, physical evidence such as diaries or letters, and so forth.

Briere and Conte (1993) described a sample of 450 male and female clinical subjects with a reported history of childhood sexual abuse. Fifty-nine percent of subjects described an inability to remember the abuse at some time during their lives. Subjects with amnesia were more likely to have had more severe, early-onset, repetitive, physically injurious abuse with multiple perpetrators and direct prohibitions of harm for disclosure. The subjects with a history of amnesia were more globally symptomatic as well. Loftus (1993) has criticized this study since the subjects were all in therapy and thus could have been influenced by the theoretical models of their therapists that "repression" of traumatic memory commonly occurs. She also criticized the wording of the question asked subjects concerning memory difficulties for abuse on the grounds that it is subject to multiple interpretations. She cites her own data that indicates that only 18% of 100 women in outpatient treatment for drug abuse who also reported a history of childhood sexual abuse claimed that they "forgot" the abuse for a period of time and then remembered it again. The Briere and Conte study presented data to suggest that the dissociation model is more robust in accounting for their data than the repression model: i.e., one based on posttraumatic alterations in memory and consciousness as opposed to a model based on intrapsychic conflict.

Ensink (1992) described 100 Dutch women who reported a history of childhood sexual abuse. They were given a large number of structured and semistructured interview and testing materials concerning life history, psychiatric symptoms, functional status, age of onset of reported trauma, number of reported perpetrators, types of reported childhood abuse (e.g., sexual, physical, neglect, witness to violence, etc.), violence of trauma, and so forth. Thirty-two subjects reported "time gaps" (i.e., amnesia), including experiences such as disremembered behavior, appearance of perplexing possessions, inexplicable changes in relationships, and fugues. Other dissociative symptoms such as spontaneous trances and depersonalization were also described. The extent of amnesia correlated most strongly with the cumulative trauma score. Ensink concluded succinctly that: "The more frequently and severely a woman as a child has been traumatized, the more frequently she tends to experience time-gaps" (pp. 104–105).

Williams (1994) followed up 129 women who had detailed, documented histories of childhood sexual abuse 17 years earlier. They had all been seen in an urban emergency room as children because of the abuse. The study compared the womens' current recollections obtained with a semistructured interview administered by "blind" interviewers with medical and other records that had been completed at the time of the initial report of the details of the abuse, including genital injury and physical trauma. Thirty-eight percent of the sample did not report the index abuse event documented in the 1970s. On the other hand, 68% of the women who did not recall the index event did describe another episode of childhood sexual abuse. These data supported the notion that these women suffered from amnesia for the abuse, not a reluctance to discuss abuse in general. The anecdotal data from the detailed individual case histories also tended to confirm this hypothesis.

Lack of memory for the abuse or accurate recall of the abuse did not follow expected age trends based on the notion of early childhood amnesia. Some individuals accurately reported documented abuse events that occurred when they were as young as 3 years old and others did not recall abuse that occurred when they were in latency or early adolescence. Subjects were less likely to recall abuse if they had had a closer relationship to the perpetrator, had more genital trauma by report in the 1970s, or had a higher "credibility rating" given at the time of the index event. Sixteen percent of those who did recall the index event retrospectively reported amnesia at some time for this event. Those with "recovered" memories were no less accurate than those who "always" remembered. There were no differences found for history of prior mental health treatment in those who always remembered compared to those with apparent amnesia. This was thought to counter the notion that reported amnesia might relate to the influence of therapists' theories about memory on the subjects. In any event, most of these women had not received much psychotherapy. They had been treated primarily for drug and alcohol abuse and severe psychiatric disorders. There were, however, higher rates of psychiatric hospitalization in those who did not recall the index event as compared to the other women.

Boon and Draijer (1993a) compared a sample of Dutch women with dissociative disorders to a sample with personality disorders, primarily borderline and histrionic personality disorders. Diagnoses were made using the SCID-D (Steinberg, 1993). A cumulative trauma score was also compiled for each subject, including data on severity and age of onset of sexual, physical, and other types of abuse. Patients with personality disorders did not differ significantly from those with dissociative disorders on a measure of depersonalization. However, dissociative disorder patients scored significantly higher on all other SCID-D subscales, including that for amnesia ($p < .0001$ for all other subscales). Trauma severity scores were also lower and trauma was of later onset in the personality disorder group as compared with the dissociative group. Table 4 summarizes findings from these studies suggesting factors that are more likely to lead to dissociative amnesia in response to traumatic circumstances.

FORENSIC ISSUES RELATED TO DISSOCIATIVE AMNESIA AND FUGUE

The problem of dissociation and the dissociative disorders has become an increasingly complex and contentious issue in civil and criminal law (Beahrs, 1994; (Coons, 1991; Lewis & Bard, 1991; Rubinsky & Brandt, 1986). Legal issues include competence to stand trial or to act as a witness in court; detection of malingered amnesia or other dissociative symptoms; responsibility for criminal behavior; and reliability of dissociated memory in the court of law in both civil and criminal matters.

From a legal standpoint, amnesia alone is not considered a sufficient factor to generate a finding of incompetence to stand trial or a verdict of not guilty by reason of insanity (Rubinsky & Brandt, 1986). Dissociative amnesia has been claimed by perpetrators in 30 to 40% of homicide cases and in a lesser percentage of other violent crimes (Kopelman, 1987a,b). Although malingering is often suspected in such cases, many of these individuals did little to avoid being charged with a crime and some even called the authorities themselves. In general, the murder cases with apparent true DA were characterized by an unpremeditated assault in a state of high emotional arousal on a victim closely related to the perpetrator (Kopelman, 1987b).

Most experts agree, however, that there is no absolute way to differentiate true DA from malingering (Schacter, 1986). Malingerers have been noted to continue their deception even during hypnotically or barbiturate-facilitated interviews

Table 4. Factors Leading to Persistent Dissociative Amnesia after Traumatic Experiences

The trauma is more likely to be caused by human assault, not natural disaster.
Repeated traumatization, not single traumatic events.
Longer duration of trauma.
Earlier age of onset of trauma.
Trauma caused by multiple perpetrators.
Fear of death or significant harm during trauma.
Threats of death or significant harm by perpetrators if victim discloses.
Violence of trauma/physical injury caused by the trauma.
Close relationship between perpetrator and victim.

(Kluft, 1988). On the other hand, in the clinical case reports, many malingerers quickly confessed their deceptions either spontanously or when confronted by the examiner. In these nonforensic reports, the malingered amnesics were frequently pathetic individuals whose deception was transparent. It was often unclear where the conscious deception began and the unconscious defenses ended (Kopelman, 1987b; Lishman, 1987; Parfitt & Carlyle-Gall, 1944).

In clinical matters, most experienced clinicians firmly hold dissociative patients responsible for their behavior despite claims of amnesia or a sense of lack of control over behavior (Beahrs, 1994). This stance is generally associated with a far better outcome clinically. Thus, it follows that a similar standard should be used in criminal matters. Under most circumstances dissociative patients know right from wrong and can modulate their conduct to conform to rules and laws (Beahrs, 1994).

Amnesia, Memory, and the Courts

A number of state legislatures have extended statutes of limitations in civil and criminal matters involving childhood abuse to permit legal actions for extended periods. Some of these statutes and legal rulings related to them have allowed extension of the statute of limitations based on return of previously dissociated or "repressed" memories of abuse (Horowitz & Bulkley, 1994). This has led to heated debate both in the media and to some extent in scholarly articles about the validity of these "recovered memories" as a basis for legal actions (see Loftus, 1993). Unfortunately, there is a dearth of research that balances the known effects of trauma on memory with the well-developed literature on the fallibility and malleability of memory under a variety of conditions.

From a clinical perspective, there is no requirement that adults who recall childhood abuse "confront" their alleged abusers or prosecute them in order to "heal." Unless carefully thought out clinically, these sorts of confrontations often result in a poor outcome at best for *both* accuser and accused (Schatzow & Herman, 1989). The long-term clinical focus is usually more appropriately placed on the patient's resolving his or her conflictual attachment to the accused abusive relative. When this is resolved, the pressure for confrontation frequently diminishes substantially, or if disclosure to family members occurs, it is handled in a way that is more likely to lead to resolution not exacerbation of difficulties (Schatzow & Herman, 1989).

Involvement of adult dissociative patients in the courts in attempts to sue or prosecute alleged abusers frequently results in clinical deterioration of the patient. This is due to the negative impact of the adversarial system on the patient who may have a highly idealized view of what will occur; an increased sense of loss of control due to the continual delays inherent in the legal process; the opening up of the patient's psychiatric history and clinical status in the courts; and the inherent difficulties in proving allegations of abuse with little evidence other than the (frequently "recovered") recollections of a patient with a history of DA and often of a significant psychiatric disturbance as well (Horowitz & Bulkley, 1994).

Clinicians should carefully review with the patient the potential clinical risks of proceeding with confrontations against alleged abusers both in and out of the courtroom. Many patients have little idea of the real implications of what will happen if they proceed in this way. Despite these cautions, some patients will proceed to confront accused abusers despite the urgings of their therapists to relent or to wait until other issues in treatment are better resolved before deciding on this course of action.

In their recent review, Horowitz and Bulkley (1994) suggest that, due to the current controversy and lack of sufficient, balanced scientific data, additional civil and criminal cases based on delayed memory should be handled on a case-by-case basis, rather than by passing new legislation. Further, they suggest that civil cases only be allowed with corroborative evidence of abuse, a higher standard of proof to "clear and convincing" evidence, and/or a limit on the number of years that the statute of limitations could be extended for civil cases involving claims of abuse. Many states have no statute of limitations for criminal matters. However, Horowitz and Bulkley (1994) argue that criminal cases involve a higher burden of proof and greater constitutional safeguards than civil ones and thus may offer greater protection to the accused.

TREATMENT

The treatment of DA and DF can be best conceptualized using a framework from the treatment of trauma disorders in general (Loewenstein, 1995). Most reviews have identified this as a phasic process characterized by at least three major epochs (Herman, 1992; van der Hart, Steele, Boon, & Brown, 1993). In the first phase, the traumatized individual is assisted to achieve safety and stability in his or her life. Once this is established, the individual may engage, if indicated, in a phase in which the focus is the processing of traumatic material in greater depth. This may involve attempts to overcome persistent amnesia symptoms as well as resolution of material that is undissociated or less completely dissociated. Finally, there is a third phase of "resolution" or "reintegration" in which the traumatized person is "reconnect[ed] to ordinary life" (Herman, 1992, p. 155). In this phase, the focus is less on the trauma per se and more on the development of a renewed, reinvigorated life apart from the symptoms of the trauma disorder and the domination of the person's psychology by issues related to traumatization.

In virtually all dynamic conceptualizations of DA, the adaptive function of the amnesia can be conceived of as a kind of "safety valve" or "circuit breaker" that reflects the patient's ability to tolerate full conscious awareness of the dissociated material. It is not only the content of the dissociated memories that is experienced as painfully intolerable, however. For the most part, it is the overwhelming affects and the personal meaning of the traumatic events that most powerfully reinforce the persistence of the amnesia (Spiegel, 1988b; Terr, 1991). Highly intense and often conflictual emotions of despair, grief, guilt, shame, rage, self-hatred, helplessness, and terror are commonly embedded in memories for which the person is amnestic. In addition, the traumatic events may cause profound shifts in the person's view of him or herself, significant others, and the nature of the world and all human relations (Briere, 1989). These posttraumatically determined aspects of the person's cognitive and assumptive world are also masked by amnesia. Without systematic clinical attention during treatment to resolution of the specific meanings of the trauma for the person, the amnestic patient usually will remain permanently symptomatic in some way (van der Hart & Brown, 1992; van der Hart et al., 1993)

Establishing Safety for the Patient with Dissociative Amnesia-Dissociative Fugue

This aspect of treatment is the most important and frequently most neglected in the treatment of trauma disorders. Patients' and clinicians' impulse to "get the memories" by intrusive means are probably shaped by the treatment literatures on the acute wartime amnesias and by the literature on "classical" acute DA-DF presentations. Generally speaking, the more acute the amnesia and the closer the patient is to the situation that generated it, the shorter the treatment time to resolution of the symptoms. However, even here, it is important to carefully stabilize acutely amnestic patients and to titrate the intensity of bringing the dissociated information into more ordinary conscious awareness (Brown, 1919; Fisher, 1943; Kardiner & Spiegel, 1947; Myers, 1916). In particular, a number of authors warn that acute amnesia and fugue states are frequently psychological alternatives to suicide (Gudjonsson & Haward, 1982). Clinical case reports have described successful suicide in amnestic patients who have not achieved adequate therapeutic stabilization before attempting to overcome amnesia or before returning to their usual life situation (Takahashi, 1988).

In cases of more long-standing or childhood-onset amnesias, attempts to rapidly uncover dissociated trauma material is usually particularly ill-advised. Attempts to uncover memories of single traumatic episodes through intrusive means, without careful prior stabilization and preparation, usually result in "retraumatization," with the patient frequently suffering from more intense intrusive PTSD symptoms accompanied by flashbacks to multiple traumatic events in addition to those of the index event (Steele & Colrain, 1990). Destabilization of the patient with acute dissociative and PTSD symptoms are common results of too rapid attempts to overcome amnesia in these cases.

In the case of the patient with acute stress disorders (American Psychiatric Association, 1994) primarily characterized by or accompanied by dissociative amnesia, the establishment of the person's physical safety is the first concern. This involves removal from the traumatizing environment such as acute combat, evaluation and treatment of medical problems including possible head injury, and provision of shelter, food, and sleep. Sedative medications such as the benzodiazepines may be indicated in some cases to assist with the latter.

The neuropsychiatric literature from World Wars I and II describe that, in many cases of acute wartime amnesias, removal of the soldier from combat and provision of food and sleep were sufficient to resolve amnesia symptoms completely. However, if these measures were insufficient to resolve symptoms, more definitive treatment was undertaken, generally after transporting the soldier away from the front (Brown, 1918; Kardiner & Spiegel, 1947; Kubie, 1943). Similar issues are important in cases of acute DA or DF presenting to civilian emergency or acute care facilities. In the series of Abeles and Schilder (1935), about 75% of their 63 cases of amnesia for personal identity were said to have had rapid spontaneous remission of amnesia once they were brought to the safety of clinical attention.

If immediate spontaneous remission does not occur in cases of acute amnesia, symptoms may abate later simply in the course of the clinician taking a psychiatric history or merely by assuring the patient that he or she *can* remember when he or she is ready and that the patient can remember at his or her own pace without the need to remember all the details or information at one time. The entire literature on DA underscores the importance of *permissive* suggestions for recall. Helping the patient experience a sense of control over the pace of recollection for dissociated information is very important during the treatment process.

Patients with long-standing, chronic amnesia presentations generally should be managed in the framework of a psychotherapy directed at resolution of the complex psychological sequelae of the events producing the amnesia, usually severe traumatization due to childhood abuse, combat, and/or other forms of adult victimization (Brende, 1985; Briere, 1993; Spiegel, 1988b; van der Kolk, 1986). Here, too, the first tasks of treatment are restoration of the patient's physical well-being and safety and establishment of a working alliance. The clinician must be prepared to intervene actively if the patient's difficulties involve suicide attempts, self-mutilation, eating disorders, alcohol or substance abuse, involvement in abusive or destructive relationships, episodes of rage or violence, abuse of the individual's own children or family members, and lack of adequate food, clothing, or shelter (Turkus, 1991). Hospitalization may be necessary to stabilize such patients, as well as referral to specialty resources such as treatment for substance abuse or eating disorders.

In individuals with severe intrusive PTSD symptoms alternating with amnesia, containment and management of intrusive recollection rather than attempts at detailed processing of trauma material is usually the goal in the stabilization phases of treatment. This may be accomplished by using supportive hypnotic techniques, pharmacotherapy, and/or cognitive therapy techniques (Colrain & Steele, 1991; Fine, 1990; Friedman, 1990; Saporta & Case, 1993; Spiegel, 1989; Steele & Colrain, 1990). There is no pharmacological agent that specifically targets DA or DF. However, treatment of the patient's PTSD, affective, dyscontrol, psychotic, obsessive-compulsive, and/or anxiety symptoms with medications may permit more focused therapeutic attention to the amnesia (Friedman, 1987, 1990; Loewenstein, 1991c; Saporta & Case, 1993).

Contraindications to a primary focus on uncovering dissociated memory material include:

> (1) Early stages of therapy; (2) an unstable therapeutic alliance; (3) current or ongoing abuse; (4) current acute external life crisis; (5) extreme age, severe physical infirmity, and/or terminal illness (abreaction may be carefully titrated in certain cases); (6) lack of ego strength, including severe borderline and psychotic states or pathological regression; (7) [in DID] uncontrolled rapid switching; (8) uncontrolled flashbacks; (9) [in DID] severe conflict and lack of cooperation in the [alter identity] system; (10) severe primary alexithymia; (11) temporary contraindications include the anticipated absence of the therapist and transitional times during the [patient's] life (Colrain & Steele, 1991, pp. 6-7)

Some severely impaired patients with PTSD and amnesia will never achieve sufficient stability to be candidates for more intensive attempts at processing dissociated memory material. Their entire treatment will consist of attempts to better assure their safety and stability. Containment and distancing of intrusive memory material and more general attempts to modulate these patients' chronic posttraumatic life maladaptations will be the goal of treatment.

Stabilization of the Patient with Dissociative Fugue

Patients with DF may present specific problems in clinical management. Most fugues are relatively brief and do not take the person far from home. However, case reports have described DF patients crossing multiple national borders during wanderings lasting for months (Fisher, 1945). DF patients may present with a range of dissociative memory disturbances including complete generalized amnesia with loss of memory for personal identity; amnesia for the entire fugue episode; a localized amnesia in which the patient believes it is a chronologically earlier time in his or her life; or, rarely, with a change in personal identity (Fisher, 1945; Fisher & Joseph, 1949; Gill & Brenman, 1959).

Some of these patients may resist uncovering their actual identity even with hypnosis or amytal narcosynthesis. Appeals through the local (or even regional) media may not alert the patient's significant others if he or she has wandered a substantial distance from home (Lyon, 1985). Also, family, sexual, occupational, and/or legal problems that were part of the original matrix that generated the fugue episode may be substantially exacerbated by the time the patient's original identity and life situation are detected.

Rarely, in the most extreme cases, the fugue patient has established a new identity, occupation, and social relationships in a different location (Hilgard, 1986). When the original identity is discovered, often by accident, there may be a variety of predicaments that ensue having to do with the real world complications of this situation. In response to this, the patient may become acutely suicidal, overwhelmed, and/or confused. Also, the patient may display more extreme or bizarre dissociative symptoms or attempt to engage in another fugue to escape the situation.

Hypnosis

Hypnosis has frequently played an important adjunctive role in the treatment of individuals with DA and DF. Hypnosis is not a treatment in itself; it is a set of adjunctive techniques that facilitate certain psychotherapeutic goals. All posttraumatic and dissociative disorders can and have been successfully treated without use of formal heterohypnosis (see, for example, Futterman & Pumpian-Mindlin, 1951).

Hypnosis can be used in a number of different ways in the treatment of DA-DF. In particular, hypnotic interventions are used to contain, modulate, and titrate the intensity of symptoms; hypnosis can be used to facilitate controlled recall of dissociated memories; hypnosis can be used supportively to provide "ego-strengthening" for the patient; and, finally, hypnosis can promote working through and integration of dissociated material (Brown & Fromm, 1986).

The clinician should be aware that use of hypnosis or drug-facilitated interviews in no way assures the veracity or lack of veracity of the information produced (Kolb, 1985; American Society of Clinical Hypnosis, 1994). In some clinical and research studies, the use of hypnosis has been associated with the production of inaccurate "memories" in whose accuracy the subject strongly believes, particularly in highly hypnotizable subjects (Laurence & Perry, 1988; McConkey, 1992). However, critical reviews have noted the complexity of this research problem, the variability in findings among studies, and the many variables related both to hypnosis and nonhypnotic factors that appear to influence this and related phenomena (McConkey, 1992). On the other hand, many studies have confirmed the essential accuracy of reports of traumatic experiences that were subject to DA, primarily involving wartime trauma, but other sorts of trauma such as childhood abuse as well (Brown, 1918; Coons & Millstein, 1986; Grinker & Spiegel, 1945; Herman & Schatzow, 1987; Kardiner & Spiegel, 1947; Terr, 1988; Williams, 1994).

Some have argued implicitly or explicitly that intensive emotional release ("abreaction") is the key therapeutic agent in the treatment of amnesia (Brown, 1920-1921; Kolb, 1985). Others have maintained that it is the integration of dissociated affects, cognitions, and self-perceptions that is essential to the resolution of symptoms in amnestic patients (van der Hart & Brown, 1992; van der Hart et al., 1993). They note that a primary treatment focus on intensive attempts to bring into awareness extreme dissociated affects frequently results in a chronic decompensation rather than in a resolution of the patient's amnesia and PTSD symptoms. It is now generally accepted that intense emotional release per se is rarely associated with positive therapeutic outcome in dissociative patients. Full therapeutic resolution of dissociated imagery, memories, affects, cognitions, and self-perceptions is a complex process that usually occurs over a number of treatment sessions.

Clinicians since World War I have recognized the importance of the patient repeatedly processing dissociated material in a number of different sessions, often at different levels of affective intensity, in order to complete the process of integration of the material (van der Hart & Brown, 1992). It is usually wise to begin working with dissociated material in a more cognitive, distanced fashion to gain an outline of the patient's history for which amnesia is present. Subsequently, the dissociated memories can be increasingly worked with and their full affective and cognitive meanings for the patient explored.

In cases of acute generalized, selective, or localized dissociative amnesia, after establishing the patient's safety and the therapeutic relationship, the next task of therapy is to help the patient regain awareness of his or her identity and general personal circumstances. Subsequent sessions then focus on the events that led to the development of the acute amnesia. The material is then reworked in greater detail in subsequent sessions. In most cases, there will be resolution of amnesia within days to a few months. However, there are cases of persistent generalized or severe localized amnesia that have required years of intensive psychotherapy to overcome (Eisen, 1989).

In the author's experience it is useful to try to account systematically for different dimensions of the dissociated, usually traumatic, experiences: sensory, affective, cognitive, and behavioral in order to assure that all key components have been identified and reconstructed (Braun, 1988; van der Hart et al., 1993). Also, it is useful to attempt to account systematically for a variety of dysphoric affects that are commonly experienced during traumatic experiences: despair, sorrow, grief, horror, shame, helplessness, rage, guilt, confusion, anguish, and so forth. Inquiry about these other affects may be quite helpful in resolving the amnesia. In particular, shame, horror, helplessness, and overwhelming confusion are emotions that patients may have the most trouble identifying without assistance from the therapist.

There is often a "core" aspect of the experience, either a specific part of the event or its meaning to the person that is central to resolving a persistent amnesia. This aspect of the recollection frequently remains dissociated despite the patient's discussing other parts of the experience. Identification of this aspect of the material and making it a focus of continued clinical attention is usually crucial to full resolution of amnesia.

RESOLUTION

In the final phases of treatment for DA, the patient is able to experience the previously dissociated material as normal autobiographical material. There should no longer be involuntary intrusions of imagery, affect, and sensation. The patient should no longer experience a conscious sense of distinct gaps in memory for life experience. Memories of the past should be experienced as parts of prior historical time, not as current "living" events. Memory experience should have a quality of voluntariness: For the most part, the patient can recollect the material or put it aside. Memories of traumatic experiences should not have a "special" quality distinct from other memory material. The patient may have the uncanny experience of actually beginning to "forget" the experiences; they are rarely called to mind as the person turns his or her attention to everyday life (Herman, 1992; van der Hart et al., 1993).

At this point, patients often experience a sense of perspective and calm about issues that seemed previously overwhelming and disruptive. The patient frequently reports greater energy for other life tasks such as relationships with others, work, or leisure activities. Some chronically traumatized individuals may experience never having lived in a calm, quiet, nontraumatized way. They may express amazement at this new "boring" way of life.

Group Psychotherapy for Amnesia

In addition to individual psychotherapy, Kardiner (1941) described the use of group psychotherapy and hypnotherapy to promote recovery in traumatic war-related amnesia. Highly supportive, structured, reassuring and "reeducative" approaches were often used by the therapist to attempt to accomplish the return of the patient to a functional status and to prevent chronic disability (Grinker & Spiegel, 1945; Kardiner, 1941; Kardiner & Spiegel, 1947).

Time-limited and longer-term group psychotherapy has been reported to be helpful treatment for many combat veterans with PTSD as well as for survivors of childhood abuse (Briere, 1989; Courtois, 1988; Goodwin & Talwar, 1989; Herman, 1992; Smith, 1985). During group sessions, some authors report that patients may recall memories for which they have had amnesia. Supportive interventions by the group members and/or group therapist may facilitate integration and mastery of the dissociated material (Goodwin & Talwar, 1989). On the other hand, clinicians working with patients at the more severe end of the dissociative spectrum have suggested that group therapy optimally should focus on "here-and-now" issues. They state that discussion of specific, detailed trauma-related material is often highly disruptive to group function and to the individual members (Coons & Bradley, 1986).

Some patients with reported histories of childhood sexual abuse have made use of self-help or 12-step groups. These groups can be highly problematic if members attempt to access or process dissociated material during sessions. Some clinicians have raised the issue of "contamination" of trauma reports among members in these groups. Although some patients report subjective benefit from such groups, clinicians should weigh carefully with the patient the potential risks and benefits for entering such a group. Indeed, some clinicians refuse to work with patients who attend self-help groups because of their potential to disrupt the patient and to confuse the therapy (R. P. Kluft, E. Frischholz, personal communications, Vancouver, Canada, May, 1994).

Somatic Therapies

There is no known pharmacotherapy for DA and DF other than drug-facilitated interviews (Perry & Jacobs, 1982; Ruedrich, Chu, & Wadle, 1985). A variety of agents have been used for this purpose including sodium amytal, pentothal, oral benzodiazepines, and amphetamines (Ruedrich et al., 1985). At the present time, there have been no adequately controlled studies to assess the efficacy of any of these agents in comparison with one another, with other treatment methods, or with placebo (Ruedrich et al., 1985).

Narcosynthesis is a term devised by Grinker and Spiegel (1945) to underscore the need for material uncovered in a drug-facilitated interview to be processed by the patient in his or her usual conscious state. Narcosynthesis continues to be used primarily to work with acute amnesias and conversion reactions, among other indications, in general hospital psychiatric services (Perry & Jacobs, 1982). There also is occasional utility for this procedure in refractory cases of chronic DA (Kolb, 1985). Some patients will only be able to overcome persistent amnesia with a drug-facilitated interview and not with other interventions.

On the other hand, these procedures must be performed where resuscitation equipment is available in case of respiratory arrest, albeit a rare complication. The interview usually must be audiotaped or videotaped to replay for the patient since amnesia generally persists for the interview. In narcosynthesis, the clinician usually can not titrate the intensity of the patient's response as in hypnotherapeutic interventions. Finally, repeated procedures are generally impractical and even may lead to a dependence on drug-facilitated interviews in the patient.

A recent case report describes amelioration of some symptoms of apparent DA with successful electroconvulsive treatment in a patient with a severe, refractory major depression (Daniel & Crovitz, 1986). Convulsive treatments with electric shock, insulin, and metrazol were occasionally prescribed for refractory combat-related disorders during World War II (Kubie, 1943), although modern military psychiatrists see no indication for such procedures (Jones & Hales, 1987). At the present time, there appears to be no indication for treatment of DA or acute or chronic posttraumatic disorders with electroconvulsive therapy.

CONCLUSIONS

The relationship of DA and DF to traumatic circumstances has been reported repeatedly for more than a century. Recent systematic studies of traumatized individuals have documented and refined this clinical observation. Further, an emerging psychobiology of trauma may permit a neurobiological understanding of the manifold memory disturbances related to overwhelming traumatic experiences. It is important that these clinical and research findings are understood by the professional community and by the public. Cognitive psychology research on the fallibility of memory needs to be informed by studies on trauma, dissociation, and dissociative amnesia just as scholarly work on dissociation needs to incorporate findings from cognitive and memory studies. Collaborative research in this area would be welcome.

The treatment of posttraumatic DA has been well described in increasingly sophisticated clinical reports that incorporate both the classical findings about these conditions as well as the data from more modern studies of the comprehensive treatment of PTSD and trauma disorders. Methodologically rigorous outcome studies still need to be performed, however, using standardized diagnostic and outcome measures.

It is unfortunate that these complex issues concerning trauma and memory are being played out in media and in the courts. The results of this process will only make more difficult the treatment of dissociative patients as well as rigorous research on the impact of traumatic experiences on memory.

REFERENCES

Abeles, M., & Schilder, P. (1935). Psychogenic loss of personal identity. *Archives of Neurology and Psychiatry, 34*, 587-604.

Akhtar, S., & Brenner, I. (1979). Differential diagnosis of fugue-like states. *Journal of Clinical Psychiatry, 40*, 381-385.

American Psychiatric Association. (1994). *Diagnostic and statistical manual of mental disorders* (4th ed.). Washington, DC: Author.

American Society of Clinical Hypnosis Committee on Hypnosis and Memory. (1994). *Guidelines for clinicians working with hypnosis and memory* and *Guidelines for the conduct of forensic hypnosis interviews*. Des Plaines, IL: American Society of Clinical Hypnosis.

Archibald, H. C., & Tuddenham, R. D. (1965). Persistent stress reaction after combat. *Archives of General Psychiatry, 12*, 475-481.

Armstrong, J. G. (1995). Reflections on multiple personality disorder as a developmentally complex adaptation. *Psychoanalytic Study of the Child, 50*, 349-364.

Beahrs, J. O. (1994). Dissociative identity disorder: Adaptive deception of self and others. *Bulletin of the American Academy of Psychiatry and the Law, 22*, 223-237.

Bernstein, E. M., & Putnam, F. W. (1986). Development, reliability, and validity of a dissociation scale. *Journal of Nervous and Mental Disease, 174*, 727-735.

Berrington, W. P., Liddell, D. W., & Foulds, G. A. (1956). A re-evaluation of the fugue. *Journal of Mental Science*, *102*, 280-286.

Boon, S., & Draijer, N. (1993a). The differentiation of patients with MPD or DDNOS from patients with Cluster B personality disorder. *Dissociation*, *6*, 126-135.

Boon, S., & Draijer, N. (1993b). Multiple personality disorder in the Netherlands: A clinical investigation of 71 patients. *American Journal of Psychiatry*, *150*, 489-494.

Bornstein, B. (1946). Hysterical twilight states in an eight-year old child. *Psychoanalytic Study of the Child*, *2*, 229-241.

Bowman, E. (1993). The etiology and clinical course of pseudoseizures: Relationship to trauma, depression and dissociation. *Psychosomatics*, *34*, 333-342.

Braun, B. G. (1988). The BASK (behavior, affect, sensation, knowledge) model of dissociation. *Dissociation*, *1*(1), 4-23.

Bremner, J. D., Davis, M., Southwick, S. M., Krystal, J. H., & Charney, D. S. (1993a). Neurobiology of posttraumatic stress disorder. In J. M. Oldham, M. B. Riba, & A. Tasman (Eds.), *American Psychiatric Association annual review of psychiatry*, (pp. 157-179). Washington, DC: American Psychiatric Press.

Bremner, J. D., Randall, P., Scott, T. M., Bronen, R. A., Seibyl, J. P., Southwick, S. M., Delaney, R. C., McCarthy, G., Charney, D. S., & Innis, R. B. (1995). MRI-based measurement of hippocampal volume in patients with combat-related posttraumatic stress disorder. *American Journal of Psychiatry*, *152*, 973-981.

Bremner, J. D., Scott, T. M., Delaney, R. C., Southwick, S. M., Mason, J. M., Johnson, D. R., Innis, R. B., McCarthy, G., & Charney, D. S. (1993b). Deficits in short-term memory in posttraumatic stress disorder. *American Journal of Psychiatry*, *150*, 1015-1019.

Bremner, J. D., Southwick, S. M., Brett, E., Fontana, A., Rosenheck, R., & Charney, D. S. (1992). Dissociation and posttraumatic stress disorder in Vietnam combat veterans. *American Journal of Psychiatry*, *149*, 328-332.

Bremner, J. D., Southwick, S. M., Yehuda, R., Johnson, D. R., & Charney, D. S. (1993c). Childhood physical abuse and combat-related posttraumatic stress disorder in Vietnam veterans. *American Journal of Psychiatry*, *150*, 235-239.

Bremner, J. D., Steinberg, M., Southwick, S. M., Johnson, D. R., & Charney, D. S. (1993d). Use of the Structured Clinical Interview for DSM-IV Dissociative Disorders for systematic assessment of dissociative symptoms in posttraumatic stress disorder. *American Journal of Psychiatry*, *150*, 1011-1014.

Brende, J. O. (1985). The use of hypnosis in post-traumatic conditions. In W. E. Kelly (Ed.), *Posttraumatic stress disorder and the war veteran patient* (pp. 193-210). New York: Brunner/Mazel.

Breslau, N., Davis, G. C., Andreski, P., & Peterson, E. (1991). Traumatic events and posttraumatic stress disorder in an urban population of young adults. *Archives of General Psychiatry*, *48*, 216-222.

Briere, J. (1989). *Therapy for adults molested as children: Beyond survival*. New York: Springer.

Briere, J. (1993). *Child abuse trauma: Theory and treatment of the lasting effects*. Newbury Park, CA: Sage.

Briere, J., & Conte, J. (1993). Self-reported amnesia for abuse in adults molested as children. *Journal of Traumatic Stress*, *6*, 21-31.

Briquet, P. (1859). *Traite de l'hysterie*. Paris: J. Bailliere.

Brown, D. P., & Fromm, E. (1986). *Hypnotherapy and hypnoanalysis*. Hillsdale, NJ: Lawrence Erlbaum.

Brown, W. (1918). The treatment of cases of shell shock in an advanced neurological centre. *Lancet*, 197-200.

Brown, W. (1919). Hypnosis, suggestion, and dissociation. *British Medical Journal*, *191*, 734-736.

Brown, W. (1920-1921). The revival of emotional memories and its therapeutic value. *British Journal of Medical Psychology*, *1*, 16-19.

Bychowski, G. (1962). Escapades: A form of dissociation. *Psychoanalytic Quarterly*, *131*, 155-173.

Cardena, E., & Spiegel, D. (1993). Dissociative reactions to the San Francisco Bay area earthquake of 1989. *American Journal of Psychiatry*, *150*, 474-478.

Carlson, E. B., & Rosser-Hogan, R. (1991). Trauma experiences, posttraumatic stress, dissociation, and depression in Cambodian refugees. *American Journal of Psychiatry*, *148*, 1548-1551.

Classen, C., Koopman, C., & Spiegel, D. (1993). Trauma and dissociation. *Bulletin of the Menninger Clinic*, *57*, 178-194.

Colrain, J., & Steele, K. (1991). Treatment protocols for spontaneous abreactive memory work. In B. G. Braun (Ed.), *Eighth international conference on multiple personality and dissociation* (p. 68). Chicago: Rush-Presbyterian St. Luke's Hospital, Department of Psychiatry.

Coons, P. M. (1991). Iatrogenesis and malingering of multiple personality disorder in the forensic evaluation of homicide defendents. *Psychiatric Clinics of North America, 14*, 757-768.

Coons, P. M., & Bradley, K. (1986). Group psychotherapy with multiple personality patients. *Journal of Nervous and Mental Disease, 174*, 715-721.

Coons, P. M., & Millstein, V. (1986). Psychosexual disturbances in multiple personality: Characteristics, etiology, and treatment. *Journal of Clinical Psychiatry, 47*, 106-110.

Coons, P. M., & Millstein, V. (1992). Psychogenic amnesia: A clinical investigation of 25 cases. *Dissociation, 5*(2), 73-79.

Courtois, C. A. (1988). *Healing the incest wound: Adult survivors in therapy*. New York: Norton.

Croft, B., Healthfield, K. W. G., & Swash, M. (1973). Differential diagnosis of transient amnesia. *British Medical Journal, 4*, 593-596.

Daniel, W. F., & Crovitz, H. F. (1986). ECT-induced alteration of psychogenic amnesia. *Acta Psychiatrica Scandinavica, 74*, 302-303.

Davidson, J. R. T., & Fairbank, J. A. (1993). The epidemiology of posttraumatic stress disorder. In J. R. T. Davidson & E. B. Foa (Eds.), *Posttraumatic stress disorder: DSM-IV and beyond* (pp. 147-169). Washington, DC: American Psychiatric Press.

Davidson, J. R. T., & Foa, E. B. (1993). *Posttraumatic stress disorder: DSM-IV and beyond*. Washington, DC: American Psychiatric Press.

Dickes, R. (1965). The defensive function of an altered state of consciousness: A hypnoid state. *Journal of the American Psychoanalytic Association, 13*, 356-403.

Eisen, M. R. (1989). Return of the repressed: Hypnoanalysis of a case of total amnesia. *International Journal of Clinical and Experimental Hypnosis, 37*, 107-119.

Ellenberger, H. F. (1970). *The discovery of the unconscious*. New York: Basic Books.

Ensink, B. J. (1992). *Confusing realities: A study on child sexual abuse and psychiatric symptoms*. Amsterdam: VU University Press.

Fine, C. G. (1990). The cognitive sequelae of incest. In R. P. Kluft (Ed.), *Incest-related disorders of adult psychopathology* (pp. 161-182). Washington, DC: American Psychiatric Press.

Fisher, C. (1943). Hypnosis in treatment of neurosis due to war and to other causes. *War Medicine, 4*, 565-576.

Fisher, C. (1945). Amnesic states in war neurosis: The psychogenesis of fugue. *Psychoanalytic Quarterly, 14*, 437-468.

Fisher, C., & Joseph, E. D. (1949). Fugue with awareness of loss of personal identity. *Psychoanalytic Quarterly, 18*, 480-493.

Fleiss, R. (1953). The hypnotic evasion. *Psychoanalytic Quarterly, 22*, 497-511.

Foy, D. W., Sipprelle, R. C., Rueger, D. B., & Carroll, E. M. (1984). Etiology of posttraumatic stress disorder in Vietnam veterans: Analysis of premilitary, military, and combat exposure influences. *Journal of Consulting and Clinical Psychology, 52*, 72-87.

Freud, S. (1893-1895). Psychotherapy of hysteria. In J. Strachey (Ed.), *The complete psychological works of Sigmund Freud* (Vol. 11, pp. 253-305). London: Hogarth Press.

Freud, S. (1910). Five lectures on psycho-analysis. In J. Strachey (Ed.), *The complete psychological works of Sigmund Freud* (Vol. 11, pp. 7-55). London: Hogarth Press.

Freud, S. (1933). New introductory lectures on psycho-analysis. In J. Strachey (Ed.), *The complete psychological works of Sigmund Freud* (Vol. 22, pp. 7-182). London: Hogarth Press.

Friedman, M. J. (1987). Toward rational pharmacotherapy for posttraumatic stress disorder. *American Journal of Psychiatry, 145*, 281-285.

Friedman, M. J. (1990). Interrelationships between biological mechanisms and pharmacotherapy of posttraumatic stress disorder. In M. E. Wolf & A. D. Mosnaim (Eds.), *Posttraumatic stress disorder: etiology, phenomenology, and treatment* (pp. 281-285). Washington, DC: American Psychiatric Press.

Futterman, S., & Pumpian-Mindlin, E. (1951). Traumatic war neuroses five years later. *American Journal of Psychiatry, 107*, 401-408.

Geleerd, E. R., Hacker, F. J., & Rapaport, D. (1945). Contribution to the study of amnesia and allied conditions. *Psychoanalytic Quarterly, 14*, 199-220.

Gill, M. M., & Brenman, M. (1959). *Hypnosis and related states*. New York: International Universities Press.

Gill, M. M., & Rapaport, D. (1942). A case of amnesia and its bearing on the theory of memory. *Character and Personality, 11*, 166-172.

Goodwin, J., & Talwar, N. (1989). Group psychotherapy for victims of incest. *Psychiatric Clinics of North America, 12*, 279-295.

Greenberg, M. S., & van der Kolk, B. A. (1986). Retrieval and integration of traumatic memories with the "painting cure." In B. A. van der Kolk (Ed.), *Psychological trauma* (pp. 191-215). Washington, DC: American Psychiatric Press.

Grinker, R. R., & Spiegel, J. P. (1945). *Men under stress*. Philadelphia: Blakiston.

Gudjonsson, G. H., & Haward, L. R. C. (1982). Hysterical amnesia as an alternative to suicide. *Medicine Science and the Law, 22*, 68-72.

Henderson, J. L., & Moore, M. (1944). The psychoneuroses of war. *New England Journal of Medicine, 230*, 273-279.

Hendin, H., Haas, A. P., Singer, P., Houghton, W., Schwartz, M., & Wallen, V. (1984). The reliving experience in Vietnam veterans with posttraumatic stress disorder. *Comprehensive Psychiatry, 25*, 165-173.

Herman, J., & Schatzow, E. (1987). Recovery and verification of memories of childhood sexual trauma. *Psychoanalytic Psychology, 4*, 1-14.

Herman, J. L. (1981). *Father-daughter incest*. Cambridge: Harvard University Press.

Herman, J. L. (1992). *Trauma and recovery*. New York: Basic Books.

Hilgard, E. R. (1986). *Divided consciousness: Multiple controls in human thought and action, expanded edition*. New York: John Wiley.

Horowitz, M. J., & Bulkley, J. A. (1994). The statute of limitations and legal remedies for adults abused as children. *The APSAC Advisor (American Professional Society on the Abuse of Children), 7*(2), 6-8.

Jaffe, R. (1968). Dissociative phenomena in former concentration camp inmates. *International Journal of Psychoanalysis, 49*, 310-312.

Janet, P. (1901). The mental state of hystericals. New York: G. P. Putnam's Sons.

Janet, P. (1907). *The major symptoms of hysteria*. New York: Macmillan.

Jones, F. D., & Hales, R. E. (1987). Military combat psychiatry: A historical review. *Psychiatric Annals, 17*, 525-527.

Kardiner, A. (1941). *The traumatic neuroses of war*. New York: Hoeber.

Kardiner, A., & Spiegel, H. (1947). *War, stress, and neurotic illness*. New York: Hoeber.

Kaszniak, A. W., Nussbaum, P. D., Berren, M. R., & Santiago, J. (1988). Amnesia as a consequence of male rape: A case report. *Journal of Abnormal Psychology, 97*, 100-104.

Kiersch, T. A. (1962). Amnesia: A clinical study of ninety-eight cases. *American Journal of Psychiatry, 119*, 57-60.

Kirshner, L. A. (1973). Dissociative reactions: An historical review and clinical study. *Acta Psychiatrica Scandinavica, 49*, 698-711.

Kluft, R. P. (1985). The natural history of multiple personality disorder. In R. P. Kluft (Ed.), *Childhood antecedents of multiple personality* (pp. 197-238). Washington, DC: American Psychiatric Press.

Kluft, R. P. (1988). The dissociative disorders. In J. A. Talbot, R. E. Hales, & S. C. Yudofsky (Eds.), *The American psychiatric press textbook of psychiatry* (pp. 557-584). Washington, DC: American Psychiatric Press.

Kluft, R. P. (1992). Discussion: A specialist's perspective on multiple personality disorder. *Psychoanalytic Inquiry, 14*, 139-171.

Kolb, L. C. (1985). The place of narcosynthesis in the treatment of chronic and delayed stress reactions of war. In S. M. Sonnenberg, A. S. Blank, & J. A. Talbott (Eds.), *The trauma of war: Stress and recovery in Vietnam veterans* (pp. 211-226). Washington, DC: American Psychatric Press.

Kopelman, M. D. (1987a). Amnesia: Organic and psychogenic. *British Journal of Psychiatry, 150*, 428-442.

Kopelman, M. D. (1987b). Crime and amnesia: A review. *Behavioral Sciences and the Law, 5*, 323-342.

Kubie, L. S. (1943). Manual of emergency treatment of acute war neurosis. *War Medicine, 4*, 582-598.

Kuch, K., & Cox, B. J. (1992). Symptoms of PTSD in 124 survivors of the Holocaust. *American Journal of Psychiatry, 149*, 337-340.

Kulka, R. A., Schlenger, W. E., Hough, R. L., Jordan, B. K., Marmar, C. R., & Weiss, D. S. (1990). *Trauma and Vietnam war generation: Report of the findings from the National Vietnam Veterans Readjustment Study*. New York: Brunner and Mazel.

Laufer, R. S., Brett, E., & Gallops, M. S. (1984). Post-traumatic stress disorder reconsidered: PTSD among Vietnam veterans. In B. van der Kolk (Ed.), *Posttraumatic stress disorder: Psychological and biological sequelae*. Washington, DC: American Psychiatric Press.

Laurence, J.-R., & Perry, C. (1988). *Hypnosis, will and memory*. New York: Guilford Press.

Leavitt, F. H. (1935). The etiology of temporary amnesia. *American Journal of Psychiatry, 91*, 1079-1088.

Lewis, D. O., & Bard, J. S. (1991). Multiple personality and forensic issues. *Psychiatric Clinics of North America, 14*, 741-756.

Lishman, W. A. (1987). *Organic psychiatry* (2nd ed.). Oxford: Blackwell Scientific.

Loewenstein, R. J. (1990). Somatoform disorders in victims of incest and child abuse. In R. P. Kluft (Ed.), *Incest-related disorders of adult psychopathology* (pp. 75-113). Washington, DC: American Psychiatric Press.

Loewenstein, R. J. (1991a). An office mental status examination for chronic complex dissociative symptoms and multiple personality disorder. *Psychiatric Clinics of North America, 14*, 567-604.

Loewenstein, R. J. (1991b). Psychogenic amnesia and psychogenic fugue: A comprehensive review. In A. Tasman & S. Goldfinger (Eds.), *American Psychiatric Press annual review of psychiatry* (Vol. 10, pp. 189-222). Washington, DC: American Psychiatric Press.

Loewenstein, R. J. (1991c). Rational psychopharmacology for multiple personality disorder. *Psychiatric Clinics of North America, 14*, 721-740.

Loewenstein, R. J. (1993). Anna O: Reformulation as a case of multiple personality disorder. In J. Goodwin (Ed.), *Rediscovering childhood trauma: Historical casebook and clinical applications* (pp. 139-167). Washington, DC: American Psychiatric Press.

Loewenstein, R. J. (1995). Dissociative amnesia and dissociative fugue. In G. O. Gabbard (Ed.), *Treatment of psychiatric disorders* (pp. 1570-1597). Washington, DC: American Psychiatric Press.

Loftus, E. F. (1993). The reality of repressed memories. *American Psychologist, 48*, 518-537.

Luparello, T. J. (1970). Features of fugue: A unified hypothesis of regression. *Journal of the American Psychoanalytic Association, 18*, 379-398.

Lyon, L. S. (1985). Facilitating telephone number recall in a case of psychogenic amnesia. *Journal of Behavior Therapy and Experimental Psychiatry, 16*, 147-149.

Marmer, S. (1980). Psychoanalysis of multiple personality disorder. *International Journal of Psychoanalysis, 61*, 439-451.

Marmer, S. (1991). Multiple personality disorder: A psychoanalytic perspective. *Psychiatric Clinics of North America, 14*, 677-693.

McConkey, K. M. (1992). The effects of hypnotic procedures on remembering: the experimental findings and the implications for forensic hypnosis. In E. Fromm & M. R. Nash (Eds.), *Contemporary hypnosis research*, (pp. 405-426). New York: Guilford Press.

McHugh, P. R. (1992). Psychiatric misadventures. *The American Scholar, 62*, 497-510.

McNally, R. J., Litz, B. T., Prassas, A., Shin, L. M., & Weathers, F. M. (1994). Emotional priming of autobiographical memory in post-traumatic stress disorder. *Cognition and Emotion, 8*, 351-367.

Menninger, K. A. (1919). Cyclothymic fugues: Fugues associated wity manic-depressive psychosis: A case report. *Journal of Abnormal Psychology, 14*, 54-63.

Myers, C. S. (1915). A contribution to the study of shell-shock. *Lancet*, 316-320.

Myers, C. S. (1916). Contributions to the study of shell-shock. *Lancet* 65-69.

Niederland, W. G. (1968). Clinical observations on the "survivor syndrome." *International Journal of Psychoanalysis, 49*, 313-315.

Ofshe, R., & Watters, E. (1994). *Making monsters: False memories, psychotherapy, and sexual hysteria*. New York: Scribners.

Orne, M. T. (1966). On the mechanisms of posthypnotic amnesia. *International Journal of Clinical and Experimental Hypnosis, 14*, 121-134.

Paley, A. N. (1988). Growing up in chaos: The dissociative response. *American Journal of Psychoanalysis, 48*, 72-83.

Parfitt, D. N., & Carlyle-Gall, C. M. (1944). Psychogenic amnesia: The refusal to remember. *Journal of Mental Science, 379*, 519-531.

Perry, J. C., & Jacobs, D. (1982). Overview: clinical applications of the amytal interview in psychiatric emergency settings. *American Journal of Psychiatry, 139*, 552-559.

Pitman, R. K. (1993). Biological findings in posttraumatic stress disorder: Implications for DSM-IV classification. In J. R. T. Davidson & E. B. Foa (Eds.), *Posttraumatic stress disorder: DSM-IV and beyond* (pp. 173-189). Washington, DC: American Psychiatric Press.

Putnam, F. W. (1985). Dissociation as a response to extreme trauma. In R. P. Kluft (Ed.), *Childhood antecedents of multiple personality* (pp. 65-97). Washington, DC: American Psychiatric Press.

Putnam, F. W. (1991). Dissociative phenomena. In A. Tasman & S. Goldfinger (Eds.), *American Psychiatric Press annual review of psychiatry* (Vol. 10, pp. 145-160). Washington, DC: American Psychiatric Press.

Rapaport, D. (1942). *Emotions and memory*. Baltimore: Williams and Wilkins.

Rivers, H. R. (1918). The repression of war experience. *Lancet* 173-177.

Ross, C. (1991). The epidemiology of multiple personality disorder and dissociation. *Psychiatric Clinics of North America, 14*, 503-517.

Ross, C., Heber, S., Norton, G., & Anderson, G. (1989). The dissociative disorders interview schedule. *Dissociation, 3*, 169-188.

Ross, C. A., Joshi, S., & Currie, R. (1990). Dissociative experiences in the general population. *American Journal of Psychiatry, 147*, 1547-1552.

Ross, D. R., & Loewenstein, R. J. (Eds.). (1992). *Perspectives on multiple personality disorder*. Hillsdale, NJ: Psychoanalytic Inquiry.

Rubin, D. C. (Ed.). (1986). *Autobiographical memory*. Cambridge: Cambridge University Press.

Rubinsky, E. W., & Brandt, J. (1986) Amnesia and the criminal law. *Behavioral Sciences and the Law, 4*, 27-46.

Ruedrich, S. L., Chu, C.-C., & Wadle, C. V. (1985). The amytal interview in the treatment of psychogenic amnesia. *Hospital and Community Psychiatry, 36*, 1045-1046.

Russell, D. E. H. (1983). The incidence and prevalence of intrafamilial and extrafamilial sexual abuse of female children. *Child Abuse and Neglect, 7*, 133-146.

Saporta, J. A., & Case, J. (1993). The role of medications in treating adult survivors of childhood trauma. In P. L. Paddison (Ed.), *Treatment of adult survivors of incest* (pp. 101-134). Washington, DC: American Psychiatric Press.

Sargent, W., & Slater, E. (1941). Amnesic syndromes in war. *Proceedings of the Royal Society of Medicine, 34*, 757-764.

Saxe, G. N., Chinman, G., Berkowitz, R., Hall, K., Lieberg, G., Schwartz, J., & van der Kolk, B. A. (1994). Somatization in patients with dissociative disorders. *American Journal of Psychiatry, 151*, 1329-1334.

Schacter, D. L. (1986). Amnesia and crime: How much do we really know? *American Psychologist, 41*, 286-295.

Schacter, D. L., & Kihlstrom, J. F. (1989). Functional amnesia. In F. Boller & J. Grafman (Eds.), *Handbook of neuropsychology* (pp. 508-514). Amsterdam: Elsevier Science Publishers.

Schacter, D. L., Wang, P. L., & Tulving, E. (1982). Functional retrograde amnesia: A quantitative study. *Neuropsychologia, 20*, 523-532.

Schacter, D. L., Kihlstrom, J. F., & Kihlstrom, L. C. (1989). Autobiobraphical memory in a case of multiple personality. *Journal of Abnormal Psychology, 98*, 508-514.

Schatzow, E., & Herman, J. L. (1989). Breaking secrecy: Adult survivors disclose to their families. *Psychiatric Clinics of North America, 12*, 337-349.

Schwartz, H. L. (1994). From dissociation to negotiation: A relational psychoanalytic perspective on multiple personality disorder. *Psychoanalytic Psychology, 11*, 189-231.

Silber, A. (1979). Childhood seduction, parental pathology, and hysterical symptomatology: The genesis of an altered state of consciousness. *International Journal of Psychoanalysis, 60*, 109-116.

Singer, J. L. (Ed.). (1990). *Repression and Dissociation: Implications for Personality Theory, Psychopathology, and Health*, Chicago: University of Chicago Press.

Smith, J. R. (1985). Rap groups and group psychotherapy for Viet Nam veterans. In S. M. Sonnenberg, A. S. Blank, & J. A. Talbott (Eds.), *The trauma of war: Stress and recovery in Vietnam veterans* (pp. 165-191). Washington DC: American Psychiatric Press.

Southard, E. E. (1919). *Shell-shock and other neuropsychiatric problems*. Boston: W. M. Leonard.

Spiegel, D. (1988a). Dissociating damage. *American Journal of Clinical Hypnosis, 29*, 123-131.

Spiegel, D. (1988b). Dissociation and hypnosis in posttraumatic stress disorders. *Journal of Traumatic Stress Studies, 1*, 17-33.

Spiegel, D. (1986). Dissociation, double binds, and posttraumatic stress. In B. G. Braun (Ed.), *The treatment of multiple personality disorder* (pp. 61-77). Washington, DC: American Psychiatric Association.

Spiegel, D. (1989). Hypnosis in the treatment of victims of sexual abuse. *Psychiatric Clinics of North America, 12*, 295-305.

Spiegel, D. (1991a). Dissociation and trauma. In A. Tasman & S. Goldfinger (Eds.), *American Psychiatric Press annual review of psychiatry* (vol. 10, pp. 261-275). Washington, DC: American Psychiatric Press.

Spiegel, D. (1991b). The dissociative disorders. In A. Tasman & S. Goldfinger (Eds.), *American Psychiatric Press annual review of psychiatry* (vol. 10, pp. 141-276). Washington, DC: American Psychiatric Press.

Steele, K., & Colrain, J. (1990). Abreactive work with sexual abuse survivors: Concepts and techniques. In M. Hunter (Ed.), *The sexually abused male* (vol. 2, pp. 1-55). Lexington, MA: Lexington.

Stein, M. B., Hannah, C., Koverola, C., & McClarty, B. (1995). Neuroanatomic and cognitive correlates of early abuse. In J. M. Oldham (Ed.), *Proceedings of the Annual Meeting of the American Psychiatric Association*, (pp. 113). Washington, DC: American Psychiatric Association.

Steinberg, M. (1993). *The Structured Clinical Interview for DSM-III-R Dissociative Disorders (SCID-D)*. Washington, DC: American Psychiatric Press.

Steinberg, M. (1994). *The Structured Clinical Interview for DSM-IV Dissociative Disorders-revised (SCID-D-R)*. Washington, DC: American Psychiatric Press.

Stengel, E. (1939). Studies on the psychopathology of compulsive wandering. *British Journal of Medical Psychology, 18*, 250-254.

Stengel, E. (1941). On the aetiology of the fugue states. *Journal of Mental Science, 87*, 572-599.

Stengel, E. (1943). Further studies on pathological wandering (fugues with the impulse to wander). *Journal of Mental Science, 89*, 224-241.

Takahashi, Y. (1988). Aokigahara-jukai: Suicide and amnesia in Mt. Fuji's black forest. *Suicide and Life Threatening Behavior, 18*, 164-175.

Terr, L. (1988). What happens to early memories of trauma? A study of twenty children under the age five at the time of documented traumatic events. *Journal of the American Academy of Child and Adolescent Psychiatry, 27*, 96-104.

Terr, L. (1991). Childhood traumas: An outline and overview. *American Journal of Psychiatry, 148*, 10-20.

Thom, D. A., & Fenton, N. (1920). Amnesias in war cases. *American Journal of Insanity, 76*, 437-448.

Tureen, L. L., & Stein, M. (1949). The base section psychiatric hospital. *Bulletin of the US Army Medical Department, 9*(suppl.), 105-137.

Turkus, J. (1991). Psychotherapy and case management for multiple personality disorder: Synthesis for continuity of care. *Psychiatric Clinics of North America, 14*, 649-660.

van der Hart, O., & Brown, P. (1992). Abreaction re-evaluated. *Dissociation, 5*, 127-140.

van der Hart, O., & Friedman, B. (1989). A reader's guide to Pierre Janet on dissociation: A neglected intellectual heritage. *Dissociation, 2*(1), 3-16.

van der Hart, O., Steele, K., Boon, S., & Brown, P. (1993). The treatment of traumatic memories: Synthesis, realization, and integration. *Dissociation, 6*, 162-180.

van der Kolk, B. (1986). *Psychological trauma*. Washington, DC: American Psychiatric Press.

van der Kolk, B. (1993). The body keeps the score: The evolving psychobiology of posttraumatic states. *Harvard Review of Psychiatry, 1*, 253-265.

van der Kolk, B. A., & Herman, J. L. (1986). Traumatic antecedents of borderline personality. In B. van der Kolk (Ed.), *Psychological trauma* (pp. 111-126). Washington, DC: American Psychiatric Association.

van der Kolk, B., & van der Hart, O. (1989). Pierre Janet and the breakdown of adaptation in psychological trauma. *American Journal of Psychiatry, 146*, 1530-1540.

Walker, E. A., Katon, W. J., Harrop-Griffiths, J., Holm, L., & Russo, J. (1988). Relationship of chronic pelvic pain to psychiatric diagnoses and childhood sexual abuse. *American Journal of Psychiatry, 145*, 75-80.

Walker, E. A., Katon, W. J., Neraas, K., Jemelka, R. P., & Massoth, D. (1992). Dissociation in women with chronic pelvic pain. *American Journal of Psychiatry*, *149*, 534-537.

Walker, E. A., Katon, W. J., Roy-Byrne, P. P., Jemelka, R. P., & Russo, J. (1993). Histories of sexual victimization in patients with irritable bowel syndrome or inflammatory bowel disease. *American Journal of Psychiatry*, *150*, 1502-1506.

Williams, L. M. (1994). Recall of childhood trauma: A prospective study of women's memories of child sexual abuse. *Journal of Consulting and Clinical Psychology*, *62*, 1167-1176.

Wilson, G., Rupp, C., & Wilson, W. W. (1950). Amnesia. *American Journal of Psychiatry*, *106*, 481-485.

Yehuda, R., Kahana, B., Binder-Barynes, K., Southwick, S. M., Mason, J. M., & Giller, E. L. (1995). Low urinary cortisol excretion in holocaust survivors with posttraumatic stress disorder. *American Journal of Psychiatry*, *152*, 982-986.

16

Dissociative Identity Disorder

Richard P. Kluft

Dissociative identity disorder (DID), formerly known as multiple personality disorder (MPD), is a complex, chronic, posttraumatic dissociative psychopathology (Kluft, 1987a; Loewenstein, 1991) characterized by disturbances of memory and identity (Nemiah, 1980). It is distinguished from other mental disorders by the ongoing coexistence of relatively consistent but alternating subjectively separate identities and either recurrent episodes of memory disruption, frank amnesia, or both, and/or amnesia for a period of noncontemporary autobiographic memory. It almost invariably emerges as the sequela of overwhelming childhood experiences (Putnam, Guroff, Silberman, Barban, & Post, 1986; Spiegel, 1984, 1991). Its childhood form is often rather simple and its traumatic antecedents frequently can be documented with facility (e.g., Fagan & McMahan, 1984; Kluft, 1984a, 1985a; Hornstein & Putnam, 1992; Coons, 1994). However, it appears that in some adult cases, secondary autonomy of the defense of alter formation and function, the development of additional complexity, and a reworking of childhood experiences occur during adolescence. By virtue of this metamorphosis, the adult form often becomes rather intricate in its structure, and adult patients' given histories demonstrate the interplay of historical events, fantasy, confabulation, postevent information, and the impact of many nontraumatic exogenous influences (Kluft, 1995, in press a).

DID IN AN HISTORICAL AND CROSS-CULTURAL PERSPECTIVE

The majority of studied societies and cultures have conditions in which another entity is understood to have taken over the body of an afflicted individual, i.e., possession states. Their common core is that

Richard P. Kluft • Dissociative Disorders Program, The Institute of Pennsylvania Hospital, Philadelphia, Pennsylvania 19139.

Handbook of Dissociation: Theoretical, Empirical, and Clinical Perspectives, edited by Larry K. Michelson and William J. Ray. Plenum Press, New York, 1996.

> An individual suddenly seems to lose his identity to become another person. His physiognomy changes and shows a striking resemblance to the individual of whom he is, supposedly, the incarnation. With an altered voice, he pronounces words corresponding to the personality of the new individual. (Ellenberger, 1970, p. 13)

Until the end of the eighteenth century, many individuals in Western society demonstrated such phenomena. They were understood, within the explanatory paradigms of their eras, to be afflicted with the various Judeo-Christian forms of possession and were treated with culturally endorsed forms of exorcism. When theological explanations of mental disease gave way to the first dynamic psychiatry, a process chronicled by Ellenberger (1970), the psychological constructs that underlay the possession states and the mental conflicts they expressed did not abruptly cease to exist. Instead, what is now called DID (and allied conditions) began to enter the literature. DID provides a secular expression of many of the same mental structures found in possession syndromes. In those societies in which indigenous possession states remain powerful and sanctioned idioms for expressing subjective experiences and conflicts, the psychopathological "niche" that DID occupies elsewhere is already filled, and DID will be quite uncommon (e.g., Adityanhjee, Raju, & Khandelwal, 1989).

Although DID was declared extinct in 1943 by Stengel, it appears to be present in most societies in which indigenous possession states have lost or are losing their cultural currency. Combining the published literature and the author's correspondence with clinical colleagues over the last quarter century, DID has been identified and treated in native-born citizens of the United States, Canada, Mexico, many Caribbean and Central American nations, over half-a-dozen South American countries, all major western European and most eastern European states, Israel, Turkey, many African countries, Australia, Japan, Korea, and several Asian nations as well (see Coons, Kluft, Bowman, & Milstein, 1991; van der Hart, 1993). Although it is still is common to hear DID referred to as a North American culture-bound syndrome (e.g., Fahy, 1988), this is not accurate. It appears to be found relatively readily whenever psychiatric patient populations are systematically studied with objective screening and diagnostic instruments. Recently Goff and Simms (1993) have repeated Fine's (1988a) demonstration that the symptomatology of DID has remained relatively constant over the centuries, notwithstanding fluctuations of the quantitative aspects of certain features, such as the number of alters.

THE HISTORY OF MULTIPLE PERSONALITY DISORDER

Although Bliss (1986) attributes a case description to Paracelsus, Petetain published the first modern descriptions of DID phenomena in 1787. The first attempt to delineate a specific syndrome or disorder consisting of these phenomena, *umgetauschte Personlichkeit* (exchanged personality), is that of Eberhardt Gmelin, in 1791. Both are described in Ellenberger (1970). Benjamin Rush described such patients early in the nineteenth century (Carlson, 1981). Thereafter numerous authorities made substantial contributions to the study of DID, most of whom are nearly forgotten by history. For example, the three Despines together saw over 40 cases; Antoine Despine, Sr., is credited with the first psychotherapeutic cure of DID, in 1836 (see Fine, 1988a). Under Charcot and Janet, many such patients were identified and treated at the Salpetriere; Janet's contributions remain fresh and relevant. In the United States, Morton Prince (1905) drew attention to the disorder and made observations of lasting importance.

The study of DID and dissociation flourished briefly and waned. Appropriate doubt was cast on many of Charcot's demonstrations (Ellenberger, 1970; McHugh, 1993). Janet left few followers; his influence was further eroded by the rise of Freudian influence. Although Freud began with a close affinity to the study of dissociation and DID [Anna O. suffered this condition (Jones, 1953)], he distanced himself from them as he developed his own models of the mind and repudiated the seduction theory. Bleuler included DID under the rubric of schizophrenia; as the diagnosis of schizophrenia rose in acceptance, the use of the diagnosis of DID dropped off precipitously (Rosenbaum, 1980). Dismissed as a subject of importance by the rising tides of psychoanalysis, descriptive-organicist psychiatry, and behaviorism, the study of dissociation and DID declined to near oblivion within a generation.

The current rise of interest in DID reflects the convergence of many influences (Kluft, 1987a). The *Diagnostic and Statistical Manual of Mental Disorders*, 3rd edition (DSM-III) (American Psychiatric Association, 1980) recognized DID as a free-standing condition and provided landmark clinical descriptions. Feminism made a most powerful impact. It sensitized the mental health professions to the hitherto unacknowledged high incidence of child abuse, incest, and the exploitation of women. Increasingly clinicians are listening to their adult patients' accounts of childhood abuse without discounting them in advance as fantasies. DID is primarily a disorder of sexually abused women; in this atmosphere, its recognition soared.

Also, there has been an explosion of interest in posttraumatic stress disorder (PTSD), which, like DID, occurs consequent to trauma and has many dissociative features (Stutman & Bliss, 1985; Spiegel, Hunt, & Dondershine, 1988). Many have noted the similarity of the two conditions, bringing credibility to DID, an appreciation of the dissociative aspects of PTSD, and an application of the treatment approaches useful for PTSD to MPD and vice versa.

Advances in psychopharmacology have encouraged greater diagnostic precision and closer scrutiny of treatment failures, a group that includes many unrecognized DID patients (Kluft, 1987a). A renaissance of interest in hypnosis is underway, and with it increased interest in dissociation. Lay attention to celebrated cases of DID and its fictional representation in the media have played a role. Schrieber's 1973 book *Sybil*, describing Cornelia B. Wilbur's work with an MPD patient, was particularly influential. Excitement was generated by studies on the psychophysiological aspects of DID (Putnam, 1984a, 1991a,b). A final influence has been the dedicated teaching efforts of many of the pioneers in field.

Before 1980-1984, clinicians' information about DID was more likely to have come from lay than professional sources. Over those 4 years, a vigorous professional literature became available and has continued to expand, bringing DID increasingly into the mainstream; 1984 marked the beginning of annual international conferences on dissociation and DID. The journal, *Dissociation: Progress in the Dissociative Disorders*, began publication in 1988; 1989 marked the publication of Putnam's masterful *Diagnosis and Treatment of Multiple Personality Disorder*, and 1993 the remarkable *Multiple Personality Disorder in the Netherlands*, by Boon and Draijer (1993a), which demonstrated the reliability and validity of the diagnosis. As of this writing, DID has become a mainstream concern of the mental health professions, albeit a controversial one. For further information about the modern history of DID, see Greaves (1993).

PHENOMENOLOGY

Diagnostic Criteria

As psychiatry moves to achieve accurate and reliable diagnostic criteria, DID has been redefined three times within a quarter century. In 1980, DSM-III proposed three criteria: (1) the existence within the individual of two or more personalities, each of which is dominant at a particular time; (2) the personality that is dominant at any particular time determines the individual's behavior; and (3) each individual personality is complex and integrated with its own unique behavior patterns and social relationships. These criteria were written as a number of new and important findings were emerging. In retrospect, they reflect the phenomenology of several classic cases that were intelligent, creative, and female, had relatively few personalities, and were not typical in all respects. They implicitly endorse a classic but superseded model of dissociation (Frischholz, 1985); that is, they rely on an all-or-none model in which what is dissociated is, for the moment, no longer a factor. In fact, the essence of dissociation is that that which is dissociated often continues to influence matters from "behind the scenes" (American Psychiatric Association, 1994; Kluft, 1987a, 1991a; Franklin, 1988; Spiegel, 1991).

With regard to criterion 1, the term *dominance* is misleading, because it implies that the relationship among the personalities is an incessant power struggle that is won completely for the moment. In fact, personalities may determine behavior from behind the scenes without emerging and may share or contend for control. Emitted behavior often is the combined vector of numerous influences, functioning as a system (Kluft, 1991a,b). Personalities commonly try to pass for one another. The same concerns apply to criterion 2. Also, recent findings indicate that contemporary cases average 13 to 15 alters (Kluft, 1984b; Putnam et al., 1986; Ross, Norton, and Wozney, 1989b; Schultz, Braun, & Kluft, 1989). Kluft (1985b) found that only about half a dozen or less of these personalities spend significant periods of time in executive control; that alters demonstrate a wide range of distinctness and complexity; and that their importance, dominance, and elaborateness may vary over time. Therefore, criterion 3 required revision.

DSM-III-R criteria were more flexible, less reified, and reflected clinical findings in the broader range of DID patients: (1) The existence within the person of two or more distinct personalities or personality states (each with its own relatively enduring pattern of perceiving, relating to, and thinking about the environment and self); and (2) at least two of these personalities or personality states recurrently take full control of the person's behavior. DSM-III-R attempted to offer a pragmatic clinical definition of the term "personality," which was a step forward. DSM-III-R depicts

DID not in reifying terms that suggest that there are many people in a single body, but indicates instead that in DID the mind is structured as a system of organizations of the self. Unfortunately, it retained the false and misleading statement that alters in control exercise complete power. Just as DSM-III drew criticism as skewed toward false-negative diagnoses, DSM-III-R, despite its consistency with the natural history of DID (Kluft, 1985b), was seen by some critics as making the diagnosis too easy to achieve and encouraging false positives. This fear has been disproven (Ross, 1989). A greater awareness of DID, rising rapidly at the time DSM-III-R was published, accounts for most of the accelerated reporting of such cases. Nonetheless, although these criteria accurately reflect a condition that can have a wide spectrum of of manifestations, they have distressed some who prefer a crisper delineation of the margins of clinical disorders.

Unlike the prior DSM committees that studied the dissociative disorders in an atmosphere of scholarly deliberation, the DSM-IV committee was polarized and contentious; consequently, the DSM-IV criteria were drafted in an adversarial atmosphere. Both the criteria and the text are a major departure from DSM-III-R and reflect a compromise between the pressures of increasing knowledge on the one hand and the power of skeptical authorities insistent on promoting their opinions in the face of that knowledge on the other. The name of the condition was changed to dissociative identity disorder, ostensibly to put to rest the controversy that surrounds MPD and to initiate a new, scientific and objective era in its study. Another rationale for the change was for uniformity in nomenclature (e.g., dissociative amnesia, dissociative fugue, dissociative identity disorder). However, depersonalization disorder was not changed, suggesting that once the name of DID had been changed, uniformity was no longer such a pressing imperative!

The DSM-IV criteria are perceived as reasonable for clinical and research usage even by those who argued bitterly over the name change (American Psychiatric Association, 1994, p. 487):

1. The presence of two or more distinct identities or personality states (each with its own relatively enduring pattern of perceiving, relating to, and thinking about the environment and self).
2. At least two of these identities or personality states recurrently take control of the person's behavior.
3. Inability to recall important personal information that is too extensive to be explained by ordinary forgetfulness.
4. Not due to the direct effects of a substance (e.g., blackouts or chaotic behavior during Alcohol Intoxication) or a general medical condition (e.g., complex partial seizures). Note: In children, the symptoms are not attributable to imaginary playmates or other fantasy play.

The decision to replace "personality" with "identity" while retaining the ambiguous and intermediate term "personality state" acknowledges the difficulties surrounding the revision of the DID section. "Personality" is admittedly a problematic term, long associated with controversy and reification, both of which the committee attempted to avoid. "Personality state" is a term introduced into DSM-III-R with the goal of discouraging reification. It is questionable whether "identity" will be confusing or clarifying. The author's reading of the literature on identity suggests that it will not be a useful heuristic, and that "self" may have been a more useful construct to explore.

There has always been considerable pressure toward including an amnesia criterion (Coons, 1984; Braun, 1986; Putnam, 1984b). However, occasional patients are encountered who have classic personalities but are without classic amnesia; DID patients frequently have periods during which their amnestic barrier becomes more permeable than usual; and many dissociative distortions of memory do not involve formal amnesia (Kluft, Steinberg, & Spitzer, 1988). Excluding patients without amnesia from the DID diagnosis will eliminate only about 5% of previously diagnosed DID patients, many of whom have progressed well enough in treatment to have achieved co-consciousness. However, it may delay the making of the diagnosis in as many as one third of them, because amnesia is not acknowledged at first interview by this percentage of patients ultimately diagnosed with DID (Putnam et al., 1986; Ross, 1989; Ross et al., 1989b). The pragmatic impact of the addition of this criterion remains to be assessed. DSM-IV wisely eliminated the word "full" in criterion 2, more accurately reflecting the function of a system of alters over time (Kluft, 1985b; Putnam, 1989).

In applying diagnostic criteria, there is some difference of opinion among experts as to whether to make the diagnosis on the basis of history, without having encountered alter personalities on one or more occasions (Coons, 1984). One does not wish to be duped by a factitious disorder patient or some other form of "wannabe." However, the overtness of DID fluctuates over time in 80% or more of DID patients (Kluft, 1985b, 1991b), and it is rather precious to withhold the diagnosis in an otherwise well-documented case with currently covert manifestations. There is much to be said for being flexible and using criteria more stringent than DSM-IV only for specialized research purposes. Often one can gain an excellent picture of the alters' presence and impact without encountering them [e.g., in the Structured Clinical Interview for DSM-IV Dissociative Disorders (SCID-D) (Steinberg, 1993)], and in some circumstances (e.g., forensic situations) making an effort to elicit an alter may diminish the credibility of the patient's condition [e.g., The "Hillside Strangler" case (Orne, Dinges, & Orne, 1984; Watkins & Watkins, 1984)].

Most DID patients do not fulfill DSM-IV criteria at all times during their illness, and there are a great many patients who suffer dissociative disorders with the structure of DID but never appear to fulfill diagnostic criteria (Kluft, 1985b; Ross et al., 1992a; Coons, 1992; Boon & Draijer, 1993a). For such patients, the diagnosis of dissociative disorder not otherwise specified (DDNOS) is technically more accurate, although for all practical therapeutic purposes they are virtually identical with DID. Two series of DDNOS patients with DID structures followed over time proved to have periods of overt DID in almost every case (Boon & Draijer, 1993b; Kluft, 1985b).

The Personalities or Identities

In the context of general psychiatry, personality is taken to mean, "the characteristic way in which a person thinks, feels, and behaves; the ingrained pattern of behavior that each person evolves, both *consciously* and *unconsciously*, as the style or way of being in adapting to the environment" (Talbott, Hales, & Yudofsky,

1988, p. 1261). Identity is understood to be "a person's global role in life and the perception of his sense of self" (Talbott et al., 1988, p. 1255). In DID, the entities in question are "here defined as a relatively enduring pattern of perceiving, relating to, and thinking about the environment and one's self that is exhibited in a wide range of social and personal contexts. Personality states differ only in that the pattern is not exhibited in as wide a range of contexts" (American Psychiatric Association, 1987, p. 269). Alter personalities are psychological structures, not separate people.

Several approaches to the issue of personality are current. Coons (1984), Kluft (1984c), and Putnam (1989) agree that the sum total of all the personalities and their interactions constitute the DID patient's personality in the more general sense. Braun (1986) has attempted to distinguish quantitatively between personalities, as defined in the above quotation, and less elaborated entities, which he terms fragments.

Putnam (1989) "conceptualize[s] the alters as highly discrete states of consciousness organized around a prevailing affect, sense of self (including body image) with a limited repertoire of behaviors and a set of state dependent memories" (p. 103). Kluft (1988, p. 51) observed:

> A disaggregate self state (i.e., personality) is the mental address of a relatively stable and enduring particular pattern of selective mobilization of mental contents and functions, which may be behaviorally enacted with noteworthy role-taking and role-playing dimensions and sensitive to intrapsychic, interpersonal, and environmental stimuli.... It has a sense of its own identity and ideation, and a capacity for initiating thought processes and actions.

Both are describing reconfigurations rather than reified divisions, emphasizing that the personalities should be understood as ways the mind may be organized rather than "pieces of a pie." From this flows an appreciation that the number of personalities can be quite large, because they constitute configurations, rather than portions of a unity.

Many skeptical of the reality of DID have argued that "we are all multiple personalities"; i.e., an individual manifests many states of mind and/or facets. Since the unity of the self is more a subjective illusion than an actuality (Hilgard, 1986), this stance has a kernel of truth. Nonetheless, clinical DID differs from such "normal multiplicity" in a number of dimensions. First, the normal individual in a wide range of situations and roles experiences no change of identity and retains a sense of continuity as to who and what he or she is. Second, one's different moods and circumstances involve no major change in self-representation. An angry normal woman does not experience herself as a large and menacing male. Third, notwithstanding the phenomena of state and mood-dependent memory (Bower, 1981), there are few major barriers in self-referential autobiographic memory across different moods, roles, and situations for the normal individual who experiences him or herself somewhat differently in various moods, roles, or situations. Fourth, there is no loss of the sense of ownership of what goes on or is done in different states of mind for the non-DID individual. For better or for worse, one's behavior (experientially) remains one's own. Therefore, the statement "we are all multiple personalities" is misleadingly reductionistic.

Although the often dramatic differences across personalities tend to arrest the attention of the observer, it is important to appreciate that their purpose is to create alternative self-structures and psychological realities within which or by virtue of which emotional survival is facilitated. A "multiple reality disorder" (Kluft, 1991a,b, 1993) is created to allow one to cope with the intolerable and is embodied within the alters to allow the enactment of alternative approaches to trying circumstances:

> For example, a young girl experiencing incest may generate an alter to hold the incest experience so that she can remain in her family without conscious awareness of what has befallen her and without being consciously burdened by the fact of her betrayal by someone on whom she remains emotionally dependent. She might create a male alter along the fantasy/wish that such a plight could not befall a boy, or that a boy could better take the pain of such encounters.
>
> The emitted observable phenomena of multiple personality disorder are epiphenomena and tools of the defensive purpose. In terms of the patient's needs, the personalities need only be as distinct, public, and elaborate as becomes necessary in the handling of stressful situations ... Anything further results from hypertrophy or secondary autonomy of these processes, and from whatever narcissistic investments and secondary gains become associated with them. (Kluft, 1991b, p. 610)

The purest form of DID is virtually isomorphic, occurring when a traumatized child creates another version of him or herself either to hold an intolerable experience or to stand for the wish to be unaffected by it. When alters can subserve their defensive purpose without emerging completely and demonstrating their separateness, they often do so, and the condition remains very covert (Kluft, 1985b, 1991b). In sum, the most important aspects of the alters are not related to their dramatic differences, which are no more than fascinating epiphenomena, but to their facilitating adaptation by segregating certain aspects of experience, self, and knowledge from one another in a relatively consistent rule-bound fashion (Kluft, 1991b; see also Spiegel, 1986).

Phenomenology of the Personalities

Several recent studies (Bliss, 1980; Boon & Draijer, 1993a; Coons & Milstein, 1986; Coons, Bowman, & Milstein, 1988; Putnam et al., 1986; Ross et al., 1989b) are largely consistent in terms of the general trends that they demonstrate. At the time of diagnosis (prior to exploration) approximately two to four personalities are in evidence. In the course of treatment an average of 13 to 15 are encountered, but this figure is deceptive. The mode in virtually all series is three, and median number of alters is eight to ten. Complex cases, with 26 or more alters (described in Kluft, 1988), constitute 15–25% of such series and unduly inflate the mean. Series currently being studied in tertiary referral centers appear to be more complex still (Kluft, Fink, Brenner, & Fine, unpublished data). This is subject to a number of interpretations. It is likely that the complexity of the more difficult and demanding cases treated in such settings may be one aspect of what makes them require such specialized care. It is also possible that the staff of such centers is differentially sensitive to the need to probe for previously undiscovered complexity in their efforts to treat patients who have failed to improve elsewhere. However, it is also possible that patients unduly interested in their disorders and who generate factitious complexity enter such series differentially, or that some factor in these units or in those who refer to them encourages such complexity or at least the subjective report thereof.

The personalities' overt differences and disparate self-concepts may be striking. They may experience and represent themselves as being different ages, genders, races, religions, and sexual orientations; they may experience themselves as having different appearances and/or hold discrepant values and belief systems. Their awareness of one another may range from complete to nil. Directionality of knowledge is almost always found among some alters, such that alter A knows of the doings of alter B, but B is unaware of the activities of A. It is not uncommon for some alters to have symptoms that others do not suffer. Psychophysiological differences (see Chapter 13, this volume) have been documented. Differences in handwriting and handedness, voice and vocabulary, accents and speech patterns, and even preferred languages are encountered. Their facial expressions and movement characteristics, both when neutral and affectively engaged, may show impressive and rather consistent differences (Kluft, Poteat, & Kluft, 1986). When the personalities have acquired separate wardrobes, followed different interests, pursued different forms of creative expression, their differences may be marked. When patients do not bring imagination and creativity to their alter systems, the differences may be muted and pallid in comparison.

Investigators have attempted to describe types of personalities (Coons et al., 1988; Putnam et al., 1986; Ross et al., 1989b). Unfortunately, their classification systems are not readily reconcilable. It appears that the picture of DID as the ongoing clash of polarized personality types (e.g., good girl–bad girl, upright citizen–sociopath) is hard to sustain, although such clashes, when they occur, arrest attention and at times become a concern of the forensic psychiatrist. Most patients have personalities that are named, but there may be those who are nameless or whose appellations are not proper names (i.e., "the slut," "rage," etc.). Child personalities, those who retain long periods of continuous awareness, those who claim to know about all of the others, and depressed personalities are the most frequent types enumerated (Putnam et al., 1986).

The classic host personality, which usually (over 50% of the time) presents for treatment, nearly always bears the legal name and is depressed, anxious, somewhat neurasthenic, compulsively good, masochistic, conscience-stricken, constricted hedonically, and suffers both psychophysiological symptoms and time loss and/or time distortion. While no personality types are invariably present, many are encountered quite frequently: childlike personalities (fearful, recalling traumata, or love-seeking), protectors, helpers–advisors, inner self-helpers (serene, rational, and objective helpers and advisors first described by Allison in 1974), personalities with distinct affective states, guardians of memories and secrets (and of family boundaries), memory traces (holding continuity of memory), inner persecutors (often based on identification with the aggressor), anesthetic personalities (created to block out pain), expressers of forbidden impulses (pleasurable and otherwise, such as defiant, aggressive, or antisocial), avengers (which express anger over abuses endured and may wish to redress their grievances), defenders or apologists for the abusers, those based on lost love objects and other introjections and identifications, specialized encapsulators of traumatic experiences and powerful affects, very specialized personalities, and those (often youthful) that preserve the idealized potential for happiness, growth, and the healthy expression of feelings (distorted by traumata) in others (Kluft, 1984b).

The often dramatic differences among the personalities are more an arresting epiphenomenon than the core of the condition. Characterological factors, cultural influences, imagination, intelligence, and creativity make powerful contributions to the form taken by the personalities. Most DID patients are rather muted compared to those cases incorrectly assumed to epitomize the condition (Kluft, 1985b). The personalities enact adaptational patterns and strategies that developed in the service of defense and survival. Once this pattern, which disposes of upsetting material and pressures rapidly and efficiently, is established, it may be repeated again and again to cope with both further overwhelming experiences and more mundane developmental and adaptational issues. Once the DID that developed in order to cope with intolerable childhood circumstances has achieved some degree of secondary autonomy, it becomes increasingly maladaptive.

The Personality System and the Inner World of the Personalities

Less compelling but far more crucial than their overt manifestations are their inner belief systems, cognitive processes, and complex interrelationships. The personalities may have considerable investment in their own separateness and may express a pseudo-delusional degree of conviction about their being separate and autonomous (Kluft, 1984b). While not formally psychotic, they may behave with the conviction that the actions that they take against the body or the other personalities will not affect them. Because the various alters have different memories, the information that they use to inform their behaviors is not uniform, nor are their modes of thinking identical. Hence, the several alters live in discrepant assumptive worlds, fail to function by uniform cognitive rules and processes, and manage identical data quite differently (Fine, 1988b). This contributes to the multiple reality disorder (Kluft, 1991a, 1993) referred to above.

The personalities may have quite a complex and subjectively compelling inner world. The alters comprise a system of mind, and not infrequently experience their interactions as if they were relationships among actual people. Unfortunately, these constellations often recapitulate, by direct imitation, symbolic representation, or by clear analogy, the relationships associated with the patient's alleged abuse experiences. Consequently, the sadomasochism of the abuse that generated the DID phenomenology is recapitulated in the profoundly dysfunctional relationships among the members of the alter system (Kluft, Braun, & Sachs, 1984; Brenner, 1994). Many of the clinical crises that so commonly are encountered in the treatment of DID are a direct consequence of the reenactments of traumatic scenarios within the patients' inner worlds.

The alters may have complex inner relationships, alliances, and hostilities; their experience of one another may resemble an inner family or society with its own rules and mores. They often try to influence one another. In this manner the alter ostensibly in control of the body may feel the impact of the others and battle or accede to their requests or find itself the recipient of passive influence experiences (Kluft, 1987b) that influence its actual behavior and feeling state. For example, most of the first-rank symptoms of schizophrenia described by Schneider (1959) are common indications of the impact of one alter upon another (Kluft, 1987b; Ross et al., 1990b). Recurrent command hallucinations were experienced by 82% of 28 DID patients; in each case the voice of a hostile alter was being heard within the head (Kluft, unpublished data). In the same series 100% experienced strong bursts of affect that were associated with alters that were not ostensibly in control at at the time, but which were reacting to inner or outer stimuli and flooding the alter that was "out" with their subjective experiences.

In such a manner alters can make an impact without emerging. This is a particularly common phenomenon with so-called inner persecutors, often based on identification with aggressors (either prior abusers or culturally sanctioned icons of malevolent intent; e.g., an abusive parent or the devil). Inner persecutors by their very nature require victim alters whom they intimidate, attack, dominate, and torment. This may take place in the inner world of the alters and never become manifest, or it may involve seizing executive control and disrupting and/or endangering the patient's life. Not infrequently the alter ostensibly in control will be bombarded by insults and threats and by command hallucinations urging it toward self-harm or suicide. Furthermore, motor control may be seized in "made" actions, so that the patient will feel himself flinging himself down the stairs without having willed such behavior or watch in terror as his or her hands steer an automobile toward an embankment, unable to regain control of his or her own limbs:

> The apparent behavior or subjective state of an MPD patient is often the vector of many interacting forces that are not apparent upon superficial exploration, or represent a series of small behaviors or subjective experiences that have occurred in rapid succession and stem from many different sources. (Kluft, 1991b, p. 612)

Aspects of Overtness

Several factors determine the likelihood that the inner structure of DID will become behaviorally manifest to the extent that it is easily detected. Resilience in the host alter makes overt switching less likely to occur, while the presence of contemporary stress and trauma makes it more likely. Greater frequency and length of alters' emergences make the DID more easily observed, while few and/or brief emergences keep it more covert. If the alters are cooperating, they may share contemporary memory, pass for one another, and switch smoothly and seamlessly in order to achieve shared goals. If they are in conflict without clear resolution, the picture may be dominated with the imposition of passive influence experiences and the patient may appear borderline or psychotic. Should the contention lead to more extreme swings of control, more overt switches may be observed.

Likewise, the manner in which alters influence one another also contributes to the likeliness of overtness. As noted above, inner dialogue, passive influence, and command hallucination will not lead to overt DID phenomena. Amnestic barriers, when strong, auger for the recognition of overtness, because if alters share memories, it is easy for their overt differences to be discounted because the patient will appear to have a continuous and ongoing life. If a patient has many similar alters, it is less likely that the switches and amnestic episodes will trigger a suspicion of DID.

Many alter systems are organized in such a way as to keep themselves secret and may become very skilled in covering over their DID phenomena. When alters assume control for very long periods of time, there may be no switches to observe for years on end.

A final series of determinants regards the alters' investment in their separateness and the narcissism across the alter system. The more pronounced the patient's creativity, the more likely the alters' differences will be pronounced and evident. Secondary gain and characterological features may have pronounced influences as well. (The above discussion is drawn largely from Kluft, 1991b.)

PSYCHOPHYSIOLOGICAL ASPECTS OF DID

It is intriguing indeed to encounter personalities with different handedness, different allergic responses (Braun, 1983), different responses to the same medication (Kluft, 1984b), requiring different eyeglass prescriptions and differing on objective ophthalmological measures (Miller, 1989), and demonstrating measurably different patterns of response to a given stimulus (Putnam, 1984a). Coons (1988) has reviewed the massive but primarily anecdotal literature in this area. Although there have been those who see such differences as proof of the "reality of DID," many thoughtful students of the field, preeminently Putnam (1984a), caution against such inferences. In sum, the phenomena that attract perhaps undue attention when they occur in the context of DID are actually expressions of more basic structures of the mind and processes in the brain; their exploration has implications far beyond the study of DID (see Spiegel, Bierre, & Rootenberg, 1989; Putnam, 1988).

THE NATURAL HISTORY OF DID

Kluft's (1985b) longitudinal study of 210 DID patients has established much of the natural history of DID and has shown that DID does not undergo spontaneous remission and rarely resolves in a treatment that fails to address it directly (Kluft, 1985b, 1993). DID has been demonstrated in children as young as 3 (Riley & Meade, 1988), but many children demonstrate rather vague dissociative features that gradually coalesce into precursors of DID (Fagan & McMahon, 1984; Braun & Sachs, 1985; Peterson, 1990, 1991) and progress into a fully structured DID condition (Kluft, 1984a, 1985a) that may become overt or remain clandestine. Although often there appears to be a clear relationship between the form taken by the DID and the developmental phases in which traumata occur (Putnam, 1991c), in others the dissociative response to trauma seems to stand aside from such considerations (Kluft, 1985a). Most children with DID or its precursors show many trancelike behaviors; fluctuations in abilities, age appropriateness, and moods; intermittent depression; amnesia; hallucinated voices; passive influence experiences; disavowed polarized behaviors; disavowed witnessed behaviors; may appear to be liars; show muted and attenuated signs of DID; have inconsistencies in school behavior; and appear to have other possible diagnoses (Kluft, 1984a). In addition, they may show suicidal or self-injurious behaviors, have imaginary companion phenomena when over 5 years of age, and show fluctuating physical symptoms (Putnam, cited in Kluft, 1984a). Children with DID or its precursors infrequently are invested in remaining divided; many can be treated rather rapidly (Kluft, 1986). Recently many investigators have expanded our appreciation of DID in childhood (Putnam, 1991c; Hornstein & Putnam, 1992; Peterson, 1990, 1991; Tyson, 1992).

In adolescence, the structure of DID usually becomes more complex and diverse and the personalities more invested in retaining their autonomy (Kluft, 1985b; Kluft & Schultz, 1993). Often the process of personality formation becomes a general way of coping with nontraumatic material as well, and specialized alters are formed in connection with new academic, social, and psychosexual challenges. Several patterns were noted in Kluft's series (1985b). One group of adolescent females appeared quite chaotic. Promiscuity, drug use, somatoform complaints, and self-injury were not uncommon. Three quarters of them switched alters quite floridly, but denied this. They usually were diagnosed as impulsive, histrionic, ictal, schizophrenic, borderline, or a combination. More recently, rapid-cycling bipolar disorder has been included in this differential. Many of these adolescents owed their confusing manifest appearance to the rapid switching of alters and to the constant inner bombardment (passive influence) of the personality ostensibly in control by the other alters. Another group of the female adolescents had a more withdrawn presentation. They had either a residual childlike form of DID or were evolving toward the classic adult presentation of a depressed and neurasthenic host with amnesias, headaches, and disremembered out-of-character behaviors. They usually were diagnosed with affective disorders, somatoform complaints, and anxiety disorders.

Adolescent males included subgroups whose confrontation with the law or school authorities were due to the actions of aggressive alters, a depressed subgroup not unlike the second subgroup of females, and a small number of individuals whose homosexual concerns dominated their presentations. The aggressive subgroup often received psychotic diagnoses on the basis of their disorganized behaviors and hallucinations, which often had a command quality.

Older adults with DID sometimes retain a rather classic presentation and simply had never been diagnosed earlier in life. Others, however, demonstrate the increased dominance of one alter over time, the others making their presence known by passive influence intrusions. Also, in many patients, the amnestic barriers begin to fray. Many have been thought to have involutional disorders, because as the barriers across the alters became more porous with age, unpleasant memories, dysphoric affects, and the overheard voices of other alters flooded the presenting personality (Kluft, 1985b).

Although approximately 20% of DID patients manifest classic phenomena over a sustained period of time, and 20% are so expert at dissimulation, so infrequent in their switching, or so covert that they rarely show diagnosable signs of DID, the remaining 60% have periods in which their psychopathology is intrusive or symptomatic and periods (sometimes a year or more) in which it is quiescent, suppressed, or readily disavowed. Hence, 80% of a series of patients known to have DSM-III DID had only certain "windows of diagnosability" during which their circumstances could be recognized with ease by an alert clinician (Kluft, 1985b,

1987c). At other times, it would have been necessary to suspect or infer their diagnosis from history or to pursue their diagnosis with systematic inquiries.

Only approximately 10% of DID patients (6% of adults and a small minority of adolescents) are exhibitionistic about their condition; in the main DID is, in Gutheil's words, "a pathology of hiddenness" (Kluft, 1985b). DID patients may show a degree of impairment that ranges from minimal to profound. Their degree of impairment may appear to fluctuate widely.

EPIDEMIOLOGY

In the mid-1980s, Coons (1984) and Worrall (unpublished data) both estimated the prevalence of DID at 1:10,000 population by comparing known cases to the population base from which they were drawn. Bliss and Jeppson (1985) screened their practices (a skewed sample) and calculated that 10% or more of their patients might suffer DID. From new cases discovered in sequential admissions to a general hospital psychiatric unit, Kluft (unpublished data) estimated 0.5–2% suffered DID. These crude efforts indicated that although its incidence and prevalence were uncertain, DID was far from rare.

More recently, three systematic studies undertaken to assess the prevalence of DID in clinical populations have demonstrated that previously undiagnosed DID patients can be identified in large number and with relative ease among hospitalized psychiatric inpatients. Ross, Anderson, Fleischer, and Norton (1991b) screened a year's sequential admissions to a university hospital in Canada, using the Dissociative Experiences Scale (DES) (Bernstein & Putnam, 1986). They excluded known DID cases and patients with organicity and followed up patients with suggestive scores with the Dissociative Disorders Interview Schedule (DDIS) (Ross, 1989), a structured diagnostic interview: 3.3% of the patients had previously unsuspected DID. Saxe et al. (1993) used a similar methodology to screen all patients in a Harvard teaching psychiatric hospital and found 4% of the patients suffered undiagnosed DID. Boon and Draijer (1993a) describe the screening of psychiatric inpatients in a Dutch teaching hospital using Dutch versions of the DES and the SCID-D (Steinberg, 1993) and found 5% of the patients suffered previously undiagnosed DID. Unpublished research reports have found similar percentages in Norwegian, German, and Turkish cohorts. Ross has done a number of studies in other clinical populations. For example, Ross et al. (1992b) found 14% of 100 adults with chemical dependency suffered DID. Studies of this nature suggest that large numbers of DID patients remain undiagnosed within psychiatric patient populations.

In nonclinical settings, Ross, Joshi, and Currie (1991c) found that 5–10% of the general population of a Canadian city had screening scores suggestive of a dissociative disorder, and in follow-up interviews (Ross, 1991) discovered 11.2% had a diagnosable dissociative disorder and 3.1% had DID. However, on follow-up Ross found that only 1.3% had clinical DID; the remainder (1.8%) were false positives. Using the Dissociative Questionnaire (DIS-Q), Vanderlinden, Van Dyck, Vandereycken, and Vertommen (1991) found that 3% of their Belgian and Dutch sample scored in the range of dissociative disorder patients and 1% scored as high as DID patients. However, no follow-up interviews were undertaken and the meaning of these findings is uncertain.

In studies completed to date, the majority of the identified patients are females: Bliss (1980), 100%; Putnam et al. (1986), 92%; Coons et al. (1988), 92%; Schultz et al. (1989), 90%; and Ross et al. (1989b), 87.7%. Their average age at diagnosis is over 30. There is widespread belief that many males with DID enter the legal rather than the psychiatric system and go unrecognized. Kluft (1985b) found that the majority of male adolescents with DID encounter difficulties with the authorities. Bliss (1986) found a high incidence of dissociative disorders among convicted sex offenders. Also, the majority of childhood DID cases reported to date are male. Taken as a whole, these findings suggest that as males with DID mature, certain aspects of their behavior may lead to their evading clinical detection, or that they may enter health care delivery systems in which the diagnosis of DID is less likely to be entertained. The nearly 9:1 female to male ratio noted above probably misrepresents the true gender distribution of DID. Recent efforts to study males with DID are demonstrating that their presentations are not that dissimilar to those of female patients (Loewenstein & Putnam, 1990; Ross & Norton, 1989) and may raise the index of suspicion for DID in those working with male populations.

Taken as a whole and placed in the context of many recent reports of the discovery of DID in more and more nations, it is clear that these studies and reports demonstrate that DID is a widespread and not uncommon condition. It appears to be a common adaptation to overwhelming childhood events and circumstances.

The occurrence of DID in several generations of the same family and in sibships has been reported (e.g., Braun, 1985; Coons, 1985; Kluft, 1984a, 1985a). In some cases it has been possible to ascertain and document an abuse history across several generations in these families. It appears that when a child has a parent modeling DID behavior, it may require less than the usual amount of abuse in order for the child to make a DID adaptation.

THE ETIOLOGY OF DID

The Role of Trauma in Inducing Dissociation

Dissociative disorders commonly are associated with substantial psychological distress or traumatic experiences (Putnam, 1985; Spiegel, 1991; Spiegel & Cardena, 1991). As Spiegel (1991, p. 261) has observed:

> Dissociative defenses, which allow individuals to compartmentalize perceptions an memories, seem to serve a dual function. They help victims separate themselves from the full impact of physical trauma while it is occurring, and, by the same token, they may delay the necessary working through and putting into perspective of these traumatic experiences after they have occurred. They help the trauma victim maintain a sense of control during an episode of physical helplessness, but then become a mechanism by which the individual feels psychologically helpless once he or she has regained physical control.

Empirical studies of dissociation following upon documented trauma in nonpatient populations have bolstered the strength of such observations (e.g., Kooper, Classen, & Spiegel, 1994).

Terr (1991) has described profiles of two types of childhood traumatizations with regard to memory. Type I follows upon the child's having experienced a single discrete traumatic event. Memory of the event is full, detailed, and "etched in." Type II occurs in the aftermath of long-standing exposure to repeated untoward events. Amnesia, self-anesthesia, and distancing with autohypnotic defenses is common, with frequent impairment of memory. Although these differentiations are not complete in the author's experience, they speak to an important distinction.

Combining the Spiegel and Terr insights, it is possible to understand that repetitive traumatizations will lead to the evoking of dissociative defenses in a manner that affects memory. Furthermore, traumatization leads to lesions of identity (Putnam, 1990). Lesions of identity and memory are the main stigmata of DID (Nemiah, 1980).

Trauma Histories Given by DID Patients

Both anecdotal reports and systematic surveys show that DID patients are universally the victims of overwhelming childhood experiences. Putnam et al. (1986) found that 97 of 100 DID patients reported having been abused as children. Interestingly, the 3% who did not were also the patients that had most recently entered treatment (Putnam, personal communication, 1986). Eighty-three percent reported sexual abuse and 68% reported incest. Repeated physical abuse was reported by 75%, 68% reported both sexual and physical abuse, and 45% stated that they had witnessed a violent death. Over 60% described severe neglect.

Ross et al. (1989b) studied 236 DID patients, claiming evidence that 88.5% had been either sexually or physically abused, with some uncertainty about whether the remainder had been abused: 74.9% alleged physical abuse, and 11.1% were unsure about this; 79.2% alleged sexual abuse, and 8.1% were uncertain as to whether this had occurred. Coons et al., (1988) found that 96% of 50 DID patients alleged abuse: 68% sexual abuse, 60% physical abuse, and 22% neglect. Schultz et al. (1989) surveyed the therapists of 355 DID patients: 86% of the patients reported sexual abuse, 82% physical abuse, and 98% one or both. Ross et al. (1990a) studied 102 structured interviews of DID patients and found that 90.2% reported sexual abuse, 82.4% physical abuse, and 95.1% one or the other.

Boon and Draijer's (1993a) studied 82 Dutch DID patients in depth and found that 65.1% reported physical and 60.3% sexual abuse, with a high prevalence of other overwhelming experiences. They believed that amnesia for childhood events led to their lower figures, because unlike most of the other investigators, they were studying a population that included many patients referred for diagnostic study whose treatments had not begun.

Although these studies did not document the abuse allegations, it is significant that Bliss (1984) documented some of the allegations of 12 of 13 DID patients. Coons and Milstein (1986) could document some allegations in 85% of a series of 20 DID patients. Dell and Eisenhower (1990) could get independent corroboration from 73% of their adolescents with DID. Coons (1994a) was able to find documentation of the abuse of 95% of 21 children and adolescents with DID and allied forms of DDNOS. Hornstein and Putnam (1992) described finding documentation of abuse in 95.3% of 64 children and adolescents with DID and allied forms of DDNOS. Kluft (1984a) documented the abuse allegations of seven of eight childhood DID patients, and Fagan and McMahon (1984) did so for the majority of their cases.

Currently it is fashionable to dispute the allegations of those who allege childhood traumatization, especially those that involve incest; here, space limitations preclude a review of this massive and contentious field. Suffice it to say that there is excellent documentation of the abuse suffered by children and adolescents with DID and excellent reason to believe that adults with DID have been traumatized. However, one should approach the precise details of the accounts of adult patients with some caution. Kluft (1984c) pointed out that in the allegations of DID patients one might encounter excellent memory, fantasy and dream material mistaken for reality, misrepresentation, contamination, and confabulation. More recently, Kluft (1994) has spoken of the metamorphosis of the childhood DID condition into the adult form of the disorder and noted the reworking and elaboration of the initial memories in that context. Consequently, it is reasonable to appreciate that DID is a complex and chronic posttraumatic condition (Loewenstein, 1991), but to bear in mind that the account that the DID patient gives of his or her traumatization may include elements of inaccuracy and distortion (Kluft, 1994, in press a,b).

Various Models of DID

A number of models have been proposed to explain and explore DID (Kluft, in press b). These are: (1) supernatural/transpersonal, (2) psychological, (3) sociological, (4) illegitimate (role-playing/malingering/iatrogenesis/social-psychological), (5) trance state/autohypnotic, (6) split brain/hemispheric laterality, (7) temporal lobe/partial complex seizure/kindling, (8) behavioral states of consciousness, (9) neural network/information processing, (10) neodissociation/ego state, and (11) basic affects (which has much in common with models 8 and 9). No one of these models precludes the operations of the other and none explains rather than illustrates a possible mechanism for the formation of DID. Space precludes any more than a cursory commentary on each.

1. Supernatural/transpersonal models hold that the alters are demons, lingering spirits, the souls of the departed, and so forth. They have a venerable history because DID is the secular expression of the form and structure of a variety of endemic possession syndromes, including the Judeo-Christian form (Ellenberger, 1970; Kluft, 1991a). Although discounted by mainstream professionals, these ideas were valued by Allison (1974, 1978) and have been the subject of a recent book (Freisen, 1991) valued by religiously oriented mental health professionals. The reader should note that recent studies (Bowman, 1993; Fraser, 1993) demonstrate that interventions of an exorcistic nature can have deleterious effects in DID patients.

2. Psychological models have been plentiful, but none had proven consistent with all known cases of DID (Kluft, 1984c, 1985b). It is impossible to summarize them succinctly. Loewenstein and Ross (1992) recently reviewed alternative psychoanalytic contributions. Many authors have thought that separation and separation-individuation concerns may form a substrate for later responses to trauma. Marmer (1980, 1991) speculates that with the failure of maternal and transitional objects, a traumatized child may take an aspect of self as self-object and initiate the experience of taking and perceiving self as object. More recently, Barach (1991) and

Liotti (1992) have offered clinical and research-based arguments that many DID concerns are consistent with the theories of Bowlby. It seems likely that the various psychological models that have been advanced will continue to explain why some DID patients behave as they do, but that the condition as a whole will elude a simple formulation.

Related to the psychological model are the many speculations that DID is a subtype of borderline personality disorder. Although many DID patients manifest borderline phenomenology, the two conditions can be distinguished, and borderline phenomena and dynamics are not intrinsic to DID (Armstrong, 1991, 1994; Boon & Drajier, 1993b; Horevitz & Braun, 1984; Kluft, 1991a).

3. Sociological models hold that dissociative phenomena may be an attempt to live, at different times, by different systems of values or in a manner that compensates for controls imposed on certain individuals or groups of individuals in various societies. This certainly is an attractive model for certain culture-bound syndromes in which the sufferer is allowed to manifest, in a dissociated state, forms of behavior proscribed for them in a rigid culture. While politically attractive to the advocates of disenfranchised persons, it cannot explain the majority of DID phenomena.

4. The illegitimate (role-playing/malingering/iatrogenesis/social-psychological) model holds that DID is not a naturalistically occurring condition, but emerges in the context of the patient's enacting a role he or she has come to understand will have beneficial consequences and/or be pleasing to someone who is encouraging such behaviors and beliefs. Hence the disorder is instigated and maintained by external contingencies and/or private motivations. Advocates of this perspective (Spanos, 1986; Spanos, Weekes, & Bertrand, 1985; Spanos, Weekes, Menary, & Bertrand, 1986; Merskey, 1992; McHugh, 1993) have been emphatic in their opinions, but have failed to prove their point. Although it is quite easy to create many of the manifestations of DID on a transient basis, the creation of the full clinical picture of DID over a sustained period of time has yet to be demonstrated. Merskey (1992) and McHugh (1993) offer their opinions on the basis of their opinions, which have been used to deny the legitimacy of DID phenomena in the first place. Their arguments are completely circular and entitle them to define any DID they encounter as iatrogenic or factitious a priori. Thereafter they allege antecedent events must have created them. Since DID cannot be legitimate, it must be artifactual, and then it is merely a matter of assigning blame for the initiation and perpetuation of the clinical picture. In the absence of a single proven case of iatrogenic DID, such allegations must be regarded with caution. However, factitious DID is not unknown and must be considered (Coons, 1994b; Kluft, 1995a). Kluft (1982, 1995b) has maintained that although iatrogenesis has not been demonstrated to cause DID, it has shown the capacity to worsen it. Kluft (1995a) argues that although the condition occurs naturalistically, in a given patient particular manifestations may be due to iatrogenesis, factitious factors, social-psychological pressures, and information absorbed from society and the media. He observes that some DID patients are not above exacting secondary gain from their illnesses, and that a therapist's fascination or ineptitude may exacerbate the baseline condition. It is helpful to bear in mind that although high hypnotizable control subjects feigning DID can show psychophysiological differences across their enacted alters, these

changes differed from the changes across alters in naturalistic DID (Putnam, Zahn, & Post, 1990).

5. Trance state/autohypnotic models are attractive because a body of research demonstrates the high hypnotizability of DID patients (Bliss, 1984; Frischholz, 1985). Bliss (1986), following the venerable hypotheses of Freud's collaborator Josef Breuer (Breuer & Freud, 1893-95), has described DID as a disorder created by the unwitting abuse of autohypnosis. Although any comprehensive model must account for the high hypnotizability of DID patients, this model does not account for the full range of DID phenomenology. In that connection, recall the Putnam et al. (1990) findings cited above.

6. Split brain/hemispheric laterality models are intellectually intriguing, but few data support them. At this point, they are no more than a potential heuristic.

7. Temporal lobe/partial complex seizure/kindling models emerged in the context of two thought-provoking articles (Schenk & Bear, 1981; Mesulam, 1981) that proposed that DID dissociative phenomena were associated with temporal lobe/partial complex seizure and their interictal manifestations. They briefly achieved a notoriety disproportionate with the strength of the data adduced to support them. Subsequent studies have failed to demonstrate a convincing correlation and have not found either epilepsy among DID patients or DID phenomena in partial complex or generalized seizure epileptics with a frequency that would suggest a strong connection (Coons et al., 1988; Devinsky, Putnam, Grafman, Bramfield, & Theodore, 1989; Loewenstein & Putnam, 1988).

8. Behavioral states of consciousness models are very powerful because they are consistent with what is known about the development of states of mind and self-structures, draw on well-studied behavioral state phenomena in infants, and are congruent with the psychophysiological studies of DID to date. Putnam (1988) has discussed this model in depth, and Braun (1984) has authored a related study. Putnam (1991b) has made this model the basis of one of the major definitions of alter personalities: "the alter personalities represent discrete behavioral states of consciousness with personality state-specific encoding of certain types of memory, behavior, and psychophysiology" (p. 499). This model is a useful heuristic and hypotheses drawn from it often are researchable.

9. Neural network/information-processing models are relatively new contenders (Andorfer, 1985; Li & Spiegel, 1992; Yates & Nasby, 1993). They offer paradigms by which the alters can be understood as related to the creation and activation of nodes in a particular neural network. The DID patient's executive consciousness at a given point in time would consist of those nodes activated above threshold at that particular moment. Stimulation and inhibition phenomena can be used to model aspects of DID structures and functions. Although in their infancy, such models have demonstrated their potential to offer hypothetical explanations for complex DID phenomena bypassed by other theory builders, and they deserve the most careful consideration in future research and theory building.

10. Neodissociation/ego state models assume that the mind may have several simultaneously ongoing and autonomous centers of cognitive activity and/or that the mind is at best a plurality of selves that, when congruent, leaves humans with the subjective illusion of unity, but when in conflict or lacking congruence and synchrony, give rise to the experience of several alternative self-structures at work

with different characteristics and the ability to influence ongoing behavior. Multiplicity, then, is a norm and pathological multiplicity occurs when the boundaries across these states or processes are sufficient to impede normal "commerce," so that parts may achieve full or partial control rather than participating in a process consistent with subjective and behavioral unity (Beahrs, 1982; Hilgard, 1986; Watkins & Watkins, 1979). These models are consistent with many laboratory and clinical findings and must be considered in any definitive conceptualization.

11. The basic affects model put forth by Nathanson (in press) applies the affect theories of the late Sylvan Tomkins and Nathanson's (1992) exegesis of them to DID. Nathanson speculates that some personalities may be organized around different basic affects and/or affect scripts. His work on shame scripts demonstrates that this model may be able to bridge the psychological and psychophysiological dimensions of DID.

In summary, while most of the above models deserve further study, an all-encompassing model will have to encompass models 5, 8, 9, 10, and possibly 11, and address 2. In any individual case, models 2 and 4 will require detailed attention.

A Pragmatic Clinical Model and Theory of DID

The etiology of DID and models for its understanding have been studied (Braun, 1984; Braun & Sachs, 1985; Kluft, 1984b; Putnam, 1989; Stern, 1984). The four-factor theory (Kluft, 1984b) encompasses most of the observations in the literature. It holds that the person who will develop DID will have (1) the capacity to dissociate, which becomes mobilized for defensive purposes in the face of (2) life experiences that traumatically overwhelm the nondissociative defenses and adaptational capacities of the child's ego; furthermore, (3) shaping influences and available substrates will determine the form taken by the dissociative defenses in the process of alter formation. Although the conjunction of these three factors is quite common and many overwhelmed children have dissociative episodes or briefly show dissociative signs, those who will develop DID also experience (4) the inadequate provision of stimulus barriers, soothing, and restorative experiences by significant others. The dissociative defenses continue to serve a purpose, and the person must fall back on aspects of her or himself to provide necessary functions and relationships.

Factor 1, dissociation potential, is the biological rather than the compliance-suggestibility component of hypnotizability (Spiegel & Spiegel, 1987). DID patients, when stable and cooperative enough for such testing, are highly hypnotizable on standard instruments (Bliss, 1984; Frischholz, 1985). It has been reported that abused populations score more highly than controls on measurements of hypnotizability and/or dissociation. High hypnotizability is present in 8-12% of the population; hypnotizability in general is highest in late childhood (see discussion in Kluft, 1986).

Overwhelming experiences, factor 2, have been discussed above. As noted by Putnam et al. (1986), 97% of North American DID patients allege histories of child abuse. The majority allege sexual abuse, usually incestuous. Child abuse is all too common, and sexual abuse may affect over one third of American women. Other common factors in dissociation were discussed by Kluft (1984c, 1986). Some who will develop DID have experienced the death or loss of significant others in childhood, witnessed deaths or the deliberate destruction of a significant other, or been exposed to dead bodies (especially being forced to touch or kiss them). Exposure to the deaths of others in the course of war, accidents, and various disasters may prove overwhelming, as may severe threats to one's survival or bodily integrity, such as in severe sustained pain, debilitating illness, or a near-death experience. Cultural dislocation, brainwashing by embattled parents, being treated as if one were a different gender, and excessive exposure to family chaos may prove decisive. Some factors seem to lower the child's defenses and render subsequent events more traumatic. These include illness and pain, unintentional physical trauma, fatigue, separation-individuation complications, and having congenital anomalies, with narcissistic hurts and body ego disturbances.

DID patients often give unsettling histories of severe and bizarre abuse experiences. Data relevant to the reality of the experiences of DID patients and the vicissitudes of memory have been discussed earlier. Although it often is possible to document allegations, often there are no surviving records or cooperative witnesses. Few abusers indict themselves by confession. Herman and Schatzow (1987) found that 74% of their 53 non-DID subjects were able to get confirmation of their memories of incest, 9% got suggestive but not definitive information, and most of the remainder actually did not pursue the inquires. It is of note that those whose abuse was most violent were most likely to have had amnesia for it prior to treatment. At this point in time it appears likely that the DID patient who alleges abuse was indeed abused, but that the precise details of the recollection are subject to all of the difficulties associated with autobiographic memory (see Kluft, 1984c, p. 14).

Factor 3, shaping influences, notes that there are many unique configurations of intrapsychic structures and dynamics and environmental influences that may converge to give rise to the phenomenological expression of DID. There are many naturally occurring phenomena that may serve as the substrates for alter formation and many environmental factors that play a role as well. These include inherent mechanisms and potentials for dividedness that may be enlisted in the presence of factors 1 and 2: dissociation per se, autohypnosis, the existence and operations of multiple systems of cognition and memory (e.g., the hidden observer phenomenon described by Hilgard, 1986), ego state phenomena (Watkins & Watkins, 1979), state- and mood-dependent memory (Bower, 1981), the many developmental lines described in the psychoanalytic literature, imaginary companionship, the processes of introjection, internalization and identification, state phenomena, protoaffect structures, and others.

Extrinsic influences play roles as well, especially those of one's culture. Those developing DID today often have alters based on television characters, an event unthinkable 50 years before. Factors of interest in childhood may be the encouragement of role-playing and acting by parents, contradictory parental demands and reinforcement systems, numerous caretakers, and identification with a DID parent among others. Certainly representations in the media and the techniques of the therapist may influence the patient's phenomenology somewhat.

The absence of soothing and restorative experiences, factor 4, relates to observations that many children with DID (Kluft, 1984a, 1985a) or incipient dissociative features (Fagan & McMahon, 1984) simply stop manifesting them when they are protected from further traumatization. If children are not subjected to conditions under which their nascent DID remains adaptive, in a substantial minority of cases there is a spontaneous remission, while in others there usually is a rapid response to treatment (Kluft, 1986).

The four-factor theory is consistent with clinical experience, but is less than satisfactory in addressing the issues raised by the psychophysiological differences across the alters (see Putnam, 1989).

COMORBIDITY

Findings Based on Phenomena at Presentation: Apparent Comorbidity

DID is usually a polysymptomatic and pleiomorphic condition, varying widely over its clinical course even within a single patient. Putnam, Loewenstein, Silberman, and Post (1984) suggest that it is best understood as a superordinate diagnosis under which a vast array of symptomatology suggestive of other diagnostic entities may be subsumed. Several investigators have described the psychopathology concomitant with DID (Bliss, 1980, 1986; Coons et al., 1988; Horevitz & Braun, 1984; Putnam et al., 1986; Ross et al., 1989b). Unfortunately, their classifications and definitions were not uniform. Therefore, although it is possible to discuss the association of certain symptoms with DID, it is far more difficult to make statements regarding actual comorbidity.

Combining data from the above sources, DID patients demonstrate anxiety symptoms (psychophysiological, 100%; phobic, 60%; panic attacks, 55%; obsessive-compulsive, 35%), affective symptoms (depressive, 90%; "highs," 15-73%), allied dissociative symptoms (amnesias, 57-100%; fugues, 48-60%; depersonalization, 38%), somatoform symptoms (all, 90%; conversion, 60%), sexual dysfunctions (60-84%), suicide attempts (60-68%), self-mutilation (34%), psychoactive substance abuse (40-45%), eating disorders (16-40%), sleep disturbance (65%), symptoms suggestive of schizophrenia (depending on symptoms, 35-73%), symptoms of PTSD (70-85%), and the stigmata of borderline personality disorder (70%).

Since the first publication of this compilation (Kluft, 1991a), a number of authorities have taken issue with the statistics, claiming that their experience indicates that certain symptoms were highly underrepresented. This criticism is no doubt correct, because certain authors reported on some symptoms and not others, and because the sources cited rarely stated their criteria for reporting. The frequency of self-mutilation is considered understated. The percentages for amnesia reflect more initial presentations than the complete symptom picture. Likewise, the low percentage for depersonalization is an artifact of the lack of systematic exploration for this symptom until quite recently.

Affective symptoms, especially depressive, are experienced by 90% or more of DID patients. However, it remains uncertain whether they suffer affective disorders, posttraumatic sequelae, the despair, despondency, and hopelessness of human misery, or combinations of the above. Many of their depressive symptoms clearly are related to the experience of rejection and guilt over responsibility they attribute to themselves. Research at the author's program is underway to explore the relationship of affective disorders and dissociative disorders.

Symptoms of PTSD often occur in DID. The conditions have similar etiologies; it is arguable that DID is a PTSD variant (e.g., Braun, 1986). Many clinicians hold that PTSD is present in 85-95% of DID patients; Loewenstein (1991) sees PTSD symptoms as a nearly universal in DID cohorts. It is not uncommon for the exploration of PTSD phenomena to lead to the DID diagnosis. As traumatic material emerges in the treatment of DID, not infrequently a delayed PTSD picture is precipitated as the patient must contend with long-dissociated traumata.

Many phenomena are shared by DID and schizophrenia, as noted above. In the modern era the coexistence of DID and schizophrenia has not yet been reported, although occasionally (in 1-2% of hospitalized cases) a coexistent schizoaffective disorder is diagnosed (Kluft, Fink, Brenner, & Fine, unpublished data).

The phenomena of borderline personality disorder (BPD) commonly co-occur with DID. DID has been considered a BPD variant, but many DID patients are without signs of BPD. Horevitz and Braun (1984) and Schultz, Kluft, and Braun (unpublished data) found that 70% of DID patients satisfied DSM-III criteria for BPD, but Horevitz and Braun (1984) found that DID and BPD were separate conditions. Those who satisfied criteria for both disorders had a far lower level of function and were more distressed. More recently Armstrong and Loewenstein (1990) and Armstrong (1991) have demonstrated that DID and BPD can be differentiated with a battery of psychological tests. Armstrong (unpublished data) found that of DID patients who appeared to have BPD as well, only 1-2% were truly BPD as well. Fink and Golinkoff (1990) also demonstrated distinguishing between DID and BPD. Boon and Draijer (1993b) were able to make a clear distinction between the two conditions by using very valid and reliable instruments.

The DID-BPD interface is quite complex. First, because BPD patients are a highly abused population, many could have a posttraumatic condition like DID. Second, Solomon and Solomon (1982) demonstrated that the core phenomena of DID led to the appearance of BPD rather than to an identical condition; i.e., DID generates a phenocopy of BPD rather than coexisting with true BPD in many instances. Third, Schultz, Kluft, and Braun (unpublished data) found that coexistent BPD features did not alter the frequency with which DID patients achieved and sustained integration, which is counterexpectational if true BPD were present. Fourth, Kluft (1991a, unpublished data) found that of treatment-adherent patients who appear to have both DID and BPD, one third rapidly ceased to show BPD features once they settled into treatment, one third lost their apparent BPD as their DID resolved, and one third retained BPD features even after integration. He concluded that DID generates a phenocopy of BPD, and that only a minority of DID patients have true BPD.

With regard to BPD and DID, often one's philosophy of diagnosis will determine whether one will decide whether a DID patient is BPD. The pure phenomenologist will be likely to diagnose both if their phenomena are present, regardless of how those phenomena came to be manifested. Conversely, the dynamicist may be inclined to disregard the surface phenomena and grapple with whether the BPD is an epiphenomenon of the DID, discarding the BPD if he or she determines that to be the source of the BPD phenomena. The author's clinical rule of thumb is that if most or all of the alters demonstrate BPD phenomena themselves, he is inclined to make both diagnoses. When the BPD phenomena emerge from the chaos of the alters and their interactions, he is inclined to omit the BPD diagnosis.

Related Findings

Ross (1989) has explored findings in DID patients and reported that as a group they are likely to believe in psychic experiences and phenomena such as extrasensory perception. These types of experiences have not received serious study in the mainstream of the mental health sciences. Kluft (1995b) has studied the suicidality of DID patients, and concluded that as a group they are among the most suicidal of all patient populations.

CONCLUSION

The study of DID has accelerated over the last 15 years. Many major discoveries have been made. Numerous advances have been achieved in understanding its phenomenology and etiology and in improving its diagnosis and treatment. At present, DID is very much in the mainstream of the American mental health professions and sciences, notwithstanding the ambivalence of its reception. Despite this progress, our present state of knowledge is only the prelude to further exciting advances.

REFERENCES

Adityanjee, Raju, G. S. P., & Khandelwal, S. K. (1989). Current status of multiple personality disorder in India. *American Journal of Psychiatry, 146,* 1607-1610.

Allison, R. B. (1974). A new treatment approach for multiple personalities. *American Journal of Clinical Hypnosis, 17,* 15-32.

Allison, R. B. (1978). A rational psychotherapy plan for multiplicity. *Svensk Tidskrift fur Hypnos, 3-4,* 9-16.

American Psychiatric Association (1980). *Diagnostic and statistical manual of mental disorders* (3rd ed.). Washington, DC: Author.

American Psychiatric Association (1987). *Diagnostic and statistical manual of mental disorders* (3rd ed., rev.). Washington, DC: Author.

American Psychiatric Association (1994). *Diagnostic and statistical manual of mental disorders* (4th ed.). Washington, DC: Author.

Armstrong, J. G. (1991). The psychological organization of multiple personality disordered patients as revealed in psychological testing. *Psychiatric Clinics of North America, 14,* 533-546.

Armstrong, J. G. (1995). Reflections on multiple personality disorder as a developmentally complex phenomenon. *Psychoanalytic Study of the Child, 49,* 349-364.

Armstrong, J. G., & Loewenstein, R. J. (1990). Characteristics of patients with multiple personality and dissociative disorders or psychological testing. *Journal of Nervous and Mental Disease, 178,* 448-454.

Andorfer, J. C. (1985). Multiple personality in the human information-processor: A case history and theoretical formulation. *Journal of Clinical Psychology, 41,* 309-324.

Barach, P. M. M. (1991). Multiple personality disorder as an attachment disorder. *Dissociation, 4,* 117-123.

Beahrs, J. O. (1982). *Unity and multiplicity: Multilevel consciousness of self in hypnosis, multiple personality, and normalcy*. New York: Brunner/Mazel.
Bernstein, E. M., & Putnam, F. W. (1986). Development, reliability, and validity of a dissociation scale. *Journal of Nervous and Mental Disease, 174*, 727-734.
Bliss, E. L. (1980). Multiple personalies: A report of 14 cases with implications for schizophrenia and hysteria. *Archives of General Psychiatry, 37*, 1388-1397.
Bliss, E. L. (1984). Spontaneous self-hypnosis in multiple personality disorder. *Psychiatric Clinics of North America, 14*, 135-148.
Bliss, E. L. (1986). *Multiple personality, allied disorders and hypnosis*. New York: Oxford.
Bliss, E. L., & Jeppson, E. A. (1985). Prevalence of multiple personality among inpatients and outpatients. *American Journal of Psychiatry, 142*, 250-251.
Boon, S., & Draijer, N. (1993a). *Multiple personality disorder in the Netherlands: A study on reliability and validity of the diagnosis*. Amsterdam: Swets & Zeitlinger.
Boon, S., & Draijer, N. (1993b). The differentiation of patients with MPD or DDNOS from patients with a cluster B personality disorder. *Dissociation, 6*, 126-135.
Bower, G. H. (1981). Mood and memory. *American Psychologist, 36*, 129-148.
Bowman, E. (1993). Clinical and spiritual effects of exorcism in fifteen patients with multiple personality disorder. *Dissociation, 6*, 222-238.
Braun, B. G. (1983). Psychophysiologic phenomena in multiple personality and hypnosis. *American Journal of Clinical Hypnosis, 26*, 124-137.
Braun, B. G. (1984). Toward a theory of multiple personality and other dissociative phenomena. *Psychiatric Clinics of North America, 7*, 171-193.
Braun, B. G. (1985). The transgenerational incidence of dissociation and multiple personality disorder: A preliminary report. In R. P. Kluft (Ed.), *Childhood antecedents of multiple personality* (pp. 127-150). Washington, DC: American Psychiatric Press.
Braun, B. G. (1986). Issues in the psychotherapy of multiple personality. In B. G. Braun (Ed.), *Treatment of multiple personality disorder* (pp. 1-28). Washington, DC: American Psychiatric Press.
Braun, B. G., & Sachs, R. G. (1985). The development of multiple personality disorder: Predisposing, precipitating, and perpetuating factors. In R. P. Kluft (Ed.), *Childhood antecedents of multiple personality* (pp. 36-54). Washington, DC: American Psychiatric Press.
Brenner, I. (1994). The dissociative character. *Journal of the American Psychoanalytic Association, 42*, 819-846.
Breuer, J., & Freud, S. (1893-95). Studies on hysteria. In J. Strachey (Ed. & Trans.), *The standard edition of the complete psychological works of Sigmund Freud* (vol. 2, pp. 1-335). London: Hogarth.
Carlson, E. T. (1981). The history of multiple personality in the United States (I): The beginnings. *American Journal of Psychiatry, 138*, 666-668.
Coons, P. M. (1984). The differential diagnosis of multiple personality. *Psychiatric Clinics of North America, 12*, 51-67.
Coons, P. M. (1985). Children of parents with multiple personality disorder. In R. P. Kluft (Ed.), *Childhood antecedents of multiple personality* (pp. 151-166). Washington, DC: American Psychiatric Press.
Coons, P. M. (1988). Psychophysiologic aspects of multiple personality disorder: A review. *Dissociation, 1*(1), 47-53.
Coons, P. M. (1992). Dissociative disorders not otherwise specified: A clinical investigation of 50 cases with suggestions for typology and treatment. *Dissociation, 5*, 187-195.
Coons, P. M. (1994). Confirmation of childhood abuse in child and adolescent cases of multiple personality disorder and dissociative disorder not otherwise specified. *Journal of Nervous and Mental Disease, 182*, 461-464.
Coons, P. M., & Milstein, V. (1994). Factitious or malingered multiple personality disorder. *Dissociation, 7*, 81-85.
Coons, P. M., & Milstein, V. (1986). Psychosexual disturbances in multiple personality. *Journal of Nervous and Mental Disease, 47*, 106-110.
Coons, P. M., Bowman, E. S., & Milstein, V. (1988). Multiple personality disorder: A clinical investigation of 50 cases. *Journal of Nervous and Mental Disease, 17*, 519-527.
Coons, P. M., Bowman, E. S., Kluft, R. P., & Milstein, V. (1991). The cross-cultural occurrence of MPD: Additional cases from a recent survey. *Dissociation, 4*, 124-128.

Dell, P. F., & Eisenhower, J. W. (1990). Adolescent multiple personality disorder: A preliminary study of eleven cases. *Journal of the American Academy of Child and Adolescent Psychiatry, 29*, 359-366.

Devinsky, O., Putnam, F. W., Grafman, J., Bramfleld, E., & Theodore, W. H. (1989). Dissociative states and epilepsy. *Neurology, 39*, 835-840.

Ellenberger, H. F. (1970). *The discovery of the unconscious*. New York: Basic Books.

Fagan, J., & McMahon, P. P. (1984). Incipient multiple personality in children. *Journal of Nervous and Mental Disease, 172*, 26-36.

Fahy, T. A. (1988). The diagnosis of multiple personality: A critical review. *British Journal of Psychiatry, 153*, 597-606.

Fine, C. G. (1988a). The work of Antoine Despine: The first scientific report on the diagnosis of a child with multiple personality disorder. *American Journal of Clinical Hypnosis, 31*, 33-39.

Fine, C. G. (1988b). Thought on the cognitive perceptual substrates of multiple personality disorder. *Dissociation, 1*(4), 5-10.

Fink, D., & Golinkoff, M. (1990). Multiple personality disorder, borderline personality disorder, and schizophrenia: A comparative study of clinical features. *Dissociation, 3*, 127-134.

Franklin, J. (1988). Diagnosis of covert and subtle signs of multiple personality disorder through dissociative signs. *Dissociation, 1*(2), 27-33.

Fraser, G. (1993). Exorcism rituals: Effects on multiple personality disorder patients. *Dissociation, 6*, 239-244.

Freisen, J. G. (1991). *Unlocking the mystery of MPD*. San Bernardino, CA: Here's Life Publishers.

Frischholz, E. J. (1985). The relationship among dissociation, hypnosis, and child abuse in the development of multiple personality disorder. In R. P. Kluft (Ed.), *Childhood antecedents of multiple personality disorder* (pp. 100-126). Washington, DC: American Psychiatric Press.

Goff, D. C., & Simms, C. A. (1993). Has multiple personality disorder remained consistent over time? A comparison of past and recent cases. *Journal of Nervous and Mental Disease, 181*, 595-600.

Greaves, G. B. (1993). A history of multiple personality disorder. In R. P. Kluft & C. G. Fine (Eds.), *Clinical perspectives on multiple personality disorder* (pp. 355-380). Washington, DC: American Psychiatric Press.

Herman, J. L., & Schatzow, E. (1987). Recovery and verification of memories of childhood sexual trauma. *Psychoanalytic Psychology, 4*, 1-14.

Hilgard, E. R. (1986). *Divided consciousness: Multiple controls in human thought and action (expanded edition)*. New York: John Wiley and Sons.

Horevitz, R. P., & Braun, B. G. (1984). Are multiple personalities borderline? *Psychiatric Clinics of North America, 7*, 69-87.

Hornstein, N., & Putnam, F. W. (1992). Clinical phenomenology of child and adolescent dissociative disorders. *Journal of the Academy of Child and Adolescent Psychiatry, 31*, 1077-1085.

Jones, E. (1953). *The life and work of Sigmund Freud* (vol. 1). New York: Basic Books.

Kluft, E., Poteat, J., & Kluft, R. P. (1986). Movement observations in multiple personality disorder: A preliminary report. *American Journal of Dance Therapy, 9*, 313-46.

Kluft, R. P. (1982). Varieties of hypnotic intervention in the treatment of multiple personality. *American Journal of Clinical Hypnosis, 24*, 230-240.

Kluft, R. P. (1984a). Multiple personality in childhood. *Psychiatric Clinics of North America, 7*, 121-134.

Kluft, R. P. (1984b). An introduction to multiple personality disorder. *Psychiatric Annals, 14*, 19-24.

Kluft, R. P. (1984c). Treatment of multiple personality disorder: A study of 33 cases. *Psychiatric Clinics of North America, 7*, 9-29.

Kluft, R. P. (1985a). Childhood multiple personality disorder: Predictors, clinical findings, and treatment results. In R. P. Kluft (Ed.), *Childhood antecedents of multiple personality* (pp. 167-196). Washington, DC: American Psychiatric Press.

Kluft, R. P. (1985b). The natural history of multiple personality disorder. In R. P. Kluft (Ed.), *Childhood antecedents of multiple personality* (pp. 197-238). Washington, DC: American Psychiatric Press.

Kluft, R. P. (1986). Treating children with multiple personality disorder. In B. G. Braun (Ed.), *Treatment of multiple personality disorder* (pp. 79-105). Washington, DC: American Psychiatric Press.

Kluft, R. P. (1987a). An update on multiple personality disorder. *Hospital and Community Psychiatry, 38*, 363-373.

Kluft, R. P. (1987b). First rank symptoms as diagnostic indicators of multiple personality disorder. *American Journal of Psychiatry, 144*, 293-298.

Kluft, R. P. (1987c). Making the diagnosis of multiple personality. In F. F. Flach (Ed.), *Diagnostics and psychopathology* (pp. 207-225). New York: Norton.
Kluft, R. P. (1988). The phenomenology and treatment of extremely complex multiple personality disorder. *Dissociation, 1*(4), 47-58.
Kluft, R. P. (1991a). Multiple personality disorder. In A. Tasman & S. M. Goldfinger (Eds.), *American Psychiatric Press review of psychiatry* (vol. 10, pp. 161-188). Washington, DC: American Psychiatric Press.
Kluft, R. P. (1991b). Clinical presentations of multiple personality disorder. *Psychiatric Clinics of North America, 14*, 605-630.
Kluft, R. P. (1993). The treatment of dissociative disorder patients: An overview of discoveries, successes, and failures. *Dissociation, 6*, 87-101.
Kluft, R. P. (1994). Ruminations on metamorphoses. *Dissociation*, 7, 135-137.
Kluft, R. P. (1995a). Reflections of current controversies surrounding dissociative identity disorder. In L. M. Cohen, M. R. Elin, & J. N. Berzoli (Eds.), *Dissociative identity disorder: Theoretical and treatment controversies* (pp. 347-377). Northvale, NJ: Aronson.
Kluft, R. P. (1995b). Suicide in dissociative identity disorder patients: A study of six cases. *Dissociation, 8*, 104-111.
Kluft, R. P. (in press a). An overview of the treatment of patients alleging that they have suffered ritualized or sadistic abuse. In G. A. Fraser (Ed.), *The phenomenon of ritualized abuse*. Washington, DC: American Psychiatric Press.
Kluft, R. P. (in press b). Multiple personality disorder: A legacy of trauma. In C. R. Pfeffer (Ed.), *Intense stress and mental disturbance in children*. Washington, DC: American Psychiatric Press.
Kluft, R. P., & Schultz, R. (1993). Multiple personality disorder in adolescence. In S. C. Feinstein & R. C. Marohn (Eds.), *Adolescent psychiary*, (Vol. 19, pp. 259-279). Chicago: University of Chicago Press.
Kluft, R. P., Braun, B. G., & Sachs, R. G. (1984). Multiple personality, intrafamilial abuse, and family psychiatry. *International Journal of Family Psychiatry, 5*, 283-301.
Kluft, R. P., Steinberg, M., & Spitzer, R. L. (1988). DSM-III-R revisions in the dissociative disorders: An exploration of their derivation and rationale. *Dissociation, 1*(1), 39-46.
Kooper, C., Classen, K., & Spiegel, D. (1994). Predictors of posttraumatic stress symptoms among survivors of the Oakland/Berkeley firestorm. *American Journal of Psychiatry, 151*, 888-894.
Li, D., & Spiegel, D. (1992). A neural network model of dissociative disorders. *Psychiatric Annals, 22*, 144-147.
Liotti, G. (1992). Disorganized/disoriented attachment in the etiology of multiple personality disorder. *Dissociation, 5*, 196-204.
Loewenstein, R. J. (1991). An office mental status examination for complex chronic dissociative symptoms and multiple personality disorder. *Psychiatric Clinics of North America, 14*, 567-604.
Loewenstein, R. J., & Putnam, F. W. (1988). A comparison study of dissociative symptoms in patients with complex partial seizures, multiple personality disorder, and posttraumatic stress disorder. *Dissociation, 1*(4), 17-23.
Loewenstein, R. J., & Putnam, F. W. (1990). The clinical phenomenology of males with multiple personality disorder: A report of 21 cases. *Dissociation, 3*, 135-143.
Loewenstein, R. J., & Ross, D. R. (1992). Multiple personality disorder and psychoanalysis: An introduction. *Psychoanalytic Inquiry, 12*, 3-48.
Marmer, S. S. (1980). Psychoanalysis of multiple personality. *International Journal of Psychoanalysis, 61*, 439-459.
Marmer, S. S. (1991). Multiple personality disorder: A psychoanalytic perspective. *Psychiatric Clinics of North America, 14*, 677-693.
Mersky, H. (1992). The manufacture of personalities: The production of multiple personality disorder. *British Journal of Psychiatry, 160*, 327-340.
Mesulam, M. M. (1981). Dissociative states with abnormal temporal lobe EEG: Multiple personality and the illusion of possession. *Archives of Neurolgy, 38*, 178-181.
Miller, S. D. (1989). Optical differences in cases of multiple personality disorder. *Journal of Nervous and Mental Disease, 177*, 480-486.
McHugh, P. R. (1993). Multiple personality disorder. *The Harvard Mental Health Letter, 10*(3), 4-6.
Nathanson, D. (1992). *Shame and pride*. New York: Norton.
Nathanson, D. (in press). A basic affects model of dissociation. *Dissociation*.

Nemiah, J. C. (1981). Dissociative disorders. In H. Kaplan, A. Freedman, & B. Sadock (Eds.), *Comprehensive textbook of psychiatry* (3rd ed., pp. 1564-1561). Baltimore: Williams and Wilkins.

Orne, M. T., Dinges, D. F., & Orne, E. C. (1984). On the differential diagnosis of multiple personality in a forensic context. *International Journal of Clinical and Experimental Hypnosis*, *32*, 118-167.

Peterson, G. (1990). Diagnosis of chidhood multiple personality disorder. *Dissociation*, *3*, 3-9.

Peterson, G. (1991). Children coping with trauma: Diagnosis of "dissociation identity disorder." *Dissociation*, *4*, 152-164.

Prince, M. (1905). *The dissocation of a personality*. New York: Longman, Green.

Putnam, F. W. (1984a). The psychophysiologic investigation of multiple personality disorder. *Psychiatric Clinics of North America*, 7, 31-40.

Putnam, F. W. (1984b). The study of multiple personality disorder: General Strategies and practical considerations. *Psychiatric Annals*, *14*, 58-62.

Putnam, F. W. (1985). Dissociation as a response to extreme trauma. In R. P. Kluft (Ed.), *Childhood antecedents of multiple personality* (pp. 65-97). Washington, DC: American Psychiatric Press.

Putnam, F. W. (1988). The switch process in multiple personality disorder. *Dissociation*, *1*(1), 24-32.

Putnam, F. W. (1989). *The diagnosis and treatment of multiple personality disorder*. New York: Guilford.

Putnam, F. W. (1990). Disturbances of "self" in victims of childhood sexual abuse. In R. P. Kluft (Ed.), *Incest-related syndromes of adult psychopathology* (pp. 113-132). Washington, DC: American Psychiatric Press.

Putnam, F. W. (1991a). Dissociative phenomena. In A. Tasman & S. M. Goldfinger (Eds.), *American Psychiatric Press review of psychiatry* (vol. 10, pp. 145-160). Washington, DC: American Psychiatric Press.

Putnam, F. W. (1991b). Recent research on multiple personality disorder. *Psychiatric Clinics of North America*, *14*, 489-502.

Putnam, F. W. (1991c). Dissociative disorders in children and adolescents: A developmental perspective. *Psychiatric Clinics of North America*, *14*, 519-532.

Putnam, F. W., Loewenstein, R. J., Silberman, E. K., & Post, R. (1984). Multiple personality disorder in a hospital setting. *Journal of Clinical Psychiatry*, *45*, 172-175.

Putnam, F. W., Guroff, J. J., Silberman, E. K., Barban, L., & Post, R. (1986). The clinical phenomenology of multiple personality disorder: Review of 100 recent cases. *Journal of Clinical Psychiatry*, *47*, 285-293.

Putnam, F. W., Zahn, T. P., & Post, R. M. (1990). Differential autonomic nervous system activity in multiple personality disorder. *Psychiatry Research*, *31*, 251-260.

Riley, R. L., & Mead, J. (1988). The development of symptoms of multiple personality disorder in a child of three. *Dissociation*, *1*(3), 41-46.

Rosenbaum, M. (1980). The role of the term schizophrenia in the decline of diagnoses of multiple personality disorder. *Archives of General Psychiatry*, *37*, 1383-1385.

Ross, C. A. (1989). *Multiple personality disorder: Diagnosis, clinical features, and treatment*. New York: Wiley.

Ross, C. A. (1991). Epidemiology of multiple personality disorder and dissociation. *Psychiatric Clinics of North America*, *14*, 503-518.

Ross, C. A., & Norton, G. R. (1989). Differences between men and women with multiple personality disorder. *Hospital and Community Psychiatry*, *40*, 186-188.

Ross, C. A., & Norton, G. R. (1990). Effects of hypnosis on the features of multiple personality disorder. *American Journal of Clinical Hypnosis*, *32*, 99-106.

Ross, C. A., Norton, G. R., & Fraser, G. A. (1989a). Evidence against the iatrogenesis of multiple personality disorder. *Dissociation*, *2*, 61-65.

Ross, C. A., Norton, G. R., & Wozney, K. (1989b). Multiple personality disorder: An analysis of 236 cases. *Canadian Journal of Psychiatry*, *34*, 413-418.

Ross, C. A., Miller, D. S., Reagor, P., Bjornson, L., Fraser, G. A., & Anderson, G. (1990a). Structured interview data on 102 cases of multiple personality disorder from four centers. *American Journal of Psychiatry*, *147*, 596-601.

Ross, C. A., Miller, D. S., Reagor, P., Bjornson, L., Fraser, G. A., & Anderson, G. (1990b). Schneiderian symptoms in multiple personality disorder and schizophrenia. *Comprehensive Psychiatry*, *31*, 111-118.

Ross, C. A., Miller, D. S., Bjornson, L., Reagor, P., Fraser, G. A., & Anderson, G. (1991a). Abuse histories in 102 cases of multiple personality disorder. *Canadian Journal of Psychiatry, 36*, 97-101.

Ross, C. A., Anderson, G., Fleisher, W. P., & Norton, G. R. (1991b). The frequency of multiple personality disorder among psychiatric inpatients. *American Journal of Psychiatry, 148*, 1717-1720.

Ross, C. A., Joshi, S., & Currie, R. (1991c). Dissociative experiences in the general population: A factor analysis. *Hospital and Community Psychiatry, 42*, 297-301.

Ross, C. A., Anderson, G., Fraser, G. A., Reagor, P., Bjornson, L., & Miller, S. D. (1992a). Differentiating multiple personality disorder and dissociative disorder not otherwise specified. *Dissociation, 5*, 87-90.

Ross, C. A., Kronson, J., Koensgen, S., Barkman, K., Clark, P., & Rockman, G. (1992b). Dissociative comorbidity in 100 chemically dependent patients. *Hospital and Community Psychiatry, 43*, 840-842.

Saxe, G. N., van der Kolk, B. A., Berkowitz, R., Chinman, G., Hall, K., Liegerg, G., & Schwartz, J. (1993). Dissociative disorders in psychiatric inpatients. *American Journal of Psychiatry, 150*, 1037-1042.

Schenk, L., & Bear, D. (1981). Multiple personality and related dissociative phenomena in patients with temporal lobe epilepsy. *American Journal of Psychiatry, 138*, 1311-1315.

Schultz, R., Braun, B. G., & Kluft, R. P. (1989). Multiple personality disorder: Phenomenology of selected variables in comparison to major depression. *Dissociation, 2*, 45-51.

Schreiber, F. R. (1973). *Sybil*. Chicago: Regnery.

Schneider, K. (1959). *Clinical psychopathology* (5th ed.). New York: Grune & Stratton.

Solomon, R. S., & Solomon, V. (1982). Differential diagnosis of multiple personality. *Psychological Reports, 51*, 1187-1194.

Spanos, N. P. (1986). Hypnosis, nonvolitional responding, and multiple personality: A social psychological perspective. *Progress in Experimental Personality Research, 14*, 1-61.

Spanos, N. P., Weekes, J. R., & Bertrand, L. D. (1985). Multiple personality: A social psychological perspective. *Journal of Abnormal Psychology, 94*, 362-376.

Spanos, N. P., Weekes, J. R., Menary, E., & Bertrand, L. D. (1986). Hypnotic interview and age regression in the elicitation of multiple personality symptoms: A simulation study. *Psychiatry, 49*, 298-311.

Spiegel, D. (1984). Multiple personality as a post-traumatic stress disorder. *Psychiatric Clinics of North America, 7*, 101-110.

Spiegel, D. (1986). Dissociating damage. *American Journal of Clinical Hypnosis, 29*, 123-131.

Spiegel, D. (1991). Dissociation and trauma. In A. Tasman & S. M. Goldfinger (Eds.), *American Psychiatric Press review of psychiatry* (vol. 10, pp. 261-276). Washington, DC: American Psychiatric Press.

Spiegel, D., & Cardeña, E. (1991). Dissociated experience: The dissociative disorders revisited. *Journal of Abnormal Psychology, 100*, 366-378.

Spiegel, D., Hunt, T., & Dondershine, H. E. (1988). Dissociation and hypnotizability in posttraumatic stress disorder. *American Journal of Psychiatry, 145*, 301-305.

Spiegel, D., Bierre, P., & Rootenberg, J. (1989). Hypnotic alteration of somatosensory perception. *American Journal of Psychiatry, 146*, 749-754.

Spiegel, H., & Spiegel, D. (1987). *Trance and treatment*. Washington, DC: American Psychiatric Press.

Steinberg, M. (1993). *The Structured Clinical Interview for DSM-IV Dissociative Disorders (SCID-D)*. Washington, DC: American Psychiatric Press.

Stengel, E. (1943). Further studies on pathological wandering (fugue with the impulse to wander). *Journal of Mental Health Science, 89*, 224-241.

Stern, C. R. (1984). The etiology of multiple personalities. *Psychiatric Clinics of North America, 7*, 149-159.

Stutman, R., & Bliss, E. L. (1985). The post-traumatic stress disorder (the Vietnam syndrome), hypnotizability, and imagery. *American Journal of Psychiatry, 142*, 741-743.

Talbott, J. A., Hales, R. E., & Yudofsky, S. C. (Eds.). (1988). *The American Psychiatric Press textbook of psychiatry*. Washington, DC: American Psychiatric Press.

Terr, L. C. (1991). Childhood traumas: An outline and overview. *American Journal of Psychiatry, 148*, 10-20.

Tyson, G. M. (1992). Childhood MPD/dissocative identity disorder. *Dissociation, 5*, 20-27.

van der Hart, O. (1993). Multiple personality disorder in Europe: Impressions. *Dissociation, 6*, 102-118.

Vanderlinden, J., Van Dyck, R., Vandereycken, W., & Vertommen, H. (1991). Dissociative experiences in the general population in the Netherlands and Belgium: A study with the Dissociative Questionnaire (DIS-Q). *Dissociation*, *4*, 180-184.

Watkins, J. G., & Watkins, H. H. (1979). The theory and practice of ego-state therapy. In H. Grayson (ed.), *Short-term approaches to psychotherapy* (pp. 176-220). New York: National Institute for the Psychotherapies and Human Sciences Press.

Watkins, J. G., & Watkins, H. H. (1984). Hazards to the therapist in the treatment of multiple personalities. *Psychiatric Clinics of North America*, 7, 111-119.

Yates, J. L., & Nasby, W. (1993). Dissociation, affect, and network models of memory: An integrative proposal. *Journal of Traumatic Stress*, *6*, 305-326.

17

Dissociative Symptoms in the Diagnosis of Acute Stress Disorder

David Spiegel, Cheryl Koopman, Etzel Cardeña, and Catherine Classen

INTRODUCTION

The proposal for a new diagnostic entity requires very careful consideration of the benefits and risks that such a decision entails. On the one hand, if a condition that is prevalent in a substantial percentage of the population goes undiagnosed or misdiagnosed, the affected individuals will lack proper diagnosis and treatment of their condition. In turn, the lack of recognition of the diagnostic entity might prevent the proper research designed to understand the condition, its treatment, and its clinical and social ramifications. On the other hand, carelessly introducing new diagnostic entities brings the risk of pathologizing what may be innocuous or even appropriate reactions to the misfortunes of life. Further, even if the symptomatology of the diagnosis can be considered "pathological," it is still incumbent upon the advocates of the diagnosis to show that their proposal will not simply add to the profusion of diagnoses, but rather that the disorder cannot be reasonably accommodated by the existing nosology.

David Spiegel, Cheryl Koopman, and Catherine Classen • Department of Psychiatry and Behavioral Sciences, Stanford University School of Medicine, Stanford, California 94305. **Etzel Cardeña** • Department of Psychiatry, Uniformed Services University of the Health Sciences, Bethesda, Maryland 20814.

Handbook of Dissociation: Theoretical, Empirical, and Clinical Perspectives, edited by Larry K. Michelson and William J. Ray. Plenum Press, New York, 1996.

Elsewhere (Koopman, Classen, Cardeña, & Spiegel, 1995; Spiegel, Koopman, & Classen, 1994), we have provided arguments for including the diagnosis of acute stress disorder (ASD) in the fourth edition of the *Diagnostic and Statistical Manual of Mental Disorders* (DSM-IV) (American Psychiatric Association, 1994). We will refer to these arguments here as they pertain to the role of dissociative responses to acute trauma. It is noteworthy that dissociative responses to trauma are required in the diagnosis of ASD even though they have not been directly mentioned in the diagnosis of posttraumatic stress disorder (PTSD). In the next pages we make the case that the emphasis on requiring three dissociative symptoms in the new diagnosis of Acute Stress Disorder in the DSM-IV is justified on empirical and theoretical grounds and fills a current vacuum that inhibits appropriate treatment and research. In particular, we examine evidence that the dissociative symptoms that comprise the disorder are directly related to the intensity of exposure to trauma and are strongly predictive of the development of later PTSD. Accurate diagnosis of this peritraumatic disorder will enhance our ability to predict and intervene with those likely to develop PTSD. Last, the adoption of this diagnosis would bring about concordance between the DSM-IV and the diagnosis of "acute stress reaction" in the International Classification of Diseases and Related Health Problems, 10th edition (ICD-10) (World Health Organization, 1990).

After giving a brief description of ASD, where the essential component is the presence of dissociative symptomatology during or shortly after traumatic events, we will briefly review the following converging lines of evidence: (1) the conceptual and empirical association between PTSD and dissociation, (2) the evidence for the presence of dissociative responses during or shortly after trauma in a substantial percentage of the population, (3) the association between level of exposure to trauma and dissociative response, and (4) the association between peritraumatic dissociative responses and later full-fledged PTSD. Thus, we will make the case that dissociative symptomatology is a frequent accompaniment of trauma that, if untreated, may lead to short- and long-term distress and malfunction.

REVIEW OF THE LITERATURE

Dissociation and PTSD: Conceptual Links

In a number of studies (e.g., Mellman, Randolph, Brawman-Mintzer, Flores, & Milanes, 1992), PTSD has been found to be the most prevalent lifetime disorder of war combatants and other individuals exposed to trauma. Although PTSD is currently included in the anxiety disorders section of DSM-III-R, we have earlier discussed the analogy between the concept of dissociation (i.e., the lack of integration of mental processes) and such PTSD phenomena as the numbing of emotional and social responsiveness and the intrusion of unbidden thoughts and feelings (Spiegel & Cardeña, 1990). This conceptual discussion has been recently supported by a number of studies showing significant correlations between standardized PTSD and dissociation inventories. In a study with 52 survivors of childhood sexual victimization, Gold and Cardeña (1993) found that dissociative symptomatology was significantly correlated with 85% of the subscales of the Mississippi Scale for

Combat-Related PTSD (Keane, Caddell, & Taylor, 1988), the Trauma Symptom Checklist-40, and the Response to Childhood Incest Questionnaire, and conclude that the boundary between PTSD and dissociation may be less evident than previously thought. Bremner and collaborators (1992) also found a significant correlation between PTSD (as measured by the Mississippi Scale) and dissociative symptoms on the Dissociative Experiences Scale (DES) (Bernstein & Putnam, 1986). These results are supported by a study with 239 male Vietnam veterans conducted by Marmar et al. (1992), who also found that dissociative (DES) and PTSD measures [Mississippi Scale; Minnesota Multiphasic Personality Inventory (MMPI) PTSD Scale; Impact of Event Scale] (Horowitz, Wilner, & Alvarez, 1979) were significantly correlated, and that this association was specific and did not reflect general psychopathology. Finally, Branscombe (1991), in a study with 35 PTSD Vietnam veterans, also found moderate to strong correlations between PTSD (the Mississippi scale) and two dissociation scales [the DES and the Perceptual Alteration Scale (PAS)]. The author also found that the DES scores of her sample were higher than those of the clinical populations of other studies with the exception of multiple personality disorder. Thus, the evidence suggests that despite the inclusion of PTSD among the stress disorders, dissociative symptomatology is commonly present among patients suffering from PTSD.

Two earlier studies showed that the hypnotizability of Vietnam veterans with PTSD was significantly higher than that of comparison psychiatric patient and normal populations (Stutman & Bliss, 1985; Spiegel, Hunt & Dondershine, 1988). Since hypnosis is a form of controlled dissociation, this line of investigation also supports the link between dissociative and PTSD symptomatology.

Dissociative Response during and Shortly after Trauma

There is accumulating anecdotal and research evidence that dissociative symptomatology occurs in a substantial proportion of the population exposed to natural and human-made disasters (cf. Cardeña, Lewis-Fernandez, Bear, Pakianathan, & Spiegel, 1995; Spiegel & Cardeña, 1991). In a programmatic series of studies, we have systematically documented the extent of dissociation occurring in individuals exposed to events such as the Loma Prieta earthquake of 1989 (Cardeña & Spiegel, 1993), the Oakland/Berkeley firestorm of 1991 (Koopman, Classen, & Spiegel, in press; Koopman, Classen & Spiegel, 1994), and in media execution witnesses (Freinkel, Koopman, & Spiegel, 1994). During and shortly after the earthquake, a normal student sample reported a significantly greater number of dissociative symptoms, compared to responses 4 months after the earthquake. These dissociative symptoms included derealization and depersonalization, time distortions, and alterations in cognition, memory, and somatic sensations. To a lesser extent they also reported significantly more anxiety and Schneiderian first-rank symptoms. We found similar results in a survey of 15 of the 18 journalists witnessing the execution of Robert Alton Harris (Freinkel et al., 1994). They endorsed on average 11.5 of 25 dissociative symptoms, with symptoms ranging from "my mind went blank" (endorsed by 27%) to "I felt distant from my emotions" (endorsed by 80%). This prevalence of reported dissociative symptoms is comparable to that seen among survivors of the recent Oakland firestorm.

From these and other studies of reactions to trauma, five kinds of dissociative symptoms have been identified: emotional numbing, derealization, depersonalization, lack of awareness of one's surroundings (stupor), and amnesia for important aspects of the traumatic event (Classen, Koopman, & Spiegel, 1993). These five kinds of symptoms may be viewed as manifestations of the lack of integration that the dissociative state entails. For example, with symptoms of depersonalization, a person lacks a sense of connection between the usual associations between his or her identity, body, and personal attributes. Similarly, with symptoms of derealization, a person does not associate the usual characteristics to the environment: it appears to be altered in some respects, perhaps temporally, spatially, and/or in other ways. One indication of derealization is when time is experienced as slowing down, as was reported by 51% of the respondents in our study of the Loma Prieta earthquake (Cardeña & Spiegel, 1993). Stupor is similar to derealization in being related to one's experience of one's environment lacking the usual associations; however, stupor constitutes a lack of awareness rather than alterations of aspects of the environment. For example, not perceiving events as they are occurring has been reported among persons held hostage (Siegel, 1984), as well as in other kinds of traumatic events. Amnesia for important aspects of the trauma shows a direct disconnection between conscious memories and earlier experience. In a recent study, 90% of Cambodian refugees who had survived the holocaust reported amnesia for past traumatic experiences (Carlson & Rosser-Hogan, 1994). Emotional numbing is a lack of feeling in response to either pleasurable or painful stimuli, revealing a disconnection of emotional responsiveness to the environment, and characterized the initial response to the Buffalo Creek disaster (Rangell, 1976). These five dissociative symptoms have been described in a number of studies of psychological reactions to acute trauma (see Koopman et al., 1995; Spiegel et al., 1994, for reviews).

Exposure to Trauma and Dissociative Response

In a study of the relation between trauma and dissociation among Cambodian refugees who had suffered considerable physical mistreatment and exposure to the elements, Carlson and Rosser-Hogan (1991) reported a significant correlation between the amount of reported trauma and scores on the DES. Similarly, Marmar and colleagues (1994) reported that retrospective accounts of peritraumatic dissociative responses were strong predictors of current PTSD symptomatology.

Peritraumatic Dissociative Responses and Later PTSD

These recent findings are consistent with inferences in the classical literature on PTSD. Lindemann (1944) noted that individuals who showed little or no initial emotional reaction to the Coconut Grove fire and did not experience acute grief over the loss of loved ones and physical injuries had extremely poor long-term prognoses. Solomon, Mikulincer, and Benbenisty's (1989) study of combat stress response in the Israeli army demonstrated that "psychic numbing" accounted for 20% of the variance in subsequent PTSD symptoms. Similarly, McFarlane (1986) observed that avoidance in the wake of the Ash Wednesday bushfires was a strong predictor of later PTSD. Thus, this literature provides convergent evidence that dissociation occurs frequently in the immediate aftermath of trauma and that in more extreme forms it predicts the development of later PTSD.

Based on these previous studies, we decided to analyze the dissociative and anxiety symptoms reported among respondents in the immediate aftermath of the 1991 Oakland/Berkeley firestorm. We had two purposes in conducting these analyses: (1) to examine differences in specific symptoms in response to varying levels of exposure to trauma (i.e., to the firestorm), and (2) to evaluate alternative combinations of symptoms that could constitute algorithms for defining ASD.

METHODS

Background

This study analyzed the symptoms reported by persons who were recruited in the immediate aftermath of the 1991 Oakland/Berkeley firestorm, which lasted two days (October 20–21) and resulted in at least 24 deaths and the destruction of 3135 homes and apartments (Taylor & Wildermuth, 1991), and was estimated to cost as much as $5 billion in damage (Marshall, 1991). After obtaining expedited approval of this study by our institutional human subjects review board, we distributed the survey October 24–31 to respondents in the Oakland/Berkeley area. Nearly all of the surveys (94%) were completed within 3 weeks after the firestorm began. Seven months after the firestorm, we mailed follow-up assessments to those 181 respondents who had provided us with contact information. Follow-up assessments were completed by 154 respondents for a follow-up rate of 82% of the original sample, 97% of whom completed these assessments by the ninth month after the firestorm.

Sample

We obtained informed consent from 187 individuals exposed to the firestorm. These were 21% of the larger number of potential respondents to whom we distributed questionnaires. Respondents received no compensation for completing the baseline assessment. Participants were recruited from sources expected to provide variation in exposure to the firestorm. These participants included: (1) 94 persons recruited in front of the Federal Emergency Management Agency providing assistance to firestorm survivors and through personal contacts with people living in neighborhoods next to the firestorm; (2) 44 University of California at Berkeley students recruited from four fraternities and sororities that were evacuated during the firestorm; and (3) 49 graduate students recruited from a professional school of psychology in Berkeley that was near the fire but was not evacuated (see Koopman et al., 1994). All participants spoke English and were at least 18 years old. This study is based on the responses of these 187 participants completing the initial assessments and also on the subset of 154 participants who completed and returned the follow-up survey sent 7 months after the firestorm, allowing a longitudinal analysis for these participants.

Immediate Aftermath of the Firestorm

Contact with the Fire. Twelve items were used to assess respondents' contact with the fire. Each item asked respondents to indicate whether or not they had experienced various effects of the fire (e.g., saw smoke, evacuated residence, lost home). A hierarchical index of contact with the fire was based on these responses, in which *high contact* was defined as losing one's residence or being injured in the fire, *medium contact* was defined as being evacuated, having trouble breathing, worrying about residence, feeling heat, or having a loss other than residence, and *low contact* was defined as seeing flames, seeing smoke, inhaling smoke, knowing someone who was a victim of the fire, assisting others, and/or fighting the fire.

Stanford Acute Stress Reaction Questionnaire (SASRQ) (Cardeña, Classen, & Spiegel, 1991). This self-report instrument provides a comprehensive assessment of dissociative and anxiety symptoms experienced during and in the weeks immediately following a traumatic event. An earlier version was developed for a study of the psychological aftermath of the 1989 Loma Prieta earthquake (Cardeña & Spiegel, 1993). The assessment that was administered immediately following the firestorm included 33 items assessing five types of dissociative symptoms: psychic numbing (4 items), depersonalization (9 items), derealization (9 items), amnesia (6 items), and stupor (5 items). It also included 34 items assessing five kinds of anxiety symptoms: intrusive thinking (11 items), somatic anxiety symptoms (17 items), hyperarousal (2 items), attention disturbance (3 items), and sleep disturbance (1 item). Each item asks about the frequency with which the respondent has experienced a particular manifestation of one of the symptoms, if at all, and provides a six-point Likert scale on which to respond as follows: "not experienced" (0); "very rarely experienced" (1); "rarely experienced" (2); "sometimes experienced" (3); "often experienced" (4); or "very often experienced" (5). This measure has been found to have high internal consistency (total dissociative symptoms, Cronbach's alpha = .90; anxiety symptoms, Cronbach's alpha = .91) and concurrent validity (r = .52–.69, $p < .001$) of both scales with scores on the avoidance and intrusion subscales of the Impact of Event Scale (Horowitz et al., 1979; Koopman et al., 1994; Spiegel, Koopman, Cardeña, & Classen, 1993).

Background Characteristics. Demographic and other background characteristics were assessed with self-report items. These items included sex, age, education, and place of residence.

Follow-up Assessments.

Civilian Version of the Mississippi Scale for Posttraumatic Stress Disorder. This scale measures posttraumatic stress symptoms among persons who have undergone a particular trauma and was originally validated and found to have high reliability with combat-related trauma (Keane, Wolfe, & Taylor, 1987; Keane et al., 1988). The instrument includes 39 Likert-style statements, to which respondents indicate their extent of agreement–disagreement with each on a 1–5 point scale. In this civilian version, for every specific reference to the trauma that respondents had undergone, we inserted the words "the firestorm." This measure is scored by first reversing the values for ten reverse-scored items and then summing the point value of all of the items. Norms have not yet been established to determine the cut-off score for diagnosing PTSD using the civilian version.

Impact of Event Scale (IES) (Horowitz et al., 1979). This instrument assesses the degree of subjective distress experienced over the past week in relation to a particular traumatic event, and contains two subscales—intrusive and avoidant experiences—two core dimensions of PTSD (Horowitz, Field, & Classen, 1993). Items assessing intrusive experience focus on having unbidden thoughts, feelings, and images of the traumatic event. Those assessing avoidant experiences focus on the extent to which respondents have tried to prevent themselves from having thoughts or reminders of the event and tried to dull their emotional response to memories of the event. Previous research has supported this measure's validity (Schwarzwald, Solomon, Weisenberg, & Mikulincer, 1987; Zilberg, Weiss, & Horowitz, 1982). Responses are scaled as follows: (0, not at all; 1, rarely; 3, sometimes; 5, often), so possible scores range from 0 to 75.

Data Analysis

To assess whether respondents experienced a particular symptom according to their responses on the SASRQ, their responses to items were recoded dichotomously as occurrence versus nonoccurrence by defining the presence of a symptom for responses of "3" or greater (meaning the symptoms occurred at least "sometimes" and not merely "rarely" indicted by a "2," or "very rarely" indicated by a "1," or even "not at all" indicated by a "0"). This was done for conceptual clarity and was found to produce similar results to that of using the continuous scale for each item.

We conducted two kinds of data analysis for this evaluation of dissociative and anxiety symptoms. First, we examined and compared the percentages of respondents who experienced each of the three levels of contact with the fire who reported each particular symptom. The purpose of these analyses was to determine whether all the symptoms varied appropriately in response to the level of trauma, with respondents in the high trauma group most frequently reporting each symptom and those in the low trauma group least frequently reporting each symptom. We conducted one-way analysis of variance to statistically test the significance of the differences between the groups.

Second, we evaluated all possible combinations of the five dissociative and five anxiety symptoms by their overall frequency in the sample (which was better if lower) and by their sensitivity and specificity in predicting the criterion group high in posttraumatic stress at the 7-month follow-up. This criterion group is comprised of 18 persons who scored within the highest 5% on any of three PTSD measures (Mississippi Civilian Version, Avoidance Subscale of the IES, Intrusion Subscale of the IES) and/or on the anxiety measure (Anxiety subscale of the SASRQ at follow-up).

RESULTS

Respondents' demographic characteristics have already been described elsewhere and were found to have little or no relationship to follow-up assessment scores on the Civilian Version of the Mississippi Scale and the IES; in contrast, their overall numbers of dissociative and anxiety symptoms appeared to be important predictors (Koopman et al., 1994). Our first step in considering these symptoms for inclusion in the diagnosis of ASD was therefore to analyze the relationship between each dissociative and anxiety symptom to the degree of trauma (contact with the fire). The results of this analysis are presented in Table 1, showing the percentages of the respondents experiencing each of the three levels of contact with the fire who reported each of the dissociative and anxiety symptoms.

The symptoms were found to vary according to degree of contact with the fire, with the respondents in the high contact group generally showing the highest percentage reporting each symptom, the respondents in the low contact group showing the lowest percentage reporting each symptom, and the respondents in the medium contact group reporting a level of symptoms inbetween the other two groups. *F*-test values are presented to show the results of using one-way analysis of variance to test the statistical significance of group differences. These differences are significant for four of the five dissociative symptoms (depersonalization, amnesia, stupor, and psychic numbing) and for three of the five anxiety symptoms (sleep disturbances, intrusive thinking, and somatic symptoms). The differences for derealization and attention problem symptoms show statistical trends ($p < .06$) in the same directions as the other symptoms. The results for hypervigilant fear did not approach significance; however, the overall pattern is similar to the results for the other symptoms.

Our second step in defining the diagnosis was then to evaluate alternative combinations of these symptoms with reference to predicting later PTSD and anxiety symptoms. This allowed us to examine the results of applying each algorithm for defining the category on frequency, sensitivity, and specificity (Kraemer, 1992). The results are shown in Table 2. In the first column are the percentages of

Table 1. Percentages of Oakland/Berkeley Fire Victims ($N = 187$) Who Experienced Symptoms Analyzed by Contact with the Fire

	Contact with the fire			
Symptom combination	Low	Medium	High	*F*-test
Dissociation				
Depersonalization	19%	33%	52%	5.24**
Amnesia	22%	23%	58%	11.29***
Numbing	34%	44%	69%	5.93**
Stupor	41%	43%	75%	8.13***
Derealization	53%	72%	77%	2.89
Anxiety				
Sleep disturbances	16%	35%	63%	10.68***
Hypervigilant fear	56%	71%	70%	0.78
Intrusive thoughts	56%	74%	83%	3.68*
Somatic symptoms	59%	78%	90%	5.23**
Attention problems	69%	76%	90%	2.86

*$P < .05$; **$P < .01$; ***$P < .001$.

Table 2. Comparing Combinations of Dissociative and Anxiety Symptoms of Oakland/Berkeley Respondents[a]

	Overall %	Sensitivity	Specificity
No dissociative symptom required			
With no anxiety symptoms required	91%	100%	0%
Plus one anxiety symptom	91%	100%	10%
Plus two anxiety symptoms	81%	100%	22%
Plus three anxiety symptoms	65%	94%	39%
Plus four anxiety symptoms	52%	89%	53%
Plus five anxiety symptoms	19%	39%	84%
Single dissociative symptom			
With no anxiety symptoms required	78%	100%	25%
Plus one anxiety symptom	77%	100%	26%
Plus two anxiety symptoms	72%	100%	32%
Plus three anxiety symptoms	59%	94%	46%
Plus four anxiety symptoms	48%	89%	57%
Plus five anxiety symptoms	18%	39%	84%
Two dissociative symptoms			
With no anxiety symptoms required	61%	100%	44%
Plus one anxiety symptom	61%	100%	45%
Plus two anxiety symptoms	58%	100%	48%
Plus three anxiety symptoms	49%	94%	57%
Plus four anxiety symptoms	39%	89%	67%
Plus five anxiety symptoms	16%	39%	87%
Three dissociative symptoms			
With no anxiety symptoms required	46%	94%	61%
Plus one anxiety symptom	46%	94%	61%
Plus two anxiety symptoms	44%	94%	64%
Plus three anxiety symptoms	38%	89%	69%
Plus four anxiety symptoms	32%	83%	75%
Plus five anxiety symptoms	14%	39%	90%
Four dissociative symptoms			
With no anxiety symptoms required	31%	94%	78%
Plus one anxiety symptom	31%	94%	78%
Plus two anxiety symptoms	31%	94%	78%
Plus three anxiety symptoms	27%	89%	81%
Plus four anxiety symptoms	26%	83%	82%
Plus five anxiety symptoms	11%	39%	93%
Five dissociative symptoms			
With no anxiety symptoms required	18%	67%	89%
Plus one anxiety symptom	18%	67%	89%
Plus two anxiety symptoms	17%	67%	90%
Plus three anxiety symptoms	15%	61%	91%
Plus four anxiety symptoms	14%	56%	91%
Plus five anxiety symptoms	5%	22%	98%

[a]These results are based on scoring a symptom as "positivie" if the respondent reported on any item measuring it that they experienced it at least "sometimes" (three or more on the 0-5 point scale).

the total sample of 147 persons who in the immediate aftermath of the Oakland/Berkeley firestorm met the criteria defined by the particular combination of dissociative and/or anxiety symptoms. In the second column of Table 2 are the sensitivity results of each combination. These are the percentages of the persons in the criterion group of 18 distressed persons in the follow-up that our algorithm with the baseline data (immediately following the firestorm) would have correctly predicted as reporting high posttraumatic stress and/or anxiety at follow-up. In the third column are the specificity results, the percentages of persons who are true negatives divided by [the number of true negatives plus the number of false positives (Kraemer, 1992). This value shows how many of those people who are not highly distressed at follow-up were accurately predicted by the algorithm to be not at risk for later distress.

These data suggest that if the algorithm for determining the disorder for DSM-IV should include at least three of the five possible dissociative symptoms plus at least one anxiety symptom. If the algorithm required the inclusion of fewer than three dissociative symptoms, it showed little impact on the criterion value of sensitivity. Alternative algorithms requiring no, one, or two dissociative symptoms accurately include everyone or nearly everyone who was in the criterion group of those reporting the greatest distress in the 7-month follow-up assessment of PTSD and anxiety symptoms, depending on the number of anxiety symptoms required. However, specificity greatly declined when fewer than three dissociative symptoms were required in the algorithm. For example, for an algorithm that included three anxiety symptoms, in combination with three dissociative symptoms the algorithm resulted in a specificity of 69%; in combination with two dissociative symptoms the algorithm declined to a specificity of 57%; in combination with one dissociative symptom the algorithm further declined to a specificity of 46%; and if no dissociative symptom was required in addition to three anxiety symptoms, the algorithm declined even further, to 39%. Alternatively, if the algorithm requires the inclusion of five dissociative symptoms, specificity went up, to 91%, but this coincided with a decline in sensitivity when compared to an algorithm requiring three dissociative symptoms in addition to three anxiety symptoms, to 61% from 89%.

So far we have discussed the results that demonstrate that requiring three dissociative symptoms in the algorithm resulted in better sensitivity and specificity. Using the data from the Oakland/Berkeley firestorm study respondents, we find that an algorithm requiring *four* dissociative symptoms produced better specificity without hurting sensitivity. In other words, for these data, requiring four symptoms in the algorithm identified fewer persons incorrectly as being in the criterion group at follow-up than did algorithms that required three symptoms, yet it was just as accurate in identifying those who did appear in the criterion group at follow-up. However, in recognition of the limitation of this data set being drawn from a study of one particular traumatic event, it is better to require three rather than four dissociative symptoms in the algorithm for making the diagnosis of ASD. Our reasoning can be illustrated with the results in Table 2; in comparison to requiring three or fewer dissociative symptoms, requiring five dissociative symptoms resulted in a substantial loss in sensitivity. It is likely that in response to other traumatic events, requiring a minimum of four dissociative symptoms in the diagnosis would also result in losing sensitivity in predicting who is at risk for later distress. Also, the presence of three of the dissociative symptoms in combination with anxiety and reexperiencing and avoiding the trauma lasting at least 2 days in the aftermath of a traumatic event seems adequately distressing and disruptive to justify this diagnosis, even if sometimes these acute symptoms decrease over time and do not result in PTSD symptoms.

DISCUSSION

The results of this analysis support the inclusion of both dissociative and anxiety symptoms in defining acute stress disorder as a new diagnostic category in the DSM-IV. We observed a systematic relationship between the percentages of persons reporting such symptoms and the level of their contact with the Oakland/Berkeley firestorm. This suggests that these symptoms are common responses to trauma and vary according to the intensity of the trauma. Furthermore, the relationships between all possible combinations of these symptoms with posttraumatic stress symptoms 7 months or more later suggest that dissociative symptoms may be especially sensitive predictors of PTSD, although including anxiety symptoms in addition to dissociative symptoms in the diagnosis improves the specificity of the diagnosis somewhat. It is indeed interesting that dissociative symptoms immediately after the trauma are such powerful predictors of later symptoms of a different but clearly related type. According to the results of this analysis, the best algorithm for defining ASD is to require a minimum of three dissociative symptoms and three anxiety symptoms, resulting in 89% sensitivity and 69% specificity in predicting later PTSD symptoms. This high number of required symptoms restricts the diagnosis to individuals who are substantially symptomatic (38% of this sample), thereby eliminating from identification as mentally ill the majority of the population who responded to the trauma with fewer symptoms and who are less at risk for later psychopathology.

This study is limited in part by its focus on a particular traumatic event, the 1991 Oakland/Berkeley firestorm. However, its results are consistent with a number of studies that similarly suggest that there are high levels of dissociative, anxiety, and other symptoms in the immediate aftermath of a variety of traumatic events, and that these symptoms are predictive of later PTSD symptoms. In particular, future research is needed to replicate the superiority of the algorithm of requiring three dissociative symptoms found in this study to predict later posttraumatic stress after a different kind of traumatic event. Although the 21% questionnaire return rate for the baseline assessments was low, more careful recruitment methodology would have delayed field recruitment and therefore the proximity of the trauma. We were careful to recruit a sample that represented substantial variation in exposure to the trauma, allowing us to examine the trauma-related sensitivity of our measures. Also, the low return rate most likely reflected the failure of the most distressed persons to complete and return questionnaires, suggesting that the symptomatology may have been even higher among the overall pool of potential respondents. Furthermore, the results of this study in conjunction with the growing body of other studies of immediate psychological reactions to trauma lend strong support to the inclusion of this diagnosis in the DSM-IV. Traumatic events continue to happen in the world, with recent years being some of the worst years for disasters in US history (e.g., Staff, 1993), and with observers remarking that traumatic events seem to be on the increase in this complex and problem-filled world (Wilkinson, 1983).

In addition to replicating the results of this research with samples of persons who have recently undergone other kinds of traumatic events, further research is needed to evaluate alternative interventions targeting persons diagnosed with ASD. The core role of dissociative symptoms in ASD suggests that interventions that will be most helpful in the immediate aftermath of trauma will draw upon approaches such as guided imagery and hypnosis exercises that draw upon the dissociative states that many trauma survivors will experience in the days following the traumatic event. Being able to diagnose this disorder is only an important first step in being able to effectively treat it.

ACKNOWLEDGMENTS. This research was supported by a contract with the Violence and Traumatic Stress Research Branch of the National Institute of Mental Health and by a grant from the John D. and Catherine T. MacArthur Foundation and the American Psychiatric Association. Helena C. Kraemer served as a consultant on the data analysis. We also wish to thank Janet Williams, Robert Matano, Terrence M. Keane, Susan Diamond, Dennis Barton, Susan Reaburn, Bita Nouriani, Jim Spira, Beverly Brock-Alexander, and the Oakland/Berkeley firestorm survivors who contributed to this research.

REFERENCES

American Psychiatric Association (1987). *Diagnostic and statistical manual of mental disorders* (3rd ed., rev.). Washington, DC: Author.

American Psychiatric Association (1994). *Diagnostic and statistical manual of mental disorders* (4th ed.). Washington, DC: Author.

Bernstein, E. M., & Putnam, F. W. (1986). Development, reliability, and validity of a dissociation scale. *Journal of Nervous and Mental Disease, 174*, 727–734.

Branscomb, L. (1991). Dissociation in combat-related post-traumatic stress disorder. *Dissociation, 4*(1), 13–20.

Bremner, J. D., Southwick, S., Brett, E., Fontana, A., Rosenheck, R., & Charney, D. S. (1992). Dissociation and posttraumatic stress disorder in Vietnam combat veterans. *American Journal of Psychiatry, 149*(3), 328–332.

Cardeña, E., & Spiegel, D. (1993). Dissociative reactions to the Bay Area earthquake. *American Journal of Psychiatry, 150*, 474–478.

Cardeña, E., Classen, C., & Spiegel, D. (1991). *Stanford Acute Stress Reaction Questionnaire*. Stanford, CA: Department of Psychiatry and Behavioral Sciences, Stanford University School of Medicine.

Cardeña, E., Lewis-Fernandez, R., Bear, D., Pakianathan, I., & Spiegel, D. (1995). Dissociative disorders. In *DSM-IV sourcebook* (pp. 973–1005). Washington, DC: American Psychiatric Press.

Carlson, E., & Rosser-Hogan, R. (1991). Trauma experiences, post-traumatic stress, dissociation, and depression in Cambodian refugees. *American Journal of Psychiatry, 148*(11), 1548–1551.

Carlson, E. B., & Rosser-Hogan, R. (1994). Cross-cultural response to trauma: A study of traumatic experiences and posttraumatic symptoms in Cambodian refugees. *Journal of Traumatic Stress, 7*(1), 43–58.

Classen, C., Koopman, C., & Spiegel, D. (1993). Trauma and dissociation. *Bulletin of the Menninger Clinic, 57*(2), 178–194.

Freinkel, A., Koopman, C., & Spiegel, D. (1994). Dissociative symptoms in media execution witnesses. *American Journal of Psychiatry, 15*(9), 1335–1339.

Gold, J. W., & Cardeña, E. (1993). Sexual abuse and combat-related trauma: Psychometric and phenomenological resemblance. Unpublished manuscript.

Horowitz, M. J., Wilner, N., & Alvarez, W. (1979). Impact of event scale: A measure of subjective distress. *Psychosomatic Medicine, 41*, 209-218.

Horowitz, M. J., Field, N. P., & Classen, C. C. (1993). Stress response syndromes and their treatment. In L. Goldberger & S. Bresnitz (Eds.), *Handbook of stress: Theoretical and clinical aspects* (2nd ed., pp. 757-773). New York: Free Press.

Keane, T. M., Wolfe, J., & Taylor, K. L. (1987). Post-traumatic stress disorder: Evidence for diagnostic validity and methods of psychological assessment. *Journal of Clinical Psychology, 43*(1), 32-43.

Keane, T. M., Caddell, J. M., & Taylor, K. L. (1988). Mississippi Scale for Combat-Related Post-traumatic Stress Disorder: Three studies in reliability and validity. *Journal of Consulting and Clinical Psychology, 56*(1), 85-90.

Koopman, C., Classen, C., & Spiegel, D. (in press). Dissociative responses in the immediate aftermath of the Oakland/Berkeley firestorm. *Journal of Traumatic Stress.*

Koopman, C., Classen, C., Cardeña, E., & Spiegel, D. (1995). When disaster strikes, acute stress disorder may follow. *Journal of Traumatic Stress, 8*(1), 29-46.

Koopman, C., Classen, C., & Spiegel, D. (1994). Predictors of posttraumatic stress symptoms among survivors of the Oakland/Berkeley, Calif., firestorm. *American Journal of Psychiatry, 151*(6), 888-894.

Kraemer, H. C. (1992). *Evaluating medical tests: Objectives and quantitative guidelines.* Newbury Park, CA: Sage.

Lindemann, E. (1944). Symptomatology and management of acute grief. *American Journal of Psychiatry, 101*, 141-148.

Marmar, C. R., Weiss, D. S., Schlenger, W. E., Fairbank, J. A., Jordan, B. K., Kulka, R. A., & Huff, R. L. (1994). Peritraumatic dissociation and posttraumatic stress in male Vietnam theater veterans. *American Journal of Psychiatry, 151*(6), 902-907.

Marshall, J. (1991, October 19). $5 billion damage estimate may be too high. *San Francisco Chronicle*, p. A19.

McFarlane, A. C. (1986). Posttraumatic morbidity of a disaster. *Journal of Nervous and Mental Disease, 174*, 4-14.

Mellman, T. A., Randolph, C. A., Brawman-Mintzer, O., Flores, L. P., & Milanes, F. J. (1992). Phenomenology and course of psychiatric disorders associated with combat-related post-traumatic stress disorder. *American Journal of Psychiatry, 149*, 1568-1574.

Rangell, L. (1976). Discussion of the Buffalo Creek disaster: The course of psychic trauma. *American Journal of Psychiatry, 133*, 313-316.

Schwarzwald, J., Solomon, Z., Weisenberg, M., & Mikulincer, M. (1987). Validation of the impact of event scale for psychological sequelae of combat. *Journal of Consulting and Clinical Psychology, 55*, 251-256.

Siegel, R. K. (1984). Hostage hallucinations: Visual imagery induced by isolation and life-threatening stress. *Journal of Nervous and Mental Disease, 172*(5), 264-272.

Solomon, Z., Mikulincer, M., & Benbenistry, R. (1989). Combat stress reaction: Clinical manifestations and correlates. *Military Psychology, 1*, 35-47.

Spiegel, D., & Cardeña, E. (1990). New uses of hypnosis in the treatment of posttraumatic stress disorder. *Journal of Clinical Psychiatry, 51*(10, suppl.), 39-43.

Spiegel, D., & Cardeña, E. (1991). Disintegrated experience: The dissociative disorders revisited. *Journal of Abnormal Psychology, 100*(3), 366-378.

Spiegel, D., Hunt, T., & Dondershine, H. E. (1988). Dissociation and hypnotizability in post-traumatic stress disorder. *American Journal of Psychiatry, 145*, 301-305.

Spiegel, D., Koopman, C., Cardeña, E., & Classen, C. (1993). *The development of a state measure of dissociative reactions to trauma.* Final report to NIMH. Stanford, CA: Department of Psychiatry and Behavioral Sciences, Stanford University School of Medicine.

Spiegel, D., Koopman, C., & Classen, E. (1994). Acute stress disorder and dissociation. *Australian Journal of Clinical and Experimental Hypnosis, 22*(1), 11-23.

Staff. (1993, January). 1992 disasters cost the U.S. $3.17 billion in emergency aid. *San Francisco Chronicle*, p. 4.

Stutman, R. K., & Bliss, E. L. (1985). Posttraumatic stress disorder, hypnotizability, and imagery. *American Journal of Psychiatry, 142*, 741-743.

Taylor, M., & Wildermuth, J. (1991, October 25). It was worst wildfire in U.S. history. *San Francisco Chronicle*, p. A1, A16.

Wilkinson, C. B., (1983). Aftermath of a disaster: The collapse of the Hyatt Regency Hotel skywalks. *American Journal of Psychiatry, 140*, 1134-1139.

World Health Organization. (1990). *International classification of diseases and related health problems* (10th ed.) Geneva: Author.

Zilberg, N. J., Weiss, D. S., & Horowitz, M. (1982). Impact of Event scale: A cross-validation study. *Journal of Consulting and Clinical Psychology, 50*, 407-414.

18

Posttraumatic Responses to Childhood Abuse and Implications for Treatment

James A. Chu

INTRODUCTION

In July 1993, the National Research Council (1993) published a comprehensive volume entitled *Understanding Child Abuse and Neglect*. In this volume, statistics from the US Department of Health and Human Services documented reports of child maltreatment in 1990 involving more than 2.7 million children. Not surprisingly, childhood trauma, usually in the form of childhood physical, sexual, or emotional abuse, or profound neglect, is a common feature in psychiatric patients. In recent years, clinical observations concerning childhood abuse and research studies have found that childhood physical and/or sexual abuse is reported in the histories of nearly two thirds of adult female psychiatric patients (Bryer, Nelson, Miller, & Krol, 1987; Chu & Dill, 1990; Surrey, Swett, Michaels, & Levin, 1990). Through clinical observations and recent research, the impact of both severe childhood abuse and the dysfunctional environments in which abuse occurs have increasingly become more clearly defined.

Childhood abuse has been correlated with a variety of nonspecific effects such as depressed mood, anxiety, self-destructive behavior, and poor self-esteem (Courtois, 1979; Finkelhor, 1984; Gelinas, 1983; Herman, 1981; Herman, Russell, &

James A. Chu • Dissociative Disorders Program, McLean Hospital, Belmont, Massachusetts 02178; and Department of Psychiatry, Harvard Medical School, Boston, Massachusetts 02115.

Handbook of Dissociation: Theoretical, Empirical, and Clinical Perspectives, edited by Larry K. Michelson and William J. Ray. Plenum Press, New York, 1996.

Portions of this chapter are reprinted from Chu (1992a) and Gunderson and Chu (1993).

Trocki, 1986; Pribor & Dinwiddie, 1992; Russell, 1986; Shapiro, 1987; Swanson & Biaggio, 1985). New research and clinical studies have suggested that severe childhood trauma is a primary etiologic factor with at least three major areas of psychological disturbance: dissociative symptoms (including dissociative identity disorder as the most severe form) (Braun, 1990; Chu & Dill, 1990; Saxe et al., 1993; Putnam, 1985), posttraumatic stress symptoms (Donaldson & Gardner, 1985; Kirby, Chu, & Dill, 1993; Pribor & Dinwiddie, 1992; Saxe et al., 1993; Ulman & Brothers, 1988; van der Kolk, 1987a), and disruption of personality development and maturation such as is seen in borderline personality disorder (Goldman, D'Angelo, DeMaso, & Mezzacappa, 1992; Herman, Perry & van der Kolk, 1989; Herman & van der Kolk, 1987; Ludolph et al., 1990; Ogata et al., 1990; Saxe et al., 1993).

The contention that this triad of areas of psychological disturbance should result from severe childhood trauma has considerable face validity. Dissociation appears to be an available psychological defense for children whose limited coping capacities are overwhelmed by extremely traumatic events (Putnam, 1985). Dissociation enables such events to be "forgotten," or at least emotionally distanced. Posttraumatic symptoms also appear to be logical consequences of childhood abuse. Freud's (1920) repetition compulsion appears to be highly applicable to repressed childhood trauma, and adults with such backgrounds evidence many different kinds of reexperiencing phenomena (Chu, 1991a; van der Kolk & Kadish, 1987) as well as avoidant symptoms and autonomic arousal (Ulman & Brothers, 1988; van der Kolk, 1987a). Finally, symptoms of borderline personality disorder—including ongoing relational disturbances, difficulty tolerating intense affects, behavioral dyscontrol, and identity diffusion—seem to be logical consequences of the failures of attachment and the inadequate care and protection that are common in dysfunctional and abusive families.

This discussion briefly examines each of the above areas of symptomatology related to early childhood abuse with a focus on dissociative syndromes that do not fall into well-defined categories and outlines a treatment model that addresses the need to prioritize and sequence treatment interventions in patients with complex posttraumatic symptomatology.

DISSOCIATION IN RELATION TO CHILDHOOD ABUSE

In early studies of multiple personality disorder, the finding of childhood abuse was nearly universal (Putnam, Guroff, Silberman, Barban, & Post, 1986), leading investigators to propose a link between dissociative symptoms and early trauma (Putnam, 1985). Other investigators, such as Terr (1991), who investigated the effects of psychic trauma on children, proposed a model in which dissociation is "learned" by children as a way of escaping overwhelming experiences. This mechanism may begin as a conscious attempt at self-hypnosis, but eventually becomes an automatic and uncontrollable response to trauma or stimulus associated with trauma. The development of dissociative defenses appears to occur more readily in childhood (Putnam, 1985), and there is increasing evidence to suggest that severe dissociative disorders are frequently linked to early childhood trauma (Kirby, Chu & Dill, 1993).

Dissociative disorders may be much more common than previously believed. Using the Dissociative Experiences Scale (DES) (Bernstein & Putnam, 1986), Chu and Dill (1990) found that 24% of consecutively admitted adult women inpatients scored above the previously established median for posttraumatic stress disorder (PTSD) and that 6% scored above the median for multiple personality disorder (MPD). In another study of inpatients, utilizing the Dissociative Disorders Interview Schedule (DDIS) (Ross, 1989), Ross, Anderson, Fleischer, & Norton (1991) found a dissociative disorder in 21% and MPD in over 5% of their subjects. The implications of these finding are at least threefold. First, dissociative disorders may be generally underdiagnosed, perhaps due to clinicians failing to ask about dissociative symptomatology. Second, MPD or dissociative identity disorder (DID) may be much more common than previously thought. Third, the majority of diagnosable dissociative disorders are *not* DID. In fact, these studies suggest that there may be three or four times as many dissociative disorders which are not DID as are DID. While some of these patients fall into recognizable categories such as dissociative amnesia, fugue, and depersonalization disorder, many others are not so easily characterized. Based on clinical experience, a very large number of patients who have a dissociative disorder, but who do not have DID, fall into the category of dissociative disorder, not otherwise specified.

Dissociative Disorder, Not Otherwise Specified

Dissociative disorder, not otherwise specified (DDNOS) is described in the DSM-IV as "disorders in which the predominant feature is a dissociative symptom (i.e., a disturbance of alteration in the normal integrative functions of identity, memory, or consciousness, memory, identity, or perception of the environment) that does not meet the criteria for any specific Dissociative Disorder" (American Psychiatric Association, 1994, p. 490). Examples include Ganser's syndrome (the giving of approximate answers to questions accompanied by dissociative and conversion symptoms), trance states, derealization unaccompanied by depersonalization, dissociation following intense coercive persuasion, and atypical fuguelike states and amnesia. In clinical experience, however, one of the most common types of patients with DDNOS are those who have extensive fragmentation of experience and identity, which resembles DID, but the fragmentation does not reach the level of severity of DID.

Braun (1986), Bernstein and Putnam (1986) and others have proposed the concept of a dissociative continuum with dissociative experiences ranging from normal to pathological. Patients who fall in the range of the dissociative continuum short of DID may, in fact, have severe dissociative symptoms including a fragmented sense of self. Such patients often describe feeling as though they are different people at different times, or that they watch themselves doing things almost as though they were outside their own bodies. However, these kinds of DDNOS patients are able to acknowledge that these alterations in sense of identity are various split-off aspects of themselves and not separate identities. Watkins and Watkins (1979) described such patients as having various "ego-states" in which they have clear changes in their sense of identity, but do not necessarily have the extreme dissociative barriers of DID. The following case example illustrates some of the features of this kind of DDNOS:

> A 32-year-old woman sought a psychiatric evaluation for chronic difficulties with relationships. It rapidly became clear that she had a history of childhood neglect and abuse, and that many of the relational issues inherent in the abuse had strongly affected her adult relationships. The patient also described very clear shifts in mood, behavior, and identity which often occurred abruptly and were out of her control. One example she gave was in the context of becoming involved in relationships. Often, as a relationship became increasingly intimate, she would experience an internal emotional shift in which she would become suddenly hostile and cold. She reported, "Sometimes I can't believe the words that are coming out of my mouth. I know it's me speaking, but I'm appalled at the kinds of things I am saying." Other instances included occasions when she would suddenly find herself crying for unknown reasons, and other times when she would feel despairing and panicky for periods lasting from a few minutes to a few hours. The patient described a life-long ability to "space out"; she would sit in one spot or lie on her bed, staring off into space, not thinking about much of anything, and feeling very far away. She described these periods as a kind of "mental vacation." During times of high stress, she also reported brief amnestic periods, and sometimes heard critical voices in her head which she recognized as her own thoughts. Although the differential diagnosis included panic disorder, affective disorder, and temporal lobe epilepsy, the initial impression that the patient's difficulties were consistent with DDNOS.

Patients with DDNOS who have major shifts in affect, identity, and behavior often have associated symptomatology including chronic depersonalization and derealization and sometimes auditory hallucinations. It should be noted that these auditory hallucinations, which are heard inside the head, are actually a kind of dissociative hallucinosis representing the thoughts of split-off parts of the self and not evidence of true psychosis (Kluft, 1987; Putman et al., 1986).

An additional problem in making accurate diagnostic assessments with patients with dissociative disorders is that the level of dissociative symptomatology is somewhat variable for many patients. For example, some patients with severe dissociative symptoms may manifest more florid symptoms under conditions of stress, sometimes to the extent of demonstrating transient but clear multiple personalities. Braun (1986, p. 20) labels such patients as having atypical MPD, and notes: "In atypical MPD, the patient initially does not appear to have multiple personalities at all. ... Under sufficient stress, the atypical MPS patient will decompensate and present as a typical MPD patient." Such patients do not consistently meet the criteria for MPD or DID, and probably should be considered as having DDNOS as in the following example from Chu (1991b, p. 201):

> A 25-year-old woman with a known history of childhood physical and sexual abuse, as well as symptoms of post-traumatic stress disorder, was admitted to the hospital after being mugged on the street in her neighborhood. While in the hospital, she showed evidence of three separate personalities, including a depleted host personality, a child personality, and an angry persecutor personality. She worked actively on issues related to the mugging and on how to maintain personal safety, and was discharged in about two weeks. On follow-up one month later, she was asked about the various personalities. She answered,

"Well, they're all a part of me now," and her outpatient therapist confirmed that there was no continuing evidence of separateness.

POSTTRAUMATIC STRESS DISORDER

One of the essential features of PTSD is a process in which overwhelming traumatic experiences are dissociated from current awareness and periodically reexperienced in various forms, e.g., flashbacks. There are particular differences in posttraumatic and dissociative symptomatology between persons who have been first traumatized as adults and those who have been traumatized as children. Because children have a greater innate dissociative capacity, as well as less mature and developed capacity to tolerate stress, severely abused children develop more dissociative symptoms including more dissociative amnesia. Several studies have demonstrated that extensive childhood abuse prior to adolescence frequently results in either partial or complete amnesia for the abusive events (Briere & Conte, 1993; Herman & Schatzow, 1987; Kirby et al., 1993). Not remembering abuse does not free persons from reexperiencing aspects of the abuse. Instead, many survivors of childhood abuse are frequently tormented by intensely dysphoric feelings such as helplessness, depression, anger, and isolation that are connected to the forgotten abuse. Moreover, since such patients are unable to report the core reasons for their distress, neither they nor clinicians are able to make sense of their painful lives. Judging from clinical experience, the reexperiencing of intense affect, bodily sensation, and behavior related to childhood abuse is extremely common, often accompanied by no awareness or only fragmentary awareness of the actual abuse.

A somewhat more subtle difficulty for persons with early childhood abuse has to do with communication. Prior to adolescence, and especially in early childhood, the primary modality of experiencing the world is not verbal and linguistic as it is in adults, but is largely sensorimotor (van der Kolk & van der Hart, 1989). Thus, traumatic events that occur early in childhood are encoded in the psyche in a modality that is primarily nonverbal. When these events are reexperienced, they have a similar nonverbal quality. In the clinical arena, it is quite striking to encounter patients who are otherwise highly intelligent, verbal, and articulate, but who literally seem to have no words to describe their childhood experiences.

Several additional concepts connected with the syndrome of PTSD are important in the treatment of survivors of childhood abuse. The biphasic response to trauma, first described by Lindemann (1944) and subsequently by Horowitz (1976) and van der Kolk (1987a), suggests that psychological trauma results in alternating phases of intrusion and numbing. Intrusive responses, as described in the DSM-IV, include distressing recollections of the traumatic events, traumatic dreams, reexperiencing of the events, and intense distress on exposure to reminders of the trauma. These alternate with the numbing responses, which include efforts to avoid thoughts, feelings, or activities associated with the traumatic events, inability to recall details of the events, diminished interest in activities, social withdrawal, emotional constriction, and a sense of foreshortened future (American Psychiatric Association, 1994). Survivors of childhood abuse may show all these features. When in the intrusive phase, they are overwhelmed and in crisis, desperate to regain a sense of control. When they are in the numbing phase, they are depressed, empty, and feel that life has no meaning. The cycle of intrusion and numbing may continue over long periods of time, with patients going through phases of intolerable crisis followed by crushing depression.

Another feature of PTSD common to survivors of childhood abuse is generalized autonomic hyperarousal manifested by chronic anxiety, panic attacks, startle responses, and disturbed sleep. These symptoms are often very distressing and respond poorly to psychological interventions such as psychotherapy. However, some partial relief can be obtained through the judicious use of medications. Benzodiazepines such as lorazepam (Ativan) or clonazepam (Klonapin) may be helpful for anxiety and panic attacks. In some cases, when patients do not respond to or become addicted to benzodiazepines, low-dose neuroleptics may also be used for extreme anxiety. Sleep disturbance in patients with PTSD stemming from early trauma is often characterized by fear of falling asleep and multiple anxious midsleep awakenings (Chu, unpublished manuscript). Low doses of sedating antidepressants such as trazodone (Desyrel), amitriptyline (Elavil and others), or doxepin (Sinequan) have sometimes been helpful with this kind of sleep disturbance.

BORDERLINE PERSONALITY DISORDER AND CHILDHOOD ABUSE

Classic psychoanalytic theories concerning borderline personality disorder (BPD) have focused on intrapsychic phenomenology such as ego strength or weakness, defenses, and developmental history. Kernberg (1967, 1968, 1970) hypothesized that there was a failure of normal psychological development early in life, particularly around the necessary integration of conflictual feelings about primary caretakers. Mahler's (1971, 1972) and Masterson's (1972) contributions point specifically to the rapprochement subphase of the separation-individuation process around the age of 18 months as a time of difficulty. They hypothesized that disruptions of attachment can occur in the mother-child relationship if a proper balance of holding and letting go does not occur.

Recent studies have demonstrated very high rates of traumatic childhood experiences in adolescent and adult patients with BPD, generally in the range of 60 to 75% (Goldman et al., 1992; Herman et al., 1989; Herman & van der Kolk, 1987; Ludolph et al., 1990; Ogata et al., 1990; Saxe et al., 1993). This growing body of evidence suggests that childhood abuse is often a significant factor in the development of borderline psychopathology, and that a shift should be made in the conceptual paradigm of BPD. Rather than only focusing on issues concerning intrapsychic structure, one must also consider the reality of the impact of cataclysmic events in molding such structures. This shift in conceptual paradigm has major implications for the treatment of borderline patients with childhood abuse (Gunderson & Chu, 1993).

In clinical experience, many patients with BPD report extensive histories of childhood emotional, physical, and sexual abuse, profound neglect, and the witnessing of violence. However, it is our contention that it is not the trauma per se that results in BPD; after all, a significant minority of patients seem to develop BPD without evidence of childhood trauma. Rather, it is the gross disruptions of familial attachments and the massive failure of adequate care and protection of the child that result in distortions of normal characterological development. Experiences of intrafamilial abuse and neglect are extreme manifestations of the failure of normal parental attachment and nurturance. In most cases, these disruptions of attachment and nurturance have been neither subtle nor circumscribed, but have existed throughout multiple phases of childhood development.

In light of evidence of a history of significant trauma in many borderline patients, borderline symptomatology has become more understandable. The intensity of the borderline patients' relationships and the wild oscillations between idealization and devaluation may well be understood as recapitulations of early abusive relationships. Their poor affect tolerance and behavioral dyscontrol, as well as self-destructive patterns of tension reduction, can be understood as the result of the failure of early care and protection and the lack of proper support of the child's ability to tolerate both internal and external experiences. Their fear of abandonment and intense anger may be understood as resulting from real abandonment and deprivation. And their persistent sense of emptiness and debased self-identity can be understood as resulting from the failure of adequate mirroring and validation and from real neglect and abuse.

In a paradigm that takes into account the actual occurrence of major trauma in the early background of borderline patients, one must move away from the prevailing view of a subtle kind of degeneracy, i.e., that borderline patients inherently have abnormal or excessive reactions to current untoward life events. Rather, one must see many patients with BPD as having adapted to overwhelming life events by developing certain patterns of relating and specific defenses and by viewing themselves and reacting to others on the basis of long-standing and unresolved traumatic experiences. These patterns of adaptation can be seen as currently dysfunctional but eminently understandable in view of past life experiences. This kind of attitudinal shift may be crucial in ameliorating the pejorative associations common to the borderline diagnosis (Vaillant, 1992) and in providing effective treatment.

A TREATMENT MODEL

Certainly not all adults with histories of significant childhood abuse experience dissociative, posttraumatic, and severe personality disorder symptoms. However, close clinical observation suggests that many individuals with psychiatric difficulties, particularly those who are the most disabled and those who are frequently hospitalized, show evidence of this triad of symptoms. These patients commonly present with a bewildering range of psychiatric symptomatology and represent diagnostic and treatment challenges. It is understandably difficult to know how to approach patients who manifest such a complex array of symptoms. Perhaps it is because of this complexity of symptoms that these patients are seen as difficult to treat, and much time and effort on the part of both the patient and therapist are often wasted in misdirected therapeutic efforts. It is a common experience for therapists to feel as though they are riding some kind of therapeutic roller coaster, with little sense of control or direction, and to have a constant feeling of impending crisis and potential danger. This discussion will examine the concepts behind the management of complex childhood abuse survivors and set out a rational paradigm for treatment (Chu, 1992a).

Clear recognition of the profound effects of early abusive experiences and the complexity of adult syndromes related to such experiences underscores the need for a sophisticated understanding of the treatment process for childhood abuse survivors. Because of the many and varied psychiatric symptoms that such individuals commonly present, clinicians need to conceptualize a hierarchy of treatment approaches designed to address specific symptomatology. Many survivors of severe childhood abuse require a lengthy period of building a psychotherapeutic foundation, so that later, more definitive abreactive work will be successful.

The therapeutic value of abreaction in adult war veterans has been described in studies using techniques that precipitate the reexperiencing of the traumatic event in a context of high social support so that the experience is tolerated, attitudinally reframed, and integrated into conscious experience (Foa, Steketee, & Rothbaum, 1989; Keane, Fairbank, Caddell, & Zimering, 1989). There are no similar studies of the use of abreactive techniques in survivors of childhood trauma. However, based on clinical experience, it is widely believed that the *eventual* reexperiencing and working through of childhood trauma has a beneficial therapeutic effect. Persons who have been able to successfully abreact abusive childhood experiences often report dramatic changes in their lives. They report changes such as a reduction in acute symptomatology, fewer and less troubling intrusions of the abusive experiences, a new sense of identity as being psychologically healthy and functionally competent, and a much improved ability to relate to others.

The clear value of abreaction of childhood trauma in some patients has led to an erroneous belief system that seems remarkably ubiquitous among many patients and their therapists. In this belief system, it is felt that in any clinical situation where childhood abuse is discovered in the history, all efforts should be made to immediately explore and abreact those abusive experiences. Moreover, many clinicians appear to feel that if current difficulties seem related to past abuse, then the treatment of choice is to abreact the etiologic abuse. Unfortunately, in the treatment of many patients, such a belief system is conceptually flawed and inappropriate and can have untoward effects such as increasing acute symptomatology and functional difficulties. Patients who have not done the necessary preliminary work are once again overwhelmed by these experiences, and the patient is actually retraumatized and there is little or no working through or resolution.

In order to be able to tolerate abreactive work, the patient must be able to utilize a high level of social and interpersonal support. Unfortunately, the ability to relate to and feel supported by others is a primary area of disability in many patients with a history of severe childhood abuse. These individuals often have acute relational difficulties that derive from their early abusive experiences. Instead of being able to trust in others to support them, they fully expect abandonment and betrayal. Characteristically, when faced with any major stressor (internal or external), severely abused patients flee into isolation as the perceived safest alternative and/or resort to ingrained solutions that are dysfunctional in their current life. Because therapy may explore past traumatic experiences, the therapist and the therapeutic process may be experienced as major stressors and may precipitate negative therapeutic reactions.

The following model divides the treatment course into early, middle, and late stages. The early stage is comprised primarily of building basic relational and coping skills. The middle stage involves exploration and abreaction of traumatic experiences. Finally, the late stage consists of stabilization of gains and increased personal growth particularly in relation to the external world. This division of the course of treatment is somewhat arbitrary, since patients generally move back and forth between stages, rather than progressing in a neat linear fashion. However, this delineation is useful in specifying the components and hierarchy of treatment.

Early-Stage Treatment: The "Safer" Model

Abreaction and resolution of early traumatic experiences are limited by the ability of childhood abuse survivors to utilize supportive relationships, including the therapeutic relationship. Abreactive work must be deferred pending the development of basic skills in terms of relating and coping. In a treatment model previously described (Chu, 1992a), five areas of focus can be identified as crucial in the early stages of treatment. These are discussed here as part of the mnemonic SAFER: self-care, acknowledgment, functioning, expression, and relationships.

Self-Care. Survivors of childhood abuse are prone to become involved in a wide variety of self-destructive and dysfunctional behaviors (van der Kolk, Perry & Herman, 1991). Self-mutilation of a nonlethal nature is extremely common (Shapiro, 1987; van der Kolk et al., 1991) and, paradoxically, is often used as a soothing and coping mechanism. Patients with histories of extensive childhood abuse often describe their nonlethal cutting or burning as tension-relieving rather than painful. Abuse survivors often have other dysfunctional behaviors such as substance abuse (National Victim Center, 1992; Pribor & Dinwiddie, 1992), eating disorders (Hall, Tice, Beresford, Wooley, & Hall, 1989), and addiction to risk-taking behaviors (van der Kolk, 1987b). Finally, revictimization is remarkably common (Chu, 1992b), including repetitions of emotional, physical, and sexual abuse. Patients' propensities toward inadequate self-care through both self-destructive behavior and vulnerability to revictimization must be controlled prior to the institution of any exploratory therapy. Failure to do so increases the likelihood of serious self-harm when traumatic material is broached. Analogous to the situation of abused children, abuse survivors must create an environment of personal safety prior to any dismantling of protective (albeit now dysfunctional) defenses.

Abuse survivors tend to be ambivalent about self-care. Perhaps one of the most damaging aspects of chronic childhood abuse is the compulsion to continue the patterns of abuse long after the original perpetrators are no longer actively abusive. In addition, a sense of inner worthlessness may make self-care seem internally inconsistent or unimportant. And perhaps most significantly, alternative coping mechanisms, which involve reliance on others, may seem extremely risky to the abuse survivors who have backgrounds of abandonment and betrayal. Nonetheless, therapists need to insist that the therapy of patients with extensive childhood abuse focus on self-care. It should be noted in the early stage of therapy that many patients will lack the strength to fully achieve self-care. In many situations, lapses will occur and patients may retreat to self-destructive behavior. However, such lapses are only acceptable when patients are able to demonstrate a commitment to the principles of self-care over time.

Acknowledgment. Although intensive exploration of past traumatic experiences may be inadvisable in the early stage of treatment, acknowledgment of the central role of the early trauma is crucial. Childhood abuse is an important determinant in the lives of trauma survivors not only in terms of posttraumatic symptomatology, but also in terms of ability to cope with normal life experiences, especially interpersonal relationships. To ignore the role of abusive experiences is to tacitly collude in patients' erroneous beliefs of inherent personal defectiveness. The simple acknowledgment of the possible role of early traumatic experiences begins the process of helping survivors to understand many of their current difficulties as being derived from extraordinarily overwhelming events.

Patients who are abuse survivors are often remarkably ambivalent about acknowledging the role of trauma in their lives. It is striking that many trauma survivors continue to minimize obviously abusive experiences and their effects, and instead insist that they are simply "crazy" or "bad" for having difficulties in their lives. In the face of backgrounds of truly abusive experiences, such denial appears to be further evidence of the extent and unbearable nature of the abuse.

Functioning. In therapy, patients who suffered early abuse often become acutely symptomatic when they are overwhelmed by the reexperiencing of their trauma. Without persistent effort on the part of both patients and their therapists to maintain some semblance of normal functioning, the reexperiences of trauma can rapidly consume every aspect of patients' lives. The syndrome of constant flashbacks, repeatedly occurring crises, desperate efforts to obtain comfort and reassurance, and dysphoric dependence on therapists is seen frequently in treatment that is out of control.

Maintaining some appropriate level of functioning is often difficult but nonetheless essential. Even if such efforts to function seem to patients to be superficial or just "going through the motions," they are important in terms of balancing the internal pull toward becoming totally immersed in past events. Therapists must emphasize the importance of maintaining both functioning and supportive relationships during the therapeutic process. Without an emphasis on functioning outside the therapy, problems such as regression and overly intense transferences are prone to flourish.

Expression. The intense affects associated with posttraumatic symptomatology must be expressed in a nondestructive and therapeutic manner. Although full exploration of the traumatic events may not be advisable in the early stage of treatment, patients do experience some of the overwhelming negative affects associated with the events such as dysphoria, panic, and anger. The nonverbal nature of these feelings and patients' ingrained but dysfunctional coping mechanisms frequently lead patients to withdraw and isolate themselves and to engage in a variety of tension-releasing and destructive activities.

Unspeakable feelings need to find expression in words. Particularly in the early stages of therapy, however, this process may be facilitated through therapeutic nonverbal expression. The expressive therapies may have a special role in permitting and encouraging appropriate nonverbal expression. In the early stage of therapy, such efforts should be directed primarily at therapeutic expression rather than exploration, and they can be powerful forces in helping patients to find words for their previously unspeakable feelings.

Relationships. Perhaps the most important task of early-stage treatment is beginning to establish patterns of interpersonal relatedness that are mutual and collaborative. Survivors of childhood abuse bring the abusive style of relating from their childhood environments into all their adult relationships, including the therapeutic relationship. Childhood abandonments, betrayals, and abuse often transform the therapeutic relationship into an emotional battlefield in which the patient and therapist alternately take the perceived role of abused and abuser. The recapitulation and reenactment of early abusive relationships makes collaborative work on resolving past traumatic experiences impossible until some semblance of mutuality is established.

In the early stage of therapy, the patient and therapist must repeatedly renegotiate the therapeutic alliance. As the patient is repeatedly unconsciously compelled to precipitate abusive reenactments within the treatment relationship, the therapist must interpret the process and help the patient in developing a sense of collaboration and mutuality. This process of disconnection and reconnection must occur on seemingly endless occasions with endless variations before a minimal sense of basic trust is formed. It is the difficulties encountered in the interpersonal process that makes the early stage of therapy long and arduous. However, the repeated disconnection and reconnection is the vehicle that provides for the patient a model of mutuality in relationships and ways to resolve conflict and ultimately provides a corrective emotional experience. Negotiation of the relationship is a necessary and prerequisite step for the eventual exploration and resolution of the actual traumatic events.

Middle-Stage Treatment

When abuse survivors have mastered the tasks of early therapy, they may then proceed to the exploration and abreactive work of the middle stage of treatment. Patients vary considerably in their ability to move beyond early-stage treatment. Some abuse survivors enter therapy with excellent coping skills and may quickly move toward middle-stage treatment. However, many others require months or even years of preliminary work. Several caveats in terms of abreaction of traumatic experiences should be noted. It is premature, at this point in time, to estimate what proportion of abuse survivors will be able to abreact and successfully work through early traumatic experiences. Clinical evidence suggests that although many are able to do so, others may be able to achieve resolution and integration of traumatic backgrounds only to a minimal or partial extent. For such patients, stabilization and symptom management remain the long-term goals of treatment.

Significant regression is commonly observed in the face of abreaction of traumatic experiences. That is, under the stress of reexperiencing early abuse, patients may return to former patterns of isolation and dysfunctional or self-destructive behavior. If and when these patterns reemerge, clinical attention should return to early-stage issues until these issues are once again mastered. Patients need to establish powerful relational bonds and be prepared to withstand extremely dysphoric affects without resorting to dysfunctional behavior in order to tolerate abreactive work. Thus, abreactive should be undertaken from a position of strength rather than vulnerability. Without adequate preparation and support, patients are prone to reexperience traumatic events once again in isolation and once again to be overwhelmed by them. Although abuse survivors may be able to vent affect and release internal tension through uncontrolled abreactions, these experiences have very little lasting therapeutic value.

For patients with complex syndromes of posttraumatic symptomatology and severe characterological difficulties, abreactive work is likely to be a series of processes rather than a single cathartic event. It is the frequent expectation of patients that traumatic events can be abreacted and worked through in a brief and dramatic fashion. However, clinical experience suggests that working through each major issue or important event may entail a prolonged process lasting days, weeks, or months. Although patterns of abreaction differ according to the individual characteristics of patients, several phases are commonly seen. These are: (1) increased symptomatology, particularly more intrusive reexperiencing, (2) intense internal conflict, (3) acceptance and mourning, and (4) mobilization and empowerment.

An increase in the reexperiencing of traumatic events—with symptoms such as nightmares and disturbed sleep, increased anxiety, dissociative experiences, and generalized hyperactivity and autonomic hyperarousal—is a common early feature of the abreactive process. These symptoms are often accompanied by the patient's efforts to deny any link to traumatic events, but denial of this type begins to break down as patients are flooded by reexperiencing.

As the abreactive process continues, patients begin to tolerate and accept the reality of past events and begin to attempt to reframe these events. With the assistance of the perspective of the therapist, the events that were originally experienced (and are being reexperienced in the present) from the perspective of a helpless abused child begin to be seen from a more adult viewpoint. This process produces intense internal conflict. As an example, patients are often unable to let go of long-held feelings of self-blame at the same time that they begin to understand that they were not responsible for their abuse. Patients may retain a sense of identification with the perpetrators of abuse even though they know that they were victimized. Abuse survivors may also experience intense shame about having "given in" to the abuse even though they understand that they had no choice.

The resolution of such conflicts involves the patient's "new," stronger, and healthier aspects understanding and having compassion for the "old" and dysfunctional aspects. That is, patients must understand and accept that they did what they had to do in response to extreme events. Acceptance of past feelings and behaviors as opposed to rejection and disavowal leads to the resolution of these internal conflicts.

Persons with unresolved abusive experiences frequently underestimate and minimize the extent of their own victimization as a way of protecting themselves from the full impact of the abuse. Despite the intense dysphoria that often accompanies fragmentary memories of the abuse, survivors are often stunned by the full realization of the extent of past abuse. As patients begin to accept their past realities, they are often overcome by the extent of their former helplessness and by the abandonment and betrayal of important people in their lives. This part of the abreactive process often leaves patients emotionally drained, analogous to survivors of a natural disaster who are just beginning to take in the extent of the devastation that surrounds them.

Full realization of the extent of their abuse and the subsequent toll it has taken on their lives allows patients to begin to mourn the losses that have resulted from the abuse. This slow and painful process may involve patients examining each significant aspect of their pasts and reframing their understanding of the events and their meaning. Patients begin to accept that they were truly not to blame for their victimization and to understand how the early abusive experiences may have made them vulnerable to later revictimization.

Supported by these insights, patients begin the process of surrendering the role of "victim" and replacing it with a sense of self as a "survivor" of abuse. Over time, the abreactive process enables abuse survivors to mobilize their strengths and to gain a sense of control. Diffuse feelings become more focused. For example, rather than feeling frightened of all men, sexual abuse survivors may be able to recognize that there were specific men responsible for the abuse. They may then be able to focus their fear, anger, and outrage on the perpetrators as opposed to displacing these feelings in a generalized fashion.

Abreaction of past trauma frees abuse survivors from fear of their own repressed memories. Their nightmarish childhood realities have lost the power to overwhelm and control them. Moreover, their sense of identity is positively enhanced by an understanding that they have been able to tolerate and overcome the reexperiencing of past abuse. An adult perspective on the childhood trauma allows abuse survivors freedom from unreasonable fear, as well as enabling them to protect themselves from future victimization.

Late-Stage Treatment

Abreaction and resolution of past abusive experiences enables trauma survivors to proceed with their lives relatively unencumbered by their pasts. Late-stage treatment is familiar to experienced therapists as the processes of healthy introspection and engagement of the external world, which is usual in the psychotherapy of nontraumatized patients. Resolution of the all-encompassing and overwhelming past events reduces survivors' narcissistic preoccupation with their symptoms and difficulties. Moreover, an empowered sense of self leads patients to have increased confidence in their abilities to participate successfully in interpersonal relationships and other interactions in ways that previously eluded them. In persons who previously have had a fragmented sense of identity, a profound sense of a new, integrated self arising from new psychic structures often emerges, which facilitates persons' ability to engage with the external world.

It should be noted that it is common for patients in the late stage of therapy to find areas of yet unresolved trauma or trauma-related issues as they proceed with their lives and encounter new situations. This process should be construed only as a need to complete further abreactive work and not as a failure of therapy. In fact, previous successful experiences with abreactive therapy facilitate and often shorten any additional similar treatment.

CONCLUSIONS

The therapy of severely traumatized patients is often extremely complex and confusing. Sophisticated understanding of both the nature of the psychological effects of trauma and of the therapeutic process of psychotherapy is necessary to design and implement a useful treatment program. When treating abuse survivors, even clinically sophisticated therapists are still prone to encounter certain common clinical dilemmas (Chu, 1988, 1992a). There appear to be particular characteristics of abuse survivors and their therapy that interfere with therapists exercising their usual clinical skills. As a result, therapists often find themselves beleaguered, emotionally drained, and uncertain of what they are doing (Chu, 1988; Kluft, 1989), which enhances their sense of riding a therapeutic roller coaster and facing a constant sense of impending peril. Clinical dilemmas are often inherently part of the treatment and must be negotiated. Common dilemmas often concern such issues as maintaining the treatment frame, sharing therapeutic responsibility, achieving control of dissociative symptoms, and managing transference-countertransference reactions (Chu, 1992a).

The profound effects of early abuse on the development of personality in terms of relatedness and coping abilities must not be overlooked in efforts to confront posttraumatic and dissociative symptomatology. Therapists must help patients address these basic characterological issues in order to lay the foundations for later abreactive work and resolution of the etiologic abuse. There are no real shortcuts in the often lengthy and arduous process of the psychotherapy of severely harmed trauma survivors. Premature efforts at abreaction are potentially dangerous in terms of the likelihood of patients' regression and increased morbidity and mortality.

Even though the treatment of severely traumatized patients requires sophisticated understandings and interventions, therapists should remember that the basic tenets of psychotherapy are applicable to these patients. In particular, the provision of a safe and containing environment is of central importance (Herman, 1992). Without a sense of safety in both the therapeutic relationship and the patient's outside life, little can be accomplished. As patients are able to experience themselves in a safe environment, they are able to move forward and progress in their treatment.

The nature of the etiologic abuse and the dysfunctional family environments in which the abuse occurred can precipitate many treatment traps, dilemmas, and potential impasses within the therapeutic arena. Even in the hands of experienced therapists, these difficulties cannot always be avoided or circumvented. In fact, the nature of successful treatment of abuse survivors demands that therapists become involved and fully appreciate the dilemmas and psychological pain that patients experience. However, an understanding of the treatment process allows therapists to be better prepared, less anxious about the treatment, and more proficient in resolving problems when they arise. Therapists must maintain clearly defined therapeutic stances in regard to such issues and must sometimes even insist that patients ally with such therapeutic stances as a condition of continuing the treatment. After all, therapists should not be placed in the position of continuing and colluding in any process that is inherently antitherapeutic and that does not have the potential for a positive therapeutic result.

The psychotherapeutic process is a powerful interpersonal tool, capable of enabling both positive therapeutic growth and psychological harm. Therapists must take seriously the potential of the psychotherapeutic process to harm patients. For example, therapists must avoid collusion with patients' ingrained debased sense of self and should help patients limit unending repetitions of reenactments of abusive relatedness. On the other hand, well-conceived psychotherapeutic efforts, used with good clinical judgment by dedicated psychotherapists, can have dramatic and positive effects. Such treatment offers abuse survivors new hope, and many patients—even those who have suffered the most horrendous childhood abuse—are able to move forward and substantially improve their lives.

REFERENCES

American Psychiatric Association (1994). *Diagnostic and statistical manual of mental disorders* (3rd ed.). Washington, DC: Author.

Bernstein, E. M., & Putnam, F. W. (1986). Development, reliability, and validity of a dissociation scale. *Journal of Nervous and Mental Disease, 174*, 727-734.

Braun, B. G. (1986). Issues in the psychotherapy of multiple personality disorder. In B. G. Braun (Ed.), *Treatment of multiple personality disorder* (pp. 1-28). Washington, DC: American Psychiatric Press.

Braun, B. G. (1990). Dissociative disorders as sequelae to incest. In R. P. Kluft (Ed.), *Incest-related syndromes of adult psychopathology* (pp. 227-246). Washington, DC: American Psychiatric Press.

Briere, J., & Conte, J. (1993). Self-reported amnesia in adults molested as children. *Journal of Traumatic Stress, 6*, 21-31.

Bryer, J. B., Nelson, B. A., Miller, J. B., & Krol, P. A. (1987). Childhood sexual and physical abuse as factors in adult psychiatric illness. *American Journal of Psychiatry, 144*, 1426-1430.

Chu, J. A. (1988). Ten traps for therapists in the treatment of trauma survivors. *Dissociation, 1*(4), 24-32.

Chu, J. A. (1991a). The repetition compulsion revisited: Reliving dissociated trauma. *Psychotherapy, 28*, 327-332.

Chu, J. A. (1991b). On the misdiagnosis of multiple personality disorder. *Dissociation, 4*, 200-204.

Chu, J. A. (1992a). The therapeutic roller coaster: Dilemmas in the treatment of childhood abuse survivors. *Journal of Psychotherapy Practice and Research, 1*, 351-370.

Chu, J. A. (1992b). The revictimization of adult women with histories of childhood abuse. *Journal of Psychotherapy Practice and Research, 1*, 259-269.

Chu, J. A. (in submission). Depressive and post-traumatic symptomatology in adults with histories of childhood abuse. Unpublished manuscript. Available through Dr. Chu, 115 Mill St., Belmont, MA 02178.

Chu, J. A., and Dill, D. L. (1990). Dissociative symptoms in relation to childhood physical and sexual abuse. *American Journal of Psychiatry, 149*, 887-893.

Courtois, C. (1979). The incest experience and its aftermath. *Victimology, 4*, 337-347.

Donaldson, M. A., & Gardner, R. (1985). Diagnosis and treatment of traumatic stress among women after childhood incest. In C. Figley (Ed.), *Trauma and its wake* (pp. 356-377). New York: Brunner/Mazel.

Finkelhor, D. (1984). *Child sexual abuse: New theory and research*. New York: Free Press.

Foa, E. B., Steketee, G., & Rothbaum, B. O. (1989) Behavioral/cognitive conceptualizations of post-traumatic stress disorder. *Behavior Therapy, 20*, 155-176.

Freud, S. (1920). Beyond the pleasure principle. In *The Complete Works of Sigmund Freud* (vol. 18, pp. 7-64). London: Hogarth Press, 1955.

Gelinas, D. J. (1983). The persisting negative effects of incest. *Psychiatry, 46*, 312-332.

Goldman, S. J., D'Angelo, E. J., DeMaso, D. R., & Mezzacappa, E. (1992). Physical and sexual abuse among children with borderline personality disorder. *American Journal of Psychiatry, 149*, 1723-1726.

Gunderson, J. G., & Chu, J. A. (1993) Treatment implications of past trauma in borderline personality disorder. *Harvard Review of Psychiatry, 1*, 75-81.

Hall, R. C., Tice, L., Beresford, T. P., Wooley, B., & Hall, A. K. (1989). Sexual abuse patients with anorexia nervosa and bulimia. *Psychosomatics, 30*, 73-79.

Herman, J. (1981). *Father-daughter incest*. Cambridge, MA: Harvard University Press.

Herman, J. L. (1992). *Trauma and recovery*. New York: Basic Books.

Herman, J. L., & Schatzow, E. (1987). Recovery and verification of memories of childhood sexual trauma. *Psychoanalytic Psychology, 4*, 1-4.

Herman, J. L., & van der Kolk, B. A. (1987). Traumatic antecedents of borderline personality disorder. In B. A. van der Kolk (Ed.), *Psychological trauma* (pp. 111-127). Washington, DC: American Psychiatric Press.

Herman, J., Russell, D., & Trocki, K. E. (1986). Long-term effects of incestuous abuse in childhood. *American Journal of Psychiatry, 143*, 1293-1296.

Herman, J. L., Perry, J. C., & van der Kolk, B. A. (1989). Childhood trauma in borderline personality disorder. *American Journal of Psychiatry, 146*, 490-495.

Horowitz, M. J. (1976). *Stress response syndromes*. New York: Jason Aronson.

Keane, T. M., Fairbank, J. A., Caddell, J. M., & Zimering, R. T. (1989) Implosive (flooding) therapy reduces symptoms of PTSD in Vietnam combat veterans. *Behavior Therapy, 20*, 245-260.

Kernberg, O. F. (1967). Borderline personality organization. *Journal of the American Psychoanalytic Association, 15*, 641-685.

Kernberg, O. F. (1968). The treatment of patients with borderline personality organization. *International Journal of Psychoanalysis, 49*, 600-619.

Kernberg, O. F. (1970). A psychoanalytic classification of character pathology. *Journal of the American Psychoanalytic Association, 18*, 800-822.

Kirby, J. S., Chu, J. A., & Dill, D. L. (1993). Severity, frequency, and age of onset of physical and sexual abuse as factors in the development of dissociative symptoms. *Comprehensive Psychiatry, 34*, 258-263.

Kluft, R. P. (1987). First rank symptoms as a clue to multiple personality disorder. *American Journal of Psychiatry, 144*, 293-298.

Kluft, R. P. (1989). The rehabilitation of therapists overwhelmed by their work with multiple personality disorder patients. *Dissociation, 2*, 244-250.

Lindemann, E. (1944). Symptomatology and management of acute grief. *American Journal of Psychiatry, 101*, 141-148.

Ludolph, P. S., Westen, D., Misle, B., Jackson, A., Wixon, J., & Wiss, F. C. (1990). The borderline diagnosis in adolescents: Symptoms and developmental history. *American Journal of Psychiatry, 147*, 470-476.

Mahler, M. S. (1971). A study of the separation-individuation process and its possible application to borderline phenomena in the psychoanalytic situation. *Psychoanalytic Study of the Child, 26*, 403-424.

Mahler, M. S. (1972). Rapprochement subphase of the separation-individuation process. *Psychoanalytic Quarterly, 41*, 487-506.

Masterson, J. (1972). *Treatment of the borderline adolescent: A developmental approach*. New York: Wiley-Interscience.

National Research Council, Commission on Behavioral and Social Sciences and Education, Panel on Research on Child Abuse and Neglect. (1993). *Understanding child abuse and neglect*. Washington, DC: National Academy Press.

National Victim Center. (1992). *Rape in America: A report to the nation*. Arlington, VA: National Victim Center.

Ogata, S. N., Silk, K. R., Goodrich, S., Lohr, N. E., Westen, D., & Hill, E. M. (1990). Childhood sexual and physical abuse in adult patients with borderline personality disorder. *American Journal of Psychiatry, 147*, 1008-1013.

Pribor, E. F., & Dinwiddie, S. H. (1992). Psychiatric correlates of incest in childhood. *American Journal of Psychiatry, 149*, 53-56.

Putnam, F. W. (1985). Dissociation as a response to extreme trauma. In R. P. Kluft (Ed.), *Childhood antecedents of multiple personality* (pp. 65-97). Washington, DC: American Psychiatric Press.

Putnam, F. W., Guroff, J. J., Silberman, E. K., Barban, L., & Post, R. M. (1986). The clinical phenomenology of multiple personality disorder: A review of 100 cases. *Journal of Clinical Psychiatry, 47*, 258-293.

Ross, C. A. (1989). *Diagnosis and treatment of multiple personality disorder*. New York: Guilford Press.

Ross, C. A., Anderson, G., Fleisher, W. P., & Norton, G. R. (1991). The frequency of multiple personality disorder among psychiatric inpatients. *American Journal of Psychiatry, 148*, 1717-1720.

Russell, D. E. H. (1986). *The secret trauma: Incest in the lives of girls and women*. New York: Basic Books.

Saxe, G. N., van der Kolk, B. A., Berkowitz, R., Chinman, G., Hall, K., Lieberg, G., & Schwartz, J. (1993). Dissociative disorders in psychiatric inpatients. *American Journal of Psychiatry, 150*, 1037-1042.

Shapiro, S. (1987). Self-mutilation and self-blame in incest victims. *American Journal of Psychotherapy, 41*, 46-54.

Surry, J., Swett, C., Michaels, A., & Levin, S. (1990). Reported history of physical and sexual abuse and severity of symptomatology in women psychiatric outpatients. *American Journal of Orthopsychiatry, 60*, 412-417.

Swanson, L., & Biaggio, M. K. (1985). Therapeutic perspectives on father-daughter incest. *American Journal of Psychiatry, 142*, 667-674.

Terr, L. C. (1991). Childhood traumas: An outline and overview. *American Journal of Psychiatry, 148*, 10-20.

Ulman, R. B., & Brothers, D. (1988). *The shattered self*. Hillsdale, NJ: Analytic Press.

Vaillant, G. E. (1992). The beginning of wisdom is never calling a patient borderline. *Journal of Psychotherapy Practice and Research, 1*, 117-134.

van der Kolk, B. A. (1987a). The psychological consequences of overwhelming life experiences. In B. A. van der Kolk (Ed.), *Psychological trauma* (pp. 1-30). Washington, DC: American Psychiatric Press.

van der Kolk, B. A. (1987b) Psychobiology of the trauma response. In B. A. van der Kolk (Ed.), *Psychological trauma* (pp. 63-79). Washington, DC: American Psychiatric Press.

van der Kolk, B. A., & Kadish, W. (1987). Amnesia, dissociation and the return of the repressed. In B. A. van der Kolk (Ed.), *Psychological trauma* (pp. 173-190). Washington, DC: American Psychiatric Press.

van der Kolk, B. A., & van der Hart, O. (1989). Pierre Janet and the breakdown of adaptation in psychological trauma. *American Journal of Psychiatry, 146*, 1530-1540.

van der Kolk, B. A., Perry, J. C., & Herman, J. L. (1991). Childhood origins of self-destructive behavior. *American Journal of Psychiatry, 148*, 1665-1671.

Watkins, J. G., & Watkins, H. H. (1979). The theory and practice of ego-state therapy. In H. Grayson (Ed.), *Short-term approaches to psychotherapy* (pp. 176-220). New York: Human Sciences Press.

Zanarini, M. C., Gunderson, J. G., & Marino, M. F. (1987). Childhood experiences of borderline patients. *Comprehensive Psychiatry, 30*, 18-25.

VI

THERAPEUTIC INTERVENTIONS

This section provides an overview of the important and emerging question of the treatment of dissociative disorders. Using a variety of perspectives, the authors examine the difficulty and complexity of treatment. One common theme found in all of the therapies is the initial establishment of safety in the therapeutic relationship. A second theme is the allowing of experiences and memories to come forth on the part of the patient rather than a search for "forgotten" events. In Chapter 19, Fine discusses a cognitive behavioral treatment for DID. The basic premise is that how one thinks will affect how one feels. As with other types of cognitive therapy, the utilization of the Socratic method lies at the basis of the work, with each identity in search of relevant cognitive schema. However, questions of control and trust are also emphasized along with the cognitive work. In Chapter 20, Barach and Comstock examine DID from a psychoanalytic perspective. One of the main foci is on reducing the need for dissociative defenses. The overall goal is to help the patient reestablish emotional connection between events in his or her life. As described in the chapter, this may also require developmental reeducation to approach development aspects of the patient's life that were not accomplished because of the psychopathology. Overall, this requires a more active therapist who is sensitive to both the type of interpretations required as well as the variety of transference relationships seen in these situations.

The next two chapters describe techniques that utilize hypnosis as a means to facilitate therapy. In Chapter 21, Watkins and Watkins develop their model of ego state therapy based on traditional psychodynamic theory. In Chapter 22, Peterson emphasizes the nature of hypnosis itself in the treatment of dissociative disorders. She begins by dispelling the popular press notion that the fundamental role of hypnosis is memory retrieval. Throughout the chapter, specific techniques are described that illustrate the treatment.

Throughout this volume, the role of trauma as precursor to dissociation has been discussed. However, in the therapy situation, the question arises as to how to work with trauma memories as they come forth. In Chapter 23, Sachs and Peterson offer insights and techniques for processing these memories. The first rule suggested is to honor the patients' defenses and allow them to process traumatic memories at their own pace. This information then needs to be worked through with the goal of achieving resolution and integration of the memories. An important point raised by Sachs and Peterson is the fact that working with these difficult cases may take its toll on the therapists themselves and they in turn often can suffer a PTSD-type reaction.

In the final three chapters of this section, the authors approach specific types of treatments for dissociative disorders: inpatient treatments, art, and psychopharmacology. Whereas all of the therapies discussed previously emphasize the need for a safe psychological environment, there are situations in which treatment must begin with a safe physical environment, in particular, an inpatient situation. In Chapter 24, Young and Young describe some of the precursors that establish the need for hospitalization for the treatment of dissociative disorders, especially DID, and the types of inpatient treatments available. They further discuss the important question of inpatient staffing and the use of adjunctive therapies. One of the adjunctive therapies is the use of art, which is described by Cohen in Chapter 25. Art has the advantage of being able to move beyond the verbal to allow for expression in a different form. Cohen suggests that art offers a fundamental way of representing one's inner world, especially important when this world contains traumatic experiences. The chapter ends by asking the provocative question of why people with severe dissociative disorders produce so much art. In the final chapter of the section, Torem overviews the uses and benefits of various psychotropic medications directed at dissociative disorders. Although there is no pharmacological cure for a dissociative disorder, Torem suggests their importance in three areas: (1) reducing debilitating symptoms; (2) improving the patient's mental state in order to benefit from psychotherapy; and (3) treating a comorbid disorder. The chapter not only overviews specific medications, but also offers some general guidelines when considering their use.

19

A Cognitively Based Treatment Model for DSM-IV Dissociative Identity Disorder

Catherine G. Fine

Dissociative identity disorder (DID) is the most recent renaming by the American Psychiatric Association (1994) of a psychiatric syndrome that has been recorded from the time of Paracelsus (sixteenth century) (Bliss, 1986; Kluft, 1991). Its recognition has waxed and waned more as a function of the socioreligious Zeitgeist and the psychological theory(ies) dominating the era than from actual variations or fluctuations of the disorder itself. The curious archivist and medical historian (Ellenberger, 1970) could readily track the various literature pools and obscure sources to shed some light on the epidemiology of dissociative disorders. More recently, clinicians with an interest in history and psychoarcheology have collected, reexamined, reviewed, and sometimes reinterpreted past misdiagnosed conditions to be dissociative ones (Goodwin, 1993). Skeptics of the existence of dissociative disorders remain: some on politicophilosophical grounds (Orne, 1984a; Orne, Dinges, & Orne, 1984), others because they have never seen them in their practice (Chodoff, 1987), and many because they are repulsed by the possibility that child abuse, which is part of the etiology of DID in 97% of the cases (Putnam, Guroff, Silberman, Barban, & Post, 1986), could be so prevalent. However, an increasing number of men and women are currently being appropriately diagnosed with DID.

DID is considered to be a chronic, complex dissociative psychopathology accompanied by disturbances of identity and memory (Kluft, 1991; Nemiah, 1991).

Catherine G. Fine • Dissociative Disorders Unit, Institute of Pennsylvania Hospital, Philadelphia, Pennsylvania 19139.

Handbook of Dissociation: Theoretical, Empirical, and Clinical Perspectives, edited by Larry K. Michelson and William J. Ray. Plenum Press, New York, 1996.

DID patients can be helpfully conceptualized as struggling with multiple reality disorder (Kluft, 1991); this means that DID patients live and function with fluctuating and alternating levels of hypnotic involvement in external and internal realities. They can be thought of as trying to maintain (hypnotic) duality with one foot (one ego state-one personality) in a social consensual reality and the other(s) in an alternate one(s). Therefore, the therapy for DID patients needs to be one that is cautiously disequilibrating and frequently restabilizing. The task of the therapist is to bring to the forefront what was hidden (i.e., the other realities, the other personalities with their concurrent experiences) and to help the patient as a whole recognize, metabolize, and reabsorb through abreaction and subsequent processing the experiences contained in the alter personalities or alternate realities. A cognitive-behavioral treatment module for DID has become a straightforward comprehensive integrationist model for the work with DID (Fine, 1991, 1992, 1993).

THE TRADITIONAL COGNITIVE–BEHAVIORAL MODEL IN THE TREATMENT OF DID

A cognitive-behavioral (CB) model for treating DID fosters a more structured, less chaotic therapy where safety, predictability, and consistency are favored. The cognitive therapy for DID values an experimental model to hypothesis test the established beliefs of the various personalities and those of the patient as a whole.

This CB model is based on the cognitive model of emotional disorder (Beck, 1976), which states that how someone thinks is going to effect how that person feels. In treating DID, helping a personality notice cognitive-perceptual-affective-behavioral incongruities and appropriately label and modify dysfunctional cognitions will impact on the personality's inner world by correcting the distorted conceptualizations and dysfunctional schemata that are the underpinnings of DID patients unchallenged affects.

Do the Same Principles of Cognitive Therapy Apply to the Dissociating as well as the Nondissociating Patient?

Even though cognitive therapy for nondissociators is typically thought of as a time-limited, brief psychotherapy geared to symptom relief through cognitive change, the cognitive therapy of a DID patient can be best conceptualized as a series of time-limited CB therapies with repeated treatment across all personalities, all themes, and all affects. The challenges to the cognitive distortions need to be about reconnecting the various parts of the mind to the current pleasant or even unpleasant reality, often to the overt objection of many personalities who prefer their dissociatively created worlds.

In the CB therapy of the DID patient the importance of the therapeutic alliance cannot be overemphasized. Because the DID patient's trust has been violated in such a profound way in childhood, appropriate respect and concern for the issue of trust and its transferential entanglements are essential. With DID patients, trust is built one step at a time, and therefore it is understood that the credibility of the therapist will be challenged repeatedly. A direct and honest therapist with firm boundaries will help the DID patient better negotiate the initial stages of the therapy, which can be particularly fraught with acting out. Furthermore, the structure of the CB therapy and the collaborative directedness of the therapist creates an environment of consistency, predictability, and safety for the DID patient in which the therapist engages each personality very directly and with no hidden agendas.

Additionally, CB therapy promotes the use of the Socratic method for problem solving through the asking of judicious questions by the therapist to each personality of the DID patient. The Socratic method is especially helpful when working with alter personalities who are resistant to any comment the therapist will make; this means that the Socratic method is particularly beneficial when working with adolescent alter personalities and those persecutor personalities who continue to identify with external abusers. Overall, DID patients struggle with control issues and mistrust. These are patients who are understandably cautious about any suggestion made by an authority figure and will often balk at the most obvious self-protective measure presented by the therapist.

The problem-solving quality of CB therapy facilitates and strengthens the therapeutic alliance, helps uncover representational schemata underlying each personality's belief system, and reveals the original and present function of each personality. Approaching the patient with a psychoeducational stance furthers their sense of budding self-efficacy and self-mastery as the therapist teaches the patient what tools to use and how to use them. In the CB therapy of the DID patient, as in any traditional CB therapy, the therapist becomes initially a role model for information seeking and information testing for the patient.

Goals of Treatment for the DID Patient

There are two nonmutually exclusive ways of explaining the goals of treatment for DID patients: (1) achievement of congruence of purpose and motivation across the different parts of the mind (Kluft, 1985); and (2) experiencing completeness of events and continuity of history over time using Braun's model of dissociation as a referent (Fine, 1990, 1991). The latter conceptualization will be explored here.

Braun's (1988) BASK (behavior, affect, sensation, knowledge) model of dissociation is conceptually synchronous with the CB therapy approach. This model has noteworthy descriptive and explanatory power. It states that people, which in a nondissociated state, experience events almost simultaneously across four dimensions: they have knowledge of events, they can associate behaviors to those events, they have sensations spanning all sensory receptors during them, and they feel affects as well. For people in a dissociated state, any or all of these interconnections can be completely or partially severed and seemingly fancifully recombined. The treatment goal for the DID patient becomes reconnecting the four dimensions of the BASK model for each event and then organizing the BASK events, life experiences, along a time line for the patient to make meaning of his or her life. Formulating the DID treatment goal in this manner helps patients renegotiate their multiple realities and move from a life that is necessarily decontextualized to one that is increasingly integrated.

Formatting Treatment for the DID Patient to Prevent Crises and Work toward Integration

The tactical integration model proposed by Fine (1991, 1992, 1993) takes into account the affective, cognitive, and perceptual struggles of the DID patient. DID patients traditionally struggle with feeling out of control and vulnerable. The tactical integration perspective focuses on establishing an increasingly stable cognitive foundation prior to the patient feeling feelings with any degree of completeness. In short, the tactical integration model helps the DID patient build up affect tolerance prior to doing abreactive work related to their experiences.

The Treatment Model. Fine's (1991, 1992, 1993) model proposes an initial suppression of affect phase in the treatment of DID. The patient learns to notice what thoughts, sensations, and incomplete affects arise in everyday life as well as in the therapy sessions. Once therapist and patient have a beginning overview of the dissociative landscape, once ego strengths are assessed and the therapeutic alliance is in process, and once a number of the personalities are actively involved in the therapy, the cognitive stabilization phase will be followed by the dilution of affect stage. This phase focuses on bringing into the cognitive narrative (i.e., the patient's reported experiences) other BASK dimensions; these dimensions will be driven particularly by the affective and sensation realms. Only then can DID patients begin to truly piece their experiences together and inquire as to how these experiences can be understood.

What Is Meant by Experience? Recent debates about normal memory, traumatic memory, clinically retrieved memories, and memories retrieved in an experimental setting could leave patients and therapists immobilized until researchers, clinical and otherwise, come to some agreed upon closure. Meanwhile, these debates, though relevant at the academic and legal levels, do very little to help the hurting individual resolve their experiences. Many DID patients quite commonly attempt to push therapists to validate memories; even though patients' reports can be extremely compelling, often therapists have very little corroborative or independent reporting available to them to even begin a constructive exchange on this topic. Additionally, in those patients where family members agree with the patient's allegations and support the patient in his or her recovery, the conflict remains and these patients can continue to deny what may already be documented in medical, court, or family records. Therefore, what is truly relevant for the patient is not that the therapist validate memories, but rather that the therapist help the patient tackle and resolve an experience that may or may not have happened, that may or may not have happened as recalled, or that may be a screen for something else or outright confabulated. Kluft (in press) effectively summarizes a neutral stance when he says that he believes *in* his patients but does not necessarily believe his patients. The patients' indignant and sometimes overtly hostile posture when a therapist chooses to not validate or invalidate what they say is often an unconscious flashback (Blank, 1985) rather than a truly examined and explored position. Therefore, the most helpful stance for the patient is that the therapist work with the material that the patient brings to treatment and work with his or her experiences as the patient understands them.

The Role of Cognitive Interventions. The work with the DID patient involves reconnecting, uniting, and processing the patient's dissociated life experiences. Established cognitive techniques can be adapted to DID patients to help them remember and assimilate previously dissociated thoughts and feelings. Adjunctive behavioral techniques can support modulation of intense affects to permit more rapid affective and behavioral change. These cognitive interventions are advanced in an atmosphere of safety and predictability in which the cognitive therapist explores with the DID patient the value of the experimental model to hypothesis test the validity of the established beliefs (Fine, 1988c, 1991).

Fine (1990, 1991, 1992) has described elsewhere how to do cognitive restructuring with DID patients by paying attention to patients' thinking and speech patterns. She has recommended addressing what they say and don't say through noticing the cognitive distortions (Fine, 1988, 1992) that they favor and overuse. Fine has discussed the importance of helping the DID patient look for alternative explanations for their thoughts rather than letting them assume that thoughts rooted in childhood trauma continue to be valid (unless of course they are legitimate—which means that the DID patient remains in abusive circumstances and may require supportive therapy to leave these conditions before getting to the dissociative work). Alternative explanations for strongly held cognitions are sought through considering with the DID patient how an outside observer would understand the held opinion. If there is agreement between what an outside observer would believe and the DID patient, the belief-cognition is more likely to be maintained; on the other hand, if there is discrepancy between these views, the thought or belief is apt to be revisited and appropriate reattribution sought.

As the therapist promotes appropriate substitution with corrected attributions, the patients' negative self-attributions and their disequilibrated worldviews are redressed. These stepwise cognitive interventions are a precursor to the DID patients' correct recontextualization of cause and effect. These interventions require careful planning as well as sensitivity when confronting the patient's false assumptions.

THE COGNITIVE MODEL REVISITED: SCHEMA-FOCUSED COGNITIVE THERAPY

Though focusing on the cognitions is understood as the beginning of helping the patient learn to contain the affect as well as explore its underpinnings, the pure CB model has a tendency to decontextualize aspects of treatment, to not provide a better frame for "why look at this particular distorted thought rather than another," and to not provide a structure within which the DID patient could with greater ease begin to regroup, reassemble, and make sense of categories of distorted cognitions. The pure CB model requires that the therapist address the distortions and elicit the underlying beliefs, but it does not necessarily contextualize the themes and therefore does not formally connect categories of distortions with categories of affective experiences.

An evolving model of CB therapy may begin to address these concerns; this model is called schema-focused cognitive therapy (SFCT) and has been proposed by Jeff Young (1990) as a way of treating personality disorders. Established cognitive therapists have come to realize what analysts have known for years: that addressing surface complaints (i.e., depression), however compelling, does little to resolve long-term issues rooted in childhood. SFCT rests on the premise that significant experiences of early life influence the formation of schemas (Young, 1990). A schema is a mental construct that represents organized knowledge and affect about a given concept or about a type of stimulus.

What Are Schemas?

Schemas underlie everyday object categories and our social categories as well (Janoff-Bulman, 1985). Schemas help individuals elucidate their position and role within established social consensual structures. But more importantly, they also underlie people's self-definitions. Schemas represent extremely strong beliefs that a person holds about themselves; the belief is so strong that the person simply assumes that it is true. A schema established in childhood reflects the perceptions and subsequent cognitions from childhood experiences. This schema may still be active and stimulated in adulthood whether or not the adult life circumstances validate it or not. The strength of the schema for Young (1990) seems connected at least heuristically to the assumption that it is bound to strong feelings because it was initially encoded with very strong affect.

This affect, like a magnet, will pull for interpretations of information that will be consistent with the schema even in the face of contradictory information. Therefore, according to SFCT, these cognitively based schemas are affectively driven themes which will be uncovered through exploration of the cognitive distortions. Fine (1988a) has discussed the parallels between the cognitive distortions of the DID patient and the depressogenic thoughts of the dysthymic patient; however resilient to elucidation depressogenic cognitive distortions appear to be, those of the DID patient are more established still.

The distortions of the DID patient are the outcome of a dual attack on the schemas of the child. The first frontal attack is on the actual formation of the schemas and the second attack is on the schemas once established whether they are distorted or not and how these schemas get broken down.

Attack on the Formation of Schemas

The evolution of perceptual-cognitive structures has been described by Piaget (1971) who addresses his heuristic of four developmentally interrelated and contiguous stages through which all children progress. He has called these stages the sensorimotor stage, the preoperational stage, the concrete operational stage, and the formal operations stage. The child masters and then progresses from each stage to the next through adaptation and organization. Adaptation for the child means having to negotiate accommodative and assimilative functions coordinated with one another by the supraordinate concept of organization. The overwhelming affect experienced by the abused child leads to the formation of "war-based" schemas that are traumatogenic in content and schemas that are themselves impacted by dissociation in their inception.

When a child develops in an abusive environment, dissociative processes are mobilized to deal with the impact of overwhelming stress imposed by violations to the self (Kluft, 1984; Spiegel, 1984). The age of onset of abuse, its intensity, and its duration will differentially affect the child's accommodative and assimilative functions. Fish-Murray et al. (1987) have reported that self-correction in abused children is difficult because their accommodative functions are impaired. Their cognitive functions are more fixed than variable and lack optimal flexibility. Abuse affects not only accommodation, but it also interferes with assimilation. If assimilation does not occur, some of the cognitive schemas may remain fixed at a previous level of ontogenic development in part or in totality. If this occurs, the schemas may remain meaningless and nonintegrated, or they may reflect a meaning acquired at a preceding developmental level and thus be incomplete or immature. These difficulties in the proper evolution of schemas will lead to the cognitive distortions discussed previously.

Young (1990) has labeled this schema-based deeper level of cognitive process early maladaptive schemas (EMS). They reflect an unconditional belief about the self, are self-perpetuating, are dysfunctional in a significant and recurrent manner, are activated by relevant events in the environment, are tied to higher levels of affect than underlying assumptions, and seem to be tied to early interrelationships with family members (Young, 1990). For the DID patient, EMS may be at the foundation of their developing perceptual cognitive structures and reflect in part the impact of dissociative intrusions on the child's evolving sense of self. However, all schemas may not be impacted by abuse; the dissociative intrusions may strike both differentially and/or opportunistically.

Attack on the Established Schemas

In Braun's (1988) BASK model of dissociation, he proposes that an event can be dissociated into its four components: behavior, affect, sensation, and knowledge. It is heuristically plausible that not only does abuse sever knowledge from the three other dimensions as described by Braun, but abuse may force the knowledge dimension to shatter into smaller units of information, into fragments of knowledge. Knowledge may not only be broken down into its schematic elements, but the schematic elements themselves may get split off.

Dissociation consequent to abuse may affect the schemas in a number of ways. The cognitive schemas may become completely segregated from one another, leading to two separate schemas encapsulating two seemingly complete but different information pools (i.e., two separate alter personalities in a patient: one who knows, for instance, that the neighbor abused him/her, the other who just knows that the neighbor was great fun). Second, the cognitive schemas may be partially severed from one another, with both overlapping and disjunctive parts leading to a common information pool and one or more divergent pools. Two personalities may know that the neighbor abused them (common information); however, one believes it was just physical abuse, whereas the other knows about some of the sexual abuse (separate information). Third, the cognitive schemas may be entirely severed in an imbalanced way, with one cognitive schema being replete with information while the other schema holds only minimal residual information. For example, one alter in a DID patient knows the whole family and is quiet in treatment, whereas another alter who vehemently claims much knowledge of family genealogy may truly know only one family member directly who so happens to be the family historian. Finally, the cognitive schema may be entirely severed from one another and forced into almost exact self-replication (cloning); this is relatively frequent in DID patients who use event-based dissociation. Regardless of how the EMSs are formed, they will have to be addressed systematically.

The Doing and Undoing of EMS

Young (1990) states that short-term cognitive therapy has been concerned with three levels of cognitive phenomena: automatic thoughts, cognitive distortions, and underlying assumptions. Fine (1991, 1992), in her adaptation of cognitive therapy to the treatment of DID, has focused on organizing the work with the DID patient to better correct the cognitive distortions through the uses of direct or indirect interventions. Knowledge of the cognition delineates the likely/plausible or at least tacit content of the schema on which both the therapist and the patient will need to focus and intervene. For those interventions to be most effective, understanding some of the processes that sustain and aid in the nonresolution of EMS is helpful.

Three processes are thought to operate on these EMS to keep them well in place: schema maintenance, schema avoidance, and schema compensation (Young, 1990).

Schema Maintenance. It is understood according to SFCT that EMSs are the cornerstone of the DID patient's self-concept. Schema maintenance refers to processes by which the EMSs are reinforced. These processes are upheld cognitively and behaviorally; they include the habitual utilization of both cognitive distortions and self-defeating behaviors. Schema maintenance processes account for the rigidity so commonly seen in DID patients' cognitive and affective realities. At the cognitive level, schema maintenance is usually accomplished by "highlighting or exaggerating information that confirms the schema, and by negating, minimizing or denying information that contradicts the schema" (Young, 1990, p. 17). The more obvious cognitive interventions that I use with DID patients (with or without formal hypnosis), such as cognitive restructuring, cognitive reframing, or facilitating perceptual shifting, focus on challenging DID patients' schema maintenance conditioning. The second process that keeps EMS active and dysfunction is schema avoidance.

Schema Avoidance. Avoiding feelings, especially avoiding certain feelings, is common in DID patients. SFCT therapists would say that when the particular EMS is triggered, the DID patient experiences a high level of ego dystonic affect, such as guilt, intense anger, profound shame, or fear. These emotions and their intensity is so overwhelming to some DID patients or to some personalities within the patient that either in or out of awareness, the DID patient avoids the triggering of the schema or the experience of affect connected to it.

Some DID patients-personalities reorganize their inner and/or their outer reality to avoid these feelings. The inner reality modification may be an inflexibility in the adult patient to accept varying configurations of personalities. The therapist can suspect active schema avoidance components when there is dysfunctional and/or rapid switching of personalities. When the DID patient tries to control external reality to avoid triggering EMSs, the patient is often obsessionally preoccupied with controlling everyday objects, occurrences, and people; the DID patient in the midst of this struggle appears paranoid, manipulative, and extremely controlling. Schema avoidance processes can be likened to aversive conditioning (Young, 1990).

One schema avoidance process is *cognitive avoidance*. This process "refers to automatic or volitional attempts to block thoughts, images that might trigger the schema" (Young, 1990, p. 16). For example a common strategy used by some DID patients to thought block is to disguise it in "amnesialike" talk where there may be little to no true amnesia, but rather a decision to not attend to drifting or stray thoughts. Two other expressions of this same phenomenon are the ongoing editing of some DID patients as well as the intentional vagueness of their responses. An example of suspicious amnesia could be:

> THERAPIST: Josie, you have given me generous amounts of data, of detail about your experiences in first grade, your teacher, your friends, your favorite games at school. What was it like at home during that same year?
> PATIENT: I don't know (rapidly).

Further exploration led to understanding that she did know some very stressful details about life at home that she justly understood as only the tip of an iceberg.

Another schema avoidance process is *affective avoidance*. This process reflects "automatic or volitional attempts to block feelings that are triggered by schemas" (Young, 1990, p. 16). In the face of distressing life events, some DID patients are fully capable of reporting their cognitions, yet deny experiencing the emotions that would normally accompany these thoughts (*belle indifference*). This affective avoidance in DID patients and/or in some of their personalities makes them appear either flat in affect or affect phobic. However, those DID patients who report little affect and who do not talk about feelings are more likely to report chronic, diffuse generalized anxiety or psychosomatic symptoms. A typical example would be the "I feel fine" DID patient who comes into your office, sits down on the couch, and either grabs a pillow that she folds and places on her abdomen "nonchalantly" or who tries to disguise a raging dissociative headache by rearranging her bangs. The third and final process proposed by Young (1990) to keep EMSs in place is schema compensation.

Schema Compensation. This refers to processes that overcompensate for EMS. Many DID patients or personalities within them may adopt cognitive-behavioral styles that are the opposite of what we would predict as the therapist comes to understand or have knowledge of the patient's EMSs. Schema compensation is functional to a certain extent. Counterphobic impulses can be advantageous.

But schema compensation is truly best understood as only a partially successful attempt by DID patients to challenge the original schema and almost always involves a failure to recognize the underlying vulnerability. For instance, one of my DID patients would walk in with leather boots, leather jacket, and "walking tough." When the time came to begin to explore childhood issues, she required increasing amounts of benzodiazepines as she slowly learned to control her acting out impulses. It took several years before she could tentatively acknowledge her helplessness; as she disclosed more of her fear, her dressing habits changed as did her walk.

In summary, SFCT supports the elicitation and restructuring of EMSs in order to reconfigure the dysfunctional belief system of the DID patient. It behooves the DID therapist to attend to all means of maintenance of EMS in the DID patient in order to disequilibrate the faulty thinking and favor integration of all parts of the mind.

TREATMENT IMPLICATIONS

The treatment of DID patients can be challenging and protracted. A traditional cognitively based model of therapy has proven helpful from the tactical integrationist perspective of work with DID patients (Fine, 1991, 1992, 1993). A more complete theoretical heuristic may allow for more thorough and rapid rectification of distorted belief systems by increased specificity of intervention.

The validity of SFCT model in the work with DID patients would be supported by recurrent and similar clinical findings across a number of personalities. Indeed, the more fragmented the DID patient, the more each personality locks into an EMS. There is no anecdotal evidence for the preferred use of one EMS over another as a function of the number of personalities. However, there is some suggestion that very fragmented DID patients demonstrate a smaller range of affect and an increased commitment to alternate realities perhaps in response to a capitulation to entrenched EMSs. If this premise is accurate, the CB interventions of choice would be geared to rectification of EMS by taking each personality through the process of exploring affect-laden schema in terms of their schema maintenance, schema avoidance, and schema compensation aspects.

Speculatively, SFCT would allow a DID patient to experience and talk about affect through a process mediated by the cognition in a schema-oriented suprastructure. This supraordinate understanding would lend itself to a heightened organizing of the therapy, increased structuring, and therefore stabilization of the work and should facilitate the recontextualization of the patients' beliefs and distorted cognitions. SFCT may allow the therapist, from treatment onset, to better focus the DID patient on an affectively based consensual reality without the downfalls of spontaneous and unwanted abreactions.

REFERENCES

American Psychiatric Association. (1994). *Diagnostic and statistical manual of mental disorders* (4th ed.). Washington, DC: Author.

Beck, A. T. (1976). *Cognitive therapy and the emotional disorders*. New York: International Universities Press.

Blank, A. S. (1985). The unconscious flashback to the war in VietNam veterans: Clinical mystery, legal defense and community problem. In S. M. Sonnenberg, A. S. Blank, & J. A. Talbott (Eds.), *The trauma of war: Stress and recovery in Vietnam veterans* (pp. 293-308). Washington, DC: American Psychiatric Press.

Bliss, E. (1986). *Multiple personality, allied disorders and hypnosis*. New York: Oxford University Press.

Braun, B. G. (1988). The BASK model of dissociation. *Dissociation, 1,* 4-23.

Chodoff, P. (1987). More on multiple personality disorder. *American Journal of Psychiatry, 144,* 124.

Ellenberger, H. F. (1970). *The discovery of the unconscious: The history and evolution of dynamic psychiatry*. New York: Basic Books.

Fine, C. G. (1988). Thoughts on the cognitive perceptual substrates of multiple personality disorder. *Dissociation, 1*(4), 5-10.

Fine, C. G. (1988c). Mood, cognition and multiplicity. Presented at the World Congress of Cognitive Therapy, Oxford, England.

Fine, C. G. (1989). Treatment errors and iatrogenesis across therapeutic modalities in MPD and allied disorders. *Dissociation, 2,* 77-82.

Fine, C. G. (1990). The cognitive sequelae of incest. In R. P. Kluft (Ed.), *Incest related syndromes of adult psychopathology* (pp. 161-182). Washington, DC: American Psychiatric Press.

Fine, C. G. (1991). Treatment stabilization and crisis prevention: Pacing the therapy of the multiple personality disorder patient. *Psychiatric Clinics of North America, 14,* 661-675.

Fine, C. G. (1992). Multiple personality disorder. In A. Freeman & F. M. Dattilio (Eds.), *Comprehensive casebook of cognitive therapy* (pp. 347-360). New York: Plenum Press.

Fine, C. G. (1993). A tactical integrationist perspective on the treatment of multiple personality disorder. In R. P. Kluft & C. G. Fine (Eds.), *Clinical perspectives on multiple personality disorder* (pp. 135-153). Washington, DC: American Psychiatric Press.

Fish-Murray, C., Koby, E., Van der Kolk, B. (1987). Evolving ideas: The affect of abuse on children's thought. In B. Van der Kolk (Ed.), *Psychological trauma* (pp. 89-110). Washington, DC: American Psychiatric Press.

Goodwin, J. M. (Ed.). (1993). *Rediscovering childhood trauma: Historical casebook and clinical applications*. Washington, DC: American Psychiatric Press.

Janoff-Bulman, R. (1985). The aftermath of victimization: Rebuilding shattered assumptions. In C. Figley (Ed.), *Trauma and its wake* (pp. 15-35). New York: Brumner-Mazel.

Kluft, R. P. (1984). Multiple personality in childhood. *Psychiatric Clinics of North America, 7,* 121-134.

Kluft, R. P. (Ed.). (1985). *Childhood antecedents of multiple personality*. Washington, DC: American Psychiatric Press.

Kluft, R. P. (1991). Multiple personality disorder. In A. Tasman & S. Goldfinger (Eds.), *American Psychiatric Press review of psychiatry* (Vol. 10, pp. 161-188). Washington, DC: American Psychiatric Press.

Kluft, R. P. (1993). The treatment of dissociative disorder patients: An overview of discoveries. *Dissociation, 6,* 87-107.

Kluft, R. P. (in press). An overview of the treatment of patients alleging that they have suffered ritualized or sadistic abuse. In G. A. Frazier (Ed.), *The phenomenon of ritualized abuse*. Washington, DC: American Psychiatric Press.

Nemiah, J. C. (1991). Dissociation, conversion and somatization. In A. Tasman & S. M. Goldfinger (Eds.), *American psychiatric press review of psychiatry* (Vol. 10, pp. 248-260). Washington, DC: American Psychiatric Press.

Orne, M. T. (1984) Forensic hypnosis. Part I. The use and misuse of hypnosis in court. In W. C. Wester & A. H. Smith (Eds.), *Clinical hypnosis: A multidisciplinary approach*. New York: Lippincott.

Orne, M. T., Dinges, D. F., & Orne, E. C. (1984) On the differential diagnosis of multiple personality disorder in a forensic context. *International Journal of Clinical and Experimental Hypnosis, 32,* 118-167.

Piaget, J. (1971). *Biology and knowledge: An essay on the relations between organic regulations and cognitive processes*. Chicago: University of Chicago Press.

Putnam, F. W., Guroff, J. J., Silberman, E. K., Barban, L., & Post, R. M. (1986). The clinical phenomenology of multiple personality disorder: A review of 100 recent cases. *Journal of Clinical Psychiatry, 47,* 285-293.

Spiegel, D. (1984). Multiple personality as a post traumatic stress disorder. *Psychiatric Clinics of North America, 7,* 000-000.

Young, J. E. (1990). *Cognitive therapy for personality disorders: A schema-focused approach*. Sarasota, FL: Practioner's Resource Series, Professional Resource Exchange.

20

Psychodynamic Psychotherapy of Dissociative Identity Disorder

Peter M. Barach and Christine M. Comstock

The tools of psychodynamic therapy serve the purpose of bringing disparate elements of the psyche together. These tools originate from a model of the psyche that highlights the symptomatic properties of unresolved and unconscious conflicts, and the tools help to bring these conflicts to awareness so that the patient may confront them. The psychodynamic approach aims to "give [the patient's] ego back its mastery over lost provinces of his mental life" (Freud, 1969, p. 30) and is well suited for the treatment of dissociative identity disorder (DID).

Although most of the literature on treating DID recommends a primarily psychodynamic approach (e.g., Kluft, 1991; Kluft & Wilbur, 1989; Putnam, 1989; Ross, 1989), writers have tended to highlight aspects of the treatment process that are other than psychodynamic. They highlight specialized techniques for dealing with alters, symptoms, and crises. They focus on the phenomenology of the disorder (Thigpen & Cleckley, 1957), the use of hypnosis by patient (Bliss, 1980) and therapist (Kluft, 1982, 1983), the healing effects of recalling the abreacting traumatic memories in the context of a nurturant therapeutic relationship (Schreiber, 1973), and the functions and interactions of the alternate personalities (Braun, 1986).

However, by focusing primarily on dissociative behaviors and specialized techniques for managing them, the therapist turns away from the psychological

Peter M. Barach and Christine M. Comstock • Horizons Counseling Services, Inc., Cleveland, Ohio 44130.

Handbook of Dissociation: Theoretical, Empirical, and Clinical Perspectives, edited by Larry K. Michelson and William J. Ray. Plenum Press, New York, 1996.

functioning of the patient as a whole. The therapist inadvertently adopts the dissociative patient's worldview, perceiving related events as separate. In contrast, an integrative psychodynamic treatment approach is more consistent with the goal of producing an integrated patient.

An integrative psychodynamic approach focuses on helping the patient alter a continued reliance on dissociative defenses. The dissociative patient maintains emotional stability by ignoring connections between events (Braun, 1988). It is as if she has been examining a halftone newspaper reproduction of a disturbing photo by holding it so close to her face that she sees only the individual dots. Psychodynamic psychotherapy enables the patient to reassociate aspects of psychological functioning that are actively being held apart. By directing the patient's attention to possible connections between emotional and behavioral events, the therapist helps the patient to associate things that have previously seemed unrelated. In effect, the therapist encourages the patient to move the photo away so that she can allow herself to see the whole picture. He does this by using familiar psychodynamic tools, such as interpretations, questions, empathic reflection, and confrontation.

Adding to the therapeutic value of specific psychodynamic interventions, the treatment setting itself provides a predictability and stability that allows the patient to encounter and eventually to integrate disavowed parts of the mind. The therapist does this without exploiting, manipulating, or attempting to control verbal expression. The therapist may be the only person in the patient's life who has tried to relate to all aspects of her personhood, allowing her the freedom to verbalize all aspects of her mental life.

A SINGLE-SELF MODEL OF DID

Psychodynamic interventions are well suited for treating DID, in which the "lost provinces" of the psyche are like walled city-states that are unaware of each other. However, DID should not be seen as a disorder of multiple selves. Many descriptions of DID seem to describe multiple selves operating as separate people. A multiple-self model is probably being used when one uses implicit spatial metaphors to describe alters, such as characterizing them as "inside," "in front of," and "layered." Multiple-self models reify the alters by depicting them as talking to, comforting, or fighting with each other.

Although the transferences, resistances, and defensive styles of DID patients have often been described as multiple (e.g., Wilbur, 1984), they can be more parsimoniously understood as aspects or facets of a single self. We understand DID as taking place within a single-self system that has access to several stable configurations of memories, cognitive styles, and emotions (Barach, 1992; Watkins & Watkins, 1993). The emotional demands of the patient's immediate situation govern which configuration is active. The patient may know each configuration as an alternate personality, experiencing mental conflicts as verbal or physical interactions between alters. These experiences may be understood as autohypnotic phenomena (Bliss, 1986) that have become elaborated over many years (Putnam, 1989). DID patients are highly hypnotizable (Frischholz, Lipman, Braun, & Sachs, 1992), and they have concretized conflicting aspects of the psyche at the hallucinatory intensity accessible to hypnotizable people in trance states. However, from the framework of a single-self model of DID, when alters are not influencing behavior, they do not exist independently, except as *potential* ego states. As symptoms, alters are compromise formations (Fenichel, 1945) between complete repression of traumatic material and emergence of that material into awareness. A single-self perspective simplifies the therapeutic task of understanding and interpreting the interactions of alters as reifications of psychic conflict.

GOALS OF PSYCHODYNAMIC PSYCHOTHERAPY FOR DID

Writers generally describe integration as an overall goal for the treatment of DID. The term makes most sense conceptually when it refers to the development of integrated psychological functioning in the patient and not to the disappearance of dissociative phenomena: "It denotes an ongoing process in the tradition of psychoanalytic perspectives on structural change" (Kluft, 1993, p. 109).

From our perspective, the establishment of truly integrated psychological functioning in a DID patient involves the resolution of developmental deficits that have resulted from repeated trauma. From a psychodynamic perspective, trauma is defined by the internal experience of the child, not by the external circumstances; it is "an influx of stimuli from within or without which wholly or partly breaks through the ego's protective shield and floods the system with excitation" (Furman, 1986, p. 192). Resolving the resulting developmental deficits can reduce the patient's need for dissociative defenses or acting out and can alleviate the asocial (or "negative") symptoms of dissociation. With treatment organized around these goals, the dissociated aspects of the mind (alters) tend to integrate spontaneously and gradually without the need for structured integration rituals.

Developmental Issues to Be Resolved

Treatment of DID best brings about integration by dealing with a number of developmental tasks that must be resolved. Psychodynamic treatment of DID goes beyond the goal of eliminating dissociative dividedness and treats the characterological and object relations difficulties that abusive and neglectful childhood experiences have created. Incest and other sexual abuse can affect many aspects of self and social development (Cole & Putnam, 1992; Putnam, 1990), the ability to protect oneself (Kluft, 1990; Wyatt, Guthrie, & Notgrass, 1992), sexual functioning (Putnam, 1990), and the ability to be a nurturant parent (Kluft, 1987). The effects of trauma on early personality development are so pervasive that DID patients never reached a state of integrated psychological functioning in childhood. If the treatment is organized around dissociative phenomena rather than psychological functioning as a whole, developmental deficits resulting from abuse and neglect are never addressed. An attempt to resolve five key developmental deficits furnishes the therapist with a set of psychodynamic goals for treating DID. These developmental issues are discussed below.

Establishment of an Internalized Secure Base of Attachment. Several authors (Alexander, 1992; Barach, 1991; Liotti, 1992) have noted that sexual abuse survivors and DID patients have difficulties in feeling a secure sense of connection to important people in their lives. Their childhood experiences with emotionally unavailable or abusive caretakers have led to dysfunctional working models of what to expect from later attachment figures (Bowlby, 1973). Two explanations have been proposed for the attachment difficulties that DID patients experience: (1) They may have detached themselves (i.e., dissociated) from awareness of their needs because often nobody responded to their attachment behaviors during early childhood (Barach, 1991); or (2) they may have developed disorganized patterns of attachment as the result of having caretakers who alternated between frightening them and being frightened by their needs (Liotti, 1992).

DID patients tend to alternate between detachment and separation anxiety (which they often manifest as *dependence*) in their relationships. The transference will, of course, reflect these patterns. During the early stages of treatment, patients often present many crises, requiring large amounts of time and attention from the therapist. From the viewpoint of attachment theory, these crises may reflect the reactivation of attachment behavior in the face of the therapist's steady responsiveness. Repressed and dissociated material has begun to come to the patient's awareness, causing a wish for safety and security. Internal signals of danger tend to trigger attachment behavior, and the patient urgently reaches out for help. However, as mentioned earlier, experiences of abuse, abandonment, and neglect have taught the patient to detach from awareness of attachment needs and caretaking figures. Internal signals of danger will periodically lead the DID patient to revert to detached states of emotional and physical numbness. The therapist will see this as a fluctuation between alters who request caretaking and alters who push away from the therapist's empathic response.

In time, the patient begins to internalize a secure sense of attachment. The therapist's physical presence or voice seems less necessary during periods of stress or emotional upset. The patient learns to retain a sense of internal connection with the therapist, and emergency calls become less frequent. This comes about when the therapist remains a steady and consistent presence to which the patient can return and when the therapist interprets attachment issues so that the patient can resolve them using the ego resources available to him as an adult. Working models based on the therapeutic relationship gradually replace working models of attachment figures based on abusive or neglectful caretakers.

Ability to Tolerate Affect. Infants who have been overwhelmingly traumatized tend to experience any affect as an unbearable reminder of their early abuse (Krystal, 1988). Thus, as adults, DID patients try to avoid any experience of affect through switching, numbing, or other dissociative sensory alterations such as depersonalization, derealization, and a loss of time sense (Terr, 1990, 1991). The inadequacy of soothing experiences during childhood (Kluft, 1984) has impaired the patient's development of the ability to soothe herself.

In contrast to the patients' parents, the therapist is nondissociative, consistent, and (generally) calm no matter what the patient expresses. Like a healthy parent, the therapist's steady and containing presence helps the patient tolerate his feelings. The patient gradually sees that the therapist does not reject or hurt him when he expresses his feelings and needs. He can then begin to allow strongly conflicting feelings and needs to cohabitate in his awareness, instead of using dissociative behaviors to keep them separate. By internalizing the containment aspects of the therapeutic setting, he finds that he can tolerate and regulate his feelings without dissociating. The patient allows himself to experience ambivalence, where earlier in treatment he would have experienced dissociation.

Formation of a Cohesive Sense of Self. DID patients display inconsistent and disconnected senses of self, echoing the inconsistent parental responses that they report. In DID, emergence of dissociated aspects of the self may bring a perceived change in identity and often amnesia. The therapist then faces the task of interpreting behavior that only one part of the patient remembers.

Dissociative patients do not experience their personality aspects as belonging to them. Therefore, they have no appreciation of why different alters seem to take control at particular times. The parade of alters and dissociative experiences seems to them as random and unpredictable as the childhood environments in which they grew up. When the therapist helps the patient to see that alters and the memories associated with them come for a reason, then the patient begins to see his mental process as a single experience, instead of as a collection of disconnected internal events and separate "people."

Once the therapist has begun to understand the functions served by each alter, she can help the patient develop a cohesive sense of self by interpreting the feelings and actions of one alter in relationship to the feelings of another. For example, the therapist may "talk to the bleachers" (Loewenstein, personal communication), inquiring about the reactions of alters who may be listening without assuming executive control. Over time, as the patient's observing ego widens its field of view to include the alters, such interventions promote self-acceptance and tolerance of conflictual feelings; the patient's sense of self becomes integrated.

Development of Coherent Object and Self Representations. Important people in the DID patient's childhood failed to provide an atmosphere in which conflicting self and object representations could be integrated. A child with predictable parents comes to understand that people who care about him will still maintain their loving feelings though they may be angry with him. If the patient experienced dissociated, confused, and often violent parenting, different aspects of the mind might contain dissociated and contradictory perceptions (i.e., cognitive schemata) (Fine, 1988) of what to expect from people. Abused children develop bizarre yet functional expectations that they use to make sense out of the way others have treated them.

From a psychodynamic perspective, the dysfunctional cognitions in the DID patient are maintained by means of the defense mechanism known as splitting. Whether or not DID is a subset of borderline personality disorder as some believe (Lauer, Black, & Keen, 1993; cf. Armstrong, 1991; Kemp, Gilbertson, & Torem, 1988; Marmer, 1991), descriptions of this defense in the literature on borderline personality disorder bear much relevance to treating DID patients. Kernberg (1984) has described how "aggressively determined" object and self representations are actively separated from equally intense "libidinally determined" self and object representations: "Because of the implicit threat to the good object relations, bringing together opposite (loving and hateful) images of the self and of significant others would trigger unbearable anxiety and guilt" (Kernberg, 1984, p. 112).

The "aggressively determined" nature of the object representations may become comprehensible if one considers that child abuse may have brought them about. Splitting enables an abused child to interact with the perpetrator(s) of the abuse during the more benign interactions that occupy much of the child's daily existence. In this way, splitting has an adaptive value: "Learning to split off bad self images and others' images minimizes awareness of the ever-constant threat from which the child cannot escape" (Perry & Herman, 1993, p. 134).

Consistent interpretation of defense mechanisms such as splitting and projective identification will eventually lead to more coherent object and self representations (Kernberg, Selzer, Koenigsberg, Carr, & Appelbaum, 1989). The therapist's consistently neutral and nonjudgmental stance, maintained in spite of powerful negative transferences and projective identifications, helps the patient to blend mixed or ambivalent feelings about another person that the patient has hitherto kept from conjoint awareness. The therapist gently undermines dissociation and splitting between contradictory object and self representations by looking for relationships. He looks for the coherence behind the seemingly puzzling sequences of personality switches and affective shifts, then points out to the patient in a tentative way how each occurrence may be related to what has come before.

Of course, as in any psychodynamic therapy, the therapist needs to choose which interpretations will be most useful to the patient at any given time, and must not overload the patient with too much at once. The usual psychodynamic principle of interpreting defense before content (Greenson, 1967) applies to DID patients. The therapist should avoid using present-day feelings and events to enlighten a patient about the content of dissociated material. Such misguided reconstructions may lead the patient to clutch at the therapist's suggestions as historical fact, thereby avoiding what was actually dissociated. Dissociative defenses are not altered by such interventions.

However, interpretation of dissociative *defenses* (rather than dissociated *content*) will gradually reduce the patient's overreliance on dissociation. For example, a child alter was about to describe an episode of sadistic abuse. Suddenly, an aggressive alter appeared and attempted to hurt herself (i.e., hurt the child alter). It would have been a technical error to tell the patient that perhaps an adult had told the child she would be hurt if she told what happened. Instead, the therapist remarked that perhaps the patient could not manage in childhood to be aware of her intense mix of anger, guilt, and shame concerning the abuse; and that she had relegated those feelings to another part of her that evolved into an aggressive alter.

This kind of defense interpretation is useful because it brings the split self-representations into the patient's awareness at the same time. In time, the patient begins to own dissociated aspects of the self, instead of seeing herself as a passive victim of their apparently independent activities. A similarly beneficial effect on the integration of split object representations will occur when the therapist can interpret that the emergence of an alter may have the purpose of reducing the anxiety engendered by holding contradictory images of another person in mind at the same time.

The Ability to Differentiate Fact from Fantasy. In contrast to patients with "good enough" parenting, DID patients do not learn to distinguish reliably between internally generated reality and external reality. The confusion is partly the result of the seeming reality of hypnotically developed internal experiences and of the seeming unreality of dissociated historical experiences. Wishes, fears, memories, fantasies, and dreams mingle together in such a way that the patient is unable to distinguish among them. The confusion often occurs in relation to present-day as well as to past experiences, and may at times reach psychotic proportions in some patients.

Several aspects of the treatment help the patient learn to differentiate between fact and fantasy. As patients become more able to tolerate intense affect without resorting to dissociation, they enter autohypnotic states less frequently. Consequently, they become more able to separate fact from fantasy in understanding their present-day experiences. Also, cognitive distortions that support their misattributions of responsibility can be confronted during the processing of abreacted or interpreted material.

Reduction of Acting Out

Acting out represents "a reenactment of a past memory. The action is a slightly disguised repetition of the past ... The patient seems intent upon acting instead of remembering; it is a defense against memory" (Greenson, 1967, pp. 259). As one would expect, therapists find considerable acting out in DID patients, who have so much they wish to forget.

Some patients will act out to destroy emerging awareness of the meanings of their feelings (Bion, 1967; Langs, 1990). They attempt to "dump" feelings and memories into the therapist by means of their behavior. No doubt DID patients experienced this sort of dumping from their caretakers, and it has therefore become a familiar mode of discharging tension.

Psychodynamic psychotherapy has a distinct advantage over more directive therapies in treating patients who chronically act out. Psychodynamic psychotherapy implicitly and explicitly communicates to the adult patient that he is responsible for all of his own present-day behavior. In contrast, more directive therapies may replicate the authoritarian atmosphere of the patient's childhood, leading the patient to expect the therapist to control her. This situation may not be helpful to DID patients who, like others who act out, already tend to view themselves as not in control of their behavior. They see their self-destructive wishes as powerful needs that demand action from themselves and others. Their actions require the therapist to set forceful limits (such as not permitting overtly sexual, violent, or self-injurious activities during therapy sessions; or arranging hospitalization).

However, acting out should be more than merely managed; it should be interpreted. Interpretation helps the patient to use her adult resources and the stability of the therapeutic setting to face experiences from which she dissociated herself when her ego resources were overwhelmed.

Acting out may convey information about traumatic experiences not only in its content, but in the feelings and actions that it elicits from other people. When acting out is viewed as a form of communication between patient and therapist, the interpersonal effects of acting out can illuminate the patient's past experiences (Chu, 1991). Acting out often brings interactional pressure on the therapist to respond in a particular way. For example, many patients will state that they must cut themselves to relieve internal emotional pressure or else they will have to kill themselves. The patient may ask the therapist to make a bargain in which a less dangerous action is "allowed" in exchange for a no-suicide promise. In this scenario, acceding to the patient's request puts the therapist in the role of the unprotecting parent who allows the abuse to continue right under his nose. The request may also induce a sense of helplessness, anger, frustration, and emotional conflict in the therapist, echoing the unvoiced feelings of the patient. The therapist can use his reactions to formulate tentative interpretations concerning the defensive function served by the acting out.

Reduction of the "Negative Symptoms" of Dissociation

By analogy with the schizophrenia literature (e.g., Strauss, Carpenter, & Bartko, 1974), the symptoms of DID can be characterized as either positive (characterized by their obvious presence) or negative (characterized by the absence of normal personality function). The positive symptoms are the focus of most of the therapy, especially in its early and middle stages. These symptoms include the presence of alters, flashbacks, suicidal or other self-destructive behavior, dissociative headaches, and autohypnotic behavior. Positive symptoms represent adaptations to experiences of intrusive abuse.

Negative symptoms may result from a combination of the psychological sequelae of childhood neglect and the biological sequelae of chronic trauma (Van der Kolk and Greenberg, 1987). Present in DID patients in varying degrees, negative symptoms include the absence of meaningful relationships, affective numbing, denial of sexual feelings, and the overall avoidance of excitement and stimulation. In the common emphasis on abreactive work to help DID patients deal with intrusive trauma, the "quiet trauma" of neglect may be overlooked. For example, patients may abreact rapes by parents, but they do not abreact directly the experience of having an emotionally absent father. Such experiences are, however, readily brought to awareness through examination of the transference.

The trauma of neglect may indirectly be reenacted during abreactive work. Focusing on the content of past trauma recalled during abreaction may cause the therapist to overlook the feelings that follow. The endpoint of each abreaction is a feeling of profound abandonment—by parents, God, the therapist, other people, and oneself. Abreactions as a whole may be the psyche's regressive attempt to cope with dissociated and repressed experiences of abandonment and neglect.

Negative symptoms respond to several aspects of psychodynamic treatment. First, the consistent, emotionally involved presence of the therapist may have a soothing effect that in time the patient can internalize, partially supplanting the chaotic internalizations made during childhood. Second, the therapist's overall interpretive stance directs the patient away from demands that the therapist take care of him when he feels abandoned and instead helps him to mourn childhood experiences of neglect. Third, interpretations may help the patient to challenge dysfunctional cognitions that discourage him from drawing more stimulation from the environment. Fourth, psychodynamic psychotherapy steers the therapist away from a directive approach that may reinforce therapist-pleasing behavior and excessive dependency. Although useful at times, a directive approach may allow patients to maintain a mental map of the world in which satisfying the needs of others continues to be a central organizing principle. Directive techniques may promote reliance on the therapist, rather than on oneself. When the therapist is willing to take a primarily directive stance, the patient has little need to learn how to manage his environment to satisfy his own needs.

TECHNICAL ASPECTS OF THE TREATMENT

Once the goals of DID are considered in psychodynamic terms, the preferred treatment framework becomes clear. Psychodynamic treatment involves a relatively nondirective therapist who creates a setting in which the patient is encouraged to put all of her needs and wishes into words. The structure of the treatment invites all aspects of the psyche to be verbalized, which eventually helps the patient to experience all aspects of the psyche in an increasingly integrated way.

Boundaries

Early in treatment, the therapist should establish clearly defined boundaries that she expects she can maintain. For DID patients, clear boundaries bring predictability, a quality that was rarely in evidence in their childhood experiences. The therapist should spell out the length and starting time of sessions, fees and how they will be paid, emergency availability, and guidelines about when it is appropriate for the patient to call. We believe that it is generally not helpful for therapists to touch DID patients, because the meaning of touch may be confusing to patients who have experienced abuse. Because previous treatment settings and approaches have sometimes included touch, and because some patients have been sexually exploited by previous therapists (Kluft, 1990), it may be necessary to state specifically that the therapist will not be touching the patient.

Although the structure of a therapy should fit the needs of the specific patient, psychodynamic therapists treating DID generally see DID patients face-to-face between one and three times a week, with sessions lasting between 45 and 90 minutes. If the patient needs an extra session during a crisis, we clearly label it as an exception to the regular schedule. When there are problems (as there usually are) in the patient's significant relationships, we prefer to have someone other than the patient's therapist meet with or treat the couple, the family, or the children. The patient is asked to authorize the various therapists to stay in communication.

Therapeutic Neutrality

A relatively neutral therapeutic stance may permit the patient to move beyond the production of material that complies with what she thinks the therapist wants to hear. Although complete neutrality is impossible, a silent, critical, or detached therapist may inadvertently replicate crucial traumatic aspects of the patient's childhood environment (Giovacchini, 1989), resulting in a therapeutic impasse.

Furthermore, a high level of therapist activity is necessary during crises, particularly early in treatment.

Management of the Transference

The presence of dissociative defenses results in some modifications in the therapist's way of working with transference. Generally, psychodynamic psychotherapists identify and interpret transference by deducing its presence from the patient's free associations, dreams, and resistances. Although these sources of information are certainly available to the therapist treating DID, transference makes itself known in some additional ways. By adopting a single-self model of DID, the therapist can identify transferential implications in the presentation, timing, and sequencing of dissociative phenomena in the therapy session. For example, a sudden switch from calm personality John to belligerent alter Rocky can signify the activation of a transference reaction. Transference reactions occur not only to the therapist's behavior, but also to the patient's feelings about the therapist's behavior. Thus, Rocky might emerge not as a defense to a perceived attack by the therapist, but to the patient's discomfort with his own loving feelings for the therapist.

The usual method of interpreting transference should be slightly modified for DID patients to allow for the presence of dissociative amnesia. Interpretation becomes difficult when the patient has amnesia for the associations the therapist is trying to interpret. However, amnestic barriers are rarely as absolute as they appear. In the preceding example, the therapist might suggest that Rocky has perhaps taken control to protect the system of personalities from frightening feelings that arose when John was "out." Once the dissociative defense has been interpreted in this way, the therapist can evoke John when Rocky is in control of behavior, asking Rocky to check "inside" and see what John might have been feeling. If Rocky cooperates, he may then experience the anxiety that occurred when loving feelings toward the therapist arose in John. The experience of sharing feelings across alters is integrative in nature and effect, and also brings memories or associations that underlie the transference to the conscious mind.

The transferences that come forward in DID patients are usually quite intense and often unmodulated in their expression. Most patients develop an aggressive transference, a caretaking transference, some form of erotized transference, and a "victim" transference (in which the therapist is consciously or unconsciously perceived as a perpetrator in the patient's abuse memories) (Loewenstein, 1993). Any of these transferences may become so strongly expressed in action as to interfere with treatment progress. For example, patients may act out sexually toward the therapist, may threaten the therapist or break things in the office, or may cower in the corner because they believe the therapist is about to hurt them. Within the limits of the therapist's tolerance, the therapist can attempt to interpret such behaviors; these responses occur in venues other than the therapist's office and may in fact have brought the patient into treatment.

Acting out in the transference can be a resistance, enabling the patient to avoid upsetting feelings and memories (Greenson, 1967), and it is profitable to explore what the acting out means. However, if it is reasonably clear that the patient is making no progress in exploring these issues or if the expression of transference is beyond the limits of the therapist's tolerance, the patient may need to be referred to another therapist or to a more structured treatment setting.

Countertransference

Although DID patients may elicit stronger countertransference than many other patients (Comstock, 1991; Wilbur, 1984), the management of countertransference feelings is no different from its management with other patients: The therapist's feelings are to be handled by the therapist. The patient may be confronted about behavior that results in negative responses from the therapist, but the patient is not "blamed" for the therapist's feelings.

When the therapist is tempted to make a treatment deviation, the temptation often arises from unresolved countertransference. As with all other feelings in a psychodynamic treatment, countertransference feelings should be examined before being acted upon.

The Role of Hypnosis

Most therapists use hypnosis in treating DID (Putnam & Loewenstein, 1993). As with any directive intervention, the therapist's use of hypnosis has transferential significance. Hypnosis tends to intensify transference (Gill & Brenman, 1959), including wishes for rescue. This effect may be especially true for dissociative patients, who already spend much of their time in spontaneous or self-induced trance (Bliss, 1986). If the therapist relies on hypnosis as an uncovering technique, he temporarily circumvents the patient's resistances to remembering and feeling, but does so at the risk of eliciting more extreme forms of dissociation and more primitive defenses to manage the resulting anxiety. Even by overpowering the patient's conscious resistance to remembering, the therapist is asserting his will over the patient's will. For example, some patients unconsciously view the hypnotic penetration of amnestic barriers as a rape. They may also consciously experience the therapist as an abuser, especially during moments when they are abreacting child abuse (Spiegel, 1993).

Therapists often use hypnosis to effect integration of alters (e.g., Kluft, 1993). However, misuse or overreliance on hypnotically facilitated integration may vitiate the special value of hypnosis in giving the patient a sense of control over the emergence of distressing feelings and memories (Spiegel, 1989).

We have come to prefer a minimal use of therapist-induced hypnosis in outpatient treatment. Knowledge of hypnosis is useful in understanding dissociative phenomena and sometimes in explaining them to the patient. Also, hypnosis can occasionally be useful in managing crises. However, we have found that psychodynamic interventions produce the desired goals without the transferential complications that hypnosis introduces.

Abreactions

Abreactions occurring within a therapy context are multidetermined. Their content may reflect past experiences of trauma. They are also stimulated by situations and feelings about the present that are represented metaphorically in the content, affective tone, and timing of the abreaction. Because the therapist cannot ascertain literal accuracy of the retrieved material, she must adopt a neutral therapeutic stance so that the patient can have the freedom to explore his own fears and certainties as he works to create a cohesive sense of his own history.

Besides conveying information about dissociated trauma, abreactions can combine elements of reenactment, resistance, and communication to the therapist about the therapeutic relationship. Abreacted material does not emerge as a chronological reconstruction of the patient's childhood, but piece by piece as it is elicited by the patient's present-day situation. As the therapist interprets the parallels between the abreacted material and the patient's present life situation, dissociated feelings concerning the present situation will come forward in tandem with their metaphorical appearance in the content of the abreaction. As the patient develops the ability to modulate affect and put her feelings into words, she begins to have associations instead of abreactions. By then, she has less need to experience feelings metaphorically by reliving them.

In contrast to some other approaches to treating DID, psychodynamic psychotherapy is not organized around the goal of "getting out the memories." Abreactive work occurs in DID patients because it is dissociative in nature. It emerges from the dissociative strategies that DID patients adopted to survive their childhoods. As the patient comes to rely less on dissociative defenses, abreactive work will become less frequent, and the patient will recall historical material by means of free association.

CASE STUDY

We present two vignettes from the treatment of a DID patient that illustrate discrete psychodynamic interventions. For reasons of confidentiality and brevity, the vignettes combine elements of many patients' therapies, selected to illustrate the process of treatment.

Diane, a 30-year-old white female, sought therapy for panic attacks and night terrors that began soon after her daughter revealed abuse by a neighbor. When Dr. Jones tried to take a history, he found that Diane had few memories before age 16. She often experienced periods of missing time, found things in her possession she did not remember buying, and sometimes found herself on the floor playing with her daughter's toys. Diane scored 35 on the Dissociative Experiences Scale (DES) (Bernstein & Putnam, 1986).

During a diagnostic interview, Diane displayed dissociative behaviors, including spontaneous trance states, brief periods of confusion, and apparent difficulty remembering what she had said earlier in the interview. When he asked her if she had experienced physical or sexual abuse in childhood, she started to hyperventilate. She stared out of the window, talked in a calm child's voice, and said, "Diane is in the corner over there in that white house. It's safe over there." "Safe from what?" "Safe from the man." Diane closed her eyes for a moment. When she opened them, she appeared dazed, and asked what had happened. Dr. Jones said, "You got panicked when I asked if you had been abused." Diane recalled the panic, but did not recall the emergence of a child ego state.

Diane began to hear the voices of children within her mind, which frightened her. She started to make frequent calls to Dr. Jones after office hours, and requested extra sessions. In session, Dr. Jones told her that he was available after hours only in the event of an emergency, which he defined as imminent suicidal or homicidal behavior. She then switched to an angry alter who said, "You don't give a damn about her. She thought you were going to help her, but it was just a trick so you could get her hooked and then dump her. Well, she won't be coming back again." Dr. Jones asked her whether there was any way he could have been more direct about his limits, and pointed out that even clear boundaries felt like a trick to her. He gradually interpreted her belligerent posture as a defense against the feelings of vulnerability displayed by the child alters that had been calling him. He pointed out that she must have had some experiences that taught her to expect that she would be let down if she needed someone. Eventually, the belligerent alter began to allow herself to feel some of the vulnerability, and the vulnerable alter began to express some of her anger about being let down.

Because Dr. Jones remained relatively steady and consistent in his response to the patient, the patient found she could hold herself together in between sessions. She began to experience periods of sadness. The sadness gradually coalesced into childhood memories of having been hit by her mother when she asked for help and then having been left alone in a closet for hours. The patient began to understand why she abruptly shifted from clinging, regressive dependency to biting sarcasm in dealing with her husband. She also began to express a sense of trust in Dr. Jones' steady availability.

This highly condensed vignette shows a patient working on several of the goals described earlier. First, Diane is working on establishing a secure base for attachment. As Diane began to feel a sense of internal danger (i.e., signal anxiety) when treatment began, she displayed separation anxiety by making frequent calls to Dr. Jones. When Dr. Jones was unwilling to be available to her whenever she wanted him, the transference probably reflected experiences of parental abandonment. Dr. Jones interpreted her defense (the appearance of a belligerent alter who represents a form of passive-into-active defense: "I'll be the one who leaves, not you"). Second, Diane is developing a more coherent object representation of Dr. Jones: He gradually becomes someone who she sees as consistently caring, even though she is disappointed that she cannot call him whenever she wants. Third, Diane began to make more gradual transitions between ego states; the belligerent and vulnerable experiences shifted from being experienced as separate people to being experienced as mixed feelings.

Interpretation was the major therapeutic intervention. The dissociated memories of abuse and neglect arose spontaneously rather than through hypnotic intervention, as the result of interpretation of the transference. As Diane became aware of how she responded to her unconscious expectations of abandonment, she engaged in the process of working through and applied her insight to her marriage. Interpretation of the connections between alters gradually led to a blurring of their differences and then to some preliminary integration.

Early in treatment, a seductive alter named Regina began to appear in sessions. Her seductiveness was at first nonverbal, but later she began to talk about how much she wanted to have sex with Dr. Jones. He told her that he would not have sex with a patient at any time during or after treatment, that a sexual relationship with a patient would be harmful as well as unethical. Regina protested that a sexual relationship with a loving man like Dr. Jones would only be good for her. Going beyond merely setting a limit, Dr. Jones also asked Regina how Little Diane (a trusting and naive child alter) would feel if she found herself having sex with Dr. Jones. Regina said, "She doesn't deal with any of that stuff." Regina went on to describe sadistic sexual abuse by a trusted uncle. The host personality had not recalled this material before this point. Regina noted how much she had enjoyed it and how Little Diane had stayed "inside," crying and screaming during the abuse.

Dr. Jones then interpreted the behavior of the two alters in relationship to each other. He said that perhaps abusive experiences like the memories concerning the uncle were what Diane (the patient as a whole) expected from men; that Little Diane had wished to trust Dr. Jones; and that perhaps Regina had come forward to cope with what Diane expected would come next: sexual abuse from Dr. Jones. Regina admitted that this was indeed what she had expected, but said that it wouldn't have been abuse because she would have enjoyed it. Dr. Jones asked her to think back to what she felt when her uncle had sex with her, and Regina noted that actually she had felt quite numb. He then asked if she would be willing to check on what Little Diane might have felt during the abuse. Regina reported that Little Diane had felt frightened and hurt.

Regina then began to abreact the abuse spontaneously, partly blending with Little Diane during the process. That is, Regina recalled numbing herself but also felt some of the fear and pain that had been relegated to Little Diane. During the abreaction, Dr. Jones let the patient know that this was not happening in the present, that she was in his office, that she could open her eyes and look around to orient herself. After the abreaction, Diane, Regina, and Little Diane all shared a common understanding of the mixture of feelings concerning the memory of abuse by her uncle.

In this session, Dr. Jones interpreted the patient's acting out in terms of the interactions among alters in response to transference. The patient then recalled dissociated material that she had unknowingly been acting out. This treatment sequence helped the patient to integrate object and self representations that had been split among several alters. As a result of many such sequences, Diane began to see herself as having complex and contradictory feelings about significant people in her lives. She began to use her associations to present-day events to understand her own reactions, and was less prone to switching.

SUMMARY

The DID patient benefits from a therapeutic outlook in which all behavior and feelings are presumed to reflect a single self. Psychodynamic psychotherapy, in contrast to approaches that emphasize directive and specialized techniques, engages the patient and therapist in the shared goal of understanding all of the patient's actions and behavior. It communicates respect for the patient's autonomy, but does not sanction the patient's unconscious attempts to get reparation for past abuse by means of acting out. Dissociative symptoms may have helped the person to survive years of neglect and abuse, but they cannot compensate for the inability of the patient to complete important aspects of psychological development. If treatment focuses on completion of important developmental tasks and avoids limiting itself to eliminating dissociative phenomena, many patients can develop a resilient integration. If treatment is integrative, the patient can integrate.

REFERENCES

Alexander, P. C. (1992). Application of attachment theory to the study of sexual abuse. *Journal of Consulting and Clinical Psychology, 60*, 185-195.

Armstrong, J. (1991). The psychological organization of multiple personality disordered patients as revealed in psychological testing. *Psychiatric Clinics of North America, 14*, 533-546.

Barach, P. M. (1991). Multiple personality disorder as an attachment disorder. *Dissociation, 4*, 117-123.

Barach, P. M. (1992). An integrative approach for understanding the clinical presentation of multiple personality disorder (Abstract). In *Proceedings of the Seventh Regional Conference on Trauma, Dissociation, and Multiple Personality* (p. 48). Akron, OH: Akron General Medical Center.

Bernstein, E. M., & Putnam, F. W. (1986). Development, reliability, and validity of a dissociation scale. *Journal of Nervous and Mental Disease, 174*, 727-735.

Bion, W. R. (1967). *Second thoughts*. New York: Jason Aronson.

Bliss, E. L. (1980). Multiple personalities: A report of 14 cases with implications for schizophrenia and hysteria. *Archives of General Psychiatry, 37*, 1388-1397.

Bliss, E. L. (1986). *Multiple personality, allied disorders, and hypnosis*. New York: Oxford University Press.

Bowlby, J. (1973). *Attachment and loss: Vol. 2: Separation: Anxiety and anger*. Middlesex, England: Penguin Books.

Braun, B. G. (1986). Issues in the psychotherapy of Multiple Personality Disorder. In B. G. Braun (Ed.), *Treatment of multiple personality disorder* (pp. 3-28). Washington, DC: American Psychiatric Press.

Braun, B. G. (1988). The BASK model of dissociation. *Dissociation, 1*(1), 4-23.

Chu, J. A. (1991). The repetition compulsion revisited: Reliving dissociated trauma. *Psychotherapy, 28*, 327-332.

Cole, P. M., & Putnam, F. W. (1992). Effects of incest on self and social functioning: A developmental psychopathology perspective. *Journal of Consulting and Clinical Psychology, 60*, 174-184.

Comstock, C. M. (1991). Countertransference and the suicidal MPD patient. *Dissociation, 4*, 25-35.

Fenichel, O. (1945). *The psychoanalytic theory of neurosis*. New York: Norton.

Fine, C. G. (1988). Thoughts on the cognitive perceptual substrates of multiple personality disorder. *Dissociation, 1*(4), 5-10.

Freud, S. (1969). *An outline of psychoanalysis*. (J. Strachey, Trans.). New York: Norton. (Original work published 1940)

Frischholz, E. J., Lipman, L. S., Braun, B. G., & Sachs, R. G. (1992). Psychopathology, hypnotizability, and dissociation. *American Journal of Psychiatry, 149*, 1521-1525.

Furman, E. (1986). On trauma: When is the death of a parent traumatic? *Psychoanalytic Studies of the Child, 41*, 191-208.

Gill, M. M., & Brenman, M. (1959). *Hypnoses and related states: Psychoanalytic studies in regression*. New York: International Universities Press.

Giovacchini, P. L. (1989). *Countertransference triumphs and catastrophes*. New York: Jason Aronson.

Greenson, R. R. (1967). *The technique and practice of psychoanalysis* (Vol. 1). New York: International Universities Press.

Kemp, K., Gilbertson, A. D., & Torem, M. (1988). The differential diagnosis of multiple personality disorder from borderline personality disorder. *Dissociation, 1*(4), 41-46.

Kernberg, O. F. (1984). *Severe personality disorders: Psychotherapeutic strategies*. New Haven, CT: Yale University Press.

Kernberg, O. F., Selzer, M. A., Koenigsberg, H. W., Carr, A. C., & Appelbaum, A. H. (1989). *Psychodynamic psychotherapy of borderline patients*. New York: Basic Books.

Kluft, R. P. (1982). Varieties of hypnotic interventions in the treatment of multiple personality. *American Journal of Clinical Hypnosis, 24*, 230-240.

Kluft, R. P. (1983). Hypnotherapeutic crisis intervention in multiple personality. *American Journal of Clinical Hypnosis, 26*, 73-83.

Kluft, R. P. (1984). Treatment of multiple personality disorder. *Psychiatric Clinics of North America, 7*, 9-29.

Kluft, R. P. (1987). The parental fitness of mothers with multiple personality disorder: A preliminary study. *Child Abuse and Neglect, 11*, 273-280.

Kluft, R. P. (1990). Incest and subsequent revictimization: The case of therapist-patient sexual exploitation, with a description of the sitting duck syndrome. In R. P. Kluft (Ed.), *Incest-related syndromes of adult psychopathology* (pp. 263-287). Washington, DC: American Psychiatric Press.

Kluft, R. P. (1991). Multiple personality disorder. In A. Tasman & S. M. Goldfinger (Eds.), *American psychiatric press review of psychiatry* (pp. 161-188). Washington, DC: American Psychiatric Press.

Kluft, R. P. (1993). Clinical approaches to the integration of personalities. In R. P. Kluft & C. G. Fine (Eds.), *Clinical perspectives on multiple personality disorder* (pp. 101-133). Washington, DC: American Psychiatric Press.

Kluft, R. P., & Wilbur, C. B. (1989). Multiple personality disorder. In *Treatments of psychiatric disorders* (Vol. 3, pp. 2197-2216). Washington, DC: American Psychiatric Press.

Krystal, H. (1988). *Integration and self-healing: Affect, trauma, alexithymia*. Hillsdale, NJ: The Analytic Press.

Langs, R. (1990). *Psychotherapy: A basic text*. Northvale, NJ: Jason Aronson.

Lauer, J., Black, D. W., & Keen, P. (1993). Multiple personality disorder and borderline personality disorder: Distinct entities of variations on a common theme. *Annals of Clinical Psychiatry, 5*, 129-134.

Loewenstein, R. P. (1993). Posttraumatic and dissociative aspects of transference and countertransference in the treatment of multiple personality disorder. In R. P. Kluft & C. G. Fine (Eds.), *Clinical perspectives on multiple personality disorder* (pp. 51-85). Washington, DC: American Psychiatric Press.

Liotti, G. (1992). Disorganized/disoriented attachment in the etiology of the dissociative disorders. *Dissociation, 4*, 196-204.

Marmer, S. (1991). Multiple personality disorder: A psychoanalytic perspective. *Psychiatric Clinics of North America, 14*, 677-693.

Perry, J. C., & Herman, J. L. (1993). Trauma and defense in the etiology of borderline personality disorder. In J. Paris (Ed.), *Borderline personality disorder: Etiology and treatment* (pp. 123-139). Washington, DC: American Psychiatric Press.

Putnam, F. W. (1989). *Diagnosis and treatment of multiple personality disorder*. New York: Guilford.

Putnam, F. W. (1990). Disturbances of "self" in victims of childhood sexual abuse. In R. P. Kluft (Ed.), *Incest-related syndromes of adult psychopathology* (pp. 113-131). Washington, DC: American Psychiatric Press.

Putnam, F. W., & Loewenstein, R. J. (1993). Treatment of multiple personality disorder: A survey of current practices. *American Journal of Psychiatry, 150*, 1048-1052.

Ross, C. A. (1989). *Multiple personality disorder: Diagnosis, clinical features and treatment*. New York: Wiley.

Schreiber, F. (1973). *Sybil*. Chicago: Regnery.

Spiegel, D. (1989). Hypnosis in the treatment of victims of sexual abuse. *Psychiatric Clinics of North America, 12*, 295-305.

Spiegel, D. (1993). Multiple posttraumatic personality disorder. In R. P. Kluft & C. G. Fine (Eds.), *Clinical perspectives on multiple personality disorder* (pp. 87-99). Washington, DC: American Psychiatric Press.

Strauss, J. S., Carpenter, W. T., & Bartko, J. J. (1974). The diagnosis and understanding of schizophrenia: III. Speculation on the processes that underlie schizophrenia. *Schizophrenia Bulletin, 11*, 61-69.

Thigpen, C., & Cleckley, H. (1957). *The three faces of Eve*. New York: McGraw-Hill.

Terr, L. C. (1990). *Too scared to cry: Psychic trauma in childhood*. New York: Harper & Row.

Terr, L. C. (1991). Childhood traumas: An outline and overview. *American Journal of Psychiatry, 148*, 10-20.

Van der Kolk, B. A., & Greenberg, M. S. (1987). The psychological consequences of overwhelming life experiences. In B. A. Van der Kolk (Ed.), *Psychological trauma* (pp. 1–30). Washington, DC: American Psychiatric Press.
Wilbur, C. B. (1984). Treatment of multiple personality. *Psychiatric Annals, 14*, 27–31.
Watkins, H. H., & Watkins, J. G. (1993). Ego-state therapy in the treatment of dissociative disorders. In R. P. Kluft & C. G. Fine (Eds.), *Clinical perspectives on multiple personality disorder* (pp. 277–299). Washington, DC: American Psychiatric Press.
Wyatt, G. E., Guthrie, D., & Notgrass, C. M. (1992). Differential effects of women's child sexual abuse and subsequent sexual revictimization. *Journal of Consulting and Clinical Psychology, 60*, 167–173.

21

Overt–Covert Dissociation and Hypnotic Ego State Therapy

John G. Watkins and Helen H. Watkins

THE ORIGIN AND DEVELOPMENT OF EGO STATES

During the past decade, the psychological process of dissociation has received an increasing amount of attention as witnessed by the contributions in this volume. However, the focus has been largely on its severe ramifications evidenced in amnesia and multiple personality disorder (MPD). Such a focus has resulted in an emphasis on its pathological effects as found in severe mental illness to the neglect of its more normal manifestations as an adaptive defense. This more normal aspect of dissociation is demonstrated in many behavioral, adjustment problems and in various neurotic and psychosomatic reactions.

The continuous nature of dissociation as a separating process has been noted by various contributors, i.e., by Braun (1988) in his BASK model (see also Chapter 5). Still, the greatest interest to date has been in the understanding and treatment of this condition as manifested in true MPD.

Ego state theory (see Spring 1993 issue of *American Journal of Clinical Hypnosis*) is an extension of the principles and findings that have been noted in the severe maladjustments of MPD—now renamed dissociative identity disorder (DID), in the current revision of the American Psychiatric Association's (1994) *Diagnostic and Statistical Manual of Mental Disorders*.

John G. Watkins and Helen H. Watkins • Department of Psychology, University of Montana, Missoula, Montana 59801.

Handbook of Dissociation: Theoretical, Empirical, and Clinical Perspectives, edited by Larry K. Michelson and William J. Ray. Plenum Press, New York, 1996.

Our ego state theory stems from writings by Paul Federn (1952) and his associate, Edoardo Weiss (1960), whose concepts we have elaborated and developed further. We have summarized this theory in a number of publications (H. Watkins, 1978, 1993; Watkins & Watkins, 1979, 1981, 1986, 1991).

Ego state therapy is a treatment methodology based on this theory and derived from both our therapy with true MPD cases and from research with normal volunteers (Watkins & Watkins, 1979-80, 1980). These studies involved replication of aspects of the "hidden observer" experiments reported by Hilgard (1986) (see also Watkins & Watkins, 1992).

Hypnosis—itself a form of controlled dissociation (Hilgard, 1986)—has been the modality within which the treatment strategy has been most expeditiously carried out—although one of us (HHW) has developed a nonhypnotic technique of ego state therapy that can be used by practitioners not skilled in hypnotherapy. Our hypnotic techniques have been described in detail (Watkins, 1987, 1992).

Other researchers and clinicians are currently showing interest in ego state therapy, and a number of contributions have appeared that extend and further apply its procedures (Edelstien, 1982; Frederick & McNeal, 1993; Frederick & Kim, 1993; Gainer & Torem, 1993; Malmo, 1991; Newey, 1986; Philips, 1993; Philips & Frederick, 1995; Torem, 1987, 1993).

Our own interest in the development of ego state therapy has been motivated by the great need for a psychodynamic therapy that could achieve significant personality reorganization in less time than required by traditional psychanalysis (Freud, 1953; Fenichel, 1945). At the present time, much of the remuneration to psychotherapists is paid by insurance companies and other third-party reimbursers. Psychoanalysts have had difficulty securing compensation since that approach requires several sessions a week, often for many years. Even the more active psychoanalytic therapies, such as those proposed by Alexander and French (1946), have not been widely followed. Psychodynamically oriented practitioners have been frustrated by their inability to receive reimbursement for the time required by such treatments.

On the other hand, briefer forms of treatment, such as behavior therapy (Wright, Thase, Beck, & Ludgate, 1993) and cognitive therapy (Spiegler & Guevremont, 1993), while operating within a much shorter time frame, do not generally achieve the more profound character reorganization that is often required for long-lasting results, especially in the treatment of MPD. And it is here, where a therapist seeks psychodynamic resolution of unconscious conflicts within a comparatively lesser number of sessions, that ego state therapy holds substantial promise. It was with this problem in mind that we have been motivated in our study of ego states and their applicability to such conditions as weight reduction, smoking cessation, improved study habits, behavior and adjustment disorders, psychosomatic symptoms, and neurotic disorders, as well as the treatment of true multiple personalities.

We have attempted to share our experiences in this endeavor with colleagues through a number of workshops that have been sponsored by universities, medical schools, and scientific societies (Steckler, 1989). The essence of ego state theory follows.

INTEGRATION AND DIFFERENTIATION

Human personality develops through two basic processes: integration and differentiation. Through integration, a child learns to put concepts together, like dog and cat, and thus to build more complex units as in that called "animals." By differentiation, the child separates general concepts into more specific meanings, such as discriminating between "good doggies" and "bad doggies." Both processes are normal and adaptive. It is normal differentiation that permits us to experience one set of behaviors at a party Saturday night and another at the office during the week. When this separating or differentiating process becomes excessive and maladaptive, we call it "dissociation." The boundaries between two or more ego states become rigid and impermeable, thus preventing communication. If this dissociation is severe enough, the individual may develop amnesias or multiple personalities.

Paul Federn (1952), a close associate of Freud's, held that personality was not simply a collection of perceptions, cognitions, and affects, but that these were organized into clusters or patterns, which he called "ego states." An ego state may be defined as an organized system of behavior and experience whose elements are bound together by some common principle, and differentiated from another by boundaries that are more or less permeable. Defined in this way, ego states subsume what we call "multiple personalities." They may or may not reach consciousness and directly affect behavior.

Ego states may be large and include all the various behaviors and experiences activated in one's occupation. They may be small like the behaviors and feelings elicited when attending a baseball game. They may represent current modes of behavior and experience, or, as in the case of hypnotic regression, include many memories, postures, feelings, and so forth, which were apparently learned at an earlier age. They may be organized in different dimensions. For example, an ego state may be built around being 6 years of age. Another one may represent patterns of behavior toward father and authority figures. These two would overlap on experiences with father at the age of 6. Obviously, different ego states may use the same English language, but with some variations in the terms and expressions spoken.

THE DEVELOPMENT OF EGO STATES

Ego states apparently develop by one or more of the following three processes: normal differentiation, introjection of significant others, and reactions to trauma. First, through normal differentiation the child learns to discriminate foods that taste good and those that do not. He or she not only makes such simple discriminations, but also develops entire patterns of behavior that are appropriate for dealing with parents, teachers, or playmates. They are adaptive for adjusting to school, the playground, and so forth. These changes are considered quite normal, yet they do represent patterns of behavior and experience that are clustered and organized under some common principle. As such, they can be considered ego states.

The boundaries between these entities are very flexible and permeable. The child in school is quite aware (or easily capable of becoming aware) of himself in a playground situation. Playground behaviors, however, are not as easily activated when at the school desk. He or she is now in a different ego state, and there is resistance at the boundaries. These less-clearly differentiated ego states are usually adaptive and are economic in providing appropriate behavior patterns when needed.

Second, through the introjection of significant others the child erects patterns of behavior which if ego-cathected become roles that he himself experiences and if object-cathected represent inner objects with whom he must relate and interact. For example, if a boy introjects a punishing parent, hence developing an ego state pattern around his perceptions of that parent, he may be constantly depressed as he tries to cope inwardly and covertly with a continuation of the accusations and abuse originally heaped on him by the real parent. However, if he ego-cathects this state (e.g., infuses it with self-energy), he will not suffer, but he will abuse his own child. We say he has identified with his bad parent. He not only introjects the abusing parent, but he also introjects the drama of the original parent–child conflict; whether he suffers from this ego state or identifies with it and inflicts suffering on others will depend on whether it is primarily object or self. In a multiple personality he may alternate between these two patterns of response. Finally, if he introjects both his mother and father and if these two parents were constantly quarreling with each other, then he will have internalized their war. This may be manifested by constant headaches of whose origin he is unaware as the two parental ego states battle with each other.

Third, when confronted with overwhelming trauma, rejection, or abuse, the child may dissociate. A lonesome youngster often removes the ego cathexis (self energy) from part of himself, reenergizes it with object cathexis (non-self energy), and creates an imaginary playmate with whom he or she can interact. Most children with imaginary playmates discard or repress these entities upon going to school. But if such an ego state is merely repressed, later conflict and environmental pressure may cause it to be reinvested with energy and to reemerge, perhaps in malevolent form as it did in the case of Rhonda Johnson, who coauthored with me (J.G.W.) her life story and treatment in *We, the Divided Self* (Watkins & Johnson, 1982), or the murdering Steve personality of Ken Bianchi, the "Hillside Strangler" (see Watkins, 1984).

Evidence has been accumulating from hypnotherapy cases involving hypermnesia and regression that differentiation, and perhaps even severe dissociation, may begin at a very early age, at least within the first few months of life and possibly even before birth. This whole issue of the veridicality of early memories is controversial today, with experimental research often in opposition to clinical findings (see Loftus, 1993; Watkins, 1989, 1993). The child knows the meaning of pain before it has developed a word for this. Later, when it has learned to attach a word to this feeling, it is in a position to report on earlier pain experiences.

A paper by Helen Watkins (1986) on "Treating the Trauma of Abortion" presented specific cases where this splitting had apparently occurred. In that paper, she also described how hypnoanalytic ego state therapy was employed in treating these dissociations.

As defense mechanisms are increasingly utilized to avoid guilt and anxiety, the individual develops more unwillingness or inability to face reality and accept the consequences of his own behavior. True dissociation involves strong avoidance of responsibility for one's own behavior and unwillingness to face the consequences of one's actions. Ego states become more sharply differentiated from one another as the separating boundaries become increasingly less permeable.

The extreme of this continuum is reached when the boundaries are so rigid and impermeable that there is little or no interaction between states. If the dissociation is quite complete, the individual, when ego state A is executive, is not conscious of the behaviors and experiences that occurred when B is "out." There is then a broad amnesia for these events (especially if they are recent), and a true multiple personality is manifested. The only way these other events can be accessed is through a complete change of ego states, or as we term it, a switching of "alters."

We use the term "ego state" to cover all of those discrete patterns of behavior and experience, which range from the simple organizational patterns in "normal" adjustment, through the intermediate ones represented by neurotic defense and true neuroses, to the severe dissociations of MPD. We reserve the term "alters," as in current usage, for those ego states involved in true MPD.

In the differentiation-dissociation continuum, normal and neurotic ego states lie between simple adaptive differentiation at the one extreme and the severe dissociation of true multiple personality at the other (see Figure 1). The variable here is the rigidity or permeability of the separating boundaries. Normal separations in everyday life are exemplified by the organization of patterns of behavior and experience dividing the average person's function while at work as contrasted with the activities and mental processes needed during periods of recreation, relationships with family, and so forth.

As adaptation to everyday problems of life become more complex and stressful, the separating boundaries between the various ego states become less permeable in order to minimize conflicts between incompatible states, which would cause increased anxiety. In the lower intermediate area, characterized in Fig. 1 as "defensive", one finds processes like rationalization, compensation, reaction formation, and other neurotic defense mechanisms. These involve a partial shielding of

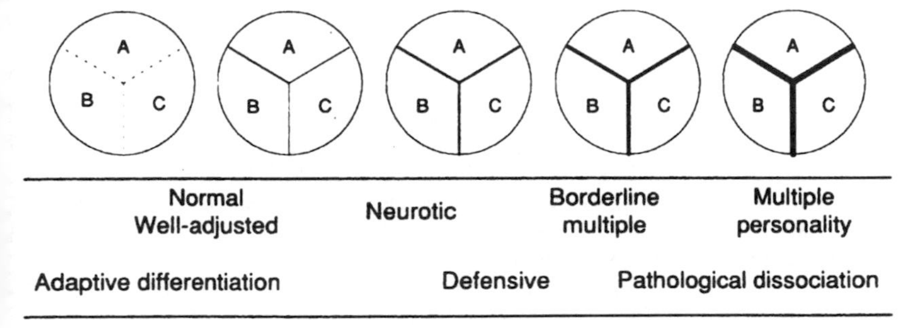

Figure 1. Differentiation-dissociation continuum.

the individual from the conflictual consequences of direct contact with unacceptable elements of mental life, such as the unwillingness to assume responsibility or guilt for misbehavior. As is well known, these mechanisms are adaptive in the sense that they keep apart incompatible elements of mental life, thus rendering the individual more free of stress. However, he or she pays a price in that behavior becomes more rigid, less geared to reality. These mechanisms are considered to be more immature and can be a step in the direction of less-adaptive behaviors. Ego states, therefore, can be normal, adaptive, defensive, or dissociative, depending on the permeability of their separating boundaries, this permeability or rigidity having been influenced by the severity of internal conflicts and the individual's perception of his or her need to escape mental "pain."

A common characteristic of ego states is, even though they are capable of growth and change, they may often be fixated at the time of their creation. Thus, a 5-year-old ego state, which was developed by a child at that age perhaps to deal with a traumatic event, may talk and act with the concrete "paralogic" typical of a 5-year-old. Understanding this point can be of great significance when a therapist is dealing with it. To resonate well with this state, the clinician needs to be able to use a child's terminology and logic, perhaps by drawing on a child ego state within him or herself. The clinician may find this difficult, since the scientific training of therapists (and even more so of researchers) emphasizes principles of Aristotelian logic.

SUBJECT–OBJECT

A fundamental distinction ever present in treating cases of dissociation, covert or overt, is recognition of just when a psychological process, act, or state is *subject* and when it is *object*. Subject means "me," "myself," and sometimes is called "ego syntonic." Object means "not me," hence, "he," "she," or "it." The determining criteria is how it is experienced by the individual.

When I move my hand up and down, the movement is by "my" hand and it is experienced as being initiated by "me." I am both conscious of the movement and of its origin within "my self." If I have been hypnotized, however, the hand is dissociated from me, followed by the suggestion that "it" will wag up and down, the movement will be experienced as "object," and hence is ego-alien. I will not perceive it as something "I" am doing, but rather as something happening to me and as if "my self" is responding to an outside force. I may be quite surprised at the experience.

Normally, a conscious thought is experienced as subject. I recognize it as my thought. However, in cases of psychosis a thought may become conscious, but actually be object. It reaches the threshold of awareness without being imbued with the sensation of "self-ness" or "me-ness." It is experienced then like a perception, and I may report that I am *seeing* my dead mother, not that I am *thinking* of her. Others say that I am having a hallucination.

This distinction between subject experiences and object experiences within the psychological life of an individual has profound significance for treatment. Too often, clinicians have described aspects of the functioning of patients without specifying and clearly describing whether the individual is experiencing the process as subject ("me") or object ("not me"). This failure to so distinguish is found frequently in clinical reports and scientific articles.

Moreover, if subject-object, like most other psychological phenomena, exists on a continuum, rather than on an either-or, we may be dealing with variability as to the *extent* to which a reported experience (or an observed behavior) is under the control of "the self," where the individual should be held responsible for it, or whether it is determined by "object, not self" processes, and hence not under the conscious "control" of the individual. This question gets us directly into the whole field of legal responsibility for thoughts or actions.

If the person's thoughts are object, experienced as perceptions, then he may be psychotic and not competent. However, where does the responsibility lie if an action is partially determined by object experiences and partially by subject ones? We have tried to address this problem in regards to certain criminal cases (see Watkins, 1976, 1978b).

FEDERN'S TWO-ENERGY THEORY

In addition to his conceptualization of ego states, Paul Federn made another significant theoretical contribution to the understanding of subject and object. Departing from Freud's term "libido" (as an erotic, object energy), he posited two kinds of psychic energy: subject, or ego cathexis, and object cathexis. Cathexis merely means a quantum of energy that activates a process. A motor is "cathected" with electricity.

The distinction here is related to the *qualitative* nature of the energy. Ego cathexis consists of "I" energy. Within it inheres the feeling of "self," or "me-ness." Any part of the body, any movement or any psychological process activated with ego cathexis will be experienced as "my" body, "my" action, or "my" thought. If a part of my body is invested with ego cathexis, like my normal hand and arm, I will experience it as "my" hand, "my arm." If I move it up and down, and it is invested with ego cathexis, I will experience it as "my" movement, "my" choice, and by "my" free will. The presence of ego-type energy determines the "me-ness" or "self" aspect.

A corollary to this might be that ego cathexis is not the energy of the the self; it *is* the self. Self is simply an energy and derives its content to be experienced as "my" memory, "my" experience, "my" motivation, body, behavior, and so on when that element is invested with ego cathexis.

If, on the other hand, the arm is not invested with ego cathexis, I will be unable to consciously move it or consciously feel it. To me, it will be as if it is anesthetized and paralyzed. If it has been hypnotically invested with object energy, then its movement will be experienced as dissociated, as ego-alien. I may be aware that "it" is wagging up and down, but not that "I" am doing it. And if a thought has reached consciousness, but is invested only with object cathexis, it will be experienced as a perception of something coming from the outside. For example, if a child ego state is activated that contains the image of being pursued by a monster, and if this state is ego-cathected, then I will experience fear. It is "my" fear. If in the same dream state the child ego state is object-cathected, then I will simply be observing the boy as "not-me." The fear is "his" fear, not mine, and I will not experience fear—except what might naturally occur through "resonance" with another person (Watkins, 1978a).

HYPNOSIS

Hypnosis is a process that involves the alteration and moving of energies, both object cathexes and ego cathexes. We can hypnotically anesthetize and paralyze a part of the body by removing its ego cathexis. It is then no longer experienced as part of the self. By investing a hysterically paralyzed arm with ego cathexis, we remove the paralysis and bring it once more within the body ego. In hypnotherapy we utilize this ability to activate and deactivate various symptoms, experiences, and behaviors. In normal differentiation and in pathological dissociation the individual initiates these same energy dispositions by himself.

Since hypnosis is a modality that can change subject into object experiences, and vice versa, then hypnosis becomes a modality for the manipulation of ego and object cathexes. With this technique a therapist can (at least temporarily and in some cases) remove hysterical paralyses, change hallucinatory experiences back into self-thoughts, activate dissociated ego states, switch MPD alters, and so forth. This appears to give the therapist great powers of manipulation. However, it is not quite that simple. Established patterns of energy interchange are not that easily altered. The many ways in which hypnosis can be employed to move cathexes have been described in detail in our two-volume work (Watkins, 1987, 1992).

It should be noted here that ego and object cathexes are theoretical concepts. They may or may not exist in reality. No experimental data are currently available to prove or disprove their existence. However, a two-energy theory does offer a rationale for many psychological phenomena such as dissociation, repression, displacement, reaction formation, and so on, which cannot be nearly as well understood through traditional "libido" theory. It also offers something tangible to the psychotherapist on which to base strategic and tactical considerations.

CONSCIOUSNESS IN EGO STATE THEORY

One other aspect of ego state theory is its suggestion for the understanding of "consciousness." An item becomes "conscious" depending on the *magnitude* of the impact of an object on "self," on an ego-cathected element or ego state. It is a question of economics. An analogy to hearing might be appropriate. If a loud noise strikes my eardrum, I will hear it, assuming that my eardrum and related sensory endings have normal sensitivity. If the noise is quite soft, I may not have the sensitivity to record it. Recording is possible if the volume of the noise is increased or if the sensitivity of the eardrum and related nerve endings are increased.

Likewise, we become conscious of an external object if the stimuli from it (auditory, visual, tactual, etc.) are strong enough to be recorded on impact with an ego, hence, self-cathected ego state. Very sensitive (highly cathected) therapists, who possess what Theodore Reik (1948) called "the third ear," can pick up nuances of communication that would not register or would do so only unconsciously to less highly energized practitioners. Since the boundary between the sleeping individual and the external world is less energized than when that person is awake, sounds and sight may impact without being felt, recorded, and perceived consciously. Repeated light stimulation, such as a prolonged tickle, may become conscious as the "self" awakens from sleep and is recathected. The treatment approach of ego state therapy is based on the foregoing theory.

EGO STATE THERAPY

Ego states that are cognitively dissonant from one another or have contradictory goals often develop conflicts with each other. If they are highly energized and have rigid, impermeable boundaries, multiple personalities develop. However, such conflicts appear between ego states that are only covert. These may be manifested by anxiety, depression, or any number of neurotic symptoms and maladaptive behaviors. For example, we have often found obesity to result from pressures on the executive personality by a disgruntled, covert ego state. Such conflicts require a kind of internal diplomacy not unlike what we do in treating true multiple personalities. However, since the contending ego states do not spontaneously appear overtly, they must generally be activated through hypnosis. We call this ego state therapy (H. Watkins, 1993).

Ego state therapy is the utilization of individual, family, and group therapy techniques for the resolution of conflicts between the different ego states that constitute a "family of self" within a single individual. It is a kind of internal diplomacy that may employ any of the directive, behavioral, cognitive, analytic, or humanistic techniques of treatment, usually under hypnosis.

TECHNIQUES OF EGO STATE THERAPY[1]

Building Trust

The first and most important task for the therapist, and a "must" before undertaking serious therapeutic work, is the establishing of trust. Every behavior, whether verbal or nonverbal, is scanned by the patient, especially by those who experienced abuse as children. The basic question for them: "Are you to be trusted?"

It is understandable that ego states might be angry at the therapist for disrupting a system that has been in operation for many years. Furthermore, they have much at stake to maintain the status quo, even if the system is damaging to psyche or soma.

When activating an ego state, it needs to be treated with courtesy, even if the

[1]The techniques presented here represent a briefer outline of procedures that are described in Watkins and Watkins (in press).

thinking seems naive or preposterous to the therapist. An ego state is not a thing or a process. It is a part-person, and as such it wants to be accorded the dignity of being heard with respect.

In establishing good relationships with each state, be sure to include the seemingly malevolent ones. Malevolent ones are often protective in origin. In their origin they were adaptive, at least temporarily. In working with such a state, it becomes essential to underscore its protective function. Perhaps then a change to more benevolent behavior is possible (Watkins and Watkins, 1988).

There are many ways to contact ego states. The most direct way is to hypnotize the patient and ask if there is a part that feels different from the main personality, or that feels an emotion the therapist knows is counter to what the patient feels in the waking state. In other words, the purpose is to find out if there is a part of the personality that is in conflict with other parts, and which is available under hypnosis. The therapist can add: "If there is such a separate part, then just say, 'I'm here.' " However, the first time this is done, it is important to add a disclaimer, as follows: "But if there is no such separate part, that's just fine," or words to that effect. The purpose is to avoid producing an artifact. It is possible for a very good hypnotic subject to produce whatever he or she thinks the therapist may want. However, an artifact will not usually last or produce meaningful results.

Another method of contacting an ego state, after the initial hypnotic induction, is to suggest descending plush-covered stairs together with the therapist. At the bottom of the stairs, it is worthwhile to suggest a room with a couch and a chair and "other furniture." To continue the fantasy, say, "As we walk into this room, you sit on the couch while I sit on the chair." In the concrete thinking of hypnosis such a statement makes clear that there is no intention of bodily harm. The therapist anticipates that several ego states might enter the scene. That anticipation will depend on knowledge obtained from previous sessions. With the setting in the hallucinated room established, it is time to evoke an ego state if one or more are available at this point in therapy. Speaking to the patient, one can say as follows:

"Please watch the door and let me know what you see. Is there someone who might come in who knows about ——?"

"Who wants to be heard?"

"Who is willing to ——?"

"Who feels different from (name of patient)?"

"But if there is no such separate part, that's just fine." The purpose of the last sentence is to obviate the possibility of artificial cooperation. If the patient reports seeing nothing, a separate ego state may still exist. It may mean one is not sufficiently formed to be a separate vocal or visual entity, because the segments of the personality are very permeable. Or it could be that no one is willing to make an appearance at this time. Separate out only those ego states pertinent to a given problem the patient wants to resolve.

Diagnostic Exploration

After the patient has indicated the presence of someone in the hallucinated room, it is time to get acquainted. Ask for:

1. *Its age and origin*: "How old was (name of patient) when you came to be?" If a specific age is given then, "What was happening at that time?" The specific age gives a clue to a possible trauma that might be abreacted at a future session.

2. *Its name*: "What name would you like me to call you?" If it resists a name, then "Is it all right if I call you by the age you gave me?" Since the ego state has appeared, it stands to reason that it wants to be heard. If the therapist expresses interest in the opinions of the ego state, then that state is most likely to agree to a word that will bring it forth under hypnosis. Persons want to be heard, even part-persons.

3. *Its needs*: "What needs do you have?" or more indirectly, "What do you want (name of patient) to do?" The satisfaction of needs are vital in ego state therapy. By satisfying needs, cooperation can be established. Needs are normal, but the internal behavior to achieve those needs can be destructive. Ego states, like whole persons, have achievement needs, play needs, dependency needs, protective needs, destructive needs, safety needs, and so forth.

4. *Its function or internal behavior*: The problem arises internally when an ego state has, for example, a strong achievement need and then nags and criticizes other states to achieve a goal that is never good enough. The surface symptom may then be in the form of depression or anxiety. An ego state is usually willing to change its internal behavior if its underlying need is being met.

5. *Its degree of permeability*: Is the ego state aware of "anyone else" within that inner world? That is to say, who knows whom, and what are the attitudes toward each other.

6. *Its gender*: Ego states are not always the same gender as the patient. If a female patient was abused by a male as a child, then at least one ego state is likely to be male. The reason is not related to sexuality per se but to the concept of strength. As one ego state said very clearly: "I have to be male; only males have strength."

7. *Nonemotional part*: Sometimes a nonemotional part of the personality is available. It has wisdom; it is nonjudgmental; it has information as to the internal landscape; and it can be a great resource for the therapist. Its inner function is to observe.

The above categories may provide understanding for the therapist on how to proceed toward the therapeutic goal. However, such information is best obtained gradually and not by a shopping list of questions at the first meeting.

Upon first meeting with an ego state the therapist's attitude sets the tone for future interaction. Since most ego states were created when the patient was a child, the best way to communicate is to think like a child.

Assume that "everyone" is listening. The therapist is less likely to make an error that will infuriate an ego state other than the one being addressed. It is a gross error to express to the one being addressed that it is more cooperative, nicer, or better in some way than other ego states. And it can be fatal to therapy to suggest that some ego state should be eliminated entirely.

Ego states and the total personality must understand that the resolution of emotional conflict lies within not outside the individual. For example, if an internal child state feels lonely and rejected because of abandonment experiences in childhood, the solution lies in someone nurturing within the system, not by a nurturing adult in the outside world. If the therapist accedes to demands for nurturance (whether explicitly or implicitly made), there is a liklihood of overdependency in the patient. Effective therapy through constructive inner change stops.

A certain degree of dependency is desirable in a good therapeutic relationship. The therapist must be willing to make a commitment to the patient and be willing to accept and tolerate a degree of dependency. If one insists on being too objective, a resentful patient may reject the therapist and terminate treatment. There is a possible dilemma here for the therapist. Both no dependency or overdependency in the therapeutic relationship may well sabotage the process. J. Watkins (1978a) in his treatise on *The Therapeutic Self* describes this conflict in considerable detail as a balance between "objectivity" and "resonance." When we are objective, we view the patient's problems like an outsider, unaffected by them emotionally. We do not contaminate our perception and understanding of the patient by our own feelings, experiences, or perhaps "transferences." When we resonate, we use our whole self through temporarily introjecting the patient and his situation, so that we can coexperience what he or she is going through. When we resonate too deeply without appropriate, objective safeguards, we encourage overdependency. The secret is to balance the two.

Internal dialoguing is the best way to understand the relationship between states. For example, if an ego state appears to a patient in the hallucinated room, then the therapist can suggest they speak to each other, silently or out loud. If the conversation is silent, the therapist can always inquire what happened. In family therapy, the therapist intervenes with one member only as long as necessary to achieve a certain change. That principle is also true for ego states. Ego states, like the less permeable alters in MPD, often contain information or feelings about past experiences that are amnestic to the main personality (the person in the waking state). In treatment we seek to make the primary person co-conscious of painful experiences currently dissociated within underlying ego states. Co-consciousness between states promotes the erosion of amnestic barriers. Such erosion opens the door to differing states understanding each other.

For example, if a "table technique" is used, the therapist can ask for everyone to enter the hypnotic room and sit at the table so that everyone can meet. Not everyone involved in the problem may come, but the scene is an opportunity for internal dialoguing, relating, and understanding. It may give evidence as to who did not come—also informational. As each ego state enters, ask each where it would like to sit and beside whom. Such a seemingly polite and social question also gives information about relationships and possible future integration or resolution. (See Fraser, 1991, for a variation of the table technique.)

Integration and Fusion

From our point of view, integration and fusion are not synonymous. Fusion suggests an amalgamation of all states into a single unit. Since we believe that the typical human being is not so fused, our goal is not fusion. Integration implies cooperation in a mutually needs-meeting resolution of differences. Sometimes two or more ego states find that their needs and the expression of those needs are so similar that it is no longer necessary or advantageous to divide their energies and be separate. They may simply decide to stay together. But that is their choice, not the therapist's.

We have been asked whether activating ego states doesn't increase dissociation. Paradoxically, ego state therapy does not increase dissociation. It decreases it. If an ego state is split off during trauma in childhood, that entity retains the feelings of the experience and the thinking of that moment in time. It does not grow up with the rest of the personality. It is as if that ego state were encased in a cocoon in which time had frozen and stood still. Communication and interaction between ego states increases boundary permeability and growth, resulting in reduced dissociation.

Dealing with Fear

Fearful states clearly need help. That can be accomplished by finding a constructive state to care for them, to play with them, or satisfy whatever need is apparent. Such a needs-meeting process, in order to be effective, must be with the consent of both parties. They need to work out the details of their "contract" with each other through internal dialoguing.

The Safe Room Technique

Using a safe room technique (Watkins, 1992) is another way to make fearful states more secure. The following is an example under hypnosis, using stairs for deepening:

"Now that we are at the bottom of the stairs, we walk along this hallway. At the end of the hallway is a door to a room of your own choosing, in which you will feel safe and comfortable. As we come close to the door, look at it carefully and describe the door for me, even the doorknob. Now I want to ask you a question. Whatever your answer, it's fine with me. Do you want me to come in with you, or do you want to go in alone?"

The answer is an index of the dependency on the therapist. If they indicate a "yes," then the therapist opens the door. If a "no," then they enter while the therapist waits outside.

"Look around this room of your own choosing in which you will feel safe and comfortable. Find a place where you can sit or lie comfortably. (Pause) Now I'd like you to search for something. What I'd like you to search for is your inner core of strength. That inner core of strength will take symbolic form. It may be part of the animal kingdom, the vegetable kingdom, or the mineral kingdom. If it is part of the animal kingdom, then it could be an animal or human form; if part of the vegetable kingdom, it could be a flower, or plant or tree; and if part of the mineral kingdom it could be an object, or maybe even an energy. I don't know what symbolic form it will take. All I know is that inner core of strength exists within you. (Whatever the response, I continue) Touch that [symbol mentioned], feel it, smell it, know it is part of you, and will help to strengthen you. This is a place to which you can return any time you wish by just closing your eyes, and walking into this room. No one else is allowed to enter here unless you specifically invite them and unless they say positive things to you." (Arousal.)

The safe room can be used for a specific ego state or for the total personality, whatever seems appropriate to do. It is also a technique that can be practiced at home. At one time a patient of mine was afraid at the door of the safe room because the "bad one is here." I said, "Don't worry. I'll hold on to him, while you run into the safe room and close the door." That maneuver worked fine.

Another technique might be providing a "cocoon" for safety:

"I'd like you to close your eyes and imagine a font of golden-white energy springing from the top of your head, moving down your body, around each arm, and around each leg, so that you are completely surrounded by this golden-white energy that lets you move about freely, is invisible to anyone else, but is strong and protects you. It protects you from hurt, from bad words someone might throw at you. If someone throws nasty words at you, it will seem like arrows coming at you, but those arrows hit the cocoon and fall off. Or maybe they stick a little, but they can't get inside. You are in control of that cocoon. If you want to take it off at night, you can. Let's try it out."

In fact, both techniques can be used with the same patient; one does not preclude the other. These methods are temporary devices. Eventually the fear needs to be ameliorated by the inside system in order to have permanent resolution.

Dealing with Critical States

In coping with critical states, the approach of choice is more likely to be confrontive, logical, or practical. Often a demanding state can be motivated to change if it really understands that a change of internal behavior is to its advantage. For example, an ego state whose need is achievement might be willing to change its nagging behavior if it can be convinced that speaking more positively, more supportively, more encouragingly to the one who is procrastinating will bring about more achievement. Sometimes it is useful to suggest trying out this kind of tactic for only a few days, allowing the critical one to determine how successful the change was. Then it has the choice of continuing the new behavior or returning to old familiar patterns. Under these circumstance it is wise for the therapist to also contact the one who is procrastinating to gain its cooperation. Giving a critical state choice to try something new has great appeal. The critical, ambitious ego state versus the internal procrastinator no doubt represents an original conflict from the patient's past.

For example, a parent long ago may have nagged the youngster to study. Unless the student was happy to do the homework, resistance will develop within the child, regardless of the actual behavior of the youngster at that time. With repeated naggings the individual will introject this drama and grow up feeling both the "should" side of itself and the "I don't want to" facet of the personality when challenged to achieve.

Resolving Internal Conflicts

In order to undo original conflicts, it is sometimes necessary to return to those experiences via hypnotic regression, perhaps to undertake an abreaction. I might have one or more of the ego states touch each other. Touch at this level can evoke all kinds of responses, including pleasure, aversion, temperature change, relief, and so on.

One ego state can converse with another, silently or out loud, either by the therapist's suggestion or spontaneously. In internal dialoguing, my most frequent statement is as follows: "Say what you want to say to (other state)." However, suggesting what one ego state should say to another is akin to directing a play. It does not spring from internal sincerity and is likely to be ineffective. Allowing the ego state to say what it wishes gives credence to what is communicated.

Communicating with Child States

Remember that states introjected in childhood and those resulting from childhood trauma think concretely like children. To think like a child becomes an asset for the therapist.

For example, one patient told me that there were some states behind the door of the hallucinated room who were afraid of me. I suggested that they could peek in from the doorway, watch and hear me while I spoke to the hypnotized patient, and then decide if I was to be feared. In that way they could gradually get used to me. Isn't that what young children do naturally with strangers?

At another time a regressed patient was afraid of monsters coming into her room. I told her I had a secret, that I knew how to get rid of monsters, and "Would you like to know my secret?" That is an irresistable question to a small child. Of course, she agreed. I continued, sitting close beside her: "Now you watch the door, and as soon as you see a monster come in, say 'Go 'way!' real loud, and the monster will go away." And, not surprisingly, she reported the monster was gone. If I had spoken to her adult self, nothing would have happened, and it would not have been helpful in allaying her fear.

Ego State "Pain"

Under hypnosis, pain within an ego state can also be drained into an adult state who agrees to accept it (Watkins & Watkins, 1990a). It is essential that both agree to the arrangement. Although it may sound strange, some ego states are reluctant to let go of the pain for fear they might disappear, die, have no power, or have no reason to exist. As one said, "My pain is me!" On the other hand, if the adult state has repressed the pain for many years, it also is reluctant to take it back. It needs to be gently persuaded along the lines of its individual logic, its individual ways of thinking, so that it will believe in the advantages of such a change. With one patient, the two states finally agreed to this process while the adult held the child in safety and love, and they were content to stay together. The result was integration.

The Use of Volunteer States

A volunteer can also be used to help out a child state, such as in the following verbalizations:

"Susie, would you look at the door of our room. I'm going to ask a volunteer to come in to help you out. It will be someone who *wants* to do this. I don't know who that might be. Let me know who comes in."

I never use this technique unless I am certain there is a nurturing aspect to the patient. If she says, "Nobody's coming," then I say, "You must *want* someone to come." That works well.

After the frightened one sees someone, one can ask for a description. Then we proceed with internal dialoguing and communication with me. The purpose is to meet the child's needs with the agreement of the volunteer.

Another method of helping a child state might be for an adult state to snatch the "child" away from an abuser. One can describe a room with a one-way vision screen where they can view what is happenening on the other side. Then the therapist may suggest a consciously recalled setting from childhood, such as when the patient was a little girl in her bedroom. "I think someone is coming into the room. Let me know what happens."

Use of an Observer State

The availability of an observer state can be of tremendous help. It can be asked to take the patient to a certain experience, or to an experience of the observer's choice. It can be consulted for advice or for an appraisal of the internal scene. After an abreaction, the observer might be able to tell the therapist how effective the abreaction was and if it needs to be repeated. Much information is possible through this entity. Finally, it must be recognized that all the transference-countertransference problems that involve interactions with a whole person can also exist between therapists and ego states (Watkins & Watkins, 1990b).

SUMMARY

Ego state therapy is an extension of understandings and procedures developed through the study of severe dissociation. It is based on the assumption that dissociation is an extreme and maladaptive splitting on a continuum, ranging from normal and adaptive differentiation, through an intermediate zone of defensive personality separation. It combines theoretical concepts originally proposed by Paul Federn with techniques of hypnoanalysis to develop a therapeutic approach that promises greater efficiency in the treatment of many normal, neurotic, and psychosomatic conditions, as well as in true multiple personality disorders.

REFERENCES

Alexander, F., & French, T. M. (1946). *Psychoanalytic therapy*. New York: Ronald Press.

American Psychiatric Association. (1994). *Diagnostic and statistical manual of mental disorders* (4th ed.). Washington, DC: Author.
Braun, B. G. (Ed.). (1988). The BASK model of dissociation: Clinical applications. *Dissociation, 1*(1), 4-23.
Edelstein, M. G. (1982). Ego state therapy in the management of resistance. *American Journal of Clinical Hypnosis, 25*, 15-20.
Federn, P. (1952). In E. Weiss (Ed.) *Ego psychology and the psychoses*. New York: Basic Books.
Fenichel, O. (1945). *The psychoanalytic theory of neuroses*. New York: Norton.
Fraser, G. A. (1991). The dissociative table technique: A strategy for working with ego states in dissociative disorders and ego state therapy. *Dissociation, 4*, 205-213.
Frederick, C., & Kim, S. (1993). Heidi and the little girl: The creation of helpful ego states for the management of performance anxiety. *Hypnosis, 20*, 49-58.
Frederick, C., & McNeal S. (1993). From strength to strength: Inner strength with immature ego states. *American Journal of Clinical Hypnosis, 35*, 250-256.
Freud, S. (1953). *The ego and the id*. New York: Norton.
Gainer, M. J., & Torem, M. (1993). Ego-state therapy for self-injurious behavior. *American Journal of Clinical Hypnosis, 35*, 257-266.
Hilgard, E. R. (1986). *Divided consciousness: Multiple controls in human thought and action*. New York: Wiley.
Loftus, P. (1993). The reality of repressed memories. *American Psychologist, 48*, 518-537.
Malmo, C. (1991). Ego-state therapy: A model for overcoming childhood trauma. *Hypnos, 28*, 39-44.
Newey, A. B. (1986). Ego state therapy with depression. In M. G. Edelstein & D. L. Araoz (Eds.), *Hypnosis: Questions and answers* (pp. 197-203). New York: Norton.
Phillips, H. (1993). The use of ego-state therapy in the treatment of post-traumatic stress disorder. *American Journal of Clinical Hypnosis, 35*, 241-249.
Philips, M., & Frederick, C. (1995). *Healing the divided self: Clinical and Ericksonian hypnotherapy for posttraumatic and dissociative conditions*. New York: Norton.
Reik, T. (1948). *Listening with the third ear*. New York: Farrar.
Spiegler, M. D., & Guevremont, D. C. (1993). *Contemporary behavior therapy* (2nd ed.). Pacific Grove, CA: Brooks/Cole.
Steckler, J. (1989). Ego state therapy: A workshop with John and Helen Watkins. *Trauma and Recovery, October*, 25-26.
Torem, M. S. (1987). Ego-state therapy for eating disorders. *American Journal of Clinical Hypnosis, 30*, 94-104.
Torem, M. S. (1993). Therapeutic writing as a form of ego-state therapy. *American Journal of Clinical Hypnosis, 35*, 267-276.
Watkins, H. H. (1978). Ego-state therapy. In J. G. Watkins (Ed.), *The therapeutic self* (pp. 360-398). New York: Human Sciences Press.
Watkins, H. H. (1986). Treating the trauma of abortion. *Pre- and Peri-Natal Psychology, 1*, 135-142.
Watkins, H. H. (1993). Ego-state therapy: An overview. *American Journal of Clinical Hypnosis, 35*, 232-240.
Watkins, H. H., & Watkins, J. G. (1993). Ego-state therapy in the treatment of dissociative disorders. In R. P. Kluft & C. G. Fine (Eds.), *Clinical perspectives on multiple personality disorder* (pp. 277-299). Washington, DC: American Psychiatric Press.
Watkins, H. H., & Watkins, J. G. (in press). *Ego states: Theory and therapy*. New York: Guilford.
Watkins, J. G. (1976). Ego states and the problem of responsibility: A psychological analysis of the Patty Hearst case. *Journal of Psychiatry and Law, Winter*, 471-489.
Watkins, J. G. (1978a). *The therapeutic self*. New York: Human Sciences Press.
Watkins, J. G. (1978b). Ego states and the problem of responsibility II: The case of Patricia W. *Journal of Psychiatry and Law, Winter*, 519-535.
Watkins, J. G. (1984). The Bianchi ("Hillside Strangler") case: Sociopath or multiple personality. *International Journal of Clinical & Experimental Hypnosis, 32*, 67-111.
Watkins, J. G. (1987). *Hypnotherapeutic techniques: Clinical hypnosis*, Vol. 1. New York: Irvington Publishers.
Watkins, J. G. (1989). Hypnotic hyperamnesia and forensic hypnosis: A cross examination. *American Journal of Clinical Hypnosis, 32*, 71-83.

Watkins, J. G. (1992). *Hypnoanalytic techniques: Clinical hypnosis*, Vol. 2. New York: Irvington Publishers.

Watkins, J. G. (1993). Dealing with the problem of "false memory" in clinic and court. *Journal of Psychiatry and Law, Fall*, 297-315.

Watkins, J. G., & Johnson, R. J. (1982). *We, the divided self.* New York: Irvington Publishers.

Watkins, J. G., & Watkins, H. H. (1979). The theory and practice of ego-state therapy. In H. Grayson (Ed.), *Short-term approaches to psychotherapy* (pp. 176-229). New York: Human Sciences Press.

Watkins, J. G., & Watkins, H. H. (1979-80). Ego states and hidden observers. *Journal of Altered States of Consciousness, 5*, 3-18.

Watkins, J. G., & Watkins, H. H. (1980). *I. Ego states and hidden observers. II. Ego-state therapy: The woman in black and the lady in white.* (Audiotape and transcript.) New York: Jeffrey Norton.

Watkins, J. G., & Watkins, H. H. (1981). Ego-state therapy. In R. J. Corsini (Ed.), *Handbook of innovative psychotherapies* (pp. 252-270). New York: Wiley.

Watkins, J. G., & Watkins, H. H. (1982). Ego-state therapy. In L. E. Abt & I. R. Stuart (Eds.), *The newer therapies: A source book.* New York: Van Nostrand Reinhold.

Watkins, J. G., & Watkins, H. H. (1986). Ego sates as altered states of consciousness. In B. B. Wolman & M. Ullman (Eds.), *Handbook of states of consciousness* (pp. 133-158). New York: Van Nostrand Reinhold.

Watkins, J. G., & Watkins, H. H. (1988). The management of malevolent ego states in multiple personality disorder. *Dissociation, 1*, 67-72.

Watkins, J. G., & Watkins, H. H. (1990a). Dissociation and displacement: Where goes "the ouch." *American Journal of Clinical Hypnosis, 33*, 1-10.

Watkins, J. G., & Watkins, H. H. (1990b). Ego-state transferences in the hypnoanalytic treatment of dissociative reactions. In M. L. Fass & D. Brown (Eds.), *Creative mastery in hypnosis and hypnoanalysis: A Festschrift for Erika Fromm.* Hillsdale, NJ: Lawrence Erlbaum.

Watkins, J. G., & Watkins, H. H. (1991). Hypnosis and ego-state therapy. In P. A. Keller & S. R. Heyman (Eds.), *Innovations in clinical practice* (pp. 23-37). Sarasota, FL: Professional Resource Exchange.

Watkins, J. G., & Watkins, H. H. (1992). A comparison of "hidden observers," ego states and multiple personalities. *Hypnos, 19*, 215-221.

Weiss, E. (1960). *The structure and dynamics of the human mind.* New York: Grune & Stratton.

Wright, J. H., Thase, M. E., Beck, A. T., & Ludgate, J. W. (Eds.). (1993). *Cognitive therapy with inpatients: Developing a cognitive mileau.* New York: Guilford Press.

22

Hypnotherapeutic Techniques to Facilitate Psychotherapy with PTSD and Dissociative Clients

Judith A. Peterson

INTRODUCTION

The inclusion of a chapter on hypnosis stems from the fact that this therapeutic phenomena falls within the body of knowledge needed to treat trauma or dissociative clients. However, the discussion about the relationship between hypnosis and dissociation is an ongoing one effectively treated in this and other books. The entire history of hypnosis is a convoluted one, and in the end relies on its advocacy by contemporary reputable therapists based on a wide variety of work that discusses its clinical applications. For those seriously interested in learning about the use of hypnosis within the therapeutic world, refer to the reference section.

Despite the fact that many therapists treating patients with dissociative disorders use hypnotherapy in their practice (and some do not), the use is still controversial, particularly because of its peculiar history. When Franz Mesmer, in the eighteenth century, "invented" hypnosis, but called it "animal magnetism," its effectiveness was discredited by the king of France (Hammond, 1992). When an English physician carried the term *hypnosis* from the Greek words for *sleep*, he

Judith A. Peterson • Phoenix Counseling, Consulting, and Forensic Services, 3303 Chimney Brook Lane, Houston, Texas 77068.

Handbook of Dissociation: Theoretical, Empirical, and Clinical Perspectives, edited by Larry K. Michelson and William J. Ray. Plenum Press, New York, 1996.

made a subtle error. The phenomena is not actually sleep (even though the phrase "deep sleep" remains in hypnotic induction vocabulary and amnesia can occur at the very deepest levels of trance), but rather it is what Hammond (1992) refers to as the ability of the individual to concentrate and focus his or her attention to self-focus inward the power of the mind (self-hypnosis).

There are a variety of ways hypnosis is used in contemporary society and it has been referred to as a "cultural creation" (Lynn and Rhue, 1991). It is some of these uses that cloud its legitimate, therapeutic use within the confines of the psychotherapeutic alliance of the patient and therapist. In fact, Spanos and Chaves (1989) claim that there is no empirical evidence to show that what occurs to hypnotic subjects is any different than what can be accomplished with nonhypnotic control subjects.

With acknowledgment of the controversy, here the subject of hypnotherapy is discussed from the perspective of personal and shared clinical practice based on years of training and use. The suggestions and conclusions found in this chapter focus more on the "how-to" than the empirical-theoretical and are based on personal practice and familiarity with the practice of many colleagues who use similar techniques.

The purpose of this chapter is to describe some of the more helpful hypnotherapeutic techniques to incorporate into psychotherapy as the clinician works with dissociative clients. The degree of dissociation, the therapeutic task at hand, and the comfort level between the therapist and the client will help determine the hypnotic techniques most useful throughout therapy. Beyond describing techniques, examples of how to use these skills with particular clients will be illustrated. Specific words for hypnotic treatment are included.

This chapter does not attempt to discuss the relationship between memory, suggestibility, and hypnosis. Instead, it is assumed that clinicians are familiar with and follow the ethical guidelines and standards of care in our field, and have received training in hypnosis followed by continual supervision and further continuing education in the areas of both hypnosis and psychotherapy with dissociative or trauma survivors. Furthermore, it is assumed that there are types, levels, and continuums of awareness, consciousness, and memory that are determined by the circumstances the client has experienced. It is also assumed that therapists know that the circumstances experienced effect memory and that all memory is inaccurate to one degree or another. These topics are covered both in other chapters in this volume and in books by Hammond (1992) and Brown, Sheflin, and Hammond (1996). Some memories are difficult to retrieve and there are those that are even irretrievable (Farthing, 1992). To put it simply, we remember and we forget. We recall some events, other events are more difficult to retrieve, and some never return to consciousness. The inaccuracy of all memory has never been questioned. Five people that witness an accident will all immediately have different perceptions of what just occurred. What is essential is that cognitive restructuring is based on the core existential crisis that the client feels. To the therapist, whether the details are accurate is irrelevant compared to the daunting task of helping a client recover from profoundly deep feelings of shame and low self-worth.

It is assumed that the clinician understands the difference between appropriate suggestion for symptom reduction, such as shame reduction or self-esteem enhancement, and inappropriate suggestions leading to conclusions that have no basis in reality or reflect the biases of the therapist more than the client. Suggestions that are made during altered states of consciousness are a fine art, used in mutual agreement between therapist and client. As a general rule, examples of appropriate suggestion during hypnosis might include some of the following: make suggestions to help build self-esteem; restructure false and negative self-perceptions or negative belief systems; suggest pain reduction images; suggest the lessening of anxiety or panic; and develop useful images such as safe places, containment of feelings, distance from frightening images, and other helpful images or metaphors.

Suggestions recommended during the processing of most memories should be restricted to helping reduce discomfort, the shortening of time (time distortion) through a difficult memory, and the suggestion of affect release if needed for symptom reduction and resolution. It is strongly suggested that any questioning during memory processing about content be restricted to simply asking "and what happened next." After the entire memory is processed, suggestions about a new way to feel about oneself and strong statements of positive affirmation would be appropriate.

Dissociative patients usually enter therapy because they have become "uncomfortable" with posttraumatic stress disorder (PTSD) symptoms such as anxiety attacks, intrusive dreams, flashbacks, severe depression, sleep disorder, night terrors, and somatization or body memories. Often clients report spontaneous abreactions, flashbacks, or some form of acting out, but the symptoms usually reflect the intrusive memories emerging through dissociative barriers. The therapist has several responsibilities. Immediate relief can begin by teaching regrounding techniques to control the flashbacks and the flood of affect. The client can be trained to use self-hypnosis to temper and control the spontaneous material. Then, later, the memories can be processed in an organized fashion. The therapist can suggest the client see a physician for medication review to assist in control of the physiological discomforts both during spontaneous flashbacks and the feelings later in therapy.

The therapist trained in clinical hypnotic techniques will find many hypnotic tools available to resolve trauma in clients who fall within any part of the continuum of posttraumatic stress disorder or dissociative disorders. A dissociative experience, of at least one aspect of the behavior, affect, sensation, knowledge (BASK) model (Braun, 1988) occurs with almost every trauma for at least a short period of time. It is hoped that the hypnotic techniques described in this chapter can help facilitate both reassociation of the dissociated material caused by severe trauma and protection of clients during memory processing in a parallel way that dissociation or altered states of consciousness were protective during the original trauma. With processing and reassociation of the memory, resolution may develop and healing may occur. The traumatic memory moves from a trauma to a normal part of narrative memory (van der Kolk, 1987).

Due to the severity of the experiences that trauma victims have frequently had, not only beginning, but much more advanced hypnotic techniques are needed to help facilitate psychotherapy. All hypnosis is a form of self-hypnosis. Self-hypnosis is a survival skill that most of these clients have used to dissociate and escape into an altered state of consciousness during the original trauma (Ludwig, 1983). Consequently, appreciating and relearning (if needed) the hypnotic skills that the clients already used (often without an awareness of their original skills) can help reassociation, can protect the clients during each phase of therapy, and can help with movement toward positive self-esteem, shame reduction, and healing.

There is a common misperception that hypnosis should or is only used for the purposes of "memory retrieval" or to "age regress" the client. In reality, hypnotherapy has many purposes in therapy. In addition, memory retrieval is normally a client-originated phenomenon that may involve spontaneously emerging fragments of memory of abuse over a lifetime, not just early childhood experiences of abuse. Often trauma victims describe an entire life history of abuse, including current abuse patterns that cause continual retraumatization. Fragments of memories are usually accompanied by intolerable, intrusive symptoms. The clients bring these fragments together to form a cohesive collection of fragments that become the "memory" of the client. The core body feelings, profound terror, and the core existential crisis need to be honored and processed. Clients need to be encouraged to balance the understanding that they have formulated as their own histories of the abuse and also encourage careful examination of the true-not true, tricks, deception, use of drugs, and suggestions from other people. The client, over time, becomes skilled at looking for the cause of current symptoms, retrieving and processing the memory, and experiencing symptom reduction.

Memories are usually chosen by clients because the client feels intolerable, intrusive symptoms. The client brings the memory to the therapist for assistance with the resolution of the memory in psychotherapy. Therefore, it is the position of this author that hypnotic techniques should not be used for simply exploring or for finding "proof" that a client has been sexually abused. "Digging" often causes symptom escalation. There are rare exceptions to this approach and the therapist is urged to use caution and seek consultation about hypnotic exploration. Successful work revolves around symptom alleviation. Clients need to be well grounded in hypnotic techniques and learn how to pace themselves to better explore their symptoms. Most clients in this population are far more involved in presenting too much intrusive material that they journal or produce in art and need to be taught how to pace their therapy. Therefore, hypnotic exploration is not often needed except in the rare case where the client has presented with symptoms over time. With no symptom alleviation, hypnotic exploration appears to be the most viable solution and is often agreed to by both client and therapist.

The reader is referred to Brown et al. (1996), Hammond (1991), Kluft (1989), and Sachs (1990), for both a history of the use of hypnosis with dissociative populations and a list of specific techniques used with this population. Hypnotherapy is helpful throughout the entire course of treatment of traumatized or dissociative clients from initial work to postintegrative session. The purpose of this chapter is to describe specific techniques that have been helpful during the various stages of therapy with dissociative clients.

DIAGNOSIS

As often as possible, diagnostic work is easier to interpret if hypnosis is not used during the diagnostic phase. Hypnosis may occur either through spontaneous trance experienced by the client or through a formal induction by the clinician. During trance, various ego states may be noted. The distinction should be made between ego states that are only available during formal hypnosis and parts that spontaneously emerge. Consistent presentation of parts that consistently have their own history and identity as separate from the part that originally presented usually indicates that the client is distinctively dissociative. Distinctive amnestic barriers are a hallmark of a classic dissociative identity disorder (DID). Hypnosis might be considered when, for example, a client may be so anxious that deep relaxation or light trance may be indicated for calming. If parts emerge during hypnosis, it is well advised to observe the phenomena of how parts emerge over several sessions, particularly sessions *without the use of hypnosis*, before making a definitive diagnosis.

UNDERSTANDING TRANCE IN THE CLIENT'S LIFE

Many therapists prefer to use the words "deep relaxation" or "guided imagery" rather than hypnosis. Actually, many words or phrases describe various levels or experiences of trance or hypnosis. While it is advisable to use a vocabulary that both client and therapist find comfortable, the client should be aware that each level of trance is a part of an experiential continuum from the absence of trance to deep trance states. Since abused clients have already used altered states of consciousness to help them tolerate the intolerable, these clients are often found to have an exceptional ability to participate in deep relaxation or guided imagery. Hypnosis can increase the capacity for building trust, building self-esteem, correcting cognitive distortions, and changing deeply embedded negative messages.

If asked, clients often describe their mental "escape route" from previous unmanageable trauma. Descriptions vary from simple to elaborate "paths" to safe places (Hilgard, 1970). The clients' gift for self-hypnosis has helped their survival in the past and can now be used to facilitate their therapeutic process in the present. Asking detailed questions about how the client experienced the dissociated state can reveal how the altered state of awareness previously occurred. Exploring further, clients can often describe how "going away" occurs and where to retreat to within a dissociative state or within the organization or system inherent in many multiples. While therapists attempt trance depth for their client's internal safety, the client is often already adept at deep trance. When the client realizes he or she possesses a beneficial tool, the client often feels empowered within the therapeutic setting. The client is able to use and reframe what was once a defense mechanism caused by abuse as the gift it is when used to manage and maintain mastery over various aspects of therapy.

Resistance to the use of hypnosis in therapy occurs when misunderstanding and misinformation leads clients to believe that hypnosis is controlling and manipulative. Clients need to understand how they have already mastered the use of hypnosis in a positive way earlier in life. Hypnosis is a fully focused attention to a selected part of the internal or external environment. Learning new hypnotic techniques in therapy actually gives them more control of their feelings and behavior. If hypnosis was used in a negative way by a perpetrator, the transference issues need to be worked through as they arise. Therapists are often perceived as having characteristics of the perpetrator and are misinterpreted in regard to the motives surrounding therapy. Hypnosis is not recommended with these clients while the transference issues are negative. Interestingly, some complex dissociatives or DIDs appear nonhypnotizable to the therapist.

Some clients have strong religious beliefs that prevent the use of hypnosis; thus, it is necessary to process that issue as a part of therapy and respect the wishes and beliefs of the client. Hypnosis is usually a point of controversy in cases that end up in court. Familiarity with the laws and court rulings of your state are recommended (Kanovitz, 1992; Sheflin, 1991).

THERAPEUTIC TASKS FOR EACH PHASE OF TREATMENT OF TRAUMA VICTIMS

Phase 1

- Build trust and establish a therapeutic relationship.
- Establish safety in present time (may start with safety in the psychotherapy session).
- Establish hypotheses about the differential diagnoses, share with the client, and take actions through appropriate interventions such as medication, working through addictions, dealing with characterological issues.
- Establish and maintain appropriate boundaries.
- Suppress spontaneous abreactions or flashbacks.
- Establish psychoeducational approach to treatment.
- Teach about the phases of treatment.
- Establish and educate the client about the combination of developmental, psychoeducational, psychodynamic and cognitive-behavioral approach to therapy.
- Promote reading of instructional, educational (not anecdotal) material.
- Teach pacing of therapy.
- Educate about medication management.
- Manage transference and countertransference issues.
- Encourage journaling.
- Encourage art therapy and self-expressive modalities.
- Master beginning hypnotic skills: safe place, containment, affect modulation, affect toleration, rapid induction, distancing, time distortion, establishing ideomotor signals, positive age progression and regression, permissive amnesia, deepening techniques, and ideomotor signals.
- Build self-esteem and overall functionality.
- Process and cognitively restructure.
- Contain memories retrieved by client outside of therapy to be processed later in therapy.
- Teach how to plan and process retrieved memories later in therapy.
- Teach internal communication if client has parts.
- Use spiritual and healing approaches to your client.

Phase 2

- Learn to plan and pace the memory processing of memories retrieved by clients.
- Teach and help client practice advanced hypnotic techniques: advanced ideomotor signals, advanced deepening techniques, mobilization of affect and cognition, penetrating or creating barriers for safety and titration, more advanced contracting for safety, combining memories, reversing the memory, dividing a memory across therapy sessions, and self-hypnosis and use of hypnotic tapes with self-esteem-building messages.
- Teach titration or fractionation of feelings or memories.
- Use cognitive restructuring to help manage shame, guilt, self-image, etc.
- Review and focus on all aspects of Phase 1 of treatment.
- Blend and integrate parts when processing memories (if client has parts).
- Use group therapy (if necessary and appropriate).
- Group psychotherapy needs to focus on present day relationships and tasks.

Phase 3

- Continue all aspects of Phases 1 and 2 as necessary.
- Begin developmental reconstructive psychotherapy.
- Use spiritual and creative therapy.
- Move into more complex memory processing if necessary.
- Continue blending and integration.
- Continue cognitive restructuring.
- Begin psychodynamic psychotherapy as a "single" personality.

Many of the hypotherapeutic techniques are described here, but this chapter is not intended to be a complete list or description of all uses of hypnosis with trauma survivors. Also, examples of PTSD and various degrees of dissociation are mixed together to help demonstate the use of all these techniques, regardless of the client's level of PTSD or dissociation.

Ideomotor Signals

The use of ideomotor signals (Cheek, 1994) provides a hypnotherapeutic method for the exploration of the parts of the ego structure that are not readily accessible at the conscious level. These signals are often finger levitations or the lifting of a finger, but also include head nods and other body movements that become nonverbal signals. Use of this as a device for communicating through hypnosis is a means to "establish a set of prearranged signals" (Putnam, 1989, p. 224) that allow a client to "tell" without speaking. Braun (1984) has described a prevalent method to teach specific signaling. Kluft (1992) has described a method for nurses and other staff in a hospital to establish and use ideomotor signals with dissociatives. The most important issue is that communication can take place with sub voce alters or parts that do not have to emerge in order to make their ideas known.

Ideomotor signals may be reliable with some clients, but not with others. With those who can use them reliably, there is a standard hypnotic induction before their use, although that is not found to be necessary with particularly highly dissociative clients. Also, after using ideomotor signals in therapy for a period of time, they are often used by the therapist and client in sessions for many reasons and no formal induction is needed.

The following instructions might be used with clients to establish ideomotor signals:

1. Tell the client that you do not expect or want a conscious, deliberate or voluntary movement of the fingers, but instead ask the client to let the unconscious mind establish a method of communication. In addition, let the client know that lifting the finger may feel like it is being tugged by a string attached to a helium balloon.
2. Ask the client if all parts of the ego structure are listening and signal when they are all listening by lifting a finger.
3. Then, ask everyone inside, or all parts of the conscious and unconscious, to let the therapist see which fingers signal "yes," "no," and "stop." Wait each time to see that a different finger makes a movement, even if subtle.
4. Then, ask questions that have a "yes" or "no" answer in order to talk to all parts of the ego structure, alters or parts about a therapeutic issue or until you have worked out safety.

As the client learns each hypnotic technique, ideomotor signals are one of the ways that the client and therapist can communicate about the progress they are together making forward jointly established goals of therapy.

Safe Place

The therapist might ask the client if there was a safe place that was used to escape from trauma (Hammond, 1990). Clients often describe safe places that they have used for years. They can continue to use these safe places in therapy. With highly dissociative clients, several safe places might have been used or will be developed during therapy. Different parts may need different types of safety. Accomplishing safety on the inside, never before achieved, can provide the potential for a positive healing place for specific parts of the ego structure. Spirituality is often incorporated into these places by these clients as new ways of comfort and healing are explored and experienced internally. This helps to establish a core sense of healing that is needed when these clients have been so profoundly assaulted.

Affect Modulation and Toleration

Trauma survivors often experience their feelings as being on or off, similar to a light switch. Since they either feel overwhelmed by their feelings (and might experience panic) or totally numb, survivors are often afraid to feel anything at all. As clients learn both affect modulation and affect toleration, these skills will help them in their daily functioning, throughout therapy, and in processing memories.

To develop modulation, clients might practice experiencing a specific feeling such as anxiety. A way to facilitate this skill is to suggest to clients to imagine a scale from 0 to 10 with 0 representing calm (an absence of anxiety) and 10 being a maximum feeling of anxiety. The therapist counts from 0 to 10 and back to 0 again. Toleration is often built by stopping at whatever number the client has difficulty with, such as 4, waiting an agreed upon time, such as 60 seconds, feeling that feeling for that time period, and then counting back down to 0. Gradually, clients can learn to build their tolerance of difficult feelings. They can learn to stop the feeling and gain a sense of mastery and control over the feeling. A concrete example to help a client begin might be to ask the client to relax the hands at the count of 0 and then progressively clench them until the count of 10. Then, slowly relax the hand until it is completely relaxed as the therapist counts back from 10 to 0. Safe emotions, such as joy, might be experimented with in this way first before attempting a more difficult emotion.

Containment Techniques

Clients find it helpful to develop containers and barriers needed to hold the different types of feelings (affective, physical, motor) that can become overwhelming before, during, or after a therapy session. One suggestion for a nonthreatening approach to the containment process is to suggest to the client that a good feeling (such as joy) can be contained in a gift box. Holding on to that positive feeling and using the pleasant and rewarding metaphor of a gift allows the client the opportunity to understand the concept of sheltering positive feelings. An added benefit to this process is that these positive feelings may be opened as a gift and experienced during difficult periods of time. Later, the client might want to use a steel vault to contain shame, guilt, or rage. Transferring the skill that the client first used for a positive feeling to the containment of a negative feeling is a practical aid in processing difficult experiences and remaining fully functional between therapy sessions. Examples of patients' creations of containment can include internal quiet rooms where alters can scream, yell, and kick. Other internal structures can provide peaceful areas to rest or sleep for alters who cannot remain in control. Even a place for "internal restraints" is effective for alters who need containing between sessions or who need to contain or restrain the body during memory processing (Young, 1986, 1991). Containers, domes, and expandable compartments are all examples of ways to place feelings within surroundings to not allow them to slip out at the wrong time. Sometimes feelings or parts of the ego structure need to be completely closed off until the next therapy session. At other times, a small, slow leak of affect is desirable to gradually allow the feeling to dissipate. Some patients build elaborate mechanisms with controls, dials, and other sophisticated metaphors to control their feelings or parts (Hammond, 1992).

Age Progression and Age Regression (Hypnotic Time Distortion)

Age progression is a form of time distortion that allows the client to move forward in time far enough to imagine the future. For example, the client can choose to look back on therapy with a sense of mastery and personal accomplishment. Hypnotically moving through time allows suggestions for a successful family life or a satisfying career, which builds self-esteem and creates a positive frame during present-day difficulties. Watkins's (1971) affect bridge can be used to move forward or backward in time. The client can focus on a positive feeling of calm and then follow that feeling of calm like a rainbow bridge to a future time and enjoy peace. The client can also follow the calm feeling to a calm past event while the therapist counts from 0 to 10 and back to 0 again.

The client can then practice experiencing a mildly positive or negative past experience while the therapist counts (an experience already known to the client). Later, when the client is prepared to work through a trauma, the practice facilitates the ease at which the client is able to return to the trauma for a very limited amount of time. The client can complete the needed work and then return to the present, using whatever containment techniques are needed.

Clients need to understand that time can be distorted, that pleasant events can be extended to feel as if they last for hours. They need to understand and experience how very difficult traumas can also be time-shortened in order to process a lengthy trauma in just a few moments. Memory processing and other aspects of therapy can become less difficult. When trauma victims were being hurt or tortured, they often felt that time stopped and that the pain went on forever. The knowledge and the experience that time is limited is crucial and comforting for these severely abused clients.

An example of words to facilitate this process:

Age Progression

I am wondering now if you can take the new insights that you have and begin to move forward in time .... past today and into the future .... and begin to feel the feelings of this new understanding as it permeates and changes your perceptions of the world around you and your relationships with people .... in the future 5 years from now .... I am going to begin counting as you feel yourself going forward in age .... perhaps imagining that you are sitting on a park bench .... or sitting on a grassy hill .... overlooking a beautiful view .... or sitting by the ocean on the sand .... watching a sunset, and further reminiscing .... as you begin to progress ahead in time .... as I count, 1, moving forward in time, 2, feeling yourself moving toward that wonderful relaxing image .... perhaps on a vacation and looking back on your therapy, 3, moving even further forward, 4 to 5, being completely there and able to look back .... and have the insight and understanding of what these new feelings and new understandings have meant to you over the last 5 years .... and letting those float down into every cell .... as you appreciate the changes .... see the differences in your life .... feel the mastery over new things .... things you enjoy now .... hobbies, work, family, looking out on that relaxing scene and feeling the peace come down over you .... and feeling that white light .... that healing light .... that at first encircled a few parts of you, and now encompasses all of you and acts as a protective shield around all of you .... around your entire body .... a wonderful sense of feeling .... a feeling of being whole .... and now it is time to go back to the present bringing with you that understanding of the future .... as I count back .... 4, 3, 2, 1.

Time distortion can also be used for a different purpose by suggesting that just a few moments of calm and healing and sleep can feel like a whole night of rest. Especially when difficult material has been processed in a therapy session, a few minutes of calm and healing peace that feels like unlimited rest can allow the client to leave the session rested and relaxed, knowing that hard work was completed and feeling mastery at the end of the session.

Hypnotic Distancing Techniques

Trance offers dissociative clients varying degrees of hypnotic distance while processing memories. Some parts need to be protected from knowing or processing specific past traumas and they ask for or require amnesia. This can be aided by hypnosis. Furthermore, parts who want to observe from a distance may do so while being protected from direct feelings through the use of trance. They may be encouraged to feel only what they are ready to feel while remaining safe. In processing sessions, distancing can help the client remain with the cognitive discussion while allowing the emotions to remain distant.

The following is one of many examples of distancing techniques. The therapist asks the client to imagine a large theater complete with stage and many rows of seats. The client is invited to be as close to or as removed from the action on the stage (the memory or the topic of discussion) as they wish to be. The therapist can suggest additional changes to decrease the intensity of the experience by changing the size of the figures on the stage or the color and backdrop of the stage. The scene can be changed from color to black and white, or changed by creating a curtain hung in front of the stage to alter the intensity of the scene. During the above process, the therapist continually assesses the client's safety. Ideomotor signals can be used to determine that all the distancing required has been successfully completed. Distancing metaphors can be changed at any time. For most clients, one can assume there is more awareness of the sessions' content than is openly acknowledged. These forms of suggestions simply offer the concept of distancing as a pacing method to allow a gradual awareness that clients can tolerate (Hammond, 1992).

MORE ADVANCED HYPNOTIC TECHNIQUES

The purpose of the more advanced hypnotic techniques described in this section is to facilitate the therapeutic process in several ways: (1) to help clients to better tolerate and safely manage the profound shame and other intense feelings, (2) to offer a safety net and helpful techniques to reduce affect overload and decrease the need for hospitalization, and (3) to help clients combine as many traumas together as possible to expedite their therapy. Advanced hypnotic techniques can particularly facilitate repair in fragmented clients with repetitive, severe abuse memories that can be processed in a single session. Clients with polyfragmentation can experience fewer difficulties with repetitive abuse memories being processed in a single session. This allows combinations of experiences to be processed at one time. This has the potential to shorten the treatment for these profoundly abused patients. In order to work with these clients, it is helpful to rely on a consistent, reliable therapeutic frame (as described earlier in this chapter) with specific boundaries that the client can depend on to facilitate processing complex work. A consistent framework for therapy is helpful in order for the client to feel safe enough to process independently retrieved complex memories.

Advanced Ideomotor Signaling

More advanced ideomotor signaling techniques include the following:

1. Ideomotor signals can help determine if containment is at a safe level for the patient to leave the office. Sometimes, with very dissociative clients, the therapist and parts in the client need to hypnotically create amnestic barriers between the host and other parts to facilitate safety. Also, barriers are often needed between a functional alter that can help the system by staying out while other parts of the system are behind protective barriers to rest or amnestic barriers. Ideomotor signals are helpful in determining if enough resolution of affect has taken place, or if enough affect has been expressed by the alters to allow the memory to be resolved.
2. The glove anesthesia technique (Hammond, 1992) might be combined with ideomotor signals at times. The therapist can ask if some of the alters or the host need to be totally unaware of the finger signals. This may be due to safety issues or due to information needed to plan therapy that the system is unable to know or it will be unsafe. The fingers can first indicate that the hand is separate from the body and then the fingers can be asked the necessary questions without the answers disturbing the system as a whole.
3. The fingers can also be asked if the body needs to be at a deeper trance level and can indicate when the body is at that deeper level. Then further questions or further therapeutic work can be asked of the system.
4. In addition, the fingers can be asked if there are alters at deeper levels that answer with the other hand or answer with the same hand only at deeper layers or systems. Often, in complex patients, both hands answer for different layers and each hand answers with different fingers to questions at different layers. For example, there might be four layers represented on the right hand and three more layers represented on the left hand.
5. Also, information about layers or alters that block can be discovered and worked through to help facilitate therapy.

Fractionation

Almost any aspect of any experience that the client is processing in therapy can be fractionated or divided up into tolerable pieces of information or feelings. A client may be prepared to process 5% of the affect or 50% of the affect or 2% of the cognition, and so on. Every aspect of the preparation for and the processing of the BASK model can be divided or titrated. The memory itself can be divided into manageable parts and worked on over several therapy sessions.

> Teresa had remembered being raped by her brother, then he and his friends, and then her father came home drunk and brutally raped her. Teresa chose to manage the rape by her brother in one session. She completed a healing piece about that part of the memory that included identification of the existential crisis and working through the cognitive restructuring related to the crisis. The next session was spent handling the gang rape of her brother's friends and the existential crises about her brother letting his friends do that to her. More healing images were used at the end of that session. The third session about this

memory included the memory of what her father did when he came home. All three parts of the memory were brought together with healing images. Blending and integration of those parts occurred.

Another advanced fractionation technique is to combine intense feelings or memories about an event, but only from the count from 0 to 10 and back to 0. Then, send the client to a calm, peaceful, safe place for the same amount of time with the hypnotic suggestion that those moments of reset feel like hours of rest. That two-part juxtaposition of intense difficult affect combined with peace and calm rest can be completed in a cycle as often as needed to dissipate the affect.

Deepening of Trance

Readers are referred to various publications including (Hammond, 1992) for various examples of both standard and rapid hypnotic inductions. Later, as work progresses, trance depth becomes more important and acts as more of a cushion. It allows an opportunity for the therapist to work with the imbedded experiences and messages caused by abusers during the existential crisis. The client has an opportunity to hear new statements that can build positive self-esteem and negate the old messages that have been so self-destructive. These new statements may positively affect core belief systems. Examples of words that might help clients move through various levels of trance depth:

> .... as you begin to float down, as you now go deeper and deeper into trance .... beginning to float like feathers that float out of a pillow .... like clouds that float down and cover quietly like a fog .... like sand that filters through water, you begin to find the natural place that allows for the protection and internal caring, that allows you to very carefully explore the memory today .... and as you float down now deeper and deeper.
> (Ideomotor signals may be used to check what is happening internally.)

In regard to using memory processing with dissociatives, PTSD, and DID, the depth of trance is extremely important and helpful. The following are suggestions that would help depending upon the patient.

- For traumatized patient with and without definitive ego states:

> Moving farther and farther down with more and more relaxation as you move deeper and deeper, moving to the depth of trance that you need today. Feeling the water as you slip over the side of the boat and begin to let yourself float down into the depths ....

Another metaphor:

> .... feeling yourself floating out into space as the earth gets smaller and smaller ....

Another metaphor:

> .... feeling that parachute billow out and begin to float you down ever so slowly .... moving even deeper to the level where all can hear and all parts can feel and see and know at whatever level you are ready to know .... in whatever way you are able to understand ....

Further suggestions:

> .... moving even deeper through the layers of the unconscious ....

- For more defined dissociation-DID who are processing a very difficult memory:

  Referring to their mapping in DIDs or layers of the unconscious:

  .... moving down through the layers ....

  or using whatever image that they have:

  .... moving beyond the layer with the triangles and shapes (previously referred to or mapped) .... moving beyond the alters that are so frightened of their memories .... moving even further down .... seeing yourself floating down .... counting down now .... down through all the layers whether I know about them or not .... whether they have engaged in therapy or not .... just moving past them without any memory of passing them ....

  permissive amnesia again:

  .... moving deeper and deeper, and then counting 1 through 10 .... with less and less memory of what you are moving deeply through ....

  using ideomotor signaling to say:

  .... and when you have reached all the way to the depths .... then let a "yes" finger float up ....

  wait now while you watch for your patient's signal:

  .... now move even deeper and deeper beyond that last layer, to a point where you can look up at the entire system .... how helpful that might be .... so unique to see yourself from an entirely different place .... like looking up from the bottom of the ocean as you float further and further down .... and can barely see the boat floating up on top of the water ....

Some abused victims need to be this deep in trance in order to do their work. This is a very somnambulistic depth from patient reports. Typically, this is more likely to occur when sufficient time has gone by and trust has developed between the therapist and the patient.

Complex, polyfragmented, multilayered DIDs often seem to have had so much experience with trance that they have their own "pathways" into trance. Exploration of former trance experience can be actively explored. Then, as the client can be encouraged to reexperience those experiences, this process can facilitate rapid movement to a very familiar deep trance level. From that deeper level of trance, even deeper levels can be achieved every time trance is facilitated through "piggybacking" on the previous experience and adding deepening images. Sometimes trance deepening occurs by moving the patient to alters formed at deeper levels of trance or by asking for certain parts to facilitate helping the system as a whole to move to a deeper level of trance.

Mobilization of Affect and Cognition

Feelings from a particular memory that have been processed can be sent throughout the system to parts that have not been in therapy yet. For example, when one part of the system experiences a terrifying memory, the therapist can help the parts transfer not only the feelings of terror, but the feelings of mastery and new insight to the alters not in therapy yet. In some systems, for example, upper alters who feel terror from being tortured may have an impact on deeper alters who considered themselves "leaders." These leaders often do not have the feelings about what has happened to the system as a whole and sometimes have been told they will never feel the feelings the upper alters have felt. The purpose of this therapeutic intervention is to help the entire system develop insight about what happened to the whole ego structure and to ultimately stay safely away from more traumatic situations through their new awareness.

> Patient, Susan, had alters who worked through all the feelings of being gang raped by perpetrators. These experiences were cognitively known by deeper alters, but the feelings were not felt. At the end of the memory, the alters who had the feelings from the gang rape decided to send feelings to the alters who continued to place the body in promiscuous situations and who had not been particularly concerned. They just thought that the job of the body was to sexually service other people. The new terrifying insights had a significant impact on these deeper alters. Behavioral changes occurred immediately with new insights beginning to occur long before those deeper alters were involved in their own memory work.

Ask the client if there are new awarenesses or ideas that the rest of the system needs to know. Sending cognitive reality throughout a system prepares the way so the therapist does not need to start over with basic concepts at every level. Often the deeper alters do not realize that the abusers have threatened and lied to the entire system.

> Patient, Carol's, alters had been told they would be arrested for pornographic experiences despite the fact that they were forced to participate. Cognitive restructuring involved processing the knowledge that the perpetrators would be implicated as criminals and their acts constituted the actual crime. This new understanding was then sent through the entire system and was powerful in freeing up the system to new truth.

With advanced hypnotic techniques, the therapist can successfully encourage change within the system. Each therapeutic intervention potentially provides a catalyst for healing beyond the specific therapy session or even beyond one particular part of the system.

Age Regression

Sometimes age regression is needed for specific reasons. The following are found to be helpful words to use in regard to age regression and moving the client directly to the beginning of the event that the client has chosen to process.

With patients that are not DID, there is more work to do with age regression. With patients who are DID, you can usually just simply ask for that alter and ask for that experience and ask for all those to be there that need to be there who remember the memory. Often that alter needs to be age-regressed to the origin of the trauma:

- Dissociatives and PTSD:

.... counting down using the elevator .... moving through the family scrapbook and feeling younger and younger .... imaging different birthday parties .... going down through the ages in regard to life experiences, such as high school and junior high and elementary school, getting younger and younger .... and letting your finger come up at the point where you are as young as you need to be ....

- For ego state and DID:

.... I am wondering if all of those that are there who are ready to begin to work on this memory can come together now with the one that remembers the beginning of the memory, in fact, to move back in time to *just before* the memory begins .... if that alter or that part could be there *now* ....

- In all patients: as you see that emerging, then *enhance* through the following:

.... I am wondering if you can remember now and be there and feel what is under your feet .... and feel what is around your body .... and smell the smells .... and hear the sounds .... as you feel yourself as much there as you need to be in order to work through this memory ....

The patient typically escalates when the reference to the different senses occurs:

.... can you begin to tell me now what happened at the beginning of your memory .... and let me know through your fingers when another part needs to be here, or there is a feeling that we need to manage the memory in a different way .... so tell me where you are now?

Using ideomotor signals helps the patient remain at a deeper level of trance, since verbalizations tend to interrupt deeper trance. Explaining what is happening might better happen later (unless necessary). Then you begin to ask:

.... and then what happened, etc? ....
.... and what happened next? ....

Do not lead the patient, but repeat the words and ask what happened next, and move the patient through the memory, using time distortion as needed. Clients are encouraged to state a cognitive part first, but some patients first express affective parts as they move through the memory. Going back to the BASK model, it is important that the therapist understand that the ultimate goal is to combine all dissociated parts. The more that can be pulled together, the more complete the experience. Sometimes you might need images such as the following:

.... it may be that you need to view it on a movie screen .... the event that you all shared in order to get through .... because of the difficulty of the memory .... and I am wondering if you would like to all see it .... and see the parts that are difficult at a very rapid rate .... and be as close or as far away from the screen as you need to be in order to view what happened ....

If you get a "yes" signal from the ideomotor signals, then the therapist might want to use the metaphor of a movie screen as a preliminary to working through the memory (Hammond, 1991). Also, when going through the memory, it might be helpful to ask:

.... are you able to handle the memory today? Does any part of you need special precautions in handling the memory? Will any part of the memory lead to feelings you will need special help with?

Often the client knows at some level how the memory is going to be managed and the therapist can use titration, containment, collapsing, or fractionation. As the client moves through the memory, as the therapist asks what is happening, and it is heard, for example, "they're on top of me, they're heavy, it's one after another." The patient may report a rape scene of one perpetrator after another. It might be helpful to again ask the fingers,

> .... can we do all of this at once ....

and most often the answer is "yes."

> .... I am going to count to 10 and I would like you to remember all the perpetration that you *need to remember* that occurred, all the physical and emotional feelings that you all need to feel by the time I count to 10 .... and I will make sure I count back to 1 to make sure that the feelings are back at a place where you can contain them and they have gone away ....

At that time, the therapist can count from 1 to 10. The patient will usually let out a lot of affect at 10. Pause there in terms of the curve of memory processing to allow for sufficient feeling to be expressed. It is important to pause, and then count back down to 1. As the client moves through processing the memory, the therapist can then continue to count from 1 to 10 whenever there is a spot where the therapist finds affect present and needing to be expressed. Then, at the end of the memory, the therapist might find it helpful to ask the patient if there is any more feeling that is needed to be expressed. If the answer is "yes":

> .... I am wondering if the body can express all the *fear* and all the *terror* that it needs to feel in order not to feel those feelings anymore in any intrusive manner .... and so I'm going to count from 1 to 10 and back down to 1 again.
>
> .... I am wondering if part of you is feeling *angry* or *rageful* ....

the answer is almost always "yes." Then ask the same questions about other feelings:

> .... Express as much feeling as you need to feel, and can contain safely with me .... To dissipate the feelings
>
> .... I'm going to begin to count down again now from 10 to 1 as every feeling that is left over that you need to be rid of melts way .... 10 .... 5 .... 1.

Penetrating or Creating Barriers in DIDs

Amnestic barriers or strong resistance can be broken through within complex systems by sending strong affect through the perceived barrier or through the resistance. This strong affect often occurs during the processing of a memory and can accelerate change in complex systems.

To work with parts who were amnestic to what had happened, the therapist might say:

> .... I am wondering if the conscious part (or host) is ready to remember what has happened? ....

If you get a "yes," it is suggested that you check about safety by asking:

.... is the conscious part or host ready for just the memory on the movie screen, or is the host ready for the entire memory including the feelings .... if the host does remember, is the host going to be harmful to herself or to other people .... are her feelings going to be very big .... or too big ....

Respond to all "yes" by modifying and containing affect until safety is established. It is important to monitor for safety before a problem develops, not after. Once safety is established and the associated part is willing to join with the dissociated part and take on this memory, then the following might be said:

.... and now I would like all of you that are going to gather around the memory, who have remembered this today, to now begin at the beginning again and send all of the perceptions of the memory (or to those parts that did not remember before) .... and allow as I count from 1 to 10 .... for that part to remember all of what happened as it moves fast forward through her mind .... all of the feelings (or as much as was agreed was safe) .... and as I count from 1 to 10 .... pause at 10 ....

Reviewing or penetrating the amnestic barrier can be extremely intense

.... and count back down to 0 ....

At this point, the patient often experiences the existential crisis of knowing or feeling something that was unknowable or unacceptable before. It is extremely important to allow that part to understand the crisis and also experiencing healing. More ego strengthening surrounding the perception of the experience occurs after you have joined together the parts that need to remember. Monitor for safety again!

Understanding the process of therapeutic healing can be enhanced with words such as:

.... the new understanding about this memory and the feelings about it are filtered throughout the mind .... some of these insights will begin to filter through whatever layers there are all the way down to wherever they need to be .... so that the new insights and understanding are available .... so you can begin to learn about what it is like to work through memories and work through feelings in an accepted and safe environment .... and achieve new understandings.

Notice the absence of leading and the permission to use the statements as they want. Sometimes to keep the client well paced (functional), there are only certain aspects of the memory that the client, host, or primary part is ready to process. Here is an example of a client who's memory might need protective barriers:

A part of the patient, Phyllis, remembered that not only was she abused by her father, but had the perception that her mother allegedly stood by watching. The intense anger from that new insight helped in therapy. But she indicated that she could not handle any negative information about mother at that time. New insights can be used as a motivator to facilitate change and speed up treatment.

Contracting for Safety

.... I would like you or everyone inside, or every part inside, to allow those barriers to come down now to protect you .... or need to have your feelings

> titrated .... slowly leaking out the feelings only as you are ready .... letting yourself be protected that were not protected before .... letting the caring and the loving and concern move throughout you .... throughout all of you .... as it has never happened before ....

and then hopefully you'll get a "yes" response:

> .... Is everyone where they need to be in order to remain protected? .... and in order to be safe outside the therapy session? (contracting for safety)

Sometimes the host in the dissociative needs to be inside, or there needs to be a part inside that is carefully cared for. The therapist might say:

> .... The parts that have especially been hurt that need to be comforted and loved .... I am wondering if those parts can stay safely within that healing light ....

or whatever healing image the patient has developed with you. Power comes from using the patient's consistent images developed during the therapy.

Look for ideomotor signals now for safety:

> .... can you stay within that healing light until your next appointment .... can the part of you that has always taken very good care of the body take very good care of the body in between sessions ....

Stop each time you don't get a "yes." Work until you have a safety agreement. For each patient it is an individual process. The therapist can begin to say:

> .... you are now free of the effects of this .... you can let go of any of those feelings from before, from long ago .... because you don't have to feel them anymore .... and all the energy that was bound up inside is now ready for you to use in a new way as you heal and develop new feelings .... you are free now of that experience .... and it will no longer be hurting you .... and the hard work you have done before to contain the feelings can now be used to help you in your therapy, until you understand what happened .... and you can feel very good about the work that you have done.

This allows for the freedom to use the energy that was bound up in "secret keeping" for other purposes. It is essential that the therapist carefully evaluate the readiness of the client's system for this and other active roles within the system.

Clients can penetrate electroshock, pain, terror, and other physical or affect memory barriers by moving the memory of that pain away to another part of the system. This allows for the processing of new information without feeling the difficult feelings until a different time.

> A complex patient determined that a pain barrier existed within her system that she described as having been caused by electroshock given to her body through wires hooked up to a generator. She then worked with her therapist to decide whether to go above or below the pain barrier and to place the physical feelings from the barrier within an internal container until they could be processed at a later time. Next, the patient chose the easiest route to move past the barrier. The alters beyond that barrier were freed up to work in therapy and the physical body memories from the electroshock were felt later.

In this way, different parts of the BASK model can be processed (such as knowledge) and other parts of the BASK model can be saved until another time. Part of the model (such as the electricity) can be saved from several memories and processed together in one memory-processing session. Hypnotic images that move from the dark, which often represents amnesia or frightening memories, into the light, which represents insight, knowledge, and mastery over fearful experiences, are consistent images that add a new dimension to the internal perceptions of the system. Ritualistic-sadomasochistic or mind control victims often report that the dark represents the perpetrators perennial power. They describe being pulled into the blackness or what they refer to as the "black hole." The power of the light as an image, sweeping like a giant flashlight, allowing vision to permeate the entire system and moving to every corner of memory, begins to erode that sense of inky black criminal power or perhaps even unconsciousness, allowing alters to see the light of day.

> A ritualistic abuse victim, Lisa, described many memories that took place in the blackness—closets, holes in the ground, a coffin. During one memory after another, the healing light that represented the normal world to her, the light of a higher power, the light of knowledge and understanding, began to permeate the blackness. Alters accelerated their process of healing by reaching out to the light. Other alters became jealous of possession of the light and wanted to complete their memory work in order to be out in the light.

COMPLEX HYPNOTIC TECHNIQUES

Processing the Memory in Reverse

Reverse memory processing allows a trauma survivor to start at the end of the memory (T + 1) and to end at the beginning of the memory, right before (T − 1). The traditional starting point and ending point of the memory are reversed. This process is especially appropriate when the following circumstances are involved. If a ritualized event has occurred over and over again for several years, it is better for the client for the memory to end at the youngest or original point rather than at the oldest or most devastating point in time. This process begins with the part of the ego that holds the memories about an event and holds the memory of when they were last abused. The information about the events is collected before the session begins. This includes what occurred at each year moving from the oldest or last memories to the earliest memories. Then, all of the alters at all ages are asked to come forward and wait their turn as the processing of the memory is begun with the oldest alters. The alters can experience the elements of the BASK model and then blend into each other, as one alter blends into the next younger set of alters.

As this process proceeds, the number of alters decreases with every year of memory that is processed. Also, as the alters decrease in age, the memory of abuse typically becomes less and less impactful or takes on a different significance. For example, at 6 years of age, the alters only remember abuse at 6 and 3 (if 3 is the youngest age of that particular abuse). At age 18, that abuse may be perceived to have happened many more times. By the time the alters move to the 3-year-old experience, the alter is only remembering the first time the abuse occurred.

Developmentally though, the impact of early rape may be more profound than later similar experiences. Then, the ego structure moves back to just before T − 1, to just before this abuse occurred. Next, this young part can begin to be comforted by the adult, and slowly, as ready, blend into the alter of origin or the host or the core of the client and can begin to grow up, through hypnotic suggestion, and blend. The oldest alters in this type of memory processing may start with sudden, very intense affect. Then, throughout the processing of the memory the affect slowly dissipates as the alters that are experiencing this abuse are younger and younger and remember less trauma. Usually, once a patient has completed this process, the patient will ask to complete work in this way as often as possible. One of the reasons is that the feeling at the end is usually that of a part that is innocent, has not been abused, and is at peace. That uninjured part can easily be blended into the host. Ego strengthening as well as cognitive restructuring techniques add to this dynamic approach to repeated abuse. This process is effective with alterations at any part of the dissociative continuum.

Combining Memories

Combinations of similar memories that are held can be combined into one memory-processing session. It is suggested that the therapist attend to the BASK model as an outline for all types of combinations of experiences that can be juxtapositioned. For example, all of the affect that is similar from some memories can be combined. All of the physical sensation that is similar can be combined.

> Kristin, a survivor with a young child, asked her system to have the alters that specifically had any information about the abuse of her son to share that knowledge. Then, that knowledge was processed and the cognitive distortions, lies, were processed and the cognitive restructuring completed. Following the knowledge of this, then the affect soon began to emerge and was managed within several sessions as it was too overwhelming to handle within one memory-processing session.

Another way to combine memories is through using the image of the reverse of the "big bang" theory. This is based on the concept that fragmentation feels like it happens at many levels of PTSD or dissociation through very profound, ego-shattering experiences such as electroshock or being forced to do something profoundly ego dystonic. Using the image of the big bang, the patient can process the feeling that the experience sent parts or fragments flying in all directions. Then, the hypnotic suggestion can be made that by starting at the point where those fragments are furthest from their point of origin and moving back to T − 1, which is the time just prior to the split, all of those fragments can come back together. An image that helps with this concept is one of the stars in the universe and how they might have resulted from an explosion and are still being propelled out into the universe. Reversing that concept and allowing for them to see themselves like the stars moving back into the original mass and then seeing the fragments moving back into the whole alter or ego state or client is a powerful image. Much healing that involves ego strengthening and cognitive reframing can then be used to facilitate the strength of that whole part.

Working with "Decision Makers"

Another more advanced technique with DIDs is to achieve a working relationship with the system leaders that are often deeply placed within the system. Consequently, the more superficial alters that might have originally presented in therapy are either near the bottom or are protected somewhere else in the system, such as in a safe place. This allows for the deepest alters to map the entire system from their knowledge and point of view, to plan therapeutic strategy with the therapist, and to complete other important therapeutic tasks at a faster pace.

> Alice, a complex, multisystemed multiple personality disorder, was finally able to have her leaders come out to work in therapy. In understanding the process by which they emerged, it became apparent that these deeper alters were used to being "out" in abusive situations and found it to be a new experience to be "out" under nonabusive and even therapeutic situations. Also, they had much more choice now than during their perpetration. Many alters were afraid of what these deeper alters would do if they were out and could just "run loose." Their description of the knowledge they had of the system, and what they could accomplish if out, led to problem solving about therapy at a new level. The alters explained to the therapist that the system "flipped" during abusive situations anyway. The deeper parts handled the abuse and protected the surface parts. The deeper alters began to learn how to function in the here and now and alters on the surface had the opportunity to observe. Therefore, she was able to move faster in therapy, the system as a whole was able to understand the feeling of being present without abuse. The sense of cognitive restructuring and healing images was not just unidirectional in source coming from the therapist, but was felt throughout the systems.

In addition, the entire system was able to benefit from the ego strength that the leaders had been using in a negative way (particularly blocking therapy). Dramatic changes appear to take place in these patients. Often this is a process that is completed time after time as each system with complex patients is ready to allow their strongest parts to be out and direct the therapist to the important issues.

Dividing a Memory through Several Therapy Sessions

Another advanced technique is to take a single memory, organize it according to which aspects of the BASK can be managed and in which order. The next step is to divide the various aspects of the memory into individual outpatient psychotherapy sessions.

> Susan had a difficult memory surrounding her perception of abuse by her parents and her brother. She had a deep knowledge of the abuse and processed the cognitive portion of the abuse. Then, she expressed her affect in the next therapy session. The third session was spent with her ego states each taking turns reading their words about their perpetrators while they imaged them in chairs in the office. Following these three sessions, she decided to feel and know completely what had happened because enough affect had been dissipated that she felt that her suicidal feelings could now be managed.

These examples of hypnotic techniques can shorten treatment, allow for the containment of affect within a therapy session, and are only limited by the therapist and client's personal creativity. These techniques also allow for as much of the ego strength of the ego system to be used as is available. Rather than having less able surface alters out, the potential is there for accessing leaders that represent strength in the system and allows the patient and therapist together to use as much of their resources as possible.

Examples of Hypnotic Techniques Found Helpful in Processing the Existential Crises and Promoting Cognitive Restructuring

- Adult frame of reference:

> .... I am wondering now, that at the same time, that the child is feeling what has happened and is confused .... that an adult part of you can be very close by and be observing what is happening from an adult's eyes ....

and look for a finger signal "yes:"

> .... from that adult point of view I am wondering if you can begin to understand and pass that understanding on to the child about whose fault it is and what choices the child really had when this memory was occurring ....

wait again for a finger signal:

> .... and I am wondering if the child then can understand what the adult is saying. The adult might need to speak in very small words, to explain to this child that very bad things happened .... that the child had no choice .... and that the child is not bad ....

- Cognitive reframing:

> .... I am wondering if you can begin to hear the things that you thought about yourself because of this memory ....

This is where you may hear, "I am bad," "I am worthless," "if I remember this I have to die," "I should have died," etc., and this is where the patient often has an existential crisis. It is important at this point to reframe that:

> .... as you hear the words now I am wondering if the adult inside can begin to say other things to the child, and if someone can begin to say the new understanding outloud ....

and hope to get a "yes" signal. What you will hear are statements like, "I am not bad," "bad things happened to me." If you don't begin to hear those you can begin to include them:

> .... I am wondering if you can hear my statements about my view of your experience in the past ....

You can then add statements:

> .... and let the feelings about what I am saying, or what the adult inside is saying, filter down now so that you are able to be aware of what is happening, begin to feel the impact of this new thinking ....

You are allowing the possibility of new insight at the moment in time when the memory is wide open. You are able to suggest a new thought, a new self-perception, and build self-esteem.

Examples of Other Special Hypnotic Techniques Found Helpful with Trauma Survivors during the Processing of a Memory

- Snapshots:

.... I would like the mind to take snapshots throughout the memory so that we have pictures that are saved .... they can be put into a book and opened up in therapy to be looked at later .... to understand exactly what happened from an adult point of view.

- For additional control of intense feelings. Add the following into your normal induction:

.... the bigger your feelings, the more angry you feel (or whatever other feeling you are concerned about) .... the heavier your limbs are going to be, and the more that they are going to feel that they cannot leave the couch, the bed, the chair (or wherever else the patient is located).

In fact, for patients where the affect is going to be fairly big:

.... it might even feel as if your hands and your wrists are tightly secured in a very safe and loving and kind manner so that they do not leave an area of safety that you find there as you feel the feeling of the couch.

- Spontaneous abreaction. It is extremely helpful to establish both a verbal and a physical cue prior to having a spontaneous reaction occur in your office, or have your patient call, or the patient's significant other call about a flashback, for example:

.... when I say the words "deep sleep," the part of you who is extremely helpful, very cognitive and understands what is happening, will be here to talk to me and explain to me what is happening inside ....

- With someone who is not a dissociative:

.... when you hear the words "deep sleep" you will move into a deep trance, deep enough that you will be able to leave the scene that troubles you and be able to move forward to the present and begin to feel where you are, and have a heightened sense of what you are touching, and holding, and hearing, and seeing, as you find yourself back in the present .... and even those words can be heard inside, as a way of beginning to help you to move forward to the present, to be in the here and now ....

- To add a physical cue:

.... when I touch your shoulder, or when I touch your hand, that will be the reminder or the cue for you or the trigger for you to then come back to the present now .... be here, clearly see me, hear me, be aware of where you are sitting or lying .... be totally aware of your environment .... alert and present and able to talk as much as you need to about what is happening inside ....

This requires practice so that you make sure you have it intact. Use it when you are in a nonemergency situation so that you can then use it with confidence when a patient is in crisis.

CONCLUSIONS

The inner world of the survivor of PTSD or complex dissociation, as a dynamic entity, can be entered and explored and choices made by the client and the therapist together as needed. Once inside that universe, for example, the therapist can help the client make choices about modulation, which memories to process, or depths to which trance might move to reduce symptoms. All of these experiences make adjustments possible in this dynamic internal world that enables the client to begin to see the world from a viewpoint beyond that of the victim. Initially, the therapist observes the client from an outside point of view. At first, the client allows only the tip of the iceberg to be known. Next, as trust develops and empathy is established, the client allows the therapist to make the therapeutic and hypnotic leap to learn about what is occurring inside. This opens the therapeutic process up to entire new vistas for the successful processing of memories, resolution of existential crises, reduction of shame, cognitive restructuring and the healing that all survivors deserve. Knowledgeable hypnotherapy is an essential ingredient in turning psychotherapy into the art that allows healing to occur and the opportunity for the victim to be come a true survivor.

REFERENCES

American Psychiatric Association. (1994). *Diagnostic and statistical manual of mental disorders* (4th ed.). Washington, DC: Author.

Braun, B. G. (1984). Hypnosis creates multiple personality: Myth or reality? *International Journal of Clinical and Experimental Hypnosis, 32*, 191-197.

Braun, B. G. (Ed.). (1986). *Treatment of multiple personality disorder*. Washington, DC: American Psychiatric Press.

Braun, B. G. (1988). The BASK (behavior, affect, sensation, knowledge) model of dissociation. *Dissociation, 1*(1), 4-23.

Brown, D. P., Sheflin, A., & Hammond, D. C., (1996). *Memory, therapy and the law*. Hillsdale, NJ: Erlbaum.

Brown, D. P., & Fromm, E. (1986). *Hypnotherapy and hypnoanalysis*. Hillsdale, NJ: Lawrence Erlbaum.

Cheek, D. B., & Le Cron, (1968). *Clinical hypnotherapy*. New York: Grune & Stratton.

Cheek, D. B. (1994). *Hypnosis: The application of ideomotor techniques*. Needham Heights, MA: Allyn & Bacon.

Diamond, M. J. (1986). Hypnotically augmented psychotherapy: The unique contributions of the hypnotically trained clinician. *American Journal of Clinical Hypnosis, 28*(4), 238-247.

Farthing, G. W. (1992). *The psychology of consciousness*. Englewood Cliffs, NJ: Prentice-Hall.

Hammond, D. C. (1988). *The integrative hypnotherapy model*. Unpublished paper. Salt Lake City, Utah.

Hammond, D. C. (1990). *Handbook of hypnotic suggestions and metaphors*. New York: Norton.

Hilgard, J. (1970). *Personality and hypnosis: A study of imaginative involvement*. Chicago: University of Chicago Press.

Kanovitz, J. (1992). Hypnotic memories and civil sexual abuse trials. *Vanderbilt Law Review, 45*(5), 1185-1262.

Kluft, R. P., (1983). Hypnotic crisis intervention in multiple personality. *American Journal of Clinical Hypnosis, 26*(2), 73-83.

Kluft, R. P. (Ed.) (1985). *Childhood antecedents of multiple personality*. Washington, DC: American Psychiatric Press.

Kluft, R. P. (1989). Playing for time: Temporizing techniques in the treatment of multiple personality disorder. *American Journal of Clinical Hypnosis, 32*(2), 90-98.

Kluft, R. P. (1992). Enhancing the hospital treatment of dissociative disorder patients by developing nursing expertise in the application of hypnotic techniques without formal trance induction. *American Journal of Hypnosis.*

Kluft, R. P. and Fine, C. J. (Eds.) (1993), *Clinical perspectives on multiple personality disorder*, Washington, DC, American Psychiatric Press.

Ludwig, A. M. (1983). The psychobiological function of dissociation. *American Journal of Clinical Hypnosis, 26*, 93-99.

Lynn, S. J. and Rhue, J. W., (1991). *Theories of hypnosis: Current models and perspectives*. New York: Guilford.

Peterson, J. A. (1991). *Advanced hypnotic techniques*. Eighth International Conference on Multiple Personality and Dissociative Disorders, Chicago, IL.

Putnam, F. W. (1989). *Diagnosis and treatment of multiple personality disorder*. New York: Guilford.

Ross, C. A. (1989). *Multiple personality disorder: Diagnosis, clinical features and treatment*. New York: John Wiley.

Sachs, R., and Peterson, J. A. (1994). *Processing memories retrieved by trauma victims and survivors: A primer for therapists*. Tyler, TX: Family Violence Institute.

Scheflin, A., Brown, D., & Hammond, D. C. (1994). *Memory therapy, and the law*. Des Plaines, IL: American Society of Clinical Hypnosis Press.

Spanos, N. P. and Chaves, J. F. (Eds.) (1989) *Hypnosis: The cognitive-behavioral perspective*. Buffalo, NH: Prometheus Books.

Van der Kolk, B. A., (1987) *Psychological trauma*. Washington, DC: American Psychiatric Press.

Watkins, J. G., (1971) *The affect bridge: A hypnoanalytic techniques. International Journal of Clinical and Experimental Hypnosis, 19*, 21-27.

Young, W. C., (1986). Restraints in the treatment of a patient with multiple personality. *American Journal of Psychotherapy, 50*, 801-806.

Young, W. C., (1991). Restraints in the treatment of dissociative disorders: A follow-up of twenty patients. *Dissociation, 4*(2), 74-76.

23

Memory Processing and the Healing Experience

Roberta G. Sachs and Judith A. Peterson

INTRODUCTION

The mental health field is in the midst of a paradigm shift. The position that Freud in 1898 was unable to sustain when he thought that the roots of mental illness were related to sexual abuse is currently being advanced by a number of researchers (van der Kolk, 1987; van der Kolk & van der Hart, 1991; van der Kolk-Perry, & Herman, 1991; Jacobsen, Koehler, & Jones-Brown, 1987; Herman, 1992; Boon & Draijer, 1993). They and others in our field are finding that this paradigm shift is occurring as research appears to link many of the symptoms of mental illness with past or present traumatic symptoms and with dysfunctional events in the lives of clients. Originally Freud was not believed. Yet, when van der Kolk (1991) asked Kernberg about the incidence of sexual abuse in the original population of clients labeled as borderline, the percentage was very high. Van der Kolk (1993) estimated that 15% of the population of the United States suffers from symptoms of posttraumatic stress disorder. Today, therapists are faced with many clients who present symptomotology resulting from trauma in childhood or adulthood.

Moreover, the psychiatric field has just recently discovered that there is a significant difference between the impact of everyday stressors and the impact of profound present or past trauma. In studying the continuum of trauma, clinicians have found that the effect of trauma is both a physiological and a psychological

Roberta G. Sachs • Highland Park Psychological Resources, 660 LaSalle Place, Highland Park, Illinois 60035. **Judith A. Peterson** • Phoenix Counseling, Consulting, and Forensic Services, Houston, Texas 77090.

Handbook of Dissociation: Theoretical, Empirical, and Clinical Perspectives, edited by Larry K. Michelson and William J. Ray. Plenum Press, New York, 1996.

phenomenon (van der Kolk, 1987b). To reduce symptoms permanently related to profound trauma, origins of the trauma need to be processed and resolved. "Traumatology" is a newly coined term describing "the study of natural and man-made trauma (from the "natural" trauma of the accidental and the geophysical, to the horrors of human inadvertent or volitional cruelty ...)" (Donovan, 1991, p. 433).

THE PURPOSE OF THIS CHAPTER

The purpose of this chapter is to offer therapists insight and specific therapeutic tools for managing the complexity of processing experiences of past trauma. As memory traces of trauma begin to emerge, both client and therapist may have concerns about how to begin this process. Therapists who have used more traditional psychotherapy may find that additional skills are necessary to manage the processing of traumatic experiences (Sachs & Peterson, 1992; Steele, 1989; Steele & Colrain, 1991).

The reason that memory processing is a key to the treatment of trauma victims is that reassociating the events that were originally dissociated during the trauma is essential for the recovery of the client. Organizing memories as they emerge and helping clients to plan memory processing sessions allows for a client's sense of mastery and permits the therapist to maintain cohesive therapeutic goals.

This chapter describes methods to facilitate planned memory processing sessions. It does not focus on methods to facilitate retrieving repressed memories of past abuse. Rather, the authors take the position of honoring the layers of defenses that the client has established to protect the ego structure, with a number of exceptions such as when clients exhibit symptoms of severe somatization, suicidality, homicidality, and protracted anxiety or depression.

Understanding the process for resolving traumatic experiences is sometimes difficult for the client. Many clients experience spontaneous abreactions and flashbacks that are painful and frightening but are common symptoms in posttraumatic stress disorder. Spontaneous abreactions may cause retraumatization, whereas planned memory processing sessions that facilitate cognitive restructuring can have a healing effect.

DESCRIPTION, PRESENTATION, AND COMPLEXITY OF TRAUMA VICTIMS

The client, whether suffering from posttraumatic stress disorder, dissociative disorder, or multiple personality disorder, seeks treatment because some aspect of his or her life situation is dysfunctional or painful. In presenting this situation and listing the symptoms, the client sometimes describes posttraumatic symptoms without any apparent awareness of trauma. Often there is no present-day explanation for symptoms, such as chronic depression, suicide attempts, self-mutilation, amnesia, anxiety, repeated nightmares, panic attacks, obsessive and intrusive thoughts, or bizarre and unexplainable behavior or flashbacks. It is widely accepted that these symptoms sometimes result from deeply embedded messages tied to an unknown earlier source. Finding the historical cause of dysfunctional symptomotology offers the opportunity for reducing these symptoms.

Conversely, those symptoms may have been caused by the repression of appropriate emotional and behavioral responses even though the client has always had detailed cognitive knowledge of the past event. Discovering the link between dysfunctional symptoms and possible trauma facilitates behavioral and affective change and growth.

Research has shown that environmental triggers with no conscious connection to known narrative history may cause the sudden emergence of memory traces of material (van der Kolk, 1987a). Basic environmental stimuli also trigger memory traces that are either sensory or affective, including sights, sounds, smells, touch, words, feelings, or pain. Basically, the authors find that when therapy focuses on processing memories as they emerge, the client is better able to maintain stability because his or her defenses remain in tact. Typical examples of possible trauma that might emerge in an adult client are: a rape as an adult or memories from a war, an accident, or a natural disaster. Sometimes memories emerge because of developmental issues. The memories may be triggered by events such as giving birth to a first child, a last child leaving home, or a child reaching a particular age when abuse has happened to the client. The age at which a trauma occurs does not determine if the memory to be processed is more or less complex to manage.

The authors refer the reader to other chapters of this book to understand the *Diagnostic and Statistical Manual of Mental Disorders*, 3rd Edition-Revised and 4th Edition (DSM-III-R and DSM-IV) categories for posttraumatic stress disorder and dissociative disorders. However, dissociative or traumatized clients present with "windows of diagnostic opportunity," since the defensive structure of the clients was in place long before they entered therapy. In fact, what the clinician sees that is diagnostic depends on what clients are able to or want to reveal at the time of the interview. What clients choose to or are ready to disclose to the clinician varies depending on many issues such as the level of trust, therapeutic alliance, presence or absence of current abuse, and degree and chronicity of abuse throughout the client's life.

A client may initially present in psychotherapy as a "whole person" and maintain that presentation throughout therapy. The therapist might believe that the client is the victim of a single traumatic episode that might have originated from childhood or adulthood. Later, as trust develops, more dissociative symptoms sometimes become apparent. However, a client may present so subtly that parts are difficult to distinguish and remain that way throughout therapy as in dissociative disorder not otherwise specified (DDNOS). On the other hand, some clients may be found to have classic dissociative identity disorder or even polyfragmented dissociative identity disorder. Thus, as therapy progresses, the diagnosis may change.

The reason it is important to know the eclectic nature of trauma victims is that the memory processing techniques needed will vary according to the (1) complexity and nature of the internal defensive structure of the client, (2) the level of internal compartmentalization, and (3) the formation and structure of amnestic barriers.

Kluft (1992) has described complex dissociative clients in detail. In addition, the authors of this chapter have found that complex dissociative victims have other characteristics that affect memory processing. These include: (1) groups of parts that are amnestic to other parts, (2) groups of parts with specific memories or jobs in common, (3) layers of parts with amnestic barriers between them, (4) multiple systems with varying degrees of amnesia, (5) mirrored or twinned systems, (6) synthetic parts (purposefully externally created parts), (7) sadomasochistic parts, or (8) system wide sociopathy.

USEFUL TERMS AND DEFINITIONS

Memory takes many forms. Some clients enter therapy reporting abuse memories they have never forgotten dating from early childhood. Others report different forms of memories including flashbacks, recurrent dreams, somatic complaints with no medical basis, and repetition-compulsions, to name a few.

Memory Retrieval

For the purposes of this chapter, the term memory retrieval will refer to the process the client uses to become aware of information about past events that they have not instinctively brought to therapy. These past events have been blocked by a defense called dissociation because part or all of the event overwhelmed the individual's adaptive capacity to process it. The authors do not recommend that therapists intentionally uncover traumas except under unusual circumstances. The following is a short list of times in treatment when it is appropriate to intentionally uncover memories.

1. In the case of a medical emergency
2. In the event of extreme, self-destructive behavior such as self-mutilation
3. In the event of potentially life-threatening symptoms such as uncontrollable choking
4. In a psychological emergency, such as the patient feeling obsessed with suicidal and/or homicidal thoughts

These examples are not frequent occurrences in the therapy of trauma survivors. Therapists are encouraged to uncover underlying psychodynamic issues, as these will frequently precede or coincide with the natural emergence of memories. If the client has retrieved a memory that is impacting his or her here-and-now functioning, then careful attention should be given to the preparation and pacing of working through this material. Rather, therapists are encouraged to pace the timing of the "working through" of traumatic material revealed by clients. Generally the authors allow the client's process to unfold gradually by honoring the dissociative defense. Therapists are encouraged to caution their clients about the unreliability of memory and to urge them to search for all possible interpretations of what they believe they have uncovered.

Abreaction

The term abreaction (coined by Viennese physician Josef Breuer who worked with clients diagnosed as suffering from "hysteria") refers to experiencing intense feelings at moments when recalling a past disturbing event that is connected to a present day neurotic symptom. During this recall, a client often momentarily reaches what Breuer referred to as "catharsis" during which original feelings of intense emotion, previously barred from current memory, reoccur.

There is a misunderstanding, however, concerning the term abreaction. Many think that abreaction causes the patient to become regressed. Therapists deserve to be criticized if therapy leads to ongoing regression. However, during memory processing the client might experience an "abreactive spike" or an emotionally "cathartic moment."

Momentary releases of affect from any trauma at any age is not regression. In addition, misunderstanding occurs when professionals assume that processing of a past experience is always a childhood memory. In many cases, the experience processed involves a trauma from teenage years or adulthood. In the past the term "abreaction" has been used within the field to describe all aspects of memory processing. Further refinement of terminology clarifies that abreaction is just one aspect of memory processing (Peterson, 1993; van der Hart et al., 1993).

Flashbacks or Spontaneous Abreactions

Many clients have flashbacks (another word for spontaneous abreactions). Flashbacks are defined as uncontrolled physiological memory loops surfacing spontaneously from implicit and explicit levels of consciousness (Graf & Schacter, 1988). These partial, traumatic memory traces can take the form of flashes of scenes, sudden body memories, intense affect such as terror or rage, suspicious smells, sounds, or tastes that become frightening, or a touch that becomes upsetting. Clients often experience spontaneous memory traces in flashbacks without any cognitive frame of reference that enables them to understand what is happening.

In 1989, Putnam listed Blank's (1955) typography (Kluft & Fine, 1993) that describes four types of flashbacks: (1) vivid dreams and nightmares of the traumatic events, (2) vivid dreams from which the dreamer awakens still under the influence of the dream content and has difficulty making contact with reality, (3) conscious flashbacks in which the subject experiences intrusive recall of traumatic events accompanied by vivid multimodal hallucinations, and may or may not lose contact with reality, and (4) unconscious flashbacks in which the individual has a sudden, discrete experience that leads to an action that recreates or repeats a traumatic event but the subject does not have any awareness at the time or later of the connection between this action and the past trauma.

Since clients cannot predict or explain the occurrence of flashbacks, they often feel overwhelmed and out of control. Their symptomotology may resemble symptoms of other psychiatric disorders and may be misinterpreted as such. Clients usually report relief when they can learn to control flashbacks and can safely explore the content of their traumas using a planned memory processing framework.

Memory Processing

Memory processing is defined as working through a past trauma from the beginning to the end of the perceived trauma with the cognitive processing and restructuring that facilitates symptom reduction and expression of whatever affect is necessary to resolve the trauma. Thorough processing of the trauma enables the client to move the experience from a traumatic remembrance to a place in narrative memory wherein the client knows it occurred in the past and has good cognitive understanding of the event. Even if the past event was unbearable, there is a recognition that it will always be a part of that individual's past. In theory, there will be a healing experience with a new understanding of that experience. When this occurs, the client has the potential to know both an inner peace and external positive change in current symptoms.

Resolution

Resolution refers to the abatement of symptoms after completion of memory processing and cognitive restructuring. Resolution is that state of co-consciousness where internal conflict and disagreement among internal parts cease. All known parts are able to function together as a team and have a different perspective about their previous roles and their relationships.

Blending

Blending is the process during which discrete internal parts or alters change their barriers, become closer in awareness, and even begin to overlap or merge.

Integration

Kluft (1993) defines integration as "an ongoing process of undoing all aspects of dissociative dividedness ... from long before reduction of numbers through fusion to a deeper level." Further, integration is "an ongoing process that follows the same processes as the tradition of psychoanalytic perspectives on structural change."

THE COMPONENTS OF MEMORY

The study of memory is complex, but Braun (1988) has created a pragmatic model to facilitate the organization or memory within a clinical setting. He identified four components necessary to completely process memory of past trauma: behavior, affect, sensation, and knowledge (BASK). His BASK model of dissociation helps therapists to understand the necessity of integrating these components completely. It is only when the four components are congruent and confluent over time that a person can be said to possibly experience a complete memory.

The question of what is true about any memory perplexes those in this difficult field. It is assumed that the therapist will explain how confusing and unreliable memory can be and that it may be several years before any clarity of memory takes place, if at all. Therefore, focus is placed on starting with the client's belief of what is true and asking the client to take the responsibility for his or her recollections. The therapist is not an investigator but a facilitator of healing.

Even though there are no well-defined stages in memory processing, the authors have found that there is a continuum in the complexity of memory processing experiences. At one end of the continuum are clients who have retrieved a memory about one trauma and are able to master processing the memory in a single therapy session. At the other end of the continuum are clients who have very complex memories involving mastery of a profound existential crisis (such as a near-death experience) and will require many sessions of therapy to complete their memory processing.

The ease with which memories are managed depends on the most basic of psychotherapeutic tasks. First, the client must attain a comfortable and assumed level of trust in the therapist; second, the client must have achieved internal trust among dissociated ego states, alters, or parts; third, the therapist should be aware that memory processing is affected by the complexity and severity of the client's previously processed trauma; fourth, therapist and client must learn and master identified therapeutic tasks; finally, the therapist should consider teaching the client hypnotic techniques that will facilitate memory processing.

Examples of the Continuum of Complexity of Memory

Case 1. A client in her 30s had always cognitively known of the inappropriate discipline she received from her foster parent who was a minister. He falsely accused her of acting out in high school and punished her by paddling her across his knees. The purpose of processing this memory was to reassociate the affective and sensory parts of these experiences with the knowledge that had always existed. In addition, the client needed empathy with regard to her shame as well as validation for her feelings, and finally cognitive restructuring to resolve this trauma.

Case 2. A client in her 40s already diagnosed as DDNOS began to have flashbacks about a date rape. She was taught containment techniques and asked to have a part that could maintain control journal as many details of the experience as could be recalled. In reading the journaling, the therapist realized that several parts were involved in this life-threatening experience. After rereading the journal, the client realized that a number of events of that night were unknown to her. Subsequently, the therapist helped the client organize all of the parts who dissociated all of the aspects of this trauma to participate in a memory processing session.

Case 3. A highly dissociative client had spontaneous cramping and hemorrhaging on her 25th birthday. After seeking treatment at the local emergency room and being told she was physically normal, she called her therapist. The client presented with extreme agitation and no conscious awareness of the reason for her symptoms. Parts emerged to tell the therapist about the birthday ritual that her father and brothers had made her participate in during childhood and adolescence. Several parts described prolonged use of intentional sadistic abuse. Many weeks were spent as the parts and host prepared for the memory processing that was needed. After the memory was processed, the physical symptoms never reoccurred.

As clients gain experience in memory processing, they tend to gain insight into how they can contain feelings both before and after the memory processing session. Also, they become better able to distinguish what core elements of the memory are really essential to process in therapy. Complex dissociative or multiple personality disorder clients often learn how to combine similar experiences in one memory processing session.

PSYCHOTHERAPEUTIC TASKS DURING THE BEGINNING PHASE OF TREATMENT

Prior to beginning planned memory processing sessions, mastery of key therapeutic tasks is helpful to establish the framework of therapy. The order of the therapeutic tasks is flexible and depends on both the client's and therapist's style. Premature and disorganized discussion or processing of traumatic experiences may be a recapitulation of the abuse. The suppression of spontaneous flashbacks is highly recommended to help avoid the reexperience of trauma. Containment techniques and cognitive processing of the event are part of the overall preparation for organized memory processing.

Mapping

Mapping is often a part of therapy for clients who have dissociative identity disorder. It is a special procedure that allows clients an external way to concretize their internal structural description (Braun & Sachs, 1986). This may be accomplished through art media, the sand tray (Sachs, 1992), occupational therapy, or journaling. Mapping involves a continuum of complexity: (1) a simple sociogram, (2) a more complex, multilayered sociogram, (3) a map depicting systems rather than distinct personalities, (4) a map depicting a combination of both individual parts and systems, or (5) a systemically layered structure.

Mapping may be used by the client to uncover data, to describe origins and alliances of parts, and to help focus and organize memory processing for therapy. The very process of mapping seems to help organize and focus chaotic and fragmented clients. In complex dissociative identity disorder clients, it may be helpful for clients to redo individual sections of their mapping in detail or expand on sections as they prepare for more advanced memory work. With complex clients, the more thorough the preparation, the greater the possibility of combining and collapsing memories in one or two memory processing sessions. Combining similar memories may also lead to a better cognitive understanding of the gestalt of the client's experience, a greater understanding of the existential crises, resolution, and eventual blending of internal parts.

PLANNED MEMORY-PROCESSING SESSIONS

The purpose of a first memory-processing experience is to practice the therapeutic tasks and to introduce a sense of mastery to clients. Therefore, the first memory processed may not have significant long-term meaning but is chosen to build skills and to ensure a mastery experience. If more difficult work is necessary later in therapy, processing less traumatic material builds the foundation for more complex work. In dissociative or highly dissociative identity disorder clients, the internal parts or alters that the therapist may not have met are watching and listening to determine whether a safe environment exists for their later therapeutic work.

Expressing the BASK Model

The different parts of the BASK model (Braun, 1988) can be expressed in memory processing by separating out the behavior, feelings, physical or body sensations, and knowledge. Whenever possible, it is advisable to attempt to work through the BASK model by beginning with the knowledge or cognitive part of the memory. Even though the acronym implies one would start with the behavior component, the recommendation is to start with knowledge. This insures that the client will maintain self-control and not be overwhelmed.

The therapist may choose to work with any one of the aspects of the BASK model during memory processing. He or she may choose to work solely on the grief from a past trauma for several memory processing sessions; the therapist may attempt to combine anger and somatic memories in one session; or the therapist may choose to fractionate the knowledge clients bring to a memory processing session to keep the total knowledge from being overwhelming. The task is to eventually bring all aspects of the BASK together and achieve congruence, cognitive restructuring, and resolution. Any initial division or fractionation of the memory is to facilitate pacing and mastery in therapy.

Hypnotic Induction or Progressive Relaxation

A rule of thumb is that the more dissociative a client, the less formal a hypnotic induction is needed or traditionally used by therapists. Therefore, a less dissociative client appears to need a more formal hypnotic induction in regular therapy sessions. But almost all dissociative clients appear to benefit strongly from a formal hypnotic induction when beginning memory-processing sessions. The purpose of hypnosis is to provide safety and facilitate processing during the session, not to retrieve memories. It is assumed that the client already has retrieved most of the content prior to this session. It is the authors' belief that if the client is suffering from posttraumatic stress disorder or from discrete dissociative episodes, the therapist needs even more formal training in hypnosis.

Memory Process with Complex Dissociatives: Helping Alters to Safe Places and Restructuring Internally Prior to Memory Processing

With highly hypnotizable clients, only a brief induction may be necessary before suggesting that they retreat to their "safe places" (see Chapter 22, this volume). With other clients, detailed hypnotic induction and deepening work may be needed to establish a safe place prior to actual memory processing work. Parts that are involved with the memory need to remain close to the surface. Parts that want or need to be amnestic can be hypnotically blocked from the processing of the memory. Furthermore, parts that want to watch from different distances still need permission to observe and at the same time feel only what they are ready to feel while they remain safe. Thus, the therapist continues to assess the client to make sure that the memory work will be as complete as possible while simultaneously ensuring the client's maintaining protection of his or her ego structure. In most systems it is a safe assumption that all parts are aware to some degree of the memory processing session.

Cognitive Narrative

The client relates the memory cognitively, that is, without sensory, somatic, or affective components. Only the knowledge component of the BASK model is utilized so that the client can practice relating the memory from beginning to end. After the cognitive summary, the therapist ascertains that all parts involved in the trauma are present and that other parts are observing at a comfortable distance. In addition, those parts unable to tolerate reassociating this memory need to be hypnotically helped to a safe place where they do not have to experience the memory-processing session.

It is important that the therapist actively listen to the cognitive narrative without adding or changing any part or detail of it. While listening to the story, the therapist looks and listens for manifestations of the other BASK components—affect, sensation and behavior. The client proceeds from $T - 1$ to $T + 1$ (Peterson, 1991), describing the beginning, middle, and end of the total memory. What the therapist hears may differ from what the client has journaled or expressed in art or the sand tray. Clients and their therapy are dynamic, not static. The therapist must be certain that the memory being processed in the cognitive narrative is the memory that the therapist and client planned to process. After the cognitive narrative has been completed, the therapist validates, reinforces mastery, and checks the safety and well-being of the client.

Identification of Existential Crisis Statements

Trauma creates existential crises that appear to affect forever how these clients feel and think about themselves. The overall goals of memory processing are to release the immense affect of the experience and to identify the existential crises that have affected these clients all their lives. When this has been completed, the therapist facilitates cognitive restructuring, mastery, and empowerment to help create long-term change. Existential crises occur when basic beliefs or assumptions about the world, reality, or sense of self are profoundly experienced as having been shattered. They may be precipitated by dramatic events as profound as rape, torture, murder, loss, or natural disaster. On the other hand, the catalyst may be as subtle as losing faith in someone who had been implicitly trusted.

These traumatic events create a loss of basic security and a disconnection from other human beings. Working through these moments of existential crisis comprise the fundamental work needed for recovery. Therapist and client alike may find it difficult to hear, to process, and to allow the expression of shame, humiliation, guilt, denigration, or hopelessness.

> The basic assumptions with which we ground our own security crumble, and we become confused and anxious. The credo shatters: I believe the world is meaningful and comprehensive; I believe the world is safe and I am invulnerable; I see myself in a positive light. I am free; I can choose. (Steele, 1989, p. 155)

The painful process of exposing and processing the cause of the overwhelming feelings of hopelessness, panic, anxiety, and low self-esteem lead to feelings of power, mastery, and hope as healing occurs. Simply exposing the feelings or hearing existential crisis statements does not help. Cognitive restructuring is necessary for the healing process to occur.

Cognitive Restructuring

Cognitive restructuring is defined as the process by which the deeply embedded negative experiences are reframed in a positive way. New positive statements about the client are then introduced to help build self-esteem, to foster a new understanding of the context of the past trauma, and to help the development of new ways of relating to others in the present.

Unless the existential crisis statements are identified and cognitive restructuring begun as memories are processed, significant change over time does not appear to occur. Affect, pain, or momentary abreaction are only by-products of the trauma. The expression of intense feelings may provide temporary relief to the client, but it does not ensure that changes will occur. Acceptance and resolution of existential crises provide the foundation for permanently changed self-perception.

Regrounding and Assessing the Client

If during a memory processing session the client appears overwhelmed, the therapist may need to interrupt the affective process even if the client does not signal "stop." When this happens, the therapist should reground the client in the present so that he or she can "metabolize" what has been overwhelming. A cognitive approach is most helpful at this time. If the client is able to easily review the narrative structure of the memory, then the therapist knows the client is managing satisfactorily. At the end of the memory-processing session it is wise for the therapist to determine whether residual body memories exist that need to be alleviated, whether the client needs to take prearranged medication, or whether the client is able to return home safely.

Healing Images

One final step in memory processing should be to suggest positive metaphoric images of increased self-esteem. A healing light is an example of a hypnotic image that can be effectively used at the end of a session. The repetition of one familiar image appears to facilitate the building of a positive sense of self from one session to the next. Once a healing image has been established, the mere mention of it may help the client return to an internal feeling of safety, peace, and a familiar place.

Finally, blending and integrating metaphors may be used to promote new ego strength. Spontaneous integration is often the result of a successful memory processing session.

Safety Contracting

Safety contracting is the last task in a memory processing session and is essential for all clients regardless of their level of dissociation. When clients have parts, the parts as well as the presenting personality need to guarantee safety. Even when safety is continually reassessed throughout the session, some dissociated parts who remained in their "safe places" may not have responded to your previous inquiries about present and future safety. If ideomotor signals are used, verbal and ideomotor contracts must be congruent to ensure the greatest possibility for ongoing safety. If there is any discrepancy between verbal and nonverbal signals concerning self-harm or harm to others, the session cannot be considered complete. More processing and negotiating with parts who are reluctant to agree to a safety contract must take place. If after a reasonable time of negotiation (a maximum of 20 minutes) there still remain actively suicidal or homicidal parts unwilling to contract for safety, hospitalization is an appropriate option and should be discussed. Therapists need to be familiar with state laws about commitment procedures for clients who are homicidal or suicidal.

The following criteria help determine if successful memory processing has been completed:

1. Has the client experienced the reduction of dysfunctional symptoms, such as those accompanying posttraumatic stress disorder, depression, anxiety, and other psychiatric disorders?
2. Has the client become aware of the existential crises and cognitively restructured the experience to allow for new insights and a different interpretation of the experience?
3. Does the client have mastery over the memory as a narrative part of his or her personal history?
4. Is the client in the process of choosing to lead a life that demonstrates reduction of retraumatizing experiences?
5. Does the client feel an increase in self-esteem and ego-strength?
6. Does the client realize the reality of positive "choices"?

ADVANCED CONCEPTS IN MEMORY PROCESSING

Combining Memories

After the client has learned how to process several individual memories, it is possible to teach him or her how to process similar abuses in one memory-processing session. Preparation involves the client retrieving one memory as a base. Ideomotor signals for dissociated parts may indicate if the patient has experienced similar abuse at other times; journaling, art, or sand tray work are also helpful indicators. The memories surrounding traumatic experiences may be assimilated by combining them so that they are processed in one session. This approach allows the opportunity for the client to learn new insights at multiple levels of consciousness.

Techniques for Management of Severe Fragmentation

Some trauma victims have experienced such severe abuse that parts simply shattered at the moment of assault. Clients describe the experience as an "explosion" inside. It is helpful to suggest to clients that through memory processing they can reverse the shattering so that parts and fragments come together as they were before the abusive event. This may be accomplished by distorting or reversing time and processing the memory backward. The client may decide to start at the end of the abusive incident (T + 1) and move backward through time until just before the abuse occurred (T − 1). At this point the client has reached the moment in time just before the shattering and that past may be experienced as a whole. Even if polyfragmentation has not occurred, this method may be helpful. An advantage to this technique is that it enables parts to know that they survived the abuse and to return to the point in time before they were abused. This technique often facilitates healing, blending, and integration.

Fractionation of a Memory or Fractionation of an Amnestic Barrier

Fractionation refers to the division of any part of the psychotherapeutic experience by the therapist into parts in order to make the process more manageable to the client. Any of the feelings, thoughts, sensations, or knowledge of memories can be separated or divided from each other to be processed individually. Other ways to fractionate include distancing the client from an event, time distorting an event, or dividing affect into portions.

With this therapeutic technique a client may be asked to imagine what 100% of the rage feels like and then decide what portion of the feeling he or she can manage to release with safety and mastery. If the client could only release 25%, then he or she would take four sessions to complete a memory. On the other hand, 100% of the feelings might be expressed in one extended session by using fractionation to pace the session.

USING OTHER THERAPEUTIC MODALITIES TO PROCESS MEMORIES

When working with dissociative disorders the expressive therapies (i.e., art, movement, occupational, and sand tray) offer numerous applications to facilitate diagnosis and treatment. Basically, the expressive therapies allow access through an indirect means to dissociated memories that are adversely affecting a client's ongoing behavior. These techniques help the client to circumvent conscious knowledge when the content is too threatening while allowing for other means of accessing memory traces of traumatic material. Moreover, the expressive therapies provide an opportunity for participating in multiple levels of communication.

One difference the authors note between dissociative disorder clients and other psychiatric populations is the concreteness with which dissociative clients use these modalities to represent their perception of the experienced trauma. The expressive therapies have been acknowledged for their contribution in the diagnosis and treatment of complex dissociative disorders (Cohen & Cox, 1989; Sachs, 1992; Fuhrman et al., 1990). Therefore, the routine use of these therapies can yield important diagnostic information; help the client become more consciously aware of memories; process the intense feelings attached to the traumatic events; facilitate the development of mastery and a unified sense of self; and provide the therapist with a unique way to monitor the progress and process of treatment.

PERSONALITY TRAITS AND CHARACTEROLOGICAL MANAGEMENT

> Personality traits are enduring patterns of perceiving, relating to and thinking about the environment and oneself, and are exhibited in a wide range of important social and personal contexts. It is only when personality traits are inflexible and maladaptive and cause either significant functional impairment or subjective distress that they constitute personality disorders. (American Psychiatric Association, 1987, p. 335)

Working with personality disorders means managing characterological issues. This involves empathy (understanding the clients' definitions, criteria, and beliefs at a cognitive and affective level), safety (establishing and maintaining psychological and physical boundaries and limits), and negotiation (presenting options that both the client and therapist can accept). Character pathology is a primary focus of treatment because adults abused as children have no sense of boundaries and/or healthy interpersonal relationships.

The authors believe that protection of the ego is the primary purpose of all clients' defensive structures. Clients who have experienced decades of profound abuse and double-bind experiences by those who should have been trustworthy experience the intense need for protection at the slightest emotional or physical threat. In addition, these victims frequently participate in unhealthy alliances, i.e., they veer from normal personality development by recreating their childhood abuse with self-destructive acts or retraumatization.

Patients may present in therapy with any number of personality disturbances. In clients with parts, one goal of therapy is to determine the difference between a general personality dysfunction and one manifested by an alter or fragment. If character pathology is not addressed, the issues surrounding this aspect of their dysfunctionality will continue even after significant trauma resolution has taken place.

Setting Limits and Boundaries

The following case studies highlight some of the more common characterological issues therapists have to manage:

Case 1. At the end of a memory-processing session, an alter refuses to guarantee safety of the body or commit to further therapy sessions. The therapist aligns himself or herself with this alter to protect the client's safety without preempting her role within the system. The therapist actually asks for advice on how they can work together, as this fosters mutuality while empowering the client. However, it is the therapist who makes sure the rules of therapy are in place.

Case 2. The client continually places emergency life-threatening calls to the therapist in the middle of the night. The therapist quickly assesses the level of the crisis to determine if the call is a manipulation. If so, the client is redirected to a hotline or other supportive resource. If the call is a genuine crisis, the therapist may attempt to resolve the issue or direct the client to the nearest emergency room.

Case 3. Within the last 5 minutes of the therapy session the patient regresses into a spontaneous abreaction or raises a major therapeutic issue. If this is the first occurrence, the therapist attempts to reground the client and cognitively process this boundary violation both in this session and the next session. If this continues to be a pattern, the therapist reminds the client that safety is always required at the end of the session and can say, "If you cannot ground yourself in the present and leave the office safely, then I will have my secretary hold your car keys while you sit in another office until you decide how to manage going home safely." As a last resort the therapist can offer to assist the client to a hospital setting by calling the paramedics.

Self-Mutilation: Chronic vs. Cyclical

In a severely traumatized population, self-mutilation, i.e., cutting and scoring various parts of the body, is a common problem serving a variety of purposes for the client: (1) to punish the self, (2) to silence alters, (3) to create physical pain to distract the client from emotional pain, (4) to feel anything in order to feel "alive," (5) to fulfill an addiction to physical pain by triggering a euphoric feeling, (6) to express automatic behavior, or (7) to express resistance (or distraction) from the therapeutic issues. All of these can be manifested on a continuum ranging from subtle to overtly dangerous behavior. Self-mutilation that is cyclical might have more to do with anniversaries of particular life experiences such as birthdays, seasons of the year, or holidays. An assessment needs to be made to determine if there is an addictive quality to the mutilation, whether chronic or cyclical. For mutilation that has an addictive quality, medication exists that has been highly effective in breaking the self-destructive cycle. Referral to a physician familiar with the medical management of these symptoms can be very helpful (van der Kolk, 1987a,b).

Sabotaging of Memory Processing

Dissociative clients who have survived profound childhood trauma often are equipped with survival skills derived from an interaction of discrete parts of the self who assume a protective role. In order to survive, clients often become as aggressive as those who harmed them. Since they have had to harm themselves or others in order to survive, their behavior in the here and now is often a recapitulation of the past.

During memory processing the hostile alters frequently act out by attempting to harm self, persecute other alters, harm the therapist, or extend limits and disregard boundaries. The client may also place the therapist in a double-bind position by saying, for example, "If you elicit this memory, I will be self-destructive; if you don't elicit and process this memory, I will continue to be self-destructive." Catherine Fine (1988), in her paper on crisis prevention at the International Society for the Study of Multiple Personality Disorder conference, stated: "The only winning move is not to play."

Therapists must show respect for the alters' protective function while challenging the perception of self-sufficiency only through self-harm. Introducing new choices about self-sufficiency, such as protecting the body, being brave enough to facilitate recovery, and so on, helps to set the stage for creating positive choices. The belief that there is only one way (usually a destructive one) for an alter to maintain safety of the body needs to be effectively challenged because it represents rigid and constrictive thinking. Careful, organized planning using hostile alters as allies will help to avoid a situation where the client may harm the body. In addition, understanding various reasons for blocking or threatening hostile behavior may further insure a client's safety.

Pacing

The goal of any kind of therapy is to provide continued mastery over memory experiences. Yet clients who have had profound abuse very often want to work through material as quickly as possible to rid themselves of the pain. When this occurs, clients often are bombarded with knowledge and affect they are unable to process, thus becoming overwhelmed and emotionally paralyzed. It is up to the therapist to educate the client about pacing therapy so as to maintain a delicate balance between client memory retrieval and processing the memories in therapy.

Blocking

When the processing of a memory is blocked for any reason, the client may be indicating the need for solving therapeutic problems, whether internal or external. Often the part of the system that emerges will directly explain what has been forgotten or what will happen if therapy proceeds. Blocking memories or engaging in resistance remains the ultimate defense mechanism for these clients. Finding the cause of this resistance, interpreting the defenses, and processing the impasse opens the door to subsequent memory retrieval. Blocking by the system is diagnostic and should be carefully explored. It may take any of the following forms: (1) an alter emerging to express hostility, (2) silence, (3) distracting statements, (4) emergence of child parts, or (5) spontaneous abreactions.

Out-of-Control or Violent Behavior

Out-of-control alters are a potential threat to the self, others, and the therapist. Understanding the client's presentation and teaching him or her to rechannel destructive energy and hostility results in more productive sessions.

When a therapist confronts a crisis, help from another therapist may be required to ensure physical control and safety. Physically restraining an out-of-control client is necessary if the client's or therapist's safety is at risk. Therefore, the therapist needs to learn appropriate and approved techniques for restraining clients. Regardless of how many safe sessions therapist and client experience, there are certain times in the therapeutic process when out-of-control behavior can be expected such as: (1) when new levels or parts of the client's system emerge, (2) when material is uncovered that triggers violent protective parts, (3) when the client has been abused in the here and now, or (4) when the client appears to exhibit compulsive or automatic behavior.

Safety limits are most often upheld and respected when the client and therapist define them. The client's unpredictable history is a precursor to the potential for unpredictable violent behavior in a therapy session. Early in therapy the client needs to understand that unsafe behavior will not be allowed. Once the client's behavior is safely under control, communication takes place with those who provoked the incident. "Talking through" the presenting part to the violent acting-out parts is the safest way to manage therapy after an explosive incident. A team approach is helpful in outpatient work. Sometimes a session's content will trigger an acting-out incident by an internal alter. Regardless of whether this is a normal psychotherapy session or a planned memory-processing session, the therapist must be aware of a client's unpredictability.

Confabulation

Confabulation is defined in Webster's dictionary as "filling in gaps in the memory with detailed, but more or less unconscious accounts of fictitious events." In dissociative patients confabulation serves a variety of purposes: (1) it helps clients hide the fact that time for them is discontinuous; (2) it helps to normalize both past and present experiences; (3) within the memory of an experience, confabulation of a less intense event can be a defense against an intolerable aspect of the event; (4) it may be used for secondary gain whether intentional or unintentional; (5) it may be used to idealize the image of a significant other; and (6) it serves to maintain the client's secrecy.

Disclosure–Recanting Cycle

Clients move through stages of belief and disbelief as a normal part of therapy. Most clients have an existential crisis surrounding the issue of never knowing with certainty about the accuracy of the details of their past. They must process the feeling of being robbed of a part of their lives through not having clear memory. Eventually the client comes to his or her own reality about what has happened. At all times therapists need to be cautious about not leading.

Often denial can turn into recanting. This is very common in many other populations of clients including criminals, child molesters, abusers, and so forth. Recanting appears to be related to several variables. Profound shame and guilt can be so overwhelming that recanting is easier than working through the feelings. Historically, sadomasochistic abusers have made victims feel that they voluntarily enjoyed perpetration. It becomes far easier to recant and/or blame the therapist for memories that are intolerable (when the system's dissociative barriers begin to break down) than to take responsibility for one's past behavior.

Terror of the consequences of "having told" in therapy is another factor in recanting. Clients fear retaliation both internally from parts that threaten to harm the body and externally through fear of harm from those who told them never to reveal the secrets. Additionally, the fear that they might be criminally charged is also significant. Returning to the belief system that accompanied the dissociation is far more psychologically comfortable than processing the tremendous pain that results from the experience of being abused or having abused others. Recanting helps clients feel more secure about their safety and quells their fears about being placed in jail or prison. While that is unlikely, reassurances about confidentiality are truly limited because knowledge of child abuse requires mandatory reporting by therapists.

Finally, the effects of the Stockholm syndrome (Ochberg, 1978) with these clients must not be overlooked. Through terror and torture these victims initially have much more alliance with their abusers (even if the abuser is dead) than with their therapist.

CONTRAINDICATIONS FOR MEMORY PROCESSING

Some clients are not suited for any memory processing work. This can often be ascertained through a full battery of psychological testing. The level of ego strength, characterological considerations, and any indications of psychotic symptoms need to be carefully assessed and fully understood before attempting memory processing even if the client is already experiencing spontaneous memory traces.

Traumatic–Psychotic Transference

Difficult negative transference issues have been described by Kluft (1984) and Spiegel (1984) as "traumatic transference" (Kluft, 1984, Loewenstein, 1993; and Spiegel, 1991). Very traumatized clients frequently view everything their therapist does, no matter how helpful it appears to be, as abusive, narcissistic, and self-fulfilling on the part of the therapist. Clients often have a very difficult time viewing any relationship as nonabusive. Parts not engaged in therapy frequently are continuing to "internally dialogue" about the supposed ulterior motives of the therapist. In addition, Spiegel has also described "flashback transference" wherein the client very literally (or with trance logic) views the therapist as a perpetrator. Furthermore, as the level of sadomasochism increases, there is a likelihood that either sadistic or masochistic transference issues will increase. While the major therapy issues are resolved by working through the negative transference, in some cases clients are simply unwilling or unable to engage in processing the shame and guilt surrounding their victim or perpetrator issues. When this occurs, therapy is stuck in a traumatic transference where personal ownership of malevolence is bestowed on the therapist. Unless a solid therapeutic alliance is available as a safety net while difficult issues are processed, it is likely that many clients will leave therapy with the perception that they were abused.

Malignant Narcissism

Malignant narcissism refers to clients who are so invested in their dissociative disorder that they may obtain secondary gain from the diagnosis or have some other reason for a lack of commitment to the therapeutic process. Achieving notoriety through media appearances, gaining special attention in the family system, being relieved of adult responsibilities, or gaining wealth from publishing a life story are examples of by-products of malignant narcissism.

Sadomasochism

Clients may be addicted to abuse or may be unwilling to break the pleasure-pain bond that has been conditioned in their everyday life. When parents and children are sadomasochistically addicted, children have no escape route. Consequently, whether adults are caught in a current sadomasochistic relationship or a child or adolescent is still living with sadomasochistic caregivers, once the therapist becomes aware of this problem, memory work is not indicated until family circumstances change.

Malignant Suicide

Clients who are malignantly suicidal truly wish to kill themselves. These clients actively manifest their death wish through severe self-mutilation, life-threatening anorexia, and other various suicidal behavior. The authors have seen both ends of a bimodal expression of this suicide phenomena. Clients who have difficulty dissociating severe trauma appear often to choose suicide as their escape. On the other end of the continuum, clients who believe they have no free will choose suicide as well.

Further contraindications for memory processing not related to psychological testing include; the client is in the early stages of therapy; the client is physically impaired, acutely ill, or terminally ill; the client is elderly and chooses not to resolve past issues; the client is currently being abused or is dangerously self-abusive; the client has no therapeutic alliance or is not capable of forming a therapeutic alliance; the client has a psychotic overlay that cannot be managed with appropriate medications; the client does not have the financial resources for continued therapy; the client's ego structure is too fragile to prevent decompensation; the client is continually being flooded with flashbacks or intense affect despite adequate attempts to teach containment techniques; or the client has a serious present-day crisis to manage (i.e., divorce, job loss). Given these difficulties, it is hoped that therapists approach clients with the concept of memory processing very carefully. In the above instances maintenance and supportive therapy is the only responsible and appropriate choice.

POSTTRAUMATIC STRESS DISORDER IN THERAPISTS

Therapists who treat dissociative disorders are often overwhelmed by the nature of the abuse their clients report. This abuse seems to exceed the scope of what is imaginable and is very difficult if not impossible for the therapist to defend against. The thoughts and emotions felt by therapists range from total denial to compelling rescue fantasies. Consequently, therapists frequently suffer from existential crises that parallel their clients' in intensity. Many therapists are experiencing the syndrome of posttraumatic stress disorder without realizing the origin of their symptomatology. Therapists need to know that these reactions are the norm and not the exception.

In a recent study (Perry, 1993), over 1000 therapists were surveyed with regard to their responses in working with this population. One half to three fourths reported that it had a significant impact on both their work and general life circumstances; relationships with both family and friends were affected. Those surveyed often withdrew from others, which led to their feeling a sense of isolation. One third reported existential crises. In addition, therapists also reported symptoms of depression, exhaustion, alienation, obsession, and paranoia. Ethical dilemmas were reported, including deciding whether to report other professionals for unprofessional behavior; reporting clients' previous criminal activity; or reporting incidents of child abuse. In addition, therapists reported emotional harassment such as clients lying about sexual molestation or clients threatening malpractice in order to discredit the therapist. Thirty-eight percent of the therapists reported being threatened physically. Safety measures listed by therapists in the study included having alarm systems, planning therapy sessions when other therapists are in the office, and taking self-defense classes.

Despite these negative results, many therapists reported enhancement in their lives from working with dissociative clients. Personal growth, increased spirituality, and close personal ties to supportive people were found to be important. Therapists reported helpful coping strategies, including a strong support system of family and colleagues; continued monitoring of their own mental health; keeping a focus on the balance between family and professional life; limiting the number of dissociatives in their practice; and proper rest, recreation, diet, and involvement in extracurricular activities.

CONCLUSION

Processing memories associated with past traumatic events is a highly complex form of therapy requiring astute timing and skilled use of specific therapeutic techniques. The concepts presented in this chapter are intended to provide therapists with an introduction to memory processing and follow-up therapy. It is important to recognize that what has been presented here is only one way of approaching memory processing, based on years of experience and our own clinical work. The order of memory processing presented here is not necessarily the order in which it takes place; depending on the client, there needs to be flexibility in managing the therapeutic process.

The authors do not believe in processing memories unless retrieved by the client. The exceptions to that are noted in the text. Currently issues about false memories, contamination, confabulation, recanting and iatrogenesis provide major controversies in the field of trauma. Sadly, these controversies are influencing the way in which both therapists and clients engage in the therapeutic process. Supportive therapy, although important, seems to be taking the place of appropriate memory processing, thus limiting therapeutic progress for this population. Finally, core existential issues remain unresolved because of clients *internal* fears of retribution and therapists and clients fears of *external* retribution.

APPENDIX: THERAPEUTIC TASKS FOR EACH PHASE OF TREATMENT OF TRAUMA VICTIMS

Phase 1

- Build trust and establish a therapeutic relationship.
- Establish safety in present time (may start with safety in the psychotherapy session).
- Establish hypotheses about the differential diagnoses.
- Establish and maintain appropriate boundaries.
- Suppress spontaneous abreactions or flashbacks.
- Establish psychoeducational approach to treatment.
- Teach about the phases of treatment.
- Promote reading of instructional, educational (not anecdotal) material.
- Teach pacing of therapy.
- Educate about medication management.
- Manage transference and countertransference issues.
- Teach journaling.
- Teach art therapy and other modalities.
- Mastery of beginning hypnotic skills: safe place, containment, affect modulation, affect toleration, rapid induction, distancing, time distortion, establish ideomotor signals, positive age progression and regression, permissive amnesia, and deepening techniques.
- Build self-esteem and overall functionality.
- Process and cognitively restructure.
- Contain memories retrieved by client outside of therapy to be processed later in therapy.
- Teach the planning and processing of retrieved memories.
- Teach internal communication if client has parts.

Phase 2

- Learn to plan and pace the memory processing of retrieved memories.
- Teach and help client practice advanced hypnotic techniques.
- Teach titration or fractionation of feelings or memories.
- Use cognitive restructuring.
- Review and focus on all aspects of Phase 1 of treatment.
- Blend and integrate parts when processing memories (if client has parts).
- Use group therapy (if necessary and appropriate).
- Group psychotherapy needs to focus on present day relationshps and tasks.

Phase 3

- Continue all aspects of Phases 1 and 2 as necessary.
- Begin developmental reconstructive psychotherapy.
- Use spiritual and creative therapy.
- Move into more complex memory processing if necessary.
- Continue blending and integration.
- Continue cognitive restructuring.
- Begin psychodynamic psychotherapy as a "single" personality.

REFERENCES

American Psychiatric Association. (1987). *Diagnostic and statistical manual of mental disorder* (3rd ed., rev.). Washington, DC: Author.

American Psychiatric Association. (1994). *Diagnostic and statistical manual of mental disorders* (4th ed.). Washington, DC: Author.

Boon, S., & Draijer, N. (1993). Multiple personality disorder in the Netherlands: A clinical investigation of 71 patients. *American Journal of Psychiatry, 159*(3), 489-494.

Braun, B. G. (Ed.). (1968). *Treatment of multiple personality disorder*. Washington, DC: American Psychiatric Press.

Braun, B. G. (1988). The BASK (behavior, affect, sensation, knowledge) model of dissociation. *Dissociation, 1*(1), 4-23.

Brown, D. P., Shelfin, A., & Hammond, D. C. (in press). *Memory, therapy, and the law*. Hillsdale, NJ: Erlbaum.

Cohen, B. M., & Cox, C. T. (1989). Breaking the code: Identification of multiplicity through art productions. *Dissociation, 2*(3), 132-137.

Donovan, D. M. (1991). Traumatology: A field whose time has come. *Journal of Traumatic Stress, 4*(3), 433-436.

Fine, C. G. (1988). Cognitive behavioral intervention in the treatment of multiple personality disorder (Abstract). In B. G. Braun (Ed.), *Dissociative disorders: 1988: Proceedings of the fifth international conference on multiple personality/dissociative states* (pp. 167). Chicago, IL:

Graf, P., & Schacter, D. L. (1989). Modality specificity of implicit memory for new associations. *Journal of Experimental Psychology: Learning, Memory and Cognition, 15*(1), 13-17.

Herman, J. L. (1992). *Trauma and recovery*. New York: Basic Books.

Jacobson, A., Koehler, J. E., & Jones-Brown, C. (1987). The failure of routing assessment to detect histories of assault experienced by psychiatric patients. *Hospital and Community and Psychiatry, 38*(4), 386-389.

Kluft, R. P. (1984). Aspects of the treatment of multiple personality disorder. *Psychiatric Annals* **14**, 19-24.

Kluft, R. P. (1991). Clinical presentations of multiple personality disorder. In R. J. Loewenstein (Ed.), *The Psychiatric Annals of North America* (pp. 605-629). Philadelphia, PA: W. B. Saunders.

Kluft, R. P. (1993). Clinical perspectives on multiple personality disorder. In R. P. Kluft & C. Fine (Eds.), *Clinical approaches to the integration of personalities* (pp. 101-133). Washington, DC: American Psychiatric Press.

Kluft, R. P., & Fine, C. G. (Eds.). (1993). *Clinical perspectives on multiple personality disorder*. Washington, DC: American Psychiatric Press.

Loewenstein, R. J. (1993). Posttraumatic and dissociative aspects of transference and countertransference in the treatment of multiple personality disorder. In R. P. Kluft & C. Fine (Eds.), *Clinical approaches to the integration of personalities* (pp. 51-85). Washington, DC: American Psychiatric Press.

Ochberg, F. M. (1978). The victim of terrorism. *The Practitioner, 220*, 293-302.

Perry, N. (1992). *Therapists' experiences of the effects of working with dissociative patients*. Paper presented at the annual meeting of the International Society for the Study of Multiple Personality and Dissociation, Chicago.

Peterson, J. A. (1991). *Advanced hypnotic techniques*. Paper delivered at the Eighth International Conference on Multiple Personality/Dissociative Disorders, Chicago, IL.

Peterson, J. A. (1993). Reply to van der Hart/Brown article. *Dissociation*, *6*(1), 74-75.

Putnam, F. W. (1989). *Diagnosis and treatment of multiple personality disorder*. New York: Guilford Press.

Sachs, R. G. (1992). *An introduction to sandtray therapy for adult victims of trauma*. Center for Psychiatric Trauma and Dissociation, Rush-Presbyterian-St. Luke's Medical Center, Chicago, IL.

Sachs, R., & Peterson, J. A. (1994). *Processing of memories retrieved by trauma survivors*. The Institute for Family Violence, Tyler, TX.

Schacter, D. L., McAndrews, M. P., & Moscovitch, M. (1988). Access to consciousness: Dissociations between implicit and explicit knowledge in neuropsychological syndromes, in L. Weiskrantz (Ed.), *Thought without language* (pp. 247-278). Oxford: Oxford University Press.

Steele, K. H. (1989a). A model for abreaction with MPD and other dissociative disorders. *Dissociation* *2*(3), 151-157.

Steele, K. H. (1989b). Sitting with the shattered soul. *Pilgrimage: Journal of Personal Exploration and Psychotherapy*, *15*(6), 19-22.

Steele, K., and Colrain, J. (1990). Abreactive work with sexual abuse survivors: Concepts and techniques. In M. A. Hunter (Ed.), *The sexually abused male: Volume 2. Application of treatment strategies* (pp. 1-55). Lexington, MA: Lexington Books.

van der Kolk, B. (1987a). *Psychological trauma*. Washington, DC: American Psychiatric Press.

van der Kolk, B. (1987b). The psychobiology of the trauma response: Hyperarousal, constriction, and addiction to traumatic re-exposure. In B. A. van der Kolk (Ed.), *Psychological trauma* (pp. 63-68). Washington, DC: American Psychiatric Press.

van der Kolk, B. (1993). *Trauma and development: Theory and treatment*. Paper presented at the annual Houston Dissociative Disorder Symposium.

van der Kolk, B., Perry, C. J., & Herman, J. (1991). Childhood origins of self-destructive behavior. *American Journal of Psychiatry*, *148*(12), 1665-1671.

van der Kolk, B., & van der Hart, O. (1991). The intrusive past: the flexibility of memory and the engraving of trauma. *American Imago*, *48*, 425-454.

van der Hart, O., and Brown, P. (1992). Abreaction revisited. *Dissociation*, *5*(3), 127-141.

van der Hart, O., and Brown, P. (1993). Author's response to Peterson, *Dissociation*, *6*(1), 76.

van der Kolk, B., Perry, C. J., & Herman, J. (1991). Childhood origins of self-destructive behavior. *American Journal of Psychiatry*, *148*(12), 1665-1671.

van der Kolk, B., & van der Hart, O. (1991). The intrusive past; The flexibility of memory and the engraving of trauma. *American Imago*, *48*, 425-454.

ADDITIONAL BIBLIOGRAPHY

Bliss, E. L. (1986). *Multiple personality, allied disorders and hypnosis*. New York: Oxford.

Boon, S., & Draijer, N. (1993). *Multiple personality disorder in the Netherlands: A study on reliability and validity of the diagnosis*. Swets & Zeitlinger.

Christianson, S.-K. (1992). Emotional stress and eyewitness memory: A critical review, *Psychological Bulletin*, *122*.

Chu, J. A. (1988). Some aspects of resistance in multiple personality disorder. *Dissociation*, *1*(2), 34-38.

Claridge, K. E. (1992). Reconstructing memories of abuse: A theory-based approach. *Psychotherapy*, *29*(2), 243-252.

Coons, P. M. (1984). The differential diagnosis of multiple personality: A comprehensive review. *Psychiatric Clinics of North America*, *7*, 51-67.

Ellenberger, H. F. (1970). *The discovery of the unconscious*. New York: Basic Books.

Fagan, J. F. (1973). Infants' delayed recognition memory and forgetting. *Journal of Experimental Child Psychology*, *16*, 424-450.

Figley, C. (1985). *Trauma and its wake*. New York: Brunner/Mazel.

Finkelhor, D., Gelles, R. J., & Hotaling, G. T. (1983). *The dark side of families*. Beverly Hills, CA: Sage Publications.

Freud, A. (1965). *Normality and pathology in childhood: Assessments of development*. New York: International Universities Press.

Goodwin, J. (1990, January). Problems of belief in approaching patients' accounts of ritual abuse. *The Advisor*, p. 6, 9.

Graf, P., & Schacter, D. L. (1989b). Unitization and grouping mediate dissociations in memory for new associations. *Journal of Experimental Psychology: Learnings, Memory and Cognition, 15*(5), 930-940.

Greenwald, A. G. (1992). New look. 3: Unconscious cognition reclaimed. *American Psychologist, 47*(6), 766-779.

Hammomnd, D. C. (1990). Facilitating a full abreaction. In *Handbook of hypnotic suggestions and metaphors* (pp. 524-525). New York: Norton.

Janoff-Bulman, R. (1985). The aftermath of victimization: Rebuilding shattered assumptions. In C. R. Figley (Ed.), *Trauma and its wake*. New York: Bruner/Mazel.

Kluft, R. P. (1984a). Treatment of multiple personality disorder: A study of 33 cases. *Psychiatric Clinics of North America*, 7, 9-29.

Kluft, R. P. (1984b). Multiple personality in childhood. *Psychiatric Clinics of North America*, 7, 121-134.

Kluft, R. P. (Ed.) (1985). *Childhood antecedents of multiple personality*. Washington, DC: American Psychiatric Press.

LeDoux, J. E. (1994). Emotion, memory, and the brain. *Scientific American*.

Levis, D. J. (1991). The recovery of traumatic memories: The etiological source of psychopathology. In R. G. Kunzendorf (Ed.), *Mental imagery* (pp. 230-240). New York: Plenum Press.

Loftus, E., Garry, M., and Feldman, J. (1994). Forgetting sexual trauma: What does it mean when 38% forget? *Journal of Counseling and Clinical Psychology, 62*, 000-000.

Masson, J. M. (1984). *The assault on truth*. Toronto: Strauss & Giroux.

Meyer, Williams, L. (1994). Recall of childhood trauma: A prospective study of women's memories of child sexual abuse. *Journal of Counseling and Clinical Psychology, 62*, 000-000.

Meyer, Williams, L. (1994). A reply to Loftus, Gar, and Feldman and What does it mean to forget child sexual abuse? *Journal of Counseling and Clinical Psychology, 62*, 000-000.

Peterson, J. A. (1992). *The effects on personality of sadomasochistic abuse*. Paper delivered at the Ninth International Conference on Multiple Personality/Dissociative Disorders, Chicago, IL.

Ross, C. A. (1989). *Multiple personality disorder: Diagnosis, clinical features and treatment*. New York: John Wiley.

Sachs, R. G. (1990). *Ethical questions in the treatment of dissociative disorders*. Paper presented at the Seventh International Conference for the Study of Multiple Personality/ Dissociative Disorders, Chicago, IL.

Schacter, D. L., McAndrews, M. P., & Moscovitch, M. (1988). Access to consciousness: Dissociations between implicit and explicit knowledge in neuropsychological syndromes. In L. Weiskrantz (Ed.), *Thought without language* (pp. 247-278). (A Fyssen Foundation symposium. Oxford: Oxford University Press.

Schacter, D. L. (1990). Perceptual representation systems and implicit memory: Toward a resolution of the multiple memory systems debate. *Annals of the New York Academy of Sciences, 608*, 543-571.

Schacter, D. L. (1992). Understanding implicit memory: A cognitive neuroscience approach. *American Psychologist, 47*(4), 559-569.

Schacter, D. L. (1992). Consciousness and awareness in memory and amnesia: Critical issues. In D. A. Milner & M. D. Rugg (Eds.), *The neuropsychology of consciousness* (pp. 179-200). London: Academic Press.

Shengold, L. (1989). *Soul murder: The effects of childhood abuse and deprivation*. New Haven, CT: Yale University Press.

Spiegel, D. (1991). Dissociation and trauma. In A. Tasman & S. M. Goldfinger (Eds.), *American Psychiatric Press review of psychiatry* (pp. 261-275). Washington, DC: American Psychiatric Press.

Stern, D. N. (1985). *The interpersonal world of the infant: A view from psychoanalysis and developmental psychology*. New York: Basic Books.

van der Kolk, B., & Ducey, C. P. (1989). The psychological processing of traumatic experience: Rorschach patterns in PTSD. *Journal of Traumatic Stress, 2*(3), 259-274.

van der Kolk, B. (1994). The body keeps the score: Memory and the evolving psychobiology of posttraumatic stress. *Harvard Review of Psychiatry*.

24

Inpatient Treatment of Dissociative Disorders

Walter C. Young and Linda J. Young

INTRODUCTION

The past two decades have seen an explosion in the diagnosis of severe dissociative disorders, including dissociative identity disorder (DID), formerly multiple personality disorder (MPD), and a variety of other related syndromes lacking the clinical specificity of dissociative identity disorder (Barkin, Braun, & Kluft, 1986; Bliss, 1986; Bliss & Jeppsen, 1985; Braun, 1986; Coons, Bowman, & Milstein, 1988; Kluft, 1984a,b, 1991a,b; Quimby, Andrei, & Putnam, 1993; Greaves, 1980, 1993; Putnam, 1986; Putnam, Guroff, Silberman, Barban, & Post, 1986; Ross, 1989, 1991; Ross, Norton, & Wozney, 1989). Fortunately, the *Diagnostic and Statistical Manual for Mental Disorders*, 4th edition (DSM-IV) (American Psychiatric Association, 1994) has renamed multiple personality disorder to dissociative identity disorder (DID), which will more accurately represent dissociative conditions as belonging to a continuum of trauma-related syndromes that disrupt normal identity formation using prominent dissociative defenses. This renaming will go a long way to end confusion that MPD is a bizarre condition in which many persons exist in a single mind and will shift clinical focus to a more traditional psychological framework where the disorder of identity reflects a dissociative elaboration that owes its complexity to early and prolonged child abuse (Coons et al., 1988; Putnam, 1985, 1989; Putnam et al., 1986; Kluft, 1984a, 1990, 1991a,b; Ross, 1989; Ross et al., 1989; Spiegel, 1984).

Walter C. Young and Linda J. Young • National Treatment Center for Traumatic and Dissociative Disorders, Del Amo Hospital, Torrance, California 90505.

Handbook of Dissociation: Theoretical, Empirical, and Clinical Perspectives, edited by Larry K. Michelson and William J. Ray. Plenum Press, New York, 1996.

DID is an inherently unstable condition, often leading to crises requiring hospitalization (Braun, 1986, 1993; Kluft, 1991b; Putnam, 1989; Ross, 1989). The most accepted theory, though controversial, is that chronic abuse in some individuals fosters the gradual evolution of dissociative states that remain separated by amnesic barriers, resulting in the failure to assimilate information and a sense of self into a unified, cohesive identity (Kluft, 1991a; Putnam, 1989; Young, 1988b). Information storage occurs within a variety of dissociative states that alternate as the individual reacts to various internal or external stimuli. Dissociated identity formation is one form of traumatic residue that leads to a diffused identity, with patients experiencing impoverished memory about significant events in their lives.

Trauma itself is highly disorganizing, leading to a variety of traumatic syndromes (Herman, 1992; Horowitz, 1986; Kluft, 1990; Kroll, 1993; Terr, 1990; van der Kolk, 1987). Important for the development and subsequent treatment of dissociative conditions is the propensity for traumatic memory to be processed pathologically, so that information and meaning of the events related to the alleged trauma remain largely unknown and thereby unmodified by new experience. Memory may be represented in a chaotic form, with severe cognitive distortions and a lack of coherent integration, which leads to a failure of the normal developmental processes that provide emotional regulation that prepares one for later life (Fine, 1988, 1990; Kluft, 1990, 1991b). Rigid, pathological defenses predominate, binding mental energy to inhibitory modes of functioning. Since the dissociative system of defenses grows out of a matrix of extensive child abuse, there are a variety of identifications reflecting persecutory, victim, counterphobic, fantasy material, and a variety of other states that intrude or disrupt smooth mental functioning (Kluft, 1991a,b; Putnam, 1989; van der Kolk, 1987; Young, 1988a). Dissociated material lacks a means of verbal expression and therefore surfaces through reenactment behaviors, flashbacks, and abreactions all accompanied by vivid emotions. Further, patients are vulnerable to crises and emotional triggering when inner or outer stimuli threaten the barriers to excessively painful material (Horowitz, 1986; Kluft, 1991b; Kroll, 1993; van der Kolk, 1987). These factors all interact to provide a psychological matrix that is unstable and disorganizing, making these patients especially vulnerable and prone to the need for hospitalization (Braun, 1986; Kluft, 1991b; Putnam, 1985; Ross, 1989).

This chapter outlines basic issues in the hospital treatment of adults with severe dissociative disorders.

INDICATIONS FOR HOSPITALIZATION

In general, the needs for hospitalization are similar to those for nondissociative conditions. Suicidality, serious danger to others, inability to use partial hospital or outpatient treatment, and grave disability are all indications for hospitalization. Further, when local communities lack the expertise to diagnose or treat dissociative conditions, referral to a center specializing in these conditions is warranted. A number of authors have discussed the indications for hospitalization and inpatient care (Braun, 1986, 1993; Kluft, 1991b; Putnam, 1986, 1989; Ross, 1989; Sakheim, Hess & Chivas, 1986). Table 1 provides a list of indications for hospitalization.

Table 1. Indications for Hospitalization

1. The applicant is actively suicidal or homicidal.
2. The applicant is too disorganized to manage outside of the hospital.
3. The material emerging requires the safety or structure of a hospital to process.
4. Outpatient treatment has been ineffective or blocked and less restricted settings have failed.
5. Medical complications require inpatient assessment.
6. There is a need for inpatient medication adjustment.
7. Diagnostic issues require inpatient observation or a specialty center.
8. There is severe, uncontrollable, destructive acting out.
9. Fugue behaviors interrupt outpatient treatment and functioning.
10. The patient risks losing a family or job during an acute crisis.
11. There is a psychotic or acute decompensation.
12. Inpatient treatment is needed to help evaluate a treatment impasse.
13. The patient is unreliable with medication.
14. Substance abuse prevents stable outpatient treatment.

GOALS OF HOSPITALIZATION

Goals for hospitalization should be clearly spelled out to correct unrealistic expectations by the patient (Braun, 1986; Kluft, 1991a,b; Putnam, 1989; Ross, 1989; Sakheim et al., 1986). Further, hospital treatment is inherently regressive for some patients so that short-term stays with a rapid assessment are preferred (Sakheim et al., 1986). Patients or therapists may have high and unachievable expectations such as full integration or excessively vague ones such as "memory work" to unearth suspected abuse memories. Overall satisfaction by both patients and therapists will be enhanced when realistic goals are defined and achievable prior to admission. Kluft (1991b) notes lengths of stay will vary and goals may need to be reassessed after a period of evaluation. Lengths of stay for discreet issues may last for 1-2 weeks or extend for several months when ego strengths are lacking and there is poor impulse control or if a personality disorder impedes effective therapeutic engagement.

When possible, the patient's principal therapist should be included in the patient's care and discharge planning (Braun, 1993; Kluft, 1991b). In addition to assessing the patient, it is critical to assess the outpatient treatment and the therapeutic relationship itself, so recommendations may be given to help referring therapists and provide them help with transference and countertransference obstacles that cause therapeutic impasses.

Despite the tendency of patients to present in states of crisis and go to press for elaboration of dissociated material, time should be taken in the early phases of treatment to ensure the patient has the capacity to manage the emotional states that occur with "memory" work. Premature efforts at retrieving dissociated information lead to further decompensation without an accompanying capacity to integrate the material usefully. In these instances patients may abreact repetitively with little improvement. Emotional homeostasis is severely disrupted when observing ego functions cannot work through emerging material (Fine, 1991; Kluft, 1991a,b). The therapist must be cognizant that reports of traumatic memories recovered in therapy are not necessarily historically accurate and may be distorted and elaborated by a variety of external and internal mental processes, yet still be perceived as real by patients.

DEVELOPING EMOTIONAL CONTAINMENT STRATEGIES

Much of the initial focus of treatment, especially with patients needing hospitalization, has to be directed toward learning to contain suicidal and destructive impulses and managing the high levels of emotional arousal that are typically released when dissociated material emerges. The destructive identifications with abusers, the masochistic behaviors arising from chronic victimization, the low self-esteem, the poorly defined internal structures that manage the pressures from internal destructive dissociative states, and the lack of impulse control during dysphoric periods all combine to make self-destructive acting out a persistent problem as psychotherapy proceeds. The learning of self-control techniques and the careful pacing of treatment then become important considerations (Fine, 1991; Kluft, 1982, 1983, 1989, 1991b; Putnam, 1989).

Hospital staff can help develop emotional containment strategies. The patient's external support systems and resources should be assessed. Family, friends, using music, art work, exercise, and other supports can all be developed. Social service, family, and staff members working with the patient can all help identify concrete external stabilizing activities.

It is equally important to develop inner coping skills to use in times of crisis. Patients need to learn that all crises are not equally threatening. Patients often react to any trigger with an all-or-none response and need to start thinking of crises as occurring along a scale of intensity that allows modified responses. Learning that states of crisis are not interminable but exist for a finite period is extremely valuable.

Using hypnotic techniques enhances the patient's capacity to channel dissociation in a healthy way (Braun, 1984; Kluft, 1982, 1983, 1991b; Putnam, 1989). Guided imagery and trance inductions with suggestions of a safe place to retreat internally can be invaluable. Alter personalities may be taught to help when the patient is overwhelmed. Establishing "inner councils" of alters or developing inner dialogue fosters greater control (Caul, 1984; Putnam, 1989). Further, hypnotic states of relaxation may be utilized to control the pace of processing dissociated information or to allow access to other internal states. Self-hypnosis can provide patients the means of using dissociation themselves and demonstrates that dissociation can be brought under their own control.

Ideomotor signals allow questioning of an entire internal dissociated system with "yes" or "no" questions. They can also be used to assess self-destructive or suicidal risks by inner states having destructive impulses of which the patient is unaware. Milieu staff can learn to "ask inside" about the safety of a patient by inquiring if there is any immediate danger or if an agreement to ask for help can be made so the patient will come to staff ahead of time to get help if he or she feels out of control. As soon as internal dialogue is established, it should replace ideomotor signals to increase the expectation of patient accountability for his or her system and to promote movement toward further integration and inner cooperation.

It should be noted that some patients cannot be trusted with ideomotor signals and they should not be relied on in these instances. Ideomotor signals should include signs for "stop" and "I don't know" to allow patients to stop proceeding if answering is not safe. "I don't know" helps preclude a demand response that may be inaccurate or misleading.

When using hypnotic techniques, staff needs to be aware of the ease with which erroneous material may be accepted by patients and elaborated on when patients are in trance states (American Medical Association, 1985; Orne, 1979; Pettinati, 1988). Direct and leading suggestions, especially when ideomotor signals are utilized or "memory" work is being done, are likely to produce artifacts. Open-ended questions are always preferable.

Within the hospital, however, developing inner containment strategies may allow staff to approach patients in crisis and reduce tension rapidly before there is a loss of control. For example, talking briefly with a patient in crisis, then having them "close down," go to a "safe place inside," or some other equivalent, lets patients know that staff is aware of the crisis and can address it later when there is time or refer it to a more appropriate person, such as a case manager or therapist.

Making a list of resources such as friends, trusted family members, support groups, and relaxing activities such as music, art work, writing, exercise, hobbies, and so on is very helpful during crises. Journaling and drawing are valuable tools to learn so that material may be disclosed in ways that are less threatening than telling a therapist "forbidden" information. In addition, patients may switch into altered states while using these media and thereby depict important information. Journaling is an important tool to use for developing internal communication between states. Patient's alters can learn to write to each other and sign their entries. There are a variety of expressive but also "closing down" and other supportive uses of a journal that exceed merely detailing traumatic events (Adams, 1990, 1993).

These internal strategies and external resources can be assessed and developed by a trained inpatient staff so that patients have specific skills that complement the primary therapist's treatment focus and prepare the patient for reprocessing dissociated traumatic material. It is helpful for patients to list their resources so they will know what they can do when they encounter a crisis. A written list helps when patients cannot think clearly and are disorganized so they can then refer to a prepared list to move through the crisis. The development of these patient coping skills becomes a key focus for a hospital team that in effect also reflects the beginning of discharge planning. Maintaining emotional equilibrium after hospitalization also requires resources outside of the hospital. Assessing these resources is a key ingredient in the hospitalized patient's treatment. Patients will be returned to an environment that may already be insufficient to meet their needs, and for the working person maintaining stability is crucial to job stability.

SPECIALTY UNITS

There are increasing numbers of hospitals offering inpatient treatment for dissociative disorders. These vary from those integrating dissociative disorders into a general milieu to those with specialty tracks to those with geographically separated units.

Presently, the authors recommend separate units rather than mixing dissociative patients with general inpatient populations. This works better for several reasons. First, many patients have difficult experiences on general units. General patients view switching, childlike behaviors, and abreactions with fear or by alienating dissociative patients. They may openly disbelieve the condition of multiplicity. These reactions are experienced abusively by dissociative patients and may be responded to by closing off further communication. Second, on general units patients often complain that the needs of dissociative patients divert staff time away from others. Third, dissociative patients are ill at ease and feel exposed and vulnerable to the scrutiny of both staff and patients who do not understand their dynamics. Last, much of the highly traumatic material dissociative patients disclose in groups disrupts or overwhelms a general population.

From a staff perspective, nursing staff may be highly skeptical and may challenge or react with negative countertransference reactions to the behaviors seen in MPD. This is demoralizing for traumatized patients who already anticipate they will be disbelieved and ridiculed (Kluft, 1991b). A staff not specifically trained may not recognize or be equipped to deal with altered states or the variety of transference paradigms and clinical pictures that present themselves. This leads to confusion, inconsistency, punitive responses, avoidance, rejection, or inappropriate curiosity and loss of boundaries.

Kluft (1991b) points out a number of advantages to special programs for dissociative conditions. He notes that staff are accustomed to the behaviors and traumatic material presented and that dissociative patients are not curiosities. A unit milieu invested in by the patients begins to develop, which fosters a milieu that overall is more therapeutic. Patients do not derive their principal sense of uniqueness and esteem through the "specialness" of their disorder. Specialty units allow the development of a closely knit team that recognizes dissociative problems, responds empathetically and appropriately, and who want to work with dissociative patients. Patient management is more consistent and staff can support one another when traumatic material or unit intensity threatens staff with burnout.

The Milieu

The ultimate function of a hospital milieu is to assess and address the dysfunctional problems that bring the patient into the hospital. It uses the unit structure to diagnose and confront behavior problems. The hospital structure provides a protective and stable environment where the patient's needs are more clearly defined and where critical problem areas requiring inpatient care are resolved. The patient's outpatient treatment is evaluated and revised so that patients can return to outpatient treatment as quickly as possible with as little regression and interference with the patient's healthier functioning as possible (Kluft, 1991b; Kroll, 1993; Putnam, 1989; Ross, 1989; Sakheim et al., 1986).

A milieu must also recognize the acuity presented by dissociative patients in a special unit. Because of their inherent instability, these patients should be considered high risks; but the least restrictive interventions should be instituted, depending on clinical situations and knowledge of the patients. If instability is ongoing, patients may require restricted privileges and have full unit privileges returned slowly, even if they appear in control by switching back to normal from a risky personality state. Despite the outward appearance of calm, patients can switch rapidly or be triggered inadvertently in therapy or group sessions into states that are highly suicidal, self-destructive, self-mutilating, assaultive, belligerent, or elopement-prone. There may be instances when a period of quiet, out-of-program time, unit or room restriction, or, in severe situations, the use of a seclusion area is needed.

Unlike many hospital patients in intensive care settings, the acute states may not be ongoing and obvious, as they are in patients with schizophrenia, impulse disorders, or bipolar conditions. Interventions may be relatively brief if the patient can switch out of these states and reestablish control. Staff needs to recognize that patients still need to be closely monitored, especially if safety agreements to come to staff are ineffective.

STAFF DEVELOPMENT

Nursing staffs will require special training when working with dissociative patients (Kluft, 1991b). First, staff will need to understand the dynamics and function of dissociation and the variety of clinical pictures presented by these patients. Second, they will need to be taught proper boundaries and limit-setting to avoid overindulgence or excessive rigidity in their therapeutic interventions. Third, they will need to implement a variety of treatment interventions that protect milieu structure and maintain milieu stability. Last, they will need an awareness of the potential for information distortion that occurs in a milieu of highly suggestible patients who may be exposed to leading questions as well as the productions of other patients. Staff needs a sound framework in which to consider the information they hear.

Dynamics

Beginning with patient dynamics, staff must be selected that are willing to work with victims of abuse. Staff must be taught that dissociative defenses serve both a defensive and a protective function. Furthermore, staff need to learn that patients do not necessarily announce their dissociative states, so that provocative behaviors may not be recognized as coming from alter personality states. Patients that switch are in distress and interventions should be geared to understanding and supporting agitated patients rather than viewing them as borderline or unmotivated. At times behavior is the only means patients have of communicating conflicts. Empathy should guide staff in knowing that patients communicate in the best way they are able. Alternative behaviors may need to be taught. Staff will also need to be supported if they are depreciated by patients as being uncaring or unhelpful.

As victims of abuse, patients may present attitudes of entitlement and revictimization. They may reenact trauma or display symptoms of profound withdrawal, regression, hyperactivity, sleep disorder, helplessness, dependency, or counterphobic behaviors that characterize variations of trauma residue (Herman, 1992; Kluft, 1990, 1991b; Kroll, 1993; van der Kolk, 1987).

Boundaries and Limits

Patients with severe behavioral disturbances and abusive histories place inordinate or inappropriate demands on staff. Staff can become confused when disruptive behaviors in some altered states are denied when the patient returns to their normal state. Often reenactment behaviors and expectations of entitlement present unrecognized invitations for inconsistent staff reactions. Staff may become overinvolved or, on the other hand, react punitively. It is imperative that clear boundaries and limits be established that guide both patient and staff expectations. Communication and training should define clear staff roles and responsibilities.

It is common for patients and staff to have differing agendas when treatment commences. On the one hand, patients may be expecting gratification of their needs or be accustomed to inappropriate indulgences by well-meaning therapists who are trying to provide caring attitudes through inappropriate nurturing experiences in a misguided effort to provide a corrective emotional environment instead of promoting a change in lifestyle and realistic expectations of others (Kroll, 1993). These agendas manifest themselves through unrecognized impulses to reenact preexisting pathological behaviors in the program milieu (Kroll, 1993; van der Kolk, 1989).

The unit, on the other hand, expects to provide support, confrontation, and interpretations to promote growth and change. While this is appropriate, it may not yet be the agreed upon understanding of patients looking for need gratification but also expecting to be reabused or to reenact abuse scenarios.

Policies that result in excessive regression and disruption of the milieu should be avoided. In the authors' experience, such practices as allowing baby bottles, holding or embracing patients, and physical soothing often feel gratifying to patients, but predictably become expectations for staff by increasing numbers of patients. This may appear to be valued by patients but serves more often to avoid confronting realistic discussion of patient needs or other difficult feelings. There are many reasons that these techniques pose problems, but they preempt the verbal expression of a patient's needs or feelings of worthlessness. Providing for physical nurturing interventions can be misunderstood by patients and lead to potential abuse by staff. They may also be requested at times when patient behaviors are inappropriate or staff is struggling with negative countertransference feelings. Maintaining good therapeutic boundaries regardless of diagnosis always remains the best rule. When staff members spend long periods of one-to-one time with patients or, on the other hand, remain aloof and distanced, an uneven distribution of staff time among patients may occur. Clear expectations should be set that allow patients to know the time available to them by staff. It is important for staff to avoid premature processing of new material when patients are not ready. This often produces emotional escalation or functional decompensation.

Milieu Structure

Turning to milieu structure, it is important that a set of unit guidelines governing expectations and behaviors on the unit be available both to staff and patients. It is advisable that these guidelines be explained simply, their rationale be clear, and whenever possible given to patients prior to their admission. When expectations are clear, the maintenance of milieu structure, safety, and consistency are enhanced. Standardized guidelines allow staff, especially pool staff, to orient to appropriate interventions and set consistent limits. They provide a predictable program that is reassuring to patients who often are still accustomed to external authority to gauge what is appropriate and who depend on staff to react with a minimum of countertransference interference.

Patients may act out in a variety of ways and verbally challenge both staff competence and empathy. They will also engage in control struggles of various kinds to deviate from unit policy. This acting out should be viewed as reenactment and behavioral communications reflecting a residual trauma effect. These behaviors are a window to important information of how patients think, process, or avoid painful material. Untrained staff may become easily engaged in power struggles and feel that patients are merely "manipulative" or "borderline," resulting in anger and potentially punitive responses. Table 2 suggests a few guidelines, but every unit will need to develop guidelines that work within their own system.

Contamination

Last, staff needs to be aware of the potential for inpatient units to generate contagion effects. The exposure of material to suggestible patients often leads to imitative behaviors or to the inadvertent absorbing of material heard on the unit, resulting in patients repressing its source and then retrieving the absorbed information and perceiving it as memories of their own. Patients may also respond when suggestions or expectations are given and produce material to please staff. This is especially true when hypnosis is used (Orne, 1979; Pettinati, 1988).

Table 2. Partial List of Suggested Patient Guidelines

1. Patients can expect to be called by their given names in the milieu.
2. Patients will not abuse each other or staff.
3. Out-of-control, overt acts of self-destructive behavior or abuse toward others will result in a modified program or may result in discharge.
4. Patients have an identified therapist avaialable to work with them upon discharge.
5. Patients felt to be a safety risk may be restricted to the unit.
6. Patient privileges will be determined by program participation and milieu behavior.
7. All medications will be kept by the nursing staff unless directed otherwise.
8. Patients should not bring valuables to prevent their inadvertent loss.
9. Patients will be held accountable for all of their behavior. If a patient is highly dissociative, the system as a whole is accountable, and reasonable therapeutic responses to the patient will be made by staff even if individual alters provoke the need for structure or control.
10. Contacts and involvement by referring therapists are encouraged.
11. Patients will participate in their treatment planning and be given informed consent if special procedures or medications are used.
12. Patients are expected to clean their rooms, make their beds, and dress appropriately.
13. Room assignments will be decided by staff.
14. Patients are expected to participate in the program designed by their treatment team.

There is a variety of contaminants that can be introduced and erroneous conclusions drawn if memories are "validated" using only the information of a few personality states without integrating the information in others. Memories often shift dramatically as more dissociated material is assimilated. It is important, then, that staff not validate material from patients unless there is clear, independent confirmation, despite patient wishes to the contrary. Premature validation can fix a patient to a particular memory and prevent their openness to alternate explanations as new information becomes available. One can, however, empathize with the patient's suffering and recognize that a clearer picture of what may have occurred can be more evident later.

PROGRAM COMPONENTS

Inpatient programs can offer a variety of therapeutic experiences. When working with severely abused patients, it is important that crucial issues around abuse and its impact on character development and cognition be well understood. While many options are considered here, each facility needs to be guided by available expertise and the logistics of the facility.

Informed Consent

Because of the nature of dissociative conditions, one cannot predict the content or course of treatment. One often finds a degree of regression and disorganization inevitable when dissociated material is surfacing. Further, it is wise to inform patients about the uncertain nature of memory itself, especially in patients with a variety of internal states containing differing and incomplete information that lacks integration and cohesion. Clinicians often have a relatively narrow understanding of the complexity of retrieved memories and the many differing ways reality may be perceived by patients. Patients may be more adequately informed as therapists learn the literature on memory, trauma, and how to consider the bizarre reports, for example, of sadistic ritual abuse (Sakheim & Devine, 1992; Young, 1992; Young, Sachs, Braun, & Watkins, 1991a). There is much to be learned from the literature of related fields, including anthropology, sociology, learning theory, hypnosis, and memory research, that will help therapists and patients alike become better informed about our evolving interpretation of dissociative disorders and dissociated material (Colligan, Pennebaker, & Murphy, 1982; Ganaway, 1989; Markush, 1973; Mulhern, 1991; Pettinati, 1988; Putnam, 1991; Sakheim & Devine, 1992; Watzlawick, 1984; Victor, 1993; Richardson, Best, & Bromley, 1991; Young et al., 1991a; Young, 1992).

Therefore, patients should be made aware of the potential sources for the contamination of memory and therapists should not attempt to establish the historical accuracy of memories as a primary therapeutic goal. Patients often seek validation from staff, which can misdirect their work into a fact-finding investigation instead of a treatment effort. Validation should be provided only when reliable corroborating data are available. When litigation is possible, hypnosis should be discussed carefully before being introduced in treatment, since in many states the use of this procedure may interfere or limit subsequent court testimony (Orne, 1979).

It is imperative that therapists working with dissociative disorders be aware of the present debate surrounding the existence of dissociative disorders and recovered memories of abuse. Much of this literature has polarized the field and taken extreme viewpoints or generalized a single representation of theory within the field as representative of what is actually a very rapidly evolving field with changing viewpoints which cannot be held accountable as a static model agreed by all within the field. Nonetheless there are important contributions from various disciplines that need to be incorporated into dissociation models as our experience develops.

This chapter cannot deal with all of these areas in depth but the reader is referred to a number of references for a more articulated discussion. Issues of validation have been approached by Coons (1994a,b), Briere & Conte (1993), Simpson (1995), Gelinas (1995), Kluft (1995), Terr (1994), and Williams (in press). Problems surrounding the use of hypnosis have wide discussions by Pettinati (1988), Mersky (1995), Lynn & Nash (1995), Yapko (1994) and American Psychiatric Association's statement on memories of sexual abuse (1993).

Numerous articles have addressed the validity of recovered memories including Loftus (1995), Koss et al. (1995), Brown (1995), Greaves (1992), Coons (1994), Spence (1994), Kihlstrom (1994), Spanos et al. (1994), and van der Kolk (1994).

A number of significant discussions are reported in related topics such as rumor panic Mulhern (1991, 1994), Victor (1993), Richardson et al. (1991), epidemic hysteria and fantasy by Wilson and Barber (1983), Collian et al. (1982), Young (1988), and Powers (1991). Several informative volumes are devoted to these discussions including Frankel & Perry (1994, 1995), American Journal of Clinical Hypnosis 36 (1994) and Cohen et al. (1995).

Appendixes 1 and 2 provide examples of informed consents used by the authors that may be adapted for individual use when treating dissociative patients or using hypnosis.

Staffing

Staffing patterns should be governed by acuity. A consistent staff should be available for adequate continuity of care and for the development of specialized skills. Four patients per staff member is a recommended when possible: preferred by the authors. Evenings may need to be staffed more intensely since evenings are likely to pose problems for individuals who were abused at night or who have sleep disturbances, and patients are more likely to be in program activity or seeing individual therapists during the day.

Social Services should be available, and a full-time person for every 10 to 12 patients is optimal. Social Services are essential to explore needed resources for patients, to communicate with referring therapists, and to assess and work with families. It is important that children be assessed or referred for evaluation when indicated, since dissociative disorders occur more frequently in family members when one member has a dissociative disorder (Braun, 1985). Further, children of abused parents are generally at higher risk of being abused. Last, the family as a whole may need support in dealing with the stress of living with a family member having a dissociative disorder (Benjamin & Benjamin, 1992; Sachs, 1986; Sachs, Frischoltz, & Wood, 1988).

Discharge Planning

This should be initiated even as hospitalization begins, with the goals for hospitalization clearly in focus. Regular treatment planning and contacts with community supports and the referring therapist are essential. A summary of treatment recommendations given to the referring therapist provides needed continuity in the transition to outpatient care.

Expressive Therapies

The use of art therapy (Cohen & Cox, 1989; Mills & Cohen, 1993), sand tray work (Sachs, 1990), movement therapy, and occupational therapy add essential dimensions to verbal work, and is discussed in more detail elsewhere in this volume (see Chapter 25). Specialized treatments should be provided by trained or certified therapists familiar with dissociation and trauma. Expressive modalities allow a broader dimension for patient work. These modalities foster a reconnection for patients with their self-expression, with their bodies, and the learning of healthy body attitudes that were distorted when their bodies were sources of pain and the objects of intrusive violations. Journaling, as previously mentioned, can be creatively used to establish inner dialogue, problem-solving skills, or exploring private information in new ways, in addition to merely maintaining a trauma diary or poems of suffering. Adams (1990, 1993) has written extensively in this area. These modalities allow a freer access to dissociated information held in other states or the representing information that is too painful or feels too forbidden to express verbally.

There are numerous clinical issues applicable to dissociative patients, and a well-rounded program establishes groups or treatment plans that address a variety of these. Table 3 gives a partial list of some problem areas that are frequently encountered in these patients.

Groups should be run by skilled therapists, and it is advisable when possible to have a cotherapist who can help maintain group focus and lend continuity if the therapist is away. Patients who are disruptive or cannot work effectively may be asked to stay out of groups until they can work effectively and stay in control. Patients should be allowed to leave groups if they are overwhelmed. If this is a regular occurrence, a reevaluation of their suitability for the troublesome groups is in order. Groups should be selectively assigned at treatment planning conferences.

When group size exceeds 10 to 12 patients, it is advisable to duplicate groups. The authors do not object if patients switch in groups as long as the patient is not a disruption and is able to make use of the group activity.

Treatment Planning

Treatment planning should include the treating therapists as well as the various clinical disciplines on the team. Weekly staffings keep everyone updated on the

Table 3. Some Suggested Topics for Program Content

1. Grief and loss
2. Coping with dissociation
3. Sexuality, gender
4. Relationships, attachment, trust, and intimacy
5. Becoming empowered, taking initiatives
6. Daily living, social and work skills
7. Women's and men's issues
8. Correcting cognitive distortions and improving reality testing
9. Eating disorders
10. Living with pain
11. Surviving incest and perpetration
12. Spirituality and existential crises
13. Crisis management
14. Marital and parenting skills
15. Substance abuse
16. Group processes and interactional skills
17. Suicidal, self-mutilating, and aggressive behaviors
18. Emotional control, impulse control, maintaining safety
19. Creativity, leisure, and fun
20. Self-esteem
21. Recognizing pathological or reenactment behaviors

patient's progress and allow a coordinated plan. Patients may attend if they assist in the planning and are not disruptive. At a minimum, they should provide input to the team and have their care plans explained to them.

When self-destructive, acting out, or abusive behaviors occur, staff needs to respond definitively. Staff may decide to alter the treatment plan, remove the patient from the general milieu, or keep them out of the regular program and provide substitute tasks that focus on understanding and controlling the aberrant behaviors. When this work is completed, the patient can reenter the program.

Aggressive Personality States

Frequently, patients harbor one or more aggressive personality states that threaten or present a history of dangerous behavior. These states often press for self-destructive, self-mutilating behaviors or suicide attempts that necessitate clinical interventions.

Aggressive personality states usually reflect an identification with alleged early perpetrators and should be understood as defensive functions that have, albeit illogically, a survival value. Patients often perceive dissociated material to be forbidden, or as children they feared retribution if they revealed their abuse. A state that induces self-destructive behavior when material surfaces assures safety by maintaining silence and keeping the patient from revealing information that in the past would have put them in danger.

In working with these states, caution should be exercised not to encourage their presenting externally until the system can assure safety. Early communications may be through writing, mediating through other alters, or by use of finger signals. An appreciation of their function should be conveyed and efforts should reflect an interest in their inclusion in the patient's whole dissociative system and not in their elimination. The patient needs to acknowledge these states and the issues that led to their particular function. These may initially be unknown by these states as well, especially as these states developed disconnected attitudes through secondary dissociations. As these states develop working alliances and work with their own issues, the internal perpetration stops and the patient starts resolving the issues underlying the development of these aggressive personality states. Aggressive personalities eventually see the dissociated issues as their own concerns, as well. It should always be recognized that each personality state's issues are, in fact, the issues of the single, whole patient being treated.

MEDICATION

There is no specific pharmacological therapy for dissociative disorders. In general, inpatient medication usage should be guided by the symptoms dominating the clinical picture (Loewenstein, 1991). Since most patients experience depression, anxiety, and posttraumatic stress symptoms, targeting these areas with established regimens is the most appropriate. Medications should be used judiciously and discontinued if not effective. Patients often end up with a potpourri of medications as one drug is added to another for persistent symptoms. It is not likely that all symptoms will be controlled as completely as desired and overmedication is a continuous hazard. Treatment is most effective if symptoms pervade most of the patient's dissociative system. Caution is warranted in patients with a history of substance abuse as they may be at risk for drug dependency. Last, the therapist needs to be aware of patient compliance and whether patients are actively suicidal and prone to overdosing.

Affective Disorders

Many patients can be expected to have a significant depressive overlay during the course of treatment. It is important to assess the patient's system as a whole. If most states show depressive features, antidepressant treatment is warranted. Adequate trials should be undertaken, and when ineffective, medications should be discontinued.

Both tricyclics and monoamine oxidase inhibitors have been effective, but one can expect that significant affective disturbance may remain while painful material continues to emerge and be processed. If they are carefully monitored, adjunctive medications such as lithium, thyroid, or psychostimulants can augment antidepressant medication. Van der Kolk (1987) has found fluoxetine useful for posttraumatic stress disorders. If agitation is severe, using more sedative drugs such as amitriptyline or trazodone may be useful and given at bedtime to enhance sleep. Newer antidepressants such as paroxetine, bupropion, and sertraline may also find their place.

Bipolar disorders should be screened as they can easily be overlooked due to the shifting clinical picture in MPD. Family history and careful monitoring may assist in diagnosis.

Dissociative patients need especially close monitoring and some personality states may harbor suicidal impulses not acknowledged in general questioning. Checking the whole "system" or some personality that knows the internal state may permit a more accurate assessment of suicidal risk and the potential for overdosing.

Anxiety

Panic and anxiety are especially common symptoms and it is often necessary to use anxiolytic medications. Patients should expect that their symptoms will not be entirely alleviated. Use of medications is directed to reducing anxiety so that patients can usefully process material as functionally as possible without overseda-tion. Judicious use of benzodiazepines can be used. Longer-acting preparations result in smoother blood levels. Several reports have shown that clonazepam is effective (Loewenstein, 1991; Loewenstein, Hornstein, & Farber, 1988). Because it is generally used in seizure disorders, informed consent should be given that it is being used for symptoms for which it was not developed.

Antipsychotic medications have not usually been effective and often produce a feeling of further depersonalization. It adds the additional risk of tardive dyskinesia. In occasional instances, especially if there are psychotic features, neuroleptic medi-cations have helped. Caution should be taken to discontinue them if there is no clinical improvement.

Braun (1990) and Barkin et al. (1986) have described the use of propranolol in large doses with careful monitoring of pulse and blood pressure. Improvement is seen in patients that experience rapid switching. Informed consent is required for non-FDA usage and one needs to watch for depressive side effects and medical contraindications when using beta blockers.

Sleep Disturbances

Many patients report insomnia and nightmares. If this is a major problem that is not controlled by other medications or hypnotic techniques, sedative medication can be helpful. When possible, antianxiety or sedating antidepressant medications can be used at bedtime to avoid adding additional medications. Otherwise, the use of sedative hypnotics may be intermittently necessary and discontinued if their effectiveness stops.

Pain Medication

Pain symptoms are a frequent and ticklish problem. Most patients suffer so-matic pains related to the emergence of dissociated material. Dissociative patients also have a high incidence of headaches. For this reason it is common for patients to request pain medications. The decision to use pain medications must be carefully measured against the potential for addiction. One general guideline used by the authors is to resist addictive pain medication in cases of somatic symptoms without demonstrable physical cause. One needs to be aware, however, that patients may actually have physical ailments, including migraine headaches, where the judicious use of pain medications is appropriate.

Excellent summaries of medications for posttraumatic stress disorder and dissociative disorders have been published by Barkin et al. (1986), Braun (1990), van der Kolk (1987), Loewenstein (1991), Loewenstein et al. (1988), Putnam (1989), and Ross (1989) and elsewhere in this volume (see Chapter 26). The clinician is encouraged to consult these.

CONCLUSION

Inpatient treatment of dissociative disorders is an interim treatment warranted to restore sufficient stability to allow continued outpatient care. Long stays should be avoided unless adequate justification is present to prevent regression and disruption in the patient's outside life. Inpatient treatment provides a valuable treatment resource when patients become overwhelmed or require a structured, safe setting for evaluation and treatment during periods when outpatient care is not sufficient.

For most effective results, hospital staff need a good understanding of the dynamics, clinical features, and problems these patients present so that they can respond appropriately and with a minimum of countertransference interference. Staff and patients should each be clear about reasonable hospital goals and the limits and boundaries of the inpatient milieu and staff treatment interventions. Staff guidelines are a major help in maintaining this consistency. A variety of evaluations and treatment approaches can be developed to educate patients and resolve inner conflicts when well-trained therapists are available.

In the current climate of shorter inpatient stays and financial cutbacks, mental health hospitals will need to be increasingly aware of useful, focused interventions that are efficient and still effective in returning patients to outpatient care. Even as our present understandings are shaping our treatment strategies, new insights are emerging that may offer even more effective interventions. Increasing communication between different treatment centers and outcome research studies are needed to document the beneficial effects of hospital care and determine which patients will benefit most from this intervention.

APPENDIX 1: INFORMED CONSENT REGARDING THE TREATMENT OF TRAUMATIC AND DISSOCIATIVE DISORDERS

This information is offered to give you important information about your treatment and provide you with an informed basis with which to understand the benefits and potential pitfalls in the treatment of traumatic and dissociative disorders. It is not meant to undermine your personal experience or make light of any work you have done. Rather, it is felt that an informed person will be able to weigh the risks and benefits of treatment and to be aware of problem areas that may have a bearing on your recovery. This can help you make the most responsible decisions about your own treatment and in the interpretation of traumatic material that may emerge as you progress.

There are many issues that you need to know about your treatment. Many patients experience a variety of problems in the course of their treatment that include flashbacks, flooding of emotions, overstimulation, nightmares, anxiety and panic attacks, suicidality, self-destructive or angry impulses, depression, increased dissociative behavior, and feelings of disorganization. There may be a need for hospital care at times. Some people may have trouble maintaining employment or have problems with their social and family relationships. It is possible to feel worse before one feels better, and some people may not feel they get better but just feel worse. Others may find they regularly feel better. Your therapy can feel demanding, and it is important that you develop friends, helpful support, activities, and other personal resources to turn to if you are in a crisis and your therapist is not available. These problems can be anticipated and discussed with your therapist.

On the other hand, most people coming into treatment are already having severe symptoms and feel they need to enter treatment because of the problems that they are already facing. In most cases, therapy may be the only way to regain a sense of balance and health. You must decide whether the risks of treatment, even if it turns out not to be helpful, is acceptable if it offers a hope for a happier and more integrated life.

The treatment of traumatic and dissociative disorders is still evolving, and it is not possible to predict what your treatment experience will be. This will also depend upon factors in you and your fit with your therapist.

Ordinarily your treatment will include a variety of components to help you gain self-control and improve your personal relationships and your functioning in the present. It will address erroneous patterns of thinking, the re-enactment of old conflicts through your behavior, and help to resolve the residuals of trauma and abuse. Treatment can take months or years for some and be much briefer for others. There is no way to predict a length of therapy. Hospitalization should be as brief as possible to prevent an interruption of your life.

There are other approaches that are available to you or that can be used simultaneously. These include a variety of traditional psychotherapies, group therapies, cognitive therapies, behavioral modification techniques, careful use of hypnosis, eye movement desensitization and reprocessing (EMDR or accelerated information processing AIP), and the use of a variety of medications. Some people feel treatment makes them feel worse and prefer to stop. You need to discuss your plan with your therapist. Consultations or a second opinion can always be requested if you feel stuck.

The mental health field is presently divided in their beliefs and understanding about dissociation and the validity of repressed memories retrieved in adulthood or during treatment. On one end of the spectrum are therapists that accept all material as accurate with no independent corroboration, and they may even suggest the presence of abuse memories based on symptoms even when memories are absent. On the other end of the spectrum are those who do not believe abuse memories are repressed, that repressed memories for severe abuse do not occur but are implanted by poorly informed therapists into unwitting, naive, or suggestible patients. Given this division, even among many credible professionals, an awareness of what we believe is exceedingly important so that your treatment leads you to your own conclusions and you are aware of alternative approaches from which to choose. It is hoped that informed decisions and an open mind will give you the best chance to heal.

Studies to date have clearly established the presence of child sexual, physical, and emotional abuse. They have also shown that a variety of adult behaviors and symptoms are correlated with a history of abuse. There are, however, instances where abuse may not always lead to significant disturbance, and simultaneously many symptomatic individuals may not have a history of severe abuse. Reports of memories for abuse do not guarantee its authenticity. Nor, on the other hand, does a failure to recall abuse mean that none was present.

Our best understanding at present is that memories of abuse may be accurate, distorted, confabulated, dissociated, or repressed from conscious recall or contaminated by a variety of other factors.

Further, memories of traumatic events may change over time as new information that is repressed or discovered becomes available. For this reason, it is wise to suspend judgement on memories until sufficient time has elapsed to allow the dissociated information to emerge and cognitive distortions to be corrected so a fuller and more accurate assimilation of retrieved material can be completed and a clearer perspective and meaning of these events can be integrated.

You should know that amnesia for traumatic events and child abuse is a regularly documented finding. What is less well known, and often objected to on the basis of its appearing to reinjure abuse survivors, is the recognition that people can under a variety of circumstances appear to remember events that, in fact, never happened. In other instances, events may have happened quite differently than they are remembered. Even inaccurate recall, however, does not mean that some kind of abuse did not occur.

Inaccurate recollections can, in some instances, be experienced as being so real and vivid and be accompanied by such significant physical sensations or body pain that they are accepted as real memories with absolute conviction.

This is not meant to discount what you know but to permit you the widest possible latitude in reconstructing your life. Memory is a complicated business. Real memory can also be recalled with intensity, vividness and physical sensations that reflect a representation of the original trauma. This is especially true with repressed memory and particularly in dissociative conditions. In dissociative conditions, the manner in which traumatic material is stored makes this problem especially difficult since both accurate, distorted and inaccurate information can be experienced similarly and believed with the same conviction.

There is no way that professionals can tell with certainty the historical accuracy of any account, and therefore it is important to know that professionals cannot validate the historical truth of any memory. The concern about being unable to validate an individual's account of their personal history is presented to help you know the limitations of therapy, and that validation would be something you would have to establish for yourself with independent corroboration or allow your therapist, if it were appropriate, to contact people in your life directly to attempt to clarify what was true, despite knowing from the literature that there is a pattern of denial in families where abuse has occurred. This would only be recommended if it were therapeutically indicated and then only with your written consent.

This information is not meant to discount the impact of your suffering, nor to suggest that you not discuss the material that emerges in your treatment. Recollections, even in people who may inadvertently have accepted inaccurate information as memories, will continue to have a significant impact on how people organize and think about their lives. These recollections, despite the issue of accuracy, are still what shape self-esteem, influence behavior, and provide meaning and perspective for people's lives. It is still important, however, that you know that severe child abuse is a known fact and that severe trauma can be forgotten and dissociated by many people and in a variety of situations.

There are times when people recall memories of things that have not occurred to them, and more problematic still are those who will purposefully present false memory for their own reasons. A professional therapist has no way of knowing the difference and must help those who may be unknowingly reporting erroneous memory by periodically challenging or trying to understand material in new ways to allow some people to arrive at different or more accurate formulations about their recollections and the impact these recollections have had.

Unfortunately we cannot distinguish malingering based only on a person's reports either. This does not take away from the seriousness of the problems faced by real survivors. Professionals have encountered memories they have not believed that subsequently turned out to be true, and similarly they have encountered memories they believed to be true that have turned out not to be. This requires that therapists and patients alike work without a pre-established bias and tolerate the ambiguity of what emerges in treatment. This will allow you to grow and resolve what you decide is true for you. The National Treatment Center and your therapist may write or use terms such as "recall," "memory," "repressed memory," "a history of," and similar terms. In the absence of external corroboration, the only responsible position for you, your treatment team, the National Treatment Center and, your therapist is to know that these terms are used for convenience in communicating and not as a statement of validation of their historical truth.

This is true not only in the treatment of trauma survivors but in the treatment of all patients where the therapist and patient work only with material that is reported. The treatment remains focused on helping to resolve the patient's suffering and not on establishing historical accuracy.

Some other possibilities suggested for contamination of memory include persuasion by therapists, hypnotic suggestibility, the unwitting recalling of someone else's experiences as one's own memories, the effects of hysterical contagion as in the spread of rumors, mistaking fantasy for reality, deception, substituting a false memory for a more painful reality, the confusion of memory that was encoded during states of disorganization when a preverbal or immature child was not capable of storing memory realistically, and a variety of other possibilities as well. Even in dissociative disorders there are a variety of coexisting yet different "realities" which are believed simultaneously.

There are a variety of explanations offered to explain false memory production. While these explanations have been hypothesized, many have not been studied. Further, there is a great deal of research information about memory that is learned from nonclinical populations that may not apply to you. Professionals still have a lot to learn about the problems of memory in nontraumatic situations and more still about the problems of processing memory in survivors of abuse. One cannot necessarily translate information about memory in nontraumatized people to those who were traumatized. It is hoped that the issue of false memories and the polarized viewpoints among professionals can be put aside so that you can receive the best possible treatment for your condition.

You also need to know that many, many people have been successfully treated and feel better after entering treatment for their traumatic and dissociative conditions. While treatment approaches may continue to change as professionals learn more, we feel that treatment results do provide a significant hope and expectation for improvement so that you can enter treatment with an understanding that many people have markedly improved or recovered.

* * * *

I have read the above information about the treatment of my condition. I have discussed questions I may have had and understand the complexities involved in my treatment and with memory in general. I understand I can assist in my treatment planning and I can discontinue treatment at any time. I agree to treatment based on my own informed with to proceed and at my own risk as well as my potential benefit.

____________________________ ____________
Patient's Signature *Date*

____________________________ ____________
Witness *Date*

APPENDIX 2: INFORMED CONSENT FOR USE OF CLINICAL HYPNOSIS

Before deciding to use clinical hypnosis, it is important that you understand the use of clinical hypnosis in the treatment of dissociative and traumatic disorders. Hypnosis is a valuable tool, but has been the subject of considerable controversy amongst clinicians in the field. For this reason, it is important that you understand some basic issues about hypnosis to be adequately informed.

Hypnosis is an altered state of consciousness which has a number of characteristics. These include a capacity for deep absorption in the hypnotic state with a reduction in the awareness of external events, an alteration in one's perception of reality and a high level of suggestibility, and a suspension of critical judgement, including the evaluation of information retrieved during the hypnotic state. These characteristics are more prominent in people who have dissociative conditions and, therefore, contaminations of memory and information retrieved in hypnotic states are more prone to occur. All of these features combine to increase the possibility of producing inaccurate, distorted or false memories. The hypnotic state can result in the confusion between reality, one's fantasy life, suggestions or demands from a therapist, and the influence of other stimuli occurring in hypnosis that may alter the realistic interpretation of retrieved information.

Research with hypnosis has demonstrated that hypnosis may enhance memory, but also distort or lead to the production of false information that is still perceived as memory. This is due to the nature of hypnosis, the demand quality inherent in some hypnotic suggestions as well as the individual's expectations of what a therapist may be wanting to discover. Further, information may be retrieved in a hypnotic state that is accompanied by high levels of intensity, body sensations and a conviction that the information is accurate, despite evidence that the information was the product of contamination or hypnotic suggestion. On the other hand, hypnosis is capable of enhancing real memory and retrieving real information which has been repressed or forgotten. Individuals in a hypnotic state may not be able to distinguish the difference between information that is accurate and information that is artifact.

Hypnotic studies, however, have not adequately studied the accuracy of hypnotic retrieval of dissociated memory for traumatic events. The uncertainty of hypnotic memory retrieval means that information retrieved in hypnosis should be accepted only with caution and a recognition that it may or may not be historically correct. There is no way of knowing whether any information that is retrieved through hypnosis is historically accurate. This can only be done by the independent validation of information that is retrieved. This is true of all memories reported in psychotherapy. These issues are particularly relevant for individuals with dissociative conditions since they are often highly suggestible and therefore, more prone to the complications of hypnosis in which the suspension of critical judgement, suggestibility, and the absorption in the experience may allow even greater degrees of distortion.

People with dissociative disorders are still more prone to accepting suggestions whether they are placed in formal hypnosis or not. Dissociative individuals are often in states of autohypnosis or self-induced trance, especially during psychotherapy sessions or periods of stress.

There are other sources of contamination. Subjects retrieving memories in hypnosis may recall information that they have heard from other sources or even of their own fears or fantasies and experience them as though they were memories. One forgets the original source of the information and subsequently feels as though it originated in oneself, attributing the emerging material to memory. This phenomena, known as source amnesia, is well known in hypnosis and can be very compelling.

Beyond the issue of memory, it is exceedingly important to be aware that in many legal jurisdictions and in different states, the use of hypnosis may have an impact in litigation. The use of hypnotically refreshed memory, for example, or simply the use of hypnosis may prevent or disqualify individuals from testifying in legal proceedings. It is important that you be aware of this in the event that you are involved in a legal action, or expect that you might utilize information that you learn in your treatment in a future legal action. Hypnosis may impede or prevent you from testifying. You may want to contact your attorney if the potential for litigation is relevant.

There are other complications that may occur with the use of hypnosis. These the include flooding of emotions, the development of flashbacks and traumatic imagery, the sudden return of highly charged traumatic memories that can lead to increased disorganization, suicidality, and self-destructive or aggressive behaviors. Hypnosis might result in premature emergence of information that you do not feel ready to manage. These problems may occur and produce the same symptoms without using clinical hypnosis.

Hypnosis, on the other hand, has many potential values. It may be used effectively for reducing anxiety, developing internal states of relaxation, or inducing guided imagery which can help during periods of crisis. Hypnosis may also help to gain information which is unavailable because it is contained in dissociated states. It may also be valuable in developing the capacity to have an internal dialogue between, or an awareness of, other internal states.

Hypnosis is not required for your treatment and many people have successfully completed treatment without it. You can utilize traditional forms of psychotherapy, groups, cognitive and behavioral techniques, the use of medications, and emotional containment strategies to develop a sense of safety in your treatment.

* * * *

I have been fully informed about the pitfalls as well as potential advantages of hypnosis. I am also aware that other forms of treatment such as psychotherapy, group therapies, cognitive therapies, and other forms of therapy are used very successfully and may reduce some of the risks surrounding memory distortion. I understand and give my consent to the utilization of hypnosis, knowing that I may discontinue it at any time.

________________________ ________________

Signed *Date*

________________________ ________________

Witness *Date*

REFERENCES

Adams, K. (1990). *Journal to the self: 22 paths to personal growth*. New York: Warner Books.

Adams, K. (1993). *The way of the journal: A journal therapy workbook for healing*. Lutherville, MD: Sidran Press.

American Medical Association (1985). Report of the American Medical Association Council on Scientific Affairs: Scientific status of refreshing recollection by the use of hypnosis. *Journal of the American Medical Association, 253*, 1918-1923.

American Psychiatric Association (1987). *Diagnostic and statistical manual of mental disorders* (3rd ed., rev.). Washington, DC: Author.

American Psychiatric Association (1994). *Diagnostic and statistical manual of mental disorders* (4th ed.). Washington, DC: Author.

Barach, P. M. (1994). *International Society for the Study of Dissociation (ISSD) guidelines for treating dissociative identity disorder (multiple personality disorder) in adults from standards of practice committee*.

Barkin, R., Braun, B. G., & Kluft, R. P. (1986). The dilemma of drug therapy for multiple personality disorder. In B. G. Braun (Ed.), *Treatment of multiple personality disorder* (pp. 107-132). Washington, DC: American Psychiatric Press.

Benjamin, L., & Benjamin, R. (1992). An overview of family treatment in dissociative disorders. *Dissociation, 5*, 236-241.

Bliss, E. L. (1986). *Multiple personality, allied disorders and hypnosis*. New York: Oxford University Press.

Bliss, E. L., & Jeppsen, E. A. (1985). Prevalence of multiple personality among inpatients and outpatients. *American Journal of Psychiatry, 142*, 250-251.

Board of Trustees, American Psychiatric Association (1993). *Statement on memories of sexual abuse*. Washington, DC: Author.

Braun, G. G. (1984). Uses of hypnosis with multiple personality disorder. *Psychiatric Annals, 14*, 34-40.

Braun, B. G. (1985). The transgenerational incidence of dissociation and multiple personality disorder: A preliminary report. In R. P. Kluft (Ed.), *Childhood antecedents of multiple personality* (pp. 127-150). Washington, DC: American Psychiatric Press.

Braun, B. G. (1986). Issues in the psychotherapy of multiple personality disorder. In B. G. Braun (Ed.), *Treatment of multiple personality disorder* (pp. 1-28). Washington, DC: American Psychiatric Press.

Braun, B. G. (1990). Unusual medication regimens in the treatment of dissociative disorder patients. Part I: Noradrenergic agents. *Dissociation, 3*, 144-150.

Braun, B. G. (1993). Aids to the treatment of multiple personality disorder on a general psychiatric inpatient unit. In R. P. Kluft, C. G. Fine (Eds.), *Clinical perspectives on multiple personality disorder* (pp. 155-178). Washington, DC: American Psychiatric Press.

Briere, J., & Conte, J. (1993). Self-reported amnesia for abuse in adults molested as children. *Journal of Traumatic Stress, 6*, 21-31.

Brown, D. (1995). Pseudomemories: The standard of science and the standard of care in trauma treatment. *American Journal of Clinical Hypnosis, 37*, 1-24.

Caul, D. (1984). Group and video tape techniques for multiple personality disorder. *Psychiatric Annals, 14*, 46-50.

Cohen, L. M., Bergoff, J. N., & Elin, M. R. (Eds.). (1995). *Dissociative identity disorder: Theoretical and treatment controversies*. Northvale, NJ: Aronson.

Cohen, B. M., & Cox, C. T. (1989). Breaking the code: Identification of multiplicity through art productions. *Dissociation, 2*, 132-137.

Colligan, M. J., Pennebaker, J. W., & Murphy, L. R. (1982). *Mass psychogenic illness: A social psychological analysis*. Hills Dale, NJ: Erlbaum.

Coons, P. M. (1994a). Confirmation of child abuse in child and adolescent cases of multiple personality disorder and dissociative disorder not otherwise specified. *Journal of Nervous and Mental Diseases, 182*, 461-464.

Coons, P. M. (1994b). Report of Satanic ritual abuse: Further implications about pseudomemories. *Perceptual and Motor Skills, 78*, 1376-1378.

Coons, P. M., Bowman, E. S., & Milstein, V. (1988). Multiple personality disorder: A clinical investigation of 50 cases. *Journal of Nervous and Mental Disease, 176*, 519-527.

Fine, C. G. (1988). Thoughts on the cognitive perceptual substrates of multiple personality disorder. *Dissociation, 1*, 5-10.

Fine, C. G. (1991). Treatment stabilization and crisis prevention: Pacing the therapy of the multiple personality disorder patient. *Psychiatric Clinics of North America, 14*, 661-675.

Frankel, F. H., & Perry, C. W. (Eds.) (1994). Special issue: Hypnosis and delayed recall: Part I. *International Journal of Clinical and Experimental Hypnosis, 42*.

Frankel, F. H., & Perry, C. W. (Eds.) (1994). Special issue: Hypnosis and delayed recall: Part II. *International Journal of Clinical and Experimental Hypnosis, 43*.

Frischholz, E. (Ed.) (1994). *American Journal of Clinical Hypnosis, 36*.

Ganaway, G. K. (1989). Historical versus narrative truth: Clarifying the role of exogenous trauma in the etiology of MPD and its variants. *Dissociation, 2*, 205-220.

Garry, M., & Loftus, E. (1994). Pseudomemories without hypnosis. *International Journal of Clinical and Experimental Hypnosis, 42*, 363-378.

Gelinas, D. J. (1995). Dissociative identity disorders and the trauma paradigm. In L. M. Cohen, J. N. Bergoff, M. R. Elin (Eds.) *Dissociative identity disorder: Theoretical and treatment controversies* (pp. 175-222). Northvale, NJ: Aronson.

Greaves, G. B. (1980). Multiple personality: 165 years after Mary Reynolds. *Journal of Nervous and Mental Disease, 168*, 577–596.

Greaves, G. B. (1992). Alternative hypotheses regarding claims of Satanic cults: A critical analysis." In D. K. Sakheim & S. F. Devine (Eds.) *Out of darkness: Exploring Satanism and ritual abuse*. New York: Lexington Books.

Greaves, G. B. (1993). A history of multiple personality disorder. In R. P. Kluft & C. G. Fine (Eds.), *Clinical perspectives on multiple personality disorder* (pp. 335–380). Washington, DC: American Psychiatric Press.

Herman, J. L. (1992). *Trauma and recovery*. New York: Basic Books.

Horowitz, M. J. (1986). *Stress response syndromes*. Northvail, NJ: Jason Aronson.

Kihlstrom, J. F. (1994). Hypnosis, delayed recall, and the principles of memory. *International Journal of Clinical and Experimental Hypnosis, 42*, 337–345.

Klein, H., Mann, D. R., & Goodwin, J. M. (1994). Obstacles to the recognition of sexual abuse and dissociative disorders in child and adolescent males. *Dissociation*, 7, 138–144.

Kluft, R. P. (1982). Varieties of hypnotic intervention in the treatment of multiple personality. *American Journal of Clinical Hypnosis, 24*, 230–240.

Kluft, R. P. (1983). Hypnotherapeutic crisis intervention in multiple personality. *American Journal of Clinical Hypnosis, 26*, 73–83.

Kluft, R. P. (1984a). Aspects of the treatment of multiple personality disorder. *Psychiatric Annals, 14*, 51–55.

Kluft, R. P. (1984b). Treatment of multiple personality: A study of 33 cases. *Psychiatric Clinics of North America*, 7, 9–29.

Kluft, R. P. (1989). Playing for time: Temporizing techniques in the treatment of multiple personality disorder. *American Journal of Clinical Hypnosis, 32*, 90–98.

Kluft, R. P. (1990). Incest and subsequent revictimization: The case of therapist-patient sexual exploitation, with a description of the sitting duck syndrome. In R. P. Kluft (Ed.), *Incest-related syndromes of adult psychopathology* (pp. 263–287). Washington, DC: American Psychiatric Press.

Kluft, R. P. (1991a). Multiple personality disorder. In A. Tasman & S. M. Goldfinger (Eds.), *American Psychiatric Press annual review of psychiatry* (Vol. 10, pp. 161–188). Washington, DC: American Psychiatric Press.

Kluft, R. P. (1991b). Hospital treatment of multiple personality disorder: An overview. *Psychiatric Clinics of North America, 14*, 695–719.

Kluft, R. P. (1994). *Editorial: Ruminations on metamorphoses. Dissociation*, 7, 138–144.

Kluft, R. P. (1995). Current controversies surrounding dissociative identity disorder. In L. M. Cohen, J. N. Bergoff, & M. R. Elin (Eds.), *Dissociative identity disorder: Theoretical and treatment controversies* (pp. 347–378). Northvale, NJ: Aronson.

Koss, M. P., Trompe, S. & Tharan, M. (1995). Traumatic memories: Empirical foundations, forensic and clinical implications. *Clinical Psychology: Science and Practice, 2*, 111–132.

Kroll, J. (1993). *PTSD/borderlines in therapy: Finding the balance*. New York: Norton.

Lanning, K. V. (1992). A law enforcement perspective on allegations of ritual abuse. In D. K. Sakheim & S. F. Devine (Eds.), *Out of Darkness: Exploring Satanism and Ritual Abuse* (pp. 109–146). New York: Lexington Books.

Loewenstein, R. J. (1991). Rational psychopharmacology in the treatment of multiple personality disorder. *Psychiatric Clinics of North America, 14*, 721–740.

Loewenstein, R. J., Hornstein, N., & Farber, B. (1988). Open trial of clonazepam in the treatment of posttraumatic stress symptoms in MPD. *Dissociation, 1*, 3–12.

Loftus, E. (1993). Reality of repressed memories. *American Psychologist, 48*, 518–537.

Loftus, E. (1995). *The myth of repressed memory: False memories and allegations of sexual abuse*. New York: St. Martin's Press.

Lynn, F. J. & Nash, M. R. (1995). Truth in memory: Ramifications for psychotherapy and hypnotherapy. *American Journal of Clinical Hypnosis, 36*, 194–208.

Markush, R. E. (1973). Mental epidemics—A review of the old to prepare for the new. *Public Health Reviews, 2*, 353–442.

Mersky, H. (1995). The manufacture of personalities: The production of multiple personality disorder. In L. M. Cohen, J. N. Bergoff, & M. R. Elin (Eds.), *Dissociative identity disorder: Theoretical and treatment controversies* (pp. 3–32). Northvale, NJ: Aronson.

Mills, A., & Cohen, B. M. (1993). Facilitating the identification of multiple personality disorder through art: The diagnostic drawing series. In E. Kluft (Ed.), *Expressive and functional therapies in the treatment of multiple personality disorder* (pp. 39-66). Springfield, IL: Charles C. Thomas.

Mulhern, S. (1991). Embodied alternative identities: Bearing witness to a world that might have been. *Psychiatric Clinics of North America, 14*, 769-786.

Mulhern, S. (1994). Satanism, ritual abuse and multiple personality disorder: A sociohistorical perspective. *International Journal of Clinical and Experimental Hypnosis, 42*, 265-288.

Nash, M. R. (1994). Memory distortion and sexual trauma: The problem of false negatives and false positives. *International Journal of Clinical and Experimental Hypnosis, 42*, 346-361.

Orne, M. T. (1979). The use and misuse of hypnosis in court. *International Journal of Clinical and Experimental Hypnosis, 27*, 311-341.

Pettinati, H. M. (Ed.). (1988). *Hypnosis and memory*. New York: Guilford Press.

Powers, F. M. (1991). Fantasy-proneness, amnesia, and the UFO abduction phenomena. *Dissociation, 4*, 46-54.

Putnam, F. W. (1985). Dissociation as a response to extreme trauma. In R. P. Kluft (Ed.), *Childhood antecedents of multiple personality disorder* (pp. 65-97). Washington, DC: American Psychiatric Press.

Putnam, F. W. (1986). The treatment of multiple personality: State of the art. In B. G. Braun (Ed.), *Treatment of multiple personality disorder* (pp. 175-198). Washington, DC: American Psychiatric Press.

Putnam, F. W. (1989). *Diagnosis and treatment of multiple personality disorder*. New York: Guilford Press.

Putnam, F. W. (1991). The satanic ritual abuse controversy. *Child Abuse and Neglect, 15*, 175-179.

Putnam, F. W., Guroff, J. J., Silberman, E. K., Barban, L. S., & Post, R. N. (1986). The clinical phenomenology of multiple personality disorder: A review of 100 recent cases. *Journal of Clinical Psychiatry, 47*, 285-293.

Quimby, L. G., Andrei, A., & Putnam, F. W. (1993). The deinstitutionalization of patients with chronic multiple personality disorder. In R. P. Kluft & C. G. Fine (Eds.), *Clinical perspectives on multiple personality disorder* (pp. 201-226). Washington, DC: American Psychiatric Press.

Richardson, J. T., Best, J., & Bromley, D. G. (1991). *The satanism scare*. New York: Aldine de Gruyer.

Ross, C. A. (1989). *Multiple personality disorder: Diagnosis, clinical features and treatment*. New York: John Wiley.

Ross, C. A. (1995). The validity and reliability of dissociative identity disorder. In L. M. Cohen, J. N. Bergoff, & M. R. Elin (Eds.), *Dissociative identity disorder: Theoretical and treatment controversies* (pp. 65-86). Northvale, NJ: Aronson.

Ross, C. A. (1991). Epidemiology of multiple personality disorder and dissociation. *Psychiatric Clinics of North America, 14*, 503-518.

Ross, C. A., Norton, G. R., & Wozney, K. (1989). Multiple personality disorder: An analysis of 236 cases. *Canadian Journal of Psychiatry, 34*, 413-418.

Sachs, R. G. (1986). The adjunctive role of social support systems in the treatment of multiple personality disorder. In E. G. Braun (Ed.), *Treatment of multiple personality disorder* (pp. 157-174). Washington, DC: American Psychiatric Press.

Sachs, R. G. (1990). The sandtray technique in the treatment of patients with dissociative disorders: Recommendations for occupational therapists. *American Journal of Occupational Therapy, 44*, 1045-1047.

Sachs, R. G., Frischoltz, E. J., & Wood, J. I. (1988). Marital and family therapy in the treatment of multiple personality disorder. *Journal of Marital and Family Therapy, 14*, 249-259.

Sakheim, D., & Devine, S. (1992). *Out of darkness—Exploring satanism and ritual abuse*. New York: Lexington Books.

Sakheim, D. K., Hess, E. P., & Chivas, A. (1986). General principles for short-term inpatient work with multiple personality disorder. *Psychotherapy, 25*, 117-124.

Simpson, M. A. (1995). Gullible's travels, or the importance of being multiple. In L. M. Cohen, J. M. Bergoff, and M. R. Elin (Eds.), *Dissociative identity disorder: Theoretical and treatment controversies* (pp. 87-134). Northvale, NJ: Aronson.

Spanos, N. P., Burgess, C. A. & Burgess, M. F. (1994). Past-life identities, UFO abductions, and satanic ritual abuse: The social construction of memories. *International Journal of Clinical and Experimental Hypnosis, 42*, 433-436.

Spence, D. P. (1994). Narrative truth and putative child abuse. *International Journal of Clinical and Experimental Hypnosis, 42*, 289-303.

Spiegel, D. (1984). Multiple personality as a post-traumatic stress disorder. *Psychiatric Clinics of North America*, 7, 101-110.

Terr, L. (1990). *Too scared to cry: Psychic trauma in childhood*. New York: Harper & Row.

Terr, L. (1994). *Unchained memories: True stories of traumatic memories, lost and found*. New York: Basic Books.

Van Benschoten, S. C. (1990). Multiple personality disorder and satanic ritual abuse: The issue of credibility. *Dissociation, 3*, 22-30.

Van der Kolk, B. A. (1987). *Psychological trauma*. Washington, DC: American Psychiatric Press.

Van der Kolk, B. A. (1989). The compulsion to repeat the trauma: Re-enactment, revictimization and masochism. *Psychiatric Clinics of North America, 12*, 389-411.

Van der Kolk, B. A. (1994). The body keeps the score: Memory and the evolving psychobiology of posttraumatic stress. *Harvard Review of Psychiatry, 1*, 253-265.

Victor, J. S. (1993). *Satanic panic: The creation of a contemporary legend*. Chicago: Open Court.

Watzlawick, P. (1984). *The invented reality: How do we know what we believe we know? Contributions to constructivism*. New York: Norton.

Williams, L. M. (in press). Adult memories of childhood abuse: Preliminary findings from a longitudinal study. *The Advisor*.

Wilson, S. C. & Barber, T. X. (1993). Fantasy-prone personality: Implications for understanding imagery, hypnosis and parapsychological phenomena. In H. A. Sheik (Ed.), *Imagery: Current Theory, Research, and Application* (pp. 340-387). New York: John Wiley.

Yapko, M. D. (1994). Suggestibility and repressed memories of abuse: A survey of psychotherapists' beliefs. *American Journal of Clinical Hypnosis, 36*, 163-171.

Young, W. C. (1988a). Observations on fantasy in the formation of multiple personality disorder. *Dissociation, 1*, 13-20.

Young, W. C. (1988b). Psychodynamics and dissociation: All that switches is not split. *Dissociation, 1*, 33-38.

Young, W. C. (1992). Recognition and treatment of survivors reporting ritual abuse. In D. Sakheim & S. Devine (Eds.), *Out of darkness—Exploring satanism and ritual abuse* (pp. 249-278). New York: Lexington Books.

Young, W. C., Sachs, R. G., Braun, B. G., & Watkins, R. T. (1991a). Patients reporting ritual abuse in childhood: A clinical syndrome. *International Journal of Child Abuse and Neglect, 15*, 181-189.

25

Art and the Dissociative Paracosm

Uncommon Realities

Barry M. Cohen

> Art must venture into areas of experience that are not yet clearly understood and perhaps never will be.
>
> MIHALY CSIKSZENTMIHALYI (1978)

INTRODUCTION

During the last decade, increasing attention has been given to the long-term sequelae of incestuous and sadistic early childhood abuse and, more specifically, the dissociative symptomatology that results (e.g., Courtois, 1988; Herman, 1992; Kluft, 1985, 1990; Loewenstein, 1991; McCann & Pearlman, 1990; Putnam, 1989; Ross, 1989). A body of research has grown to complement the observations of practitioners and their eminent predecessors, such as Janet and Prince, regarding the variform trauma in young children and the development of chronic posttraumatic dissociation (Boon & Draijer, 1993; Herman, Perry, & van der Kolk, 1989; Loewenstein, 1993; Putnam, 1991).

Those who have chosen to study and treat this complex and demanding population are aware that voluminous creative productions can be generated by many of these clients (Coons, 1988). When such productions are brought into the treatment context, their mere presence has galvanized some psychotherapists into incorporating art into therapy without training themselves in the therapeutic use of art. This is certainly tempting, and at first seems expeditious; the art is visually and

Barry M. Cohen • P.O. Box 9853, Alexandria, Virginia 22304.

Handbook of Dissociation: Theoretical, Empirical, and Clinical Perspectives, edited by Larry K. Michelson and William J. Ray. Plenum Press, New York, 1996.

emotionally compelling and contains important information about its makers and their personal worlds. Further, therapists often feel deskilled at one point or another during the course of treatment, and some have responded to this phenomenon by consciously or unwittingly engaging in unconventional practices (professional and/or personal) that they would not consider with nondissociative clients (Fine, 1990). It is the author's observation that therapists who make the choice to treat this segment of the traumatized population are typically (or fancy themselves) highly creative persons, and so may consider art to be their lingua franca. Recognizing the potential for therapeutic misadventures arising from this situation, Frye and Gannon (1990) devised excellent guidelines for clinicians not trained as art therapists.

In the past several years, however, a small body of literature has been published concerning the informed use, based on formal training, of expressive arts modalities with adults who have severe dissociative conditions. Most of it can be found or referenced in a few books and certain professional journals (Cohen, Barnes, & Rankin, 1995; Cohen & Cox, 1995; Kluft, 1993; Simonds, 1994); one comprehensive review of the audio literature on this subject is also available (Mills, 1992a).

This chapter, unlike the aforementioned literature, is not concerned with approaches to treatment or differential diagnosis of this population through art. Its purpose is primarily theoretical: to explore the relationships among visual art, traumatic experience, therapeutic art-making, and the internal worlds of people suffering from complex posttraumatic dissociation. Using clients diagnosed with dissociative identity disorder (DID) (formerly multiple personality disorder) as a focus, the author hopes to reveal the extraordinary kinship between the *dissociative reality* and the *art reality*, and to clarify the rationale for the well-informed use of art therapy in treating survivors of severe early trauma.

ESTABLISHING REALITY

> In vain do we ever say what we see; what we see never resides in what we say.
>
> MICHEL FOUCAULT (1982)

Each of us has unique perceptions of the world, based largely on our personal, psychological, sociocultural, and physiological experiences. For instance, two adults from similar backgrounds, of the same gender, with identical demographics can look at the same stimulus and each see different things, as any visit to an art gallery will confirm. Nearly all psychology students have seen the simple black and white design that shifts between the image of a chalice (in the center) and two profiles facing each other (at the sides); M. C. Escher's graphic oeuvre, with its bird and fish motifs, so familiar to millions, is rooted in this perceptual challenge. Individuality dictates reality at even the most basic levels (Tyler, 1978). The German expressionist artist, Max Beckmann, said, "It may sound paradoxical, but it is, in fact, reality which forms the mystery of our existence" (cited in Rose, 1987, p. vi).

Traditionally, psychotherapy requires patients to rely on verbal language to both express their feelings and communicate their thoughts and experiences—their inner realities. In order to be able to participate effectively in psychotherapy, clinicians must learn to apprehend the complexities of interpersonal expression by attending to both verbal and nonverbal cues. It is not sufficient, for instance, to merely comprehend the words that a client uses to recount her story. The way in which the words are spoken—volume, tone, enunciation, and emphasis, as well as facial expression, posture, and gesticulations of the speaker—must be noted.

Supportive-expressive treatment, for instance, a method of psychoanalytic psychotherapy, has four phases: listening, understanding, responding, and return to listening (Luborsky, 1984). The therapist is challenged to comprehend what the patient says and actively comment on it in order to provide clarification. In the best of circumstances, the individuality of both clinician and patient, as well as the limitations of verbal communication, can hamper effective listening, accurate understanding, and skillful responding within the dyad. Furthermore, the name "supportive-expressive" promises two experiences. It is certainly possible to provide verbal support in this format, but can psychotherapy be truly *expressive* when language is its primary vehicle?

To take this questioning a bit further, is it possible to make sense of an unfamiliar spoken language? Is it possible to communicate linguistically without the benefit of a shared vocabulary and syntax? In such a circumstance, it seems doubtful that one could deduce or assume meaning and expect it to be accurate. This impasse in communication has profound implications for the treatment of survivors of abuse. The severely traumatized client frequently communicates in a personal language that often seems foreign, even to the seasoned mental health professional.

In order to engage a dissociative survivor of childhood abuse in psychotherapy, one must use a language that the client finds effective; the interaction between language and individuality already poses an obstacle to effective communication. Because visual and sensorimotor functions are critical in the storage, coding, and recall of traumatic events, one must be willing to learn about the impact of trauma on imagery and how they manifest through art-making. Art therapy naturally facilitates the externalization of most of the aspects and outcomes of traumatic experience and clinicians can benefit from familiarity with the theories of this discipline (Cohen, 1993).

DISRUPTION AND DISCONTINUITY

> What we cannot speak about we must pass over in silence.
>
> LUDWIG WITTGENSTEIN

The relationship between art activity and the transformation of trauma can be simply illustrated through the theoretical model that uses schemas as a metaphor for the organization of various internalized constructs. Schemas are patterns of experience that help us comprehend and organize our existence; they frame issues such as safety, trust, independence, and power. Schemas are developed in response to the process of living. McCann and Pearlman (1990), in their constructivist self-development theory, describe schemas as "assumptions, beliefs, and expectations about self and world" (p. 57).

As new experiences are tested against one's existing expectations, they may be found to be congruent with each other, or not. It is theorized that those experiences that are found to be congruent with existing schemas can be internalized in such a way that the related images can be easily translated into word representations and later coded to facilitate storage in memory (Horowitz, 1970). These coded perceptions of experience are the basis of narrative memory. Narrative memory allows us to tell our experiences to others—communicate socially with them—and helps us to make sense of, accommodate, and work through experiences by recounting them (van der Kolk & van der Hart, 1991).

When experiences are found to be overwhelming, unexpected, or undesirable, they cannot be adequately processed. Because they are incongruent with our existing patterns and cannot be translated into language (Horowitz, 1970), these disrupted schemas are stored in short-term memory, primarily on an iconic (visual) and sensorimotor (body) level, and form the basis of traumatic memory. Wordless—and sometimes meaningless—this type of memory cannot be easily communicated. Its contents remain rigid and immutable despite the passage of time (van der Kolk & van der Hart, 1991).

Although some experiences succeed in entering cognition through image formation, others directly enter the lexical system. The presence of conflict, as in traumatic situations, may serve to inhibit integration of these two components, therefore preventing the development of a sense of meaning related to the experience. In the absence of meaningful connections, available images of these events might be regarded by the traumatized individual as puzzling. Maintaining traumatic images out of awareness, however, guards against the rekindling of intense emotions through connection with other unpleasant or unresolved schemas (Horowitz, 1970).

Even when they cannot be adequately processed, traumatic memories continue to manifest themselves in several ways: somatic sensations (body memories), which recur spontaneously or as a result of an environmental cue and typically revive unpleasant physiological phenomena; behavioral reenactments (repetition compulsion) in which the person participates unknowingly either as victim or perpetrator in situations reminiscent of the original trauma; and nightmares and flashbacks (intrusive revisualization) in which visual fragments or "trauma replays" arise unbidden (Brett & Ostroff, 1985).

Repetition of traumatic material "is generally understood as an attempt to come to terms with, or to integrate, the strong affects and somatic sensations invoked by the trauma into the fabric of one's life experience" (Greenberg & van der Kolk, 1987, p. 191). For the incestuously victimized child, however, demands for secrecy, coupled with potent threats, increase the likelihood of amnesia regarding these psychologically undigestible episodes.

Stored images that continue to press toward revisualization until translation is complete are often reflected in artwork as themes (repeated over a lifetime) or as perseveration in a single work of art. Magritte, the Belgian surrealist, created a series of paintings in which the broken shards of a window pane lie on the floor (Calvocoressi, 1979). Each piece of glass retains a part of the image of the scene which can also be viewed through the window. Although the image through the window is not traumatic per se, the window pane nonetheless continues to reflect the moment of the trauma. These paintings illustrate the lasting effects of unprocessed traumatic memory, which, carried in visual and somatic fragments, is more difficult to resurrect than the more complete gestalts of verbally processed narrative memory.

Spiegel (1991) defines trauma as a "sudden discontinuity in physical and psychological experience" in which the discontinuity is both a defense by the victim against the traumatic input (flight from harm), as well as a reflection of it (schema shifts and dissociation). Thus, abusive behavior induces various types of discontinuous experiences in its targets. The victim shifts states of consciousness in order to avoid pain, separates any previous positive connection with the perpetrator from awareness, and becomes a thing instead of a person—a creation of the abuser in the form of the abuse. This moment of disparity and despair facilitates a hypnoid or trance state in the victim that fosters the creation of arational, atemporal, and nonlinear constructs (Horowitz, 1970). The response to this state of overwhelming experience has been described as "speechless terror," since information can neither be fully assimilated nor accommodated (van der Kolk & van der Hart, 1991).

In this state of consciousness, incoming bits of information may be associated into discrete ego centers or, in the case of DID, alter personalities. Trauma often causes the inadvertent association of disparate stimuli; some forms of sexual abuse, for example, pair pleasure with pain. In childhood incest, maintaining secrecy obliges the victim to pair the actuality of the assault with the enforced facade of the happy family; thus, she is required to maintain long-term cognitive dissonance. Since the ability to retrieve information in a manner in which it can be translated into words depends on compatibility with or similarity to current cues, modalities that access material associated visually, kinesthetically, or through the senses offer great rewards in the healing process (Crabtree, 1992; Simonds, 1994).

Van der Kolk and van der Hart (1991) suggest that the traumatized individual lives in two different worlds: the realm of the trauma (past) and the realm of "ordinary" life (present). The realm of the trauma is internal reality—a world that is repetitive, solitary, and, very importantly, timeless. One needs to be more adaptable to "ordinary" life, on the other hand, because it is more unpredictable and contextual. Further, these are two "utterly incompatible worlds" (1991, p. 448). Disparity, like disruption and discontinuity, becomes all too familiar in the lives of those who have experienced chronic trauma. This explains in part why traumatized individuals crave metaphor and imagery in treatment to make sense of their worlds (Rose, 1987). The art reality offers a relatively safe parallel realm in which these disrupted schemas can be recalled, explored, and transformed.

THE ART REALITY

> Art does not render what is visible, it renders visible.
>
> PAUL KLEE

Nelson Goodman (1978) described art as a "fundamental way of knowing the world" because of the potential it holds as a vehicle for and process of communication. Several key qualities contribute to the unique nature of what is herein referred to as the art reality. Isomorphism is the central concept in the psychology of art and the expressive arts therapies. It derives from Gestalt psychology and refers to the similarity in structure between a person's internal state and its external expression (Arnheim, 1969). Body language, for instance, is a "pop" application of the isomorphism concept. It is isomorphism that allows us to feel the curving reverberations of Munch's ubiquitous expressionist icon, "The Scream" (1895), which reflects the artist's inner state of tension and, at the same time, induces a similar state in the viewer. "Whoever paints a figure," wrote Dante, "unless he can be it, cannot set it down."

In communicating their messages to viewers, artists use certain techniques that pertain to the arrangement, clarity, manipulation, and interrelationship of pictorial elements (Cohen & Cox, 1995; Dondis, 1973). Styles in the art are patterns of picture-making behavior that are constructed from clusters of these techniques. There are several styles in the modern history of art that are essential components of the art reality. These styles help to highlight some of the inherent qualities of art that allow for its characterization as an uncommon reality.

Cubism, the earliest of abstract styles, was a manipulation of form and space that afforded a view of a subject from multiple vantage points; thus we see sides, front, and back simultaneously. The surrealists were also interested in space, but, unlike the cubists, focused on internal rather than external space. In keeping with their fascination with the irrational, they sought to create accurate depictions of imaginary or dream space. "Pure psychic automatism" in surrealism, according to its founder, Andre´ Breton (cited in Crofton, 1988, p. 181), was intended to express the true process of thought, free from the exercise of reason. Surrealist compositions feature the trance logic of the hypnoid state, including its distortions of time. Surrealist artist Salvador Dali manipulated time and space in his paintings through the use of complex juxtaposition, distorted scale, and mixed perspectives. His early work is typified by the painting, "Illumined Pleasures" (1929), which is compositionally devised in such a way that several scenarios are perceived by the viewer to be occurring simultaneously; violent, sexual, and symbolic/oneiric themes are freely mixed with the banal.

Aesthetic forebears of the surrealists, the dadaists bestowed upon them a love for juxtaposing elements in novel and unexpected combinations. The dada work that best illustrates the power of juxtaposition is the provocative mixed media assemblage by Meret Oppenheim, "Object (Breakfast in Fur)" (1936), a fur-covered teacup and spoon, which incites a veritable sensory riot by the joining of two ordinary items from our everyday reality. Associating images that have no apparent connection by bringing them together in a single work enables the artist to generate new connections and meanings that reason alone is unlikely to anticipate (Rose, 1987). In the same way, disparate schemas that have been associated during traumatic experience can be effectively retrieved through an isomorphic process in art.

Expressionism externalizes affect through intense color, distorted form, and gestural movement. Foreshadowed by the late works of Van Gogh, developed by the Germans early in this century, and epitomized by the New York School of abstractionists such as DeKooning, Kline, and Pollock, the externalization of raw feeling in expressionist art is frequently paralleled in the artwork of traumatized persons.

Futurism, a relatively little-known style, developed in Italy during the same years cubism was evolving in France. Its proponents strove to engage the viewer in active participation through the visual evocation of dynamic movement. Marcel Duchamp, though primarily known as a dadaist, painted an example of futurism known to all students of twentieth-century art. His "Nude Descending a Staircase" (1912) attempts to record a figure moving through space, using abstract form to convey its narrative; the effect is of a strobelike pattern. It is difficult to avoid physical empathy with such an image; in this way, art can elicit motor responses through visual and kinesthetic cuing.

The attributes of the art reality enable the wordless image to work its way out in "a continuous process of concretion" (Cassirer, 1953, p. 184) without the necessity of language. There is no mandate for sequential thought in the nonverbal mind; art carries information differently than language—in visual images rather than in words. These images need not themselves be narrative because form in art *is* content; it alone can communicate. "Form is ... most associated with consciousness, judgement, control, and other ego attributes" (Storr, 1993, p. 224).

Gertrude Stein, a contemporary of the cubists, developed a literary style that was essentially cubist in nature and did not rely on narrative. The following is an excerpt from her word portrait of a Spanish dancer, written in 1913 (cited in Haas, 1976, p. 57):

> Sweet sweet sweet sweet sweet tea.
> Susie Asado
> Sweet sweet sweet sweet sweet tea.
> Susie Asado
> Susie Asado which is a told tray sure.
> A lean on the shoe this means slips slips hers.
> When the ancient light grey is clean it is yellow, it is a silver seller.
> This is a please this is a please there are the saids to jelly ...

When the narrative content is taken out of written communication, as in the Stein poem, words are distilled into sounds and rhythm, and meaningful references are lost. In visual art, however, form, color, movement, and composition remain to express the artist's intent, even if the narrative has been obscured or removed. Take, for example, Picasso's portraits in the analytical cubist style which shatter the subject's image into many small planes of color and light. At first one might see only the paint, or the complex design, but soon the image coalesces in the viewer's mind's eye and the figure can be discerned.

"Language is simply unable to capture the quality of visual truth; it muddies as much as it mediates" (Rose, 1987, p. 176). This is because words, the primary means of conveying images in spoken and written communication, have been arbitrarily assigned meaning for the things to which they refer; what does "chair" have to do with the actual object on which one sits, for instance? How many referents are ascribed to the sound "bow"? Where, exactly, is "over there"? When you hear or see the word "pipe," do you think of smoking or plumbing? Why?

The Belgian surrealist Magritte created sophisticated paradoxes that force us to confront the uneasy relationship between words, images, and consensual reality (Handler-Spitz, 1987). "This is not a pipe," inscribed in French on a painting that clearly depicts a pipe used for smoking, is a well-known example of his work. Magritte uses the combination of writing and painting in this piece to create an especially complex disparity. Of course this is not a pipe—it is a painting of a pipe (Foucault, 1982).[1] The semiotic dilemma here is not very different from the untrained nonspecialist introducing art into the trauma therapy context. "Seeing an artwork without knowing it is an artwork, is like experiencing print before being able to read" (Dissanayake, 1991, p. 183).

The capacity of visual language to convey feeling, meaning, psychological time and space and to invoke sensation, movement, and cognitive connections commends art reality as an important correlate in communicating with traumatized people.

THE DISSOCIATIVE REALITY

> When you own the shop and there are no customers, you can do anything you want.
>
> COLIN MARTINDALE (1990)

The dissociative reality, which thrives on the disrupted schemas of the traumatic realm, extends the challenges regarding individuality and interpersonal communication in psychotherapy to even more complex levels. People with DID usually manifest the most complicated psychopathology that characterizes this uncommon reality. A chronic complex form of posttraumatic stress, DID features frequent periods of dissociative amnesia during which alternate personalities take executive control of behavior.

For those who do not live it, it is nearly impossible to truly understand dissociative reality or effectively describe it. What words can one use to adequately communicate phenomena like switching, co-consciousness, a system of highly particularized alters, or internal safe places? Both patients and therapists frequently develop exquisitely refined (although somewhat rigid and unidimensional) verbal metaphors to describe these aspects of the dissociative reality. The visual image is, however, more immediate and more directly attuned to individual needs than is any verbal metaphor because art allows us "to visualize, not merely to conceptualize" (Cassirer, 1944, p. 216).

The discontinuity and disparity that are engendered by childhood abuse foster the development of pathological levels of dissociation in the young victim striving for survival. As a result, the severely abused child begins the self-hypnotic process of establishing an internal reality that differs radically from consensual reality. Silvey and MacKeith (1988) referred to elaborate invented realities of childhood as para-

[1]It is interesting to note how thoroughly many of Magritte's images have been adopted into popular culture. I believe the proliferation of surrealist imagery, which flourished after World War I—and Magritte's imagery in particular—on album covers, window dressing, greeting cards, T-shirts, and the like is a reflection of society's craving for disparity and discontinuity. The public *needs* these elements concretized and externalized for them and the surrealists provided just such a service. The daily news confirms that there is rampant trauma in all our lives. However, many people participate in a consensual trance in which certain kinds of trauma do not really exist—witness surveys regarding doubt that the Holocaust actually happened.

cosms. Paracosms are spontaneously created, systemized private worlds. Sustained over an appreciable length of time, they are internally consistent and deeply significant to the individual. The dissociative reality is essentially a posttraumatic paracosm in which discretely organized constructs and affects are elaborated into adaptive metaphorical and/or pathological realms. These internal worlds usually reflect the magical thinking of early childhood and, unlike the delusional reality of psychotics, are self-referential.

It has been suggested that alter personalities are constructs developed in an attempt to master a variety of very intense affects (Nathanson, 1993). Ross (1989) compared them to theatrical devices. The alter personalities that reside in dissociative paracosms may also be likened to styles in art, in that they represent distinct patterns of behavior that are visually distinguishable by their characteristic communication techniques; some alters may also be identified by their function within the personality system. Typically, this environment is inhabited by perpetrator introjects with cognitively distorted agendas (Ross & Gahan, 1988). In addition, unprocessed remnants of the trauma itself tend to resurface spontaneously—pressing for revisualization. For these reasons, not all posttraumatic paracosms are safe places to be.

Paracosms should not be confused with system pictures, which depict the organization of the alter personalities (Cohen & Cox, 1989), nor should they be confused with system maps (Putnam, 1989), which are typically transitory relational diagrams of the internal cast of characters. Paracosms, on the other hand, include the internal reality's environment, architecture, rules, culture, and constituents. It is in this realm, deep beneath the chaos shown outwardly to the world, that the unity beneath the patient's multiplicity might be examined (Braude, 1992). Because paracosms are so elaborate, one is more likely to glimpse different aspects of a single example across a number of art productions by a given client than to see one represented in a single art production.

In addition to these idiosyncratic imaginal realities, people with DID seem to have their own linguistic system (Greaves, 1992). It includes the use of such phrases as "the body," "the mother," and the omission of pronouns in order to avoid committing to "I" or "we" statements or indicating ownership statements with the words "my" or "mine." Kluft has informally referred to this idiosyncratic style of thinking and communicating as "multiplese." Listening to multiplese can be disorienting, but not nearly as difficult as having to make sense of the dissociative reality (with its cubist-futurist-surrealist and time-space distortions) without the help of art reality.

The dissociative reality derives from several negative constructs that are the direct result of trauma. These constructs reflect discontinuity and disparity in schemas related to identity, awareness, responsibility, and time. A patient's dissociative reality may be summed up by the following:

- not me—disavowal-dissociation of part selves
- not now—inability to remain in or experience the present
- not then—disavowal-dissociation of personal history
- not ever—lack of hope or future orientation

UNCOMMON REALITIES: A KINSHIP

... the urgent need in everyone to give form to his or her life.

Rollo May

As strong kinship exists between the art reality and the dissociative reality; inherent qualities of both realms parallel one another. The therapist's ability to capitalize on this affinity makes communication and therefore treatment easier and more effective than the use of language alone.

Bisociation refers to the pairing of habitually incompatible elements during the creative process (Koestler, 1964). As mentioned earlier, this occurs naturally in the context of trauma, when incongruent ideas or experiences are powerfully associated during an altered state. Dali's work perhaps best illustrates this quality in art. His famous portrait of Mae West (1934), in which the subject is depicted as a brothel parlor with her cascading hair as the drapery and her ruby lips as a sofa, provides an elegant example of bisociation. Dali created a trancelike reality in his painting through the trancelike process of art-making and invites the viewer to join him in it.

Plasticity is the inherent quality of art that facilitates the malleability of form, time, and space; it maximizes the effects of visual communication. In the dissociative patient's experience, the plasticity of trance logic allows for the simultaneous or consecutive experiencing of past and present time within a spatially variable posttraumatic paracosm. Plasticity is the phenomenon that enables the patient to continually reperceive herself in her various dissociated identities. Dali unwittingly illustrated plasticity as a function of both art reality and dissociative reality in a single work of art; his emblematic surrealist painting of melting watches in a timeless landscape is, ironically, titled "The Persistence of Memory" (1931).

Absorption is another key factor in the kinship between art reality and dissociative reality. It is the intensely focused state of consciousness accessible to both the artist and the highly hypnotizable person. As Storr (1993), states, "creative people are often astonished by what they have produced, and treat it ... as if someone else has produced it" (p. 219). An example of absorption during the creative process, this description is remarkably similar to the dissociative amnesia of DID patients who create art in their various alter personality states. Properly structured, art-making can engage dissociative clients in a pleasurable activity that channels their propensity for absorption.

Multileveledness suggests that several distinct levels of meaning can be comprehended in a single work of art and further that there is no hierarchy of importance among these various levels (Kreitler & Kreitler, 1972). Cohen and Cox (1989) have pointed out art's efficiency in allowing for the simultaneous revealing and concealing of information regarding abuse, dissociation, or multiplicity, which is derived from this phenomenon. Art's multileveled quality promotes repeated examinations by the viewer of a single work. Similarly, the variety and stratification of alters in a DID system invites ongoing reexamination by the therapist. This intriguing quality can sometimes offset the difficulties of working with such complex persons and case material.

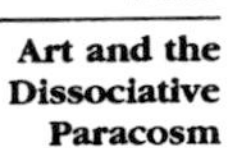

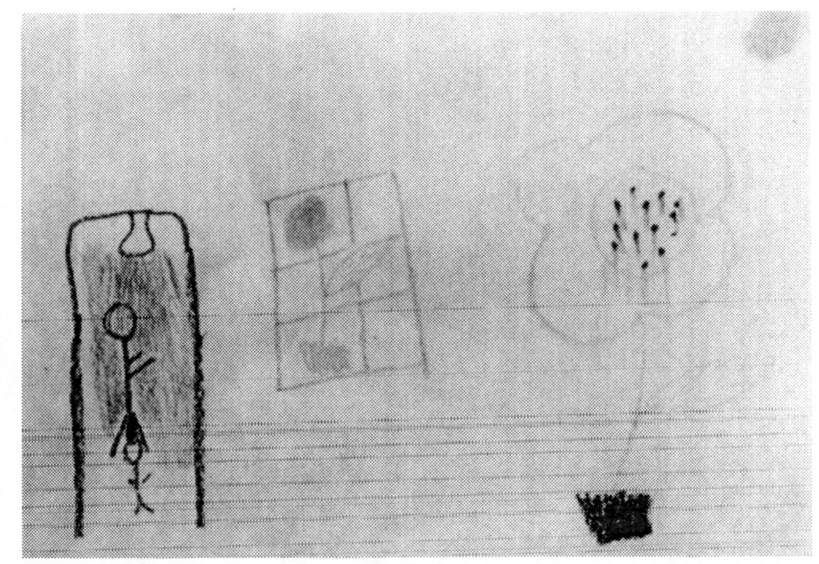

Figure 1. In this drawing by a woman with DID, the childhood experience associated with the showerhead becomes graphically signified by the crying sunflower.

For the child fellating the adult in the shower on the left side of the drawing in Figure 1, drawn by a woman with DID, the pouring shower head is equated with the bright yellow image of a sunflower on the right. The child could only allow herself to cry in the shower where her tears would be washed away undetected, hence the crying sunflower. Once this association is concretized, future drawings that may refer to knowledge of this incident or the dissociated affective and sensory responses related to it may be simply signified by the sunflower. The sunflower is a schema—in this case, an art term meaning a basic pattern or configuration that is used repeatedly to denote something (Lowenfeld & Brittain, 1975).

A flower schema is employed again in Figure 2, also drawn by a DID patient. In this image, it suggests a system and an internal threat. If trauma creates disrupted mental schemas that need to be externalized in order to effect healing, and art activity is the most effective way to accomplish this externalization, then graphic schemas are the royal road to enhancing the therapeutic outcome in the treatment of severely traumatized clients.

According to Csikszentmihalyi (1978), "Art is an adaptive tool by which we master forces in the environment in order to survive in it" (p. 125). Picture-making, like hypnosis, provides a directable shift in consciousness to an image-based construct (Kingsbury, 1988). In this way, art can offer an escape from the chaos of life to another, more comfortable, realm. Martindale (1990) has pointed out that if you do something useful, you yourself can become a tool. The all-too-usable victimized

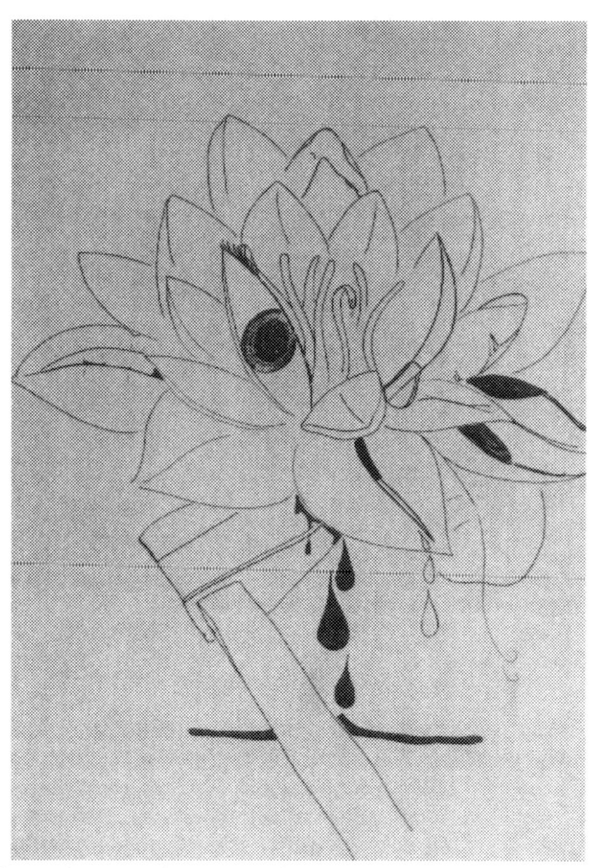

Figure 2. A flower schema is used to represent the internal personality system, which is under attack.

child adopts art as an activity of survival because it is not at all useful to the abuser and is, therefore, use-less. A child can express her internal or external reality through art in ways "that could not be expressed, and therefore controlled, by other means" (Csikszentmihalyi, 1978, p. 120).

Like any aspect of human behavior, art can be analyzed or interpreted according to any number of constructs. Likewise, art therapy approaches correspond to various schools of psychological theory. Differing outlooks on art therapy practice can be sought elsewhere in the professional literature (e.g., Landgarten, 1987; Lusebrink, 1990; McNiff, 1981; Moon, 1990; Naumburg, 1966; Rhyne 1973; Robbins & Sibley, 1976; Rubin, 1984; Schaverien, 1992; Wadeson, Durkin, & Perach, 1989).

I hear and I forget, I see and I remember, I do and I understand.

PROVERB

Art therapy is frequently misunderstood by non-art therapists as a method of creative-expressive exorcism. This misconception most likely stems from the haphazard introduction of art activity by untrained practitioners into the context of verbal psychotherapy, where cuing of undigested traumatic material has triggered posttraumatic stress disorder symptoms and heightened affective responses in clients. Performed skillfully, however, art therapy can provide a structured transformation of imagery and energy through the triadic relationship between therapist, client, and the art product (Schaverien, 1992).

Art therapy as treatment for people with severe dissociative disorders engages cognition, affect, sensation, and motor behavior. It helps to order and complete fragmented and discontinuous gestalts. Art-making externalizes visually encoded images and long-standing idiosyncratic inner realms. It gives the maker an opportunity to work through unresolved life issues in order to reach a new equilibrium. Art therapy teaches coping skills that can be used to structure time and provide a tangible reminder of the therapeutic work. It bridges two otherwise incompatible realities: the posttraumatic-dissociative and the everyday-ordinary. These are substantial rewards in working with DID clients; the potential benefits of art therapy are, however, even more extensive (Mills, 1992b).

One particularly important feature of art-making for individuals who have severe dissociative disorders is that the artist is both the maker and the observer of the image. Although art is about making messages from oneself to oneself, people who experience substantial amnesia have even more to learn from within than those who do not. Therapeutic art activity provides the client with evidence that the healing is coming from within her (Schaverien, 1992).

One practical model for structuring the art therapy process that minimizes the risk of regression with regard to the treatment of dissociative disorder clients has been discussed by Cohen (1992). His framework for the thoughtful and disciplined practice of art therapy with this population is based on the integration of the BASK model (Braun, 1988a,b), which posits a theory of dissociation and a model for its treatment, with the expressive therapies continuum (ETC) (Kagin & Lusebrink, 1978), which organizes theories of the creative process into a model for planning interventions in the expressive arts therapies.

The BASK model suggests that when behavior, affect, sensation, and knowledge (BASK) are congruent with each other and confluent over time, there is mental health (Braun, 1988a). Any or all of the BASK levels can be separated or dissociated from the others in the course of daily life. The same phenomenon holds true in art, as is illustrated in the work of DID clients who frequently feature one of the four BASK levels in their graphic expressions, to the exclusion of the others (Fuhrman, 1993).

The ETC assists the art therapist in the selection of media and tasks appropriate to the client's needs, strengths, and treatment goals. The ETC delineates the facets of the art-making process as: kinesthetic-sensory, perceptual-affective, cognitive-symbolic, and creative. One can readily see the four BASK levels paralleled in this model. The ETC suggests that art media requiring physical energy to manipulate, applied with tools that offer physical separation between the materials and the proprioceptive system, structured by tasks that employ a number of steps to complete, facilitate appropriate cognitive distance during the creative process to enhance ego function and hinder regression (Lusebrink, 1990).

Figures 3 through 6, drawn by women diagnosed with multiple personality disorder, each illustrate one BASK level. Although any art-making activity engages *all* levels of the ETC, those ETC levels that correspond to the BASK levels illustrated by these figures are indicated in parentheses.

- *Behaviors* are often depicted in drawings, such as the one reproduced in Figure 3, as self-destructive reenactments of trauma. If one perceives drawing behavior as a sublimation of the impulse to act, then—in this case—art is highly preferable to its alternative. (kinesthetic, creative).
- Art objectifies *affect* by giving it form. A pervasive and uneasy feeling is expressed in Figure 4. Amorphous shape and a murky use of color poignantly convey the essence of sexual shame in this watercolor painting. (perceptual, affective)
- *Sensation* images, such as the one in Figure 5, trigger a visceral response in the viewer, as conveyed by the maker. To avoid this isomorphic response, one would have to dissociate. It is rather unusual that such a naturalistic, narrative technique be employed to depict a sensory experience; painful sensations are more typically portrayed expressionistically through heightened color and movement. In

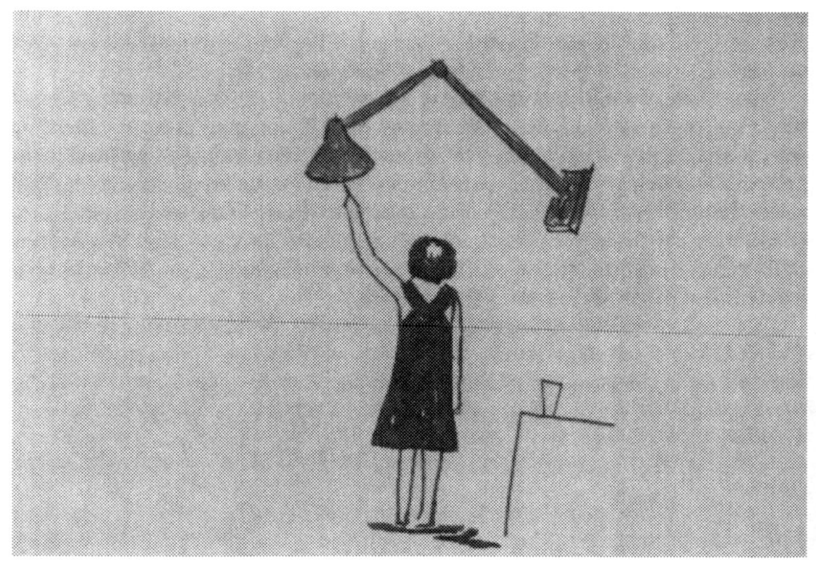

Figure 3. Impulsivity can be communicated and behavior sublimated through art-making.

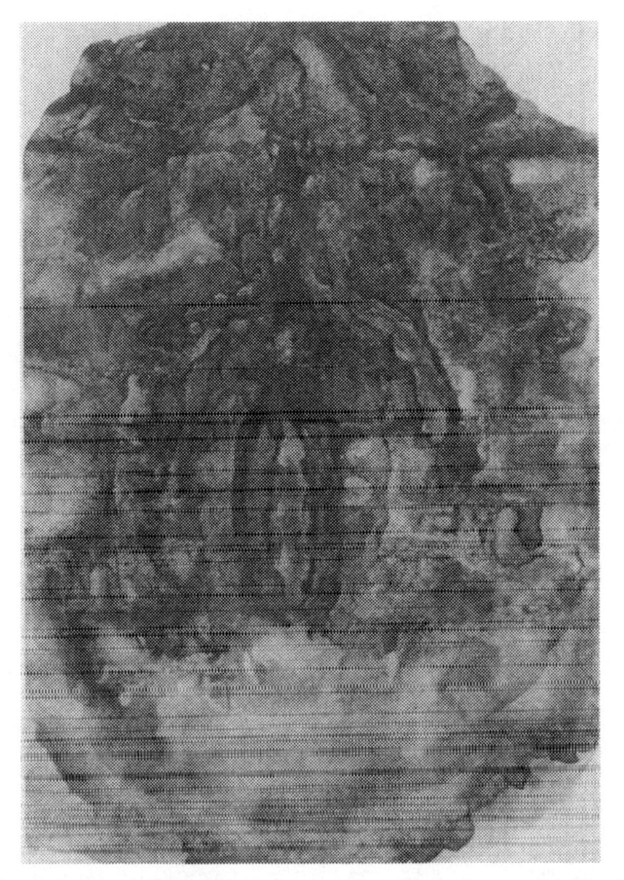

Figure 4. Color and form effectively externalize affect and convey it to the viewer.

this image, distortion and exaggeration give the grimacing face its visual impact. (sensory)

• Collage requires the maker to engage in a kind of spatial organization that serves to structure cognition; this process helps clients work with the ***knowledge*** component of experience. Since the images used in collage have been appropriated from an external source (such as a magazine), adequate emotional distance can be maintained; thus, this technique fosters containment and control within the client. The collage shown in Figure 6 is titled, "Tools of the Trade." The making of this piece helped the client to organize the chaos of a physically abusive childhood into a manageable space; once accomplished, she could begin to redefine her relationship with the everyday items represented in the collage which were previously known to her as weapons for punishment. (cognitive, symbolic)

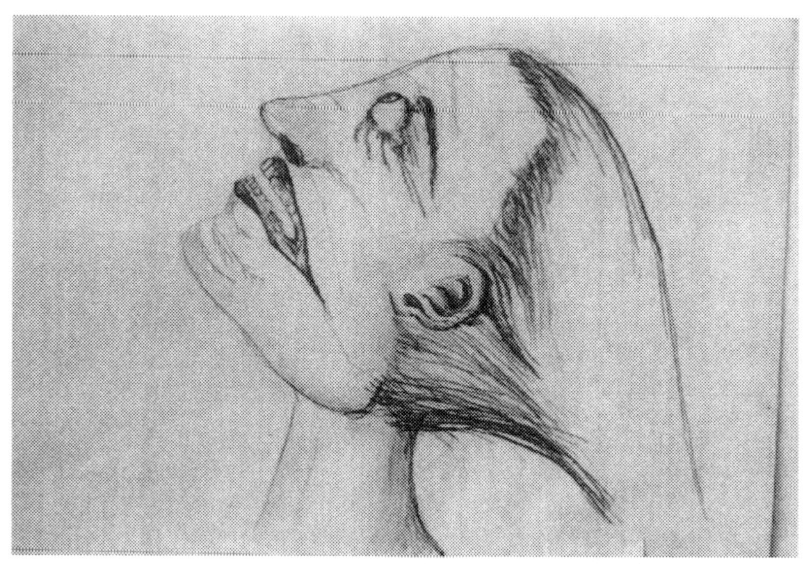

Figure 5. The impact of intense sensation is conveyed by distortion and exaggeration in this image.

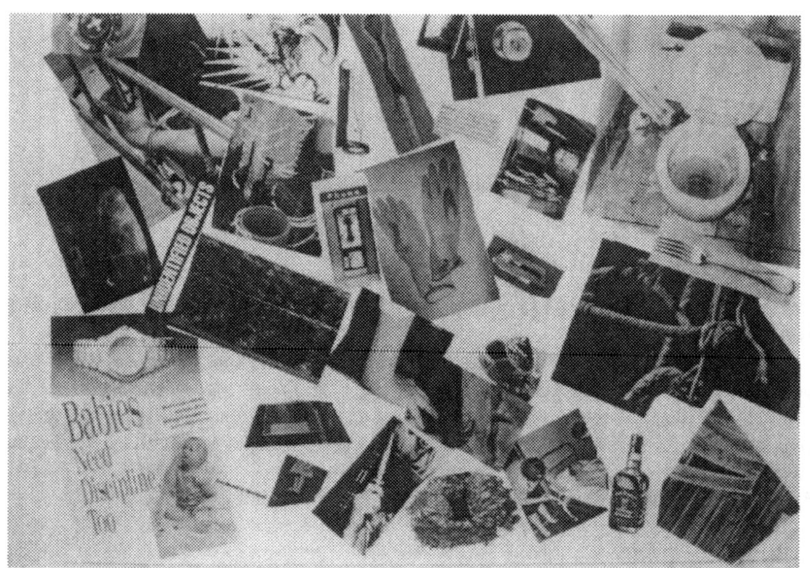

Figure 6. Collage, a popular art-making technique, can enhance knowledge by encouraging the maker to organize and define pictorial elements.

Art therapy's function in the treatment of dissociative disorders can be summed up by the following effects, each of which is associated with one or more of the BASK levels essential for the transformation of nonverbally encoded or dissociated material:

- The *restorative effect* of art therapy refers to the attainment of mastery over the past. It recovers visually stored, unprocessed representations and restores them to consciousness. Anxiety-provoking material is externalized and concretized in a tolerable or pleasurable way. (affect and sensation)
- The *orientative effect* of art therapy communicates new information about the person and her world and suggests ways for the integration of disparity within each. It deals with revealing a previously discontinuous narrative in the present. Once an issue is externalized and concretized, an appropriate resolution may be attempted. (knowledge)
- The *preparative effect* of art therapy provides for rehearsal of upcoming events and reinforcement of control in the present. It is about practicing for the future and facing challenges in a planned, methodical way. (behavior)

CONCLUSION

> We talk too much; we should talk less and draw more.
>
> GOETHE

Relying solely on verbal communication in the psychotherapy of people with severe dissociative disorders limits the possibilities for discovery, understanding, and growth. This is true, in part, because verbal psychotherapy is not an isomorphically advantageous vehicle for accessing the trauma-based constructs that constitute dissociative paracosms. Therapy with persons who have survived severe trauma must focus on the externalization of those traumatic experiences in order to adjust the anomalous constructs formed in trauma's wake. According to Herman (1992), "Creating pictures may represent the most effective initial approach to these 'indelible images' " (p. 177). Before attempting to introduce art into psychotherapy with those who were severely abused in childhood, however, it is essential that therapists be fully aware of the training necessary to effectively negotiate the complexities of graphic communication and be mindful of the option to refer or consult with a specialist for this aspect of the treatment.

Art reality and the dissociative reality have a variety of attributes in common that favor the spontaneous making of art and facilitate the use of art therapy in addressing the cognitive, emotional, behavioral, biological, and interpersonal consequences of trauma. These qualities can readily be observed in the characteristics of art movements that have spanned the last 100 years; the very same century since the development of Janet's landmark theory of dissociation.

For patients who consider themselves to be literally invisible, not worth taking up any space, or utterly powerless, engaging in art therapy can be an assertion that they are not simply a physiological entity, but rather a physical and psychological force in the universe. The artist's ability to make her mark on the world, simply by poking the clay or making a mark on paper, can be existentially fulfilling (Csikszentmihalyi, 1978).

Why do people with severe dissociative disorders produce so much art? In order to communicate. Through art, the patient is saying to the viewer, "Please listen. This happened to me. No one would believe me. I cannot remember, yet I cannot forget."

Why do people with severe dissociative disorders produce so much art? In order to exist. Through art, the patient is saying to the viewer, "I learned quickly not to feel, not to be. I went away; now I am back, taking control ... yet stuck between two realities."

ACKNOWLEDGMENTS. Portions of this chapter were previously presented at the Fifth Annual Eastern Regional Conference on Abuse and Multiple Personality, Alexandria, Virginia, June 5, 1993. The author wishes to express his thanks to Anne Mills, M.A., A.T.R., for her invaluable assistance during all phases in the preparation of this chapter.

REFERENCES

Arnheim, R. (1969). *Visual thinking*. Berkeley: University of California Press.

Boon, S., & Draijer, N. (1993). *Multiple personality disorder in the Netherlands: A study on reliability and validity of the diagnosis*. Amsterdam: Swets & Zeitlinger.

Braude, S. E. (1992). *First person plural: Multiple personality and the philosophy of mind*. London: Routledge.

Braun, B. G. (1988a). The BASK model of dissociation. *Dissociation*, *1*(1), 4-23.

Braun, B. G. (1988b). The BASK model of dissociation: Part II—Treatment. *Dissociation*, *2*(1), 16-23.

Brett, E. A., & Ostroff, R. (1985). Imagery and posttraumatic stress disorder: An overview. *American Journal of Psychiatry*, *142*, 417-424.

Calvocoressi, R. (1979). *Magritte*. London: Phaidon Press.

Cassirer, E. (1953). *An essay on man*. Garden City: Doubleday.

Cohen, B. M. (Speaker). (1992). *The expressive therapies continuum and the dissociative spectrum* (Cassette Recording No. 34). Cuyahoga Falls, OH: Dove Enterprises.

Cohen, B. M. (Speaker). (1993). *Art and MPD: Uncommon realities* (Cassette Recording No. 13-834-93). Alexandria, VA: Audio Transcripts.

Cohen, B. M., Barnes, M. M., & Rankin, A. B. (1995). *Managing traumatic stress through art: Drawing from the center*. Lutherville, MD: Sidran Press.

Cohen, B. M., & Cox, C. T. (1989). Breaking the code: Identification of multiplicity through art productions. *Dissociation*, *2*(3), 132-137.

Cohen, B. M., & Cox, C. T. (1995). *Telling without talking: Art as a window into the world of multiple personality*. New York: Norton.

Coons, P. (1988). The use of patient art productions in the diagnosis and treatment of patients with multiple personality/dissociative states (summary). In B. G. Braun (Ed.), *Proceedings of the 5th international conference on multiple personality/dissociative states* (p. 175). Dissociative Disorders Program, Department of Psychiatry, Rush University, Chicago, IL.

Courtois, C. (1988). *Healing the incest wound*. New York: Norton.

Crabtree, A. (1992). Dissociation and memory: A two-hundred-year perspective.*Dissociation*, *5*(3), 150-154.

Crofton, I. (1988). *A dictionary of art quotations*. New York: Schirmer Books.

Csikszentmihalyi, M. (1978). Phylogenetic and ontogenetic functions of artistic cognition. In S. S. Madeja (Ed.), *The arts, cognition, and basic skills* (pp. 114-127). St. Louis: CEMREL.

Dissanayake, E. (1991). *What is art for?* Seattle: University of Washington Press.

Dondis, D. A. (1973). *A primer of visual literacy*. Cambridge, MA: The MIT Press.
Fine, C. (Speaker). (1990). *Boundaries, limits, contracts, and mistakes* (Cassette Recording No. 569-90-30). Alexandria, VA: Audio Transcripts.
Foucault, M. (1982). *This is not a pipe*. Berkeley: University of California Press.
Frye, B., & Gannon, L. (1990). The use, misuse, and abuse of art with dissociative/multiple personality disorders. *Occupational Therapy Forum, 5*(24), 1, 3-5, 8.
Fuhrman, N. L. (1993). Art and multiple personality disorder: A developmental approach to treatment. In E. S. Kluft (Ed.), *Expressive and functional therapies in the treatment of multiple personality disorder* (pp. 23-37). Springfield, IL: Charles C Thomas.
Goodman, N. (1978). *Ways of worldmaking*. Indianapolis: Hackett Publishing Company.
Greaves, G. (1992). The language of dissociation (Summary). In B. G. Braun & E. B. Carlson (Eds.), *Proceedings of the 9th international conference on multiple personality/dissociative states* (p. 10). Dissociative Disorders Program, Department of Psychiatry, Rush University, Chicago, IL.
Greenberg, M. S., & van der Kolk, B. A. (1987). *Retrieval and integration of traumatic memories with the "painting cure."* In B. A. van der Kolk (Ed.), *Psychological trauma* (pp. 191-215). Washington, DC: American Psychological Press.
Haas, R. B. (1976). *A primer for the gradual understanding of Gertrude Stein*. Santa Barbara: Black Sparrow Press.
Handler-Spitz, E. (Speaker). (1987). *Magritte: Psychoanalytic and other perspectives—Mazes of meaning* (Cassette Recording No. T292-44). Garden Grove, CA: Infomedix.
Herman, J. (1992). *Trauma and recovery*. New York: Basic Books.
Herman, J., Perry, J., & van der Kolk, B. A. (1989). Childhood trauma in borderline personality disorder. *American Journal of Psychiatry, 146*, 490-495.
Horowitz, M. J. (1970). *Image formation and cognition*. New York: Appleton-Century Crofts.
Kagin, S., & Lusebrink, V. (1978). The expressive therapies continuum. *The Arts in Psychotherapy, 5*, 171-180.
Kingsbury, S. J. (1988). Hypnosis in the treatment of PTSD: An isomorphic intervention. *American Journal of Clinical Hypnosis, 31*(2), 81-90.
Kluft, E. S. (Ed.). (1993). *Expressive and functional therapies in the treatment of multiple personality disorder*. Springfield, IL: Charles C Thomas.
Kluft, R. P. (Ed.). (1985). *Childhood antecedents of multiple personality disorder*. Washington, DC: American Psychiatric Press.
Kluft, R. P. (Ed.). (1990). *Incest-related syndromes of adult psychopathology*. Washington, DC: American Psychiatric Press.
Koestler, A. (1964). *The act of creation*. New York: Dell Publishing.
Kreitler, H., & Kreitler, S. (1972). Psychology of the arts. Durham, NC: Duke University Press.
Landgarten, H. B. (1981). *Clinical art therapy*. New York: Brunner/Mazel.
Loewenstein, R. J. (Ed.). (1991). *The psychiatric clinics of North America: Multiple personality disorder*. Philadelphia: W. B. Saunders Company.
Loewenstein, R. J. (1993). Current research on multiple personality disorders: The validity of MPD. In B. G. Braun & E. B. Carlson (Eds.), *Proceedings of the 10th international conference on multiple personality dissociative states* (p. 174).
Lowenfeld, V., & Brittain, W. L. (1975). *Creative and mental growth*. New York: Macmillan.
Luborsky, L. (1984). *Principles of psychoanalytic psychotherapy: A manual for supportive-expressive treatment*. New York: Basic Books.
Lusebrink, V. B. (1990). *Imagery and visual expression in therapy*. New York: Plenum Press.
Martindale, C. (1990). *The clockwork muse: The predictability of artistic change*. New York: Basic Books.
McCann, I. L., & Pearlman, L. A. (1990). *Psychological trauma and the adult survivor*. New York: Brunner/Mazel.
McNiff, S. (1981). *The arts and psychotherapy*. Springfield, IL: Charles C Thomas.
Mills, A. (1992a). *A time line on art therapy with MPD*. (Available from A. Mills, P.O. Box 9853, Alexandria, Virginia 22304.)
Mills, A. (Speaker) (1992b). Benefits of art therapy with MPD. In M. L. Jacobson & A. Mills, *A survey of art therapy in the identification and treatment of MPD* (Cassette Recording No. 34-742-92A, B). Alexandria, VA: Audio Transcripts.

Moon, B. L. (1990). *Existential art therapy: The canvas mirror*. Springfield, IL: Charles C Thomas.

Nathanson, D. (Speaker). (1993). *Affect theory and the treatment of MPD* (Cassette Recording No. 834-93-14). Alexandria, VA: Audio Transcripts.

Naumburg, M. (1966). *Dynamically oriented art therapy: Its principles and practices*. New York: Grune & Stratton.

Putnam, F. W. (1989). *Diagnosis and treatment of multiple personality disorder*. New York: Guilford Press.

Putnam, F. W. (1991). Recent research on multiple personality disorder. In R. J. Loewenstein (Ed.), *The psychiatric clinics of North America: Multiple personality disorder* (pp. 489–502). Philadelphia: W. B. Saunders Company.

Rhyne, J. (1973). *The Gestalt art experience*. Monterey, CA: Brooks/Cole Publishing Company.

Robbins, A., & Sibley, L. B. (1976). *Creative art therapy*. New York: Brunner/Mazel.

Rose, G. J. (1987). *Trauma and mastery in life and art*. New Haven: Yale University Press.

Ross, C. A. (1989). *Multiple personality disorder: Diagnosis, clinical features, and treatment*. New York: John Wiley & Sons.

Ross, C. A., & Gahan, P. (1988) Cognitive analysis of multiple personality disorder. *American Journal of Psychotherapy*, *42*, 229–239.

Rubin, J. (1984). *The art of art therapy*. New York: Brunner/Mazel.

Schaverien, J. (1992). *The revealing image: Analytical art psychotherapy in theory and practice*. London: Tavistock/Routledge.

Silvey, R., & MacKeith, S. (1988). The paracosm: A special form of fantasy. In D. C. Morrison (Ed.), *Organizing early experience: Imagination and cognition in childhood* (pp. 173–197). Amityville, NY: Baywood Publishing.

Simonds, S. L. (1994). *Bridging the silence: Nonverbal modalities in the treatment of adult survivors of childhood sexual abuse*. New York: Norton.

Spiegel, D. (Speaker). (1991). *Dissociation during trauma: Borrowing from the future to pay for the past* (Cassette Recording No. 1A-683-91). Alexandria, VA: Audio Transcripts.

Storr, A. (1993). *The dynamics of creativity*. New York: Atheneum.

Tyler, L. E. (1978). *Individuality: Human possibilities and personal choice in the psychological development of men and women*. San Francisco: Jossey-Bass Publishers.

van der Kolk, B. A., & van der Hart, O. (1991). The intrusive past: The inflexibility of memory and engraving of trauma. *American Imago*, *48*(4), 425–454.

Wadeson, H., Durkin, J., & Perach, D. (1989). (Eds.). *Advances in art therapy*. New York: John Wiley & Sons.

26

Psychopharmacology

Moshe S. Torem

INTRODUCTION

This chapter provides a review of the various psychotropic medications and benefits of their use in the treatment of patients with dissociative identity disorder (DID). Psychopharmacology in the broad perspective includes the study of the effects of psychoactive drugs on the human mind, including the patient's thoughts, feelings, physical sensations, fantasies, activities and behavior applied in day-to-day living. In general, it is important to state that currently there is no one specific medication or combination of medications that cure patients with a dissociative disorder. However, the use of psychotropic medications can be quite helpful by providing the following benefits:

1. Reduce the intensity of debilitating symptoms such as anxiety, depression, poor concentration, insomnia, restlessness, nightmares, panic states, exaggerated startle response, and phobias.
2. Improve the patient's mental state and attention focus to be more amenable and ready to benefit from psychotherapeutic interventions.
3. Provide the benefit of psychopharmalogical interventions in patients who have the comorbidity of a dissociative disorder with another psychiatric disorder such as major depression, bipolar disorder, panic disorder, obsessive-compulsive disorder, and so forth.

The primary treatment for patients with dissociative disorders is psychotherapy using a psychodynamic approach with adjunctive use of hypnosis when

Moshe S. Torem • Department of Psychiatry and Behavioral Sciences, Akron General Medical Center, Akron, Ohio 44307; and Department of Psychiatry, Northeastern Ohio Universities College of Medicine, Akron, Ohio 44272.

Handbook of Dissociation: Theoretical, Empirical, and Clinical Perspectives, edited by Larry K. Michelson and William J. Ray. Plenum Press, New York, 1996.

indicated (Kluft, 1984, 1985, 1989; Braun, 1986; Coons, 1986; Putnam, 1986, 1989; Ross, 1989). However, I believe that a comprehensive integrative approach is more effective and commonly used by many practicing psychotherapists. Such a psychotherapeutic approach integrates psychodynamic, behavioral, existential, and cognitive modalities. The relationship between the patient and the therapist is of paramount importance in creating a partnership whereby the patient is empowered to make choices, report on the use or misuse of medications, and participate in the evaluation of a desired outcome, whether it is the alleviation of symptoms, the improvement in functioning with the activities of daily living, or both.

MEDICATIONS AND PSYCHOTHERAPY: GENERAL CONSIDERATION

Physicians are traditionally exposed in their training to the idea that medications are an important part of any general clinical practice. Nonmedical therapists need to educate themselves on the special meaning and use of psychotropic medications and their place in the psychotherapy of patients with dissociative disorders.

The outcome effects in using psychotropic medications are highly influenced by the nature of the relationship between the patient and the treating clinician, especially the one who prescribes the medications. This has been scientifically recognized and has been termed the placebo effect to include expectations of outcome as perceived by the patient as well as the therapist and not just the direct influence of the active chemical ingredient in the prescribed drug. This is so important that it has become a standard in the efficacy evaluation of new medications to include double-blind studies so that neither the patient nor the prescribing physician know which drug is the placebo and which is the one with the tested active chemical ingredient. The placebo effect is a phenomenon that occurs regularly when the patient uses medications. The placebo effect may enhance the direct therapeutic effect of the chemical ingredient in the medication, which is termed the positive placebo effect. On the other hand, the negative placebo effect refers to a phenomenon that diminishes the therapeutic efficacy of the chemical ingredient in the prescribed medication. At times, the negative placebo effect can be so powerful that it not only eliminates any potential therapeutic effect of the chemical ingredient, but may also produce undesirable and noxious side effects (Plotkin, 1985; Evans, 1985; Shapiro, 1960, 1968; Shapiro & Morris, 1978).

The purpose of the prescribing clinician is to do everything possible to enhance the possible placebo effect to maximize the therapeutic efficacy of the prescribed medication. Enhancing the positive placebo effect involves the utilization of the patient's positive transference relationship to the doctor and the patient's belief that the prescribed medication is going to have the desired therapeutic effect, as well as believing in the curative powers of the physician. On the physician's side, it involves the belief in his or her skills and knowledge in treating the patient's condition, the belief that the prescribed medication is in fact going to work in a positive therapeutic manner, and the belief that the patient receiving the prescribed medication is in fact someone who can be trusted to benefit from the medication and has hope for healing and recovery.

It's important to remember that any time the patient swallows the prescribed medication, he or she will symbolically incorporate and internalize their image of the doctor, including what took place in the previous session. This internalization when the medication is swallowed is extremely important to remember since the very relationship with the prescribing doctor is an essential part of practicing rational psychopharmacotherapy. Well-trained and skillful doctors know this, and therefore spend at least 20 to 30 minutes and at times up to an hour with a patient even though the primary therapist of the patient is at times another clinician who sees the patient weekly and whose focus is on psychotherapy. It is also important to emphasize that the nonmedical therapist can enhance the efficacy of the prescribed medications by positively endorsing the prescribing physician and his or her therapeutic knowledge, experience, and skill in the field of dissociative disorders and previous successes with other patients.

In hospitalized patients, additional members of the team that influence this process should not be ignored. They are the nurse and the nursing assistant, as well as occupational therapist, art therapist, social workers, and pharmacist who may endorse the efficacy and positive therapeutic expectations of the prescribed medication and the positive reputation of the prescribing physician or they may criticize and question the wisdom of using the prescribed medication, and thus diminish its therapeutic efficacy.

All of the above-mentioned factors may explain the high degree of variability of results in using psychotropic or other medications in patients with dissociative disorders.

MEDICATIONS AND PSYCHOTHERAPY: SPECIFIC CONSIDERATION FOR DISSOCIATIVE DISORDERS

Patients with dissociative disorders deserve specific considerations in using psychopharmacotherapy. The following points are important to remember:

1. Patients with dissociative disorders usually have a history of past trauma and may have a tendency to express their unresolved trauma by repeating and reenacting the traumatic event in the relationship with the doctor. This in itself may involve an expectation that the doctor looks and behaves in a nice way but in fact may end up hurting the patient just as it happened in the past. Spiegel (1986) called this phenomenon the traumatic transference. This phenomenon originates from the double binds and dysfunctional families common in these patients' childhood memory. Spiegel cautioned that the doctor must be aware of it and its potential to sabotage and undermine any therapeutic intervention, including pharmacotherapy.
2. Patients with dissociative disorders frequently dissociate during the session and may have amnesia for certain parts or the whole session. This may interfere with the patient's compliance and understanding in the proper use of the prescribed medications.

3. In patients with dissociative identity disorder (DID), it is vitally important to recognize that alter personality states, even though hidden, obscure, and not directly involved in the dialogue that takes place between the doctor and patient, may still sabotage and undermine the desirable therapeutic outcome of prescribed medications. This may take place in a variety of ways, such as hiding the medications while in an altered ego state and later having amnesia to it, enhancing undesirable side effects, taking higher than prescribed doses, and so forth.

4. Patients with dissociative disorders at times may be highly suggestible and could use what Orne (1959) termed "trance logic." In this type of logic, the patient's thinking is rather concrete and devoid of the ability for abstraction.

5. In patients with DID, the prescribing doctor may face the phenomenon of one personality state being depressed, anxious, or even psychotic and requiring pharmacotherapy with a specific medication. On the other hand, other personality states may be in a quiet, relaxed, and neutral state of mind, not needing any medications. The dilemma for the doctor is to choose the most appropriate and efficacious therapeutic intervention. Should the medications be prescribed for the patient as a whole only when the specific symptoms are shared by all the personalities, or is it legitimate to prescribe medications when the dominant personality states suffer from certain dysfunctional symptoms?

6. The issue of comorbidity is also very important since patients with dissociative disorders may also suffer from other psychiatric disorders such as major affective disorders, anxiety disorders, attention deficit hyperactivity disorder, alcoholism, obsessive-compulsive disorder, as well as a variety of different personality disorders, such as borderline personality disorder, narcissistic personality disorder, histrionic personality disorder, dependent personality disorder, avoidant personality disorder, and so forth. It is certainly legitimate to use pharmacotherapy for a dissociative patient who has comorbidity with another psychiatric disorder.

7. The phenomenon of dissociation in itself is many times associated with a variety of physical signs and symptoms such as changes in heart rate, perspiration, breathing, blood pressure, blurred vision, numbness, intestinal hyperperistalsis, urinary frequency, urinary urgency, dry mouth, and so forth. All these may be difficult to differentiate from potential side effects of a given medication or the coexistence of a medical illness.

8. A variety of medications can act as triggers for dissociative episodes. These are medications used in the general practice of medicine, such as the decongestant Sudafed; the antihypertensive nifedipine; anti-inflammatory agents, such as ibuprofen; cortical steroids, such as dexamethasone; antibiotics, such as norfloxacin and ofloxacin; and antiparkinsonian agents, such as benztropine.

REVIEW OF THE LITERATURE

Loewenstein (1991) provides good basic guidelines for the use of rational psychopharmacology in the treatment of patients with DID. He mentioned several ground rules. The first is that the use of medications for multiple personality disorder (MPD) patients must be understood in the context of the total treatment of MPD, pointing out that it is important to establish clear reasoning for the expected benefits of the medications and to have clinical criteria for assessment as to whether the medication is beneficial. The second rule states that most problems in the treatment of MPD patients are not solvable with medications and have to be addressed in a broader context of psychotherapy done in a trustful therapist–patient relationship. Loewenstein's third guideline has two parts to it: (1) The doctor must attempt to treat symptoms in MPD that are valid psychopharmacological targets; and (2) The doctor must target symptoms that are present across the whole person and not those localized in separate alter personalities, i.e., are the result of dissociative switching.

Kluft (1985) pointed out that the presence of valid medication-responsive symptoms are very important before the decision to use medication is enacted. Nonpharmacological interventions have to be utilized for the same symptoms in order to enhance the potential positive response from the psychotropic medications. The physician prescribing the medications should have a trustful relationship with the patient and understand the patient as a whole, including the history of previous experiences with psychotropic medications. Some clinical trials reported partial success in individual cases with dissociative disorders using a variety of medications such as antidepressants, benzodiazepines, beta-blockers, clonidine, or low-dose neuroleptics (Barkin, Brown, Kluft, 1986; Braun, 1990; Fichtner, Kuhlman, & Gruenfeld, 1990; Loewenstein, Hornstein, & Farber, 1988; Ross, 1989).

Loewenstein et al. (1988) reported on a systematic study of pharmacotherapy for patients with MPD. Loewenstein and his colleagues reported moderate improvement with the use of clonazepam in some posttraumatic stress disorder (PTSD) symptoms and in five MPD patients in an open-label, nonblind clinical trial. The patients showed sustained improvement over 6 to 12 months in the continuity of sleep and lessening severity of nightmares and flashbacks. The patients maintained a stable clonazepam dose.

Braun (1990) reported on the use of clonidine and high doses of propranolol for the treatment of hyperarousal, anxiety, poor impulse control, disorganized thinking, and rapid switching in patients with dissociative disorders.

Many patients with DID suffer from the typical posttraumatic stress symptoms such as heightened sympathetic arousal, exaggerated startle response, disrupted sleep, and disrupted dreaming. These symptoms have been studied extensively in the Veterans Administration with posttraumatic stress disorder. Friedman (1988, 1991, 1993, 1994) noted that there is a serious shortage of double blind drug trials in the pharmacotherapy of patients with posttraumatic stress disorder, as is true for patients with dissociative identity disorder. However, from the available research it is clear so far that neuroleptics are not a first-line choice for PTSD symptoms. Neuroleptic drugs should be used only briefly to control severe agitation. If other drugs, such as anxiolytics and antidepressants have not worked, neuroleptic may be added for a more extended use.

Antikindling Agents

Kindling is a neurobiological phenomenon that occurs following exposure to traumatic stress. Kindling involves a hypersensitivity of certain parts in the limbic system of the brain. Chronic high intensity of sympathetic arousal is mediated by the locus coeruleus frequently releasing norepinephrine thus kindling the limbic system nuclei. This produces a stable persistence neurobiological abnormality. Van der Kolk (1987) and Friedman (1988) have independently suggested that the chronic central nervous system sympathetic arousal associated with PTSD produced an endogenous state that optimized conditions for limbic system kindling. The increased arousal is characterized by symptoms of insomnia, nightmares, flashbacks, impulsivity, affective storms, aggressivity, and acting out a compulsion to repeat the trauma. For these symptoms, antikindling drugs have been found somewhat effective. The antikindling agents most studied are: carbamazepine (Tegretol) and valproate (Depakote). Carbamazepine has been studied by Lipper et al (1986), who observed a reduction in the intensity and frequency of nightmares, flashbacks, and intrusive recollections. Valproate was studied by Fesler (1991) who showed that this drug can produce an alleviation of hyperarousal, as well as an alleviation in the avoidant numbing symptoms in patients with PTSD.

PHARMACOTHERAPY FOR SPECIFIC SYMPTOMS

Anxiety

Anxiety is a very common symptom in patients with dissociative disorders. It may be expressed with a sense of subjectiveness, restlessness, the feeling that some disastrous event may take place, loss of control, agitation, and a variety symptoms such as shortness of breath, blurred vision, urinary frequency, urinary urgency, diarrhea, tension headaches, poor concentration, dispepsia, and parastesias (peripheral numbness). The following groups of medications can be used for the control of anxiety: benzodiazepines, sedative antihistamines, buspirones, betablockers, as well as small doses of certain neuroleptics.

Benzodiazepines. Benzodiazepines are relatively safe anxiolytic medications. They can be classified into three major subgroups: short-acting, intermediate, and long-acting (as shown in Table 1). The two drugs in the short-acting group, i.e., midazolam and triazolam, are not recommended for use with dissociative disorders. From the intermediate group, the most often used have been lorazepam and alprazolam. And from the long-acting subgroup, the most commonly used have been clonazepam, diazepam, chlordiazepoxide, and clorazepate. Generally speak-

Table 1. Benzodiazepines: Comparative Action Time

Short-acting	Midazolam (Versed)	Long-acting	Chlordiazepoxide (Librium)
	Triazolam (Halcion)		Clonazepam (Klonopin)
Intermediate-acting	Alprazolam (Xanax)		Clorazepate (Tranxene)
	Halazepam (Paxipam)		Diazepam (Valium)
	Lorazepam (Ativan)		Estazolam (ProSom)
	Oxazepam (Serax)		Flurazepam (Dalmane)
	Temazepam (Restoril)		Prazepam (Centrax)
			Quazepam (Doral)

ing, all benzodiazepines are well absorbed from the intestines after all administration. There is no significant correlation between plasma concentration and clinical effects, so plasma level monitoring has no clinical benefit. The duration of action is determined mainly by the distribution and not by the rate of elimination. The major metabolism of these medications is done in the liver through microsomal oxidation and demethylation. Patients with liver disease may have trouble metabolizing these medications.

Potential Side Effects. Relatively, these medications are very well tolerated with few side effects, which disappear with dose adjustment. The most common side effects are oversedation, fatigue, drowsiness, nystagmus, anterograde amnesia (most likely with high potency agents), and confusion and disorientation (mostly in elderly patients). In some patients, paradoxical agitation may take place in the form of insomnia, hallucinations, nightmares, and rage reactions. All of these are likely to occur in patients with a previous history of aggressive behavior.

Withdrawal. Abrupt discontinuation of a benzodiazapine may produce the following symptoms:

1. Withdrawal: This occurs within 1 to 2 days in the short-acting group, 3 to 4 days in the intermediate-acting group, and 5 to 10 days in the long-acting group. Common symptoms include insomnia, agitation, anxiety, changes in perception, dysphoria, gastrointestinal distress, and even severe reactions such as hallucinations, seizures, and coma.
2. Rebound: Rebound occurs hours to days after medication withdrawal. Symptoms of anxiety may be similar or more intense than those originally reported by the patient.
3. Relapse: Symptoms may occur weeks to months after the medication was discontinued, and the symptoms are similar to the original anxiety present prior to the use of the medication.

Withdrawal Protocol. To withdraw patients from benzodiazepine, use an equivalent dose of diazepam as a substitute (for equivalent doses, see Table 2). The withdrawal should be done according to the following protocol:

1. Reduce diazepam by 10 mg daily until a total daily dose of 20 mg is reached.
2. Then continue to reduce by 5 mg daily to an end point of total abstinence.
3. Consider propranolol to aid in the withdrawal process.
4. Alprazolam requires a special protocol that includes the following steps:
   - Reduce alprazolam by 0.5 mg/week; quicker withdraw may result in delirium and seizures.

Table 2. Benzodiazepines: Comparative Equivalent Doses

Alprazolam (Xanax)	0.5 mg
Chlordiazepoxide (Librium)	25.0 mg
Clonazepam (Klonopin)	0.25 mg
Diazepam (Valium)	5.0 mg
Lorazepam (Ativan)	1.0 mg

- Carbamazapine in therapeutic doses may aid in the withdrawal process.
- An alternative to the above method is to substitute alprazolam with an equal dose of clonazepam in divided doses and then decrease the clonazepam by 1 mg/day.

Special Precautions for All Benzodiazepines

- Do not use on patients with sleep apnea disorders.
- Administer with extreme caution to patients who perform hazardous tasks that require mental alertness and physical coordination.
- Benzodiazepines lower tolerance to alcohol and high doses may produce mental confusion similar to alcohol intoxication.
- Physical and psychological dependence, tolerance, and withdrawal symptoms may be produced by all benzodiazepines. These are correlated with the dose and the duration of use.
- Abrupt withdrawal following prolonged use may produce seizures.

Toxicity. Overdose with these medications is rarely fatal if taken alone. However, it may be lethal when the overdose is taken in combination with other drugs, such as alcohol and barbiturates. Symptoms of overdose may include hypotension, depressed breathing, and coma. Pregnant women must be cautioned that benzodiazepines freely cross the placenta and may accumulate in the fetus. Data regarding the issue of teratogenicity are inconclusive.

Special Instructions to Patients

- Consumption of caffeinated beverages may counteract the therapeutic effects of the prescribed medication.
- The dose should be maintained as prescribed. Do not increase the dose without consulting your physician.
- Driving a car or operating other machinery should be avoided until a response to the drug is determined.
- Avoid the use of alcohol since it may enhance the effects of these medications, as well as alcohol side effects.
- Avoid abrupt stopping of these medications.

Drug Interactions

- Caffeine may counteract sedation and increase insomnia.
- Cimetidine may decrease the metabolism of benzodiazepines.
- Antihistamines may increase central nervous system depression, as well as coma and respiratory depression in high doses.
- Barbiturates may cause the same drug interactions as antihistamines.
- Alcohol may cause the same drug interactions as antihistamines.
- Estrogens (including oral contraceptives) may decrease the metabolism of benzodiazepines, and thus increase its plasma levels as well as its duration in the body.
- Propoxyphene (Darvon) may decrease the metabolism of benzodiazepines.

Comparing Various Benzodiazepines (See Table 3)

1. Alprazolam (Xanax)
   - Reaches a peak plasma level within 1-2 hours of administration.
   - Half-life elimination is reached between 9 and 20 hours.

Table 3. Benzodiazepine Trade Names and Dosage Ranges

Generic name	Trade name	Usual adult dosage range (mg/day)	Adult single dose range (mg)
Alprazolam	Xanax	0.5–6	0.25–1
Chlordiazepoxide[a]	Librium	15–100	5–25
Clonazepam	Klonopin	1.5–10	0.5–2
Clorazepate	Tranxene	7.5–60	3.25–22.5
Diazepam[a]	Valium	2–60	2–10
Flurazepam[b]	Dalmane	15–30	15–30
Halazepam	Paxipam	60–160	20–40
Lorazepam	Ativan	2–6	0.5–2
Oxazepam	Serax	30–120	10–30
Prazepam	Centrax	20–60	10–20
Quazepam[b]	Doral	7.5–30	7.5–30
Temazepam[b]	Restoril	15–30	15–30
Triazolam[b]	Halcion	0.125–0.5	0.125–0.5

[a]Also available for parenteral administration. Diazepam is available for IV administration in 5 mg/ml syringes. Lorazepam is available for IM administration in 2 and 4 mg/ml syringes.
[b]FDA approved for use as a hypnotic.

- It is rapidly and completely absorbed by most patients. Increasing the speed of absorption can be achieved by using it sublingually.
- It is effective in patients with panic attacks and as an adjunct in the treatment of depression.
- Dosing: Starting dose 0.25 mg three times a day; usual daily dose 1–5 mg/day; maximum daily dose 10 mg/day.
- Please note special precautions on withdrawal.
- Effects on sleep: Decreases stages I, IV, and REM sleep; increases stage II sleep.

2. Chlordiazepoxide (Librium)
   - 25 mg of chlordiazepoxide is equivalent to 0.5 mg of alprazolam.
   - Peak plasma level is reached through oral administration in 1–4 hours.
   - Elimination half-life is 4–29 hours of the parent drug and 28–100 hours of the active metabolites.
   - Oxazepam (Serax) is one of chlordiazepoxide's active metabolites.
   - Avoid use by intramuscular injections since the absorption is erratic and unpredictable.
   - Most commonly used in patients with alcohol withdrawal to preventing delirium tremens.
   - Antacids decrease the absorption rate from the gastrointestinal tract.
   - Dosing: Starting dose 5 mg three times a day; usual daily dose 15–100 mg/day; maximum daily dose is 300 mg/day.
3. Clonazepam (Klonopin)
   - 0.25 mg of clonazepam is equivalent to 0.5 mg of alprazolam or 25 mg of chlordiazepoxide.
   - Clonazepam is quickly and completely absorbed through the intestine and reaches a peak plasma level within 1–4 hours. However, it has a slow onset of activity.

- Elimination half-life is 19-60 hours.
- It has no active metabolites.
- It has strong anticonvulsant effects.
- It is commonly used for the treatment and prevention of panic attack and is also effective in patients in a manic episode.
- It is effective in controlling aggressive behavior
- It is also effective in controlling symptoms of akathisia

4. Diazepam (Valium)
   - Equivalent dose: 5 mg of diazepam are equivalent to 0.5 mg of alprazolam, 0.25 mg of clonazepam, or 25 mg of chlordiazepoxide.
   - It has a rapid onset of action and reaches the peak plasma level within 1-2 hours of oral administration.
   - Elimination half-life is 14-70 hours for the parent drug and 30-200 hours for its metabolites.
   - It is metabolized in the liver and has active metabolites such as oxazepam and temazepam.
   - Males have a shorter half-life and higher clearance rate than females.
   - Chronic use causes accumulation in fat tissue.
   - Heavy smoking is associated with higher clearance.
   - Especially effective as an anticonvulsant, in alcohol withdrawal and akathisia, and as muscle relaxant.
   - Effects on sleep: Decreases stages I, IV, and REM sleep.
5. Lorazepam (Ativan)
   - Equivalent dose: 1 mg of lorazepam is equivalent to 0.25 mg of clonazepam, 0.5 mg of alprazolam, 5 mg of diazepam, or 25 mg of chlordiazepoxide.
   - It is well absorbed with oral administration, including sublingually.
   - Peak plasma level is reached within 2 hours by oral administration, within 45-75 minutes by intramuscular injection, within 5-10 minutes by intravenous injection, and within 60 minutes with sublingual administration.
   - Elimination half-life is 8-24 hours.
   - It has no active metabolites.
   - It has a slow onset of action.
   - Dosing: Starting dose 0.5 mg twice a day; usual daily dose 2-6 mg/day; maximum daily dose 10-20 mg/day.
   - It is a good muscle relaxant.
   - It is effective for akathisia and acute dystonia.
   - It has significant anterograde amnesia which does not correlate directly with the sedative potency.
   - Withdrawal symptoms appear sooner than with long-acting drugs.
   - Effects on sleep: Decreases stage I and REM sleep; increases stage II of sleep.

Alprazolam and clonazepam are relatively more potent for panic and somewhat less potent with generalized anxiety.

Sedative Antihistamines. In this group, I mention two examples: hydroxyzine (Vistaril, Atarax) and diphenhydramine (Benadryl). These medications do have some antianxiety effects. They have no muscle-relaxing features. There is no potential abuse or habituation. They have some antiemetic features.

Hydroxyzine has few side effects. Its sedation when used for longer periods of time loses its effect because patients develop tolerance. Starting dose is 10 mg three times a day; usual dose 25 mg three times a day; maximum dose is 400 mg/day.

Diphenhydramine is available over the counter in the United States in a variety of cough syrups, as well as decongestant agents. It depresses the REM sleep in doses of 50 mg and higher. Starting dose is 25 mg twice daily; usual daily dose is 25 mg four times a day or every 4-6 hours as needed; maximum dose is 500 mg per day.

Side Effects and Toxicity. These include drowsiness and dry mouth, and they may cause urinary retention in high doses. Antihistamines should be avoided in patients with asthma, glaucoma, emphysema, chronic pulmonary disease, or shortness of breath. Alcohol should be avoided since it will increase the drowsiness.

Buspirone. Buspirone (BuSpar) is a relatively new selective anxiolytic medication which is not a benzodiazepine. It has no anticonvulsant features nor is it a muscle relaxant. On the other hand, this medication does not develop any tolerance or habituation. It is believed that it works on the central nervous system by decreasing the noradrenergic and dopaminergic activity. Long-term administration of buspirone may cause a down-regulation of the serotonin type II receptors. This medication is specifically effective where sedation is desired without causing any psychomotor impairment in functioning. Patients with a history of alcohol and substance abuse benefit from buspirone rather than benzodiazepines. It has also been used for the augmentation of antidepressant medications, and some claim (Jacobsen, 1991) that buspirone also has its own antidepressant effect when given in doses of 40-80 mg/day. may also potentiate antiobsessional effects of fluoxetine, sertraline, or paroxetine.

Dosage. Starting dose is 5 mg two times a day; usual daily dose is 10 mg three times a day; and the maximum dose is 60-80 mg/day. Clinical efficacy begins within 1-2 weeks of administering the usual dose of 30 mg per day. This medication is not useful on an as-needed basis. The maximum effect is usually seen in 3-4 weeks from the onset of administration. Food may reduce the rate of absorption. Peak plasma takes place between 0.7 and 1.5 hours. Elimination half-life is 1-11 hours. The drug has one active metabolite.

Potential Side Effects and Toxicity. The following side effects have been reported with buspirone: headaches, dizziness, light-headedness, fatigue, numbness, and upset stomach. Withdrawal effects have not been reported. There is no cross-tolerance with benzodiazepines, barbiturates, or alcohol.

It is a relatively safe medication and no deaths have been reported in people who overdose on buspirone. Toxic effects in cases of overdose include dizziness, nausea, and vomiting. Use during pregnancy in terms of safety has not been determined. However, both buspirone and its metabolites are excreted in the mother's milk.

Drug Interactions. Haloperidol may be inhibited in its metabolism when given in combination with buspirone, and thus plasma levels may stay higher for a longer time. Fluoxetine and monoamine oxydase inhibitors, when used in combination with buspirone, may cause high blood pressure and also potentiate antiobsessional effects. Buspirone may cause an increase in the serum level of diazepam.

Wise Tip. The antianxiety effects of buspirone are gradual, and signs of improvement may begin within 7-10 days after starting the medication, reaching a peak of improvement in 2-4 weeks.

Beta-Blockers. These agents, such as propranolol (Inderal), are most effective in the treatment of the autonomic symptoms of anxiety. This medication blocks the beta-adrenergic receptor sites, and thus prevents the natural neurotransmitters of norepinephrine and epinephrine from taking effect. Since the 1960s, they have been used for the treatment of anticipatory anxiety, such as performance during tests, public speeches, the theater, interviews, and so forth. The starting dose of propranol is 10 mg three times a day; usual daily dose is 20 mg three times a day; and the maximum dose is 240 mg/day. Braun (1990) reported on the experimental use of higher doses of propranolol in patients with MPD in order to reduce rapid switching. However, the control of anxiety is not a primary indication and does not appear in the Physicians Desk Reference nor is it specifically approved by the Food and Drug Administration for this specific purpose.

Side Effects. These include bradycardia, hypotension, light-headedness, dizziness, and occasionally fainting. It may also cause mental depression.

Neuroleptics. Some patients with severe anxiety to the point of agitation, impulsivity, and aggressivity may respond better to small doses of sedative neuroleptics, such as perphenazine (Trilafon), 2 mg three times a day up to 4 mg four times a day; thioridazine (Mellaril), 10 mg three times a day up to 25 mg four times day; and chlorprothixene (Taractan), 10 mg three times a day up to 50 mg four times a day. Some patients with very severe agitation respond better to an intramuscular injection of droperidol (Inapsine), 2.5-5.0 mg, which produces sedation and sleep lasting between 1 to 3 hours, following which the patient wakes up relaxed with no agitation (see Table 4).

Side Effects. Neuroleptic drugs have a variety of side effects ranging from drowsiness to extrapyramidal-parkinsonian reactions such as akinesia, rigidity and tremor, akathisia, acute dystonia, acute dyskinesia, and the late-appearing tardive dyskinesia. Many patients develop autonomic nervous system symptoms such as dry mouth, tachycardia, blurred vision, nasal congestion, and orthostatic hypotension. Some patients may develop agranulocytosis, dermatitis, jaundice, purpura, and even a malignant neuroleptic syndrome.

Depression

Depression associated with feelings of helplessness, hopelessness, futurelessness, and anhedonia is a common symptom in patients with dissociative disorder. Some patients may have the comorbidity of a major depression, a dysthymic disorder, or bipolar disorder. These should be treated accordingly as indicated in the standards of practice for mood disorders.

Antidepressant medications are currently available in the following groups:

tricyclic antidepressants, monoamine oxidase inhibitors, selective serotonin reuptake inhibitors, and miscellaneous antidepressants. In selecting the use of an antidepressant medication, I use the following guidelines:

1. *Safety.* It is of paramount importance to emphasize the fact that some depressed patients may be very impulsive and can act out on an instant urge in a self-destructive way. Prescribing the patient with an antidepressant medication that potentially can be overdosed by the patient must be considered in terms of the medication's safety profile. The wider the gap between the therapeutic dose and the toxic lethal dose, the safer the medication. In that sense, the tricyclic antidepressants and the monoamine oxidase inhibitors are the least safe, while the new generation of antidepressants such as the selective serotonin reuptake inhibitors are the safest; such medications as trazodone and bupropion are significantly safer than the tricyclics but not as safe as the selective serotonin reuptake inhibitors.

2. *Symptom Profile.* Some patients who have depression may slow down and withdraw emotionally and physically, have increased sleep (hypersomnia), increased eating (hyperphagia), generalized fatigue, and low energy level. This subgroup of patients responds well to antidepressant medications that not only alleviate the patient's mood but also have an energizing effect by suppressing the appetite and decreasing the patient's need to sleep. Medications that belong to this group include fluoxetine (Prozac), paroxetine (Paxil), bupropion (Wellbutrin), protriptyline (Vivactil), and, to a lesser extent, desipramine (Norpramin) and tranylcypromine (Parnate). On the other hand, there is another subgroup of patients who experience depression associated with psychomotor agitation and restlessness. Such patients also experience insomnia, anxiety, poor appetite at times associated with weight loss, and a feeling of aimless energy. These patients respond better to antidepressants that have a sedating effect, which improves their sleep and reduces the patient's level of anxiety and agitation. The following medications belong to this group: trazodone (Desyrel), amitriptyline (Elavil), doxepin (Sinequan), trimipramine (Surmontil), and maprotiline (Ludiomil).

3. *Side Effect Profile*

- *Anticholinergic.* Some patients are particularly sensitive to anticholinergic side effects such as dry mouth, blurred vision, constipation, and delayed micturition (urinary retention). Antidepressants that are highly potent in their anticholinergic side effects are the following: amitriptyline, clomipramine, doxepin, maprotiline, and amoxapine. On the other hand, the following antidepressants have the least anticholinergic side effects: desipramine, nortriptyline, trazodone, fluoxetine, sertraline, and paroxetine.
- *Cardiovascular Side Effects.* Cardiovascular side effects such as orthostatic hypotension, dizziness, tachycardia, and cardiac arrhythmias are not uncommon with antidepressant medications. The following antidepressants have the least cardiovascular side effects: fluoxetine, sertraline, paroxetine, and nortriptyline. The antidepressants with a higher frequency for cardiovascular side effects include amitriptyline, clomipramine, and imipramine.
- *Extrapyramidal Side Effects.* Amoxapine is the antidepressant most commonly related to these specific side effects due to a metabolite resembling the neuroleptic drugs.

• *Epileptic Seizures*. These have been reported in maprotiline in doses above 225 mg/day and in bupropion in doses of 450 mg/day and higher.

• *Weight Gain*. The issue of weight gain is extremely sensitive in our culture. Many patients will not cooperate in taking certain medications if it is associated with weight gain. The following antidepressants are associated with a weight gain of 10 pounds or more: amitriptyline, doxepin, and maprotiline. Those associated with the least weight gain are fluoxetine, sertraline, paroxetine, bupropion, protriptyline, and tranylcypromine.

4. *Concomitant Medical Conditions*. Some patients suffer from narrow-angle glaucoma, which is relatively well managed with eye drops. Such patients should not be given antidepressants that have anticholinergic effects since it may exacerbate a state of acute glaucoma requiring emergency intervention. Other patients may have benign hypertrophy of the prostate gland, which makes them more sensitive to developing urinary retention with medications that have anticholinergic effects.

5. *Previous Experience with a Certain Antidepressant*. Patients who had a positive previous experience with a certain antidepressant prefer to use it again if faced with the choice of taking one. Prescribing clinicians should be sensitive to this issue and inquire as to the patient's previous experience with certain antidepressants. A simple guideline is, "What worked before has a good chance of working again." The opposite of that is also true. The patient's negative experience with a certain antidepressant will diminish the chances of its efficacy even if everything else is compatible.

6. *Previous Familiarity with a Certain Antidepressant*. Some patients are familiar with certain antidepressants based on their positive efficacy with a family member, friend, or from their own reading about it. Such information should be elicited from the patient since it potentiates the positive placebo effect and improves the chances of a positive therapeutic outcome providing the rest is compatible and there is no contraindication.

7. *Timing*. Many antidepressants can be given in one dose and this will be sufficient for 24 hours. Most patients with insomnia will benefit from a once a day dose given at bedtime, thus promoting the patient's sleep, in addition to the antidepressant effects. This will also increase the patient's compliance in using the medication.

8. *Patient Choice*. Some patients with dissociative disorders detest being controlled and dictated to by the medical profession or any other authority figures. It is extremely important to incorporate the patient's need for empowerment and mastery into the prescribing skills of the doctor. I ask the patient to choose their own time when they wish to take their medication, whether it is before meals or after meals, in a once-a-day dose or in divided doses, providing everything else is equal. This increases the patient's sense of partnership in the decision process and improves the chances for cooperation in taking the prescribed medication.

9. *Age*. Elderly patients are more sensitive to hypotensive side effects of any medications, including antidepressants. Therefore, they should be given antidepressants with the least hypotensive side effects and should be educated as to measures to prevent orthostatic hypotension.

10. *Cost*. High cost of an antidepressant that is beyond the patient's economic affordability will reduce the chances of the patient's cooperation in taking

the prescribed medication. Physicians should be sensitive to the issue of cost and educate themselves as to the financial impact that a specific medication may have on the patient's weekly and monthly budget. This issue should be included in the discussion with the patient prior to choosing a specific antidepressant.

For specific daily doses of antidepressant medications, look for details in Table 4.

Flashbacks and Poor Impulse Control

These symptoms are quite common in patients with dissociative disorders. The following medications have been found to provide some relief of the intensity of these symptoms: perphenazine, chlorprothixene, haloperidol, and droperidol. It is important to note that such medications should be used with great caution and in low doses. Once the symptom has been significantly reduced, every attempt should be made to decrease and discontinue the specific neuroleptic medication used. Droperidol is available only by injection for intramuscular or intravenous use. In dissociative patients, it should be used only as an intramuscular injection in extreme states of high agitation with flashbacks, confusion, and destructive acting out. Droperidol has been found to be very helpful in doses of 2.5 to 5 mg every 4 to 6 hours. The therapeutic response takes place within 15-30 minutes. Many patients fall asleep and wake up in a different state of mind, more relaxed, mature, and appropriate. For specific daily doses of these medications, see Table 5.

Rapid Switching

This symptom is not easy to control. Braun (1990) reported on the use of propranolol and clonazepam with limited success in reducing rapid switching. My experience involved the use of Inderal in doses of 60-240 mg a day, as well as clonazepam in doses of 6-16 mg a day. The success rate improves with the utilization of hypnotherapeutic centering techniques (Torem & Gainer, 1993, 1995).

Table 4. Daily Dosages of Antidepressant Medications

Generic name	Trade name	Starting dose (mg/day)	Usual dose (mg/day)	Maximum dose (mg/day)
Nortriptyline	Pamelor	10-25	75-100	150
Amitriptyline	Elavil	10-75	100-150	300
Imipramine	Tofranil	10-50	100-150	300
Protriptyline	Vivactil	5-10	30-45	60
Trimipramine	Surmontil	25-50	100-150	300
Doxepin	Sinequan	25-50	100-150	300
Amoxapine	Asendin	50-100	100-200	600
Maprotiline	Ludiomil	25-50	75-125	225
Fluoxetine	Prozac	10-20	20-40	80
Sertraline	Zoloft	25-50	100-150	200
Paroxetine	Paxil	10-20	20-40	50
Trazodone	Desyrel	25-75	100-250	600
Bupropion	Wellbutrin	75-100	150-300	450
Tranylcypromine	Parnate	10-20	20-40	60

Table 5. Daily Dosages of Neuroleptics

Generic name	Brand name	Starting dose	Commonly used dose	Maximum dose (mg/day)
Perphenazine	Trilafon	2 mg TID[a]	4 mg/QID	24-30
Chlorprothixene	Taractan	10 mg TID	50 mg QID	300
Thioridazine	Mellaril	10 mg TID	25 mg QID	100
Droperidol	Inapsine	1.25 mg TID	2.5 mg TID	10

[a]TID, three times a day; QID, four times a day.

In two patients, there was a moderate response to the use of the antiepileptic and mood stabilizer carbamazepine in doses of 100 mg, three times a day, up to 200 mg, four times a day. Therapeutic serum levels for carbamazepine should be in the range of 4-12 μg/ml.

New Released Medications

The following medications have recently been released by the Food and Drug Administration for the use with a variety of psychiatric conditions and may also be helpful in patients with DID: fluvoxomine, naltrexone, nefazodone, risperidone, and venlafaxine.

Table 6 provides basic information regarding the drugs' primary indications, postulated mechanisms of action, and the various appropriate doses.

Fluvoxomine. Fluvoxomine is a selective seratonin reuptake inhibitor (SSRI). In that sense, it is quite similar to others in the SSRI group, such as fluoxetine, sertraline, and paroxetine. Even though the medication is particularly indicated in the treatment of patients with obsessive-compulsive disorder, it has also been known to have antidepressant features similar to the other SSRIs. So far, I have only limited experience in the use of this medication, and I have found it helpful in DID patients who have roominating thoughts, various obsessions, and compulsions, as well as in cases of DID patients who have a concurrent diagnosis of obsessive-compulsive disorder. For further information on this newly released medicine, please refer to the articles by John Griest et al. (1995). However it may be important to note here that fluvoxemine inhibits the activity of cytochrome P450 isozymes 1A2, 2C9 and 3A4, thereby slowing down the metabolism of other medications that are taken concurrently by the patient. It delays the clearance and increases serum concentration of the following drugs: alprazolam, propranolol, terfenadine, astemizole, and some of the tricyclic antidepressants. Dissociative identity disorder patients who concurrently suffer from drug addiction and are receiving methadone treatment may have increase plasma concentrations of methadone if they concurrently take fluvoxamine. In addition, fluvoxamine and MAO inhibitors should not be taken within two to three weeks of each other.

Naltrexone. This medication has been found helpful in DID patients who suffer from a concurrent diagnosis of alcohol dependence and opiate addiction.

Table 6. Newly Released Drug Names and Dosage Ranges

Generic name	Brand name	Indication	Average adult dose range (mg/day)	Adult single dose range (mg/day)
Fluvoxomine	Luvox	OCD	100-200	50-300
Naltrexone	ReVia	Alcoholism/narcotic dependence	50-100	25-150
Nefazodone	Serzone	Antidepressant	200-300	200-600
Risperidone	Risperdal	Antipsychotic	2-4	2-8
Venlafaxine	Effexor	Antidepressant	100-125	75-225

Naltrexone is an opiate antagonist, and animal studies have shown that opiate antagonists will decrease the animal's drinking of alcohol and craving for opiate-type drugs. In 1990, Braun reported some success in the use of naltrexone in the treatment of DID patients. Dr. Braun believes that some of the DID patient's symptoms can be understood in terms of the brain's addiction to its own internal opiates, i.e., the beta endorphins. Beta endorphins may be stimulated for increase in higher amounts at the time of repeated abreactions and repeated self-injurious behavior, which, according to Braun, are analogous to a drug addict's dependence on opiates. Dr. Braun reported on a trial of naltrexone for the control of such self-injurious behaviors as self-mutilation, binging and purging, compulsive sexuality, and compulsive exercising. However, this was a non-blind trial. So far, I have not had any experience in my practice with the use of this medication. Its place and efficacy in the treatment of DID patients remains to be seen in further research.

Nefazodone. This drug is chemically related to trazodone. It is an antidepressant and works by blocking the re-uptake of norepinepherine, serotonin, and dopamine. One of the effects of nefazodone is somnolence, which makes it best to be used at bedtime and perhaps an effective drug in the treatment of insomnia since it does not interfere with the patient's REM sleep. My experience in using this new drug with DID patients is rather limited, however, it may have a special place in the treatment of DID patients who suffer from depression associated with severe insomnia, since this drug does not reduce the patient's REM sleep and, in fact, according to a recent study by Sharpley et al. (1992), may increase REM sleep.

Risperidone. Risperidone is a newly-released neuroleptic classified as an atypical antipsychotic medication which is claimed not to have any extrapyramidal side effects and no tardive dyskinesia side effects. Apparently its mechanism of action may be mediated by blocking the receptors for dopamine type 2 (D2) and serotonin type 2 receptors. It also blocks alpha 1 and alpha 2 adrenergic receptors, as well as histaminergic receptors. My clinical experience with risperidone in DID patients has been limited to several severe cases dominated by symptoms of rapid switching, severe flashbacks, and other PTSD-intrusive symptoms such as severe anxiety, panic, and agitation. A dose of 0.5-3.0 mg, twice a day, was found to be highly effective in diminishing flashbacks, nightmares, agitation, and rapid switching. I have heard similar reports on the success in using this medication for DID patients with the above symptoms from other clinicians, such as Dr. James Chu, from McLean Hospital in Boston, Massachusetts (1995) and Dr. Richard Wolin from Buffalo, New York (1994).

Further research and clinical trials need to be done to have a better assessment on the efficacy and usefulness of this medication with DID patients.

Venlafaxine. Venlafaxine is a newly released antidepressant whose mechanism of action is believed to be the inhibition of reuptake of serotonin and norepinephrine. It is also a weak inhibitor of dopamine reuptake. Chemically, it is unrelated to tricyclics or other known antidepressant agents. The drug is reported to have no anticholinergic side effects. It should not be used in conjunction with MAO inhibitors. Venlafaxine is metabolized in the liver by the Cytochrome P450IID6 system. So any drugs that inhibit the effectiveness of this system will increase the plasma level of venlafaxine. The major side effects of this medication are nausea (37%), headaches (25%), and somnalence (23%). The usual dosing begins with 25 mg, three times a day, gradually increasing up to a maximum dose of 225 mg/day. My experience with the use of this medication in DID patients is rather limited, and I have reserved its use for those DID patients who suffer from depression as a major dysfunctional symptom and have not responded to other well-known antidepressants. For further information on venlafaxine, see Montgomery (1993).

Moclobemide. Moclobemide is a reversible monoamine oxidose inhibitor type-A. It is focused on affecting the central nervous system rather than the periphery. Amrein et al. (1989) pointed out that this drug has more potency in vivo than in vitro, suggesting that it is most likely metabolized to a different chemical form with higher affinity for the MAO-A than the parent compound. Moclobemide has also been shown *not* to have the increased inhibition of monoamine oxidaze by repeated administration of the drug, which does occur with the irreversible MAO inhibitors. The half-life of moclobemide is about 12 hours. This drug has been found effective in patients with all types of depression, including psychotic and bipolar depression. It is expected that this drug will be effective in the treatment of patients with bulimia, panic disorder, and posttraumatic stress disorder, as well as patients with dissociative disorders. Some of these effects have been shown by Versiana et al. (1992), Larsen et al. (1991), and Rossel and Moll (1990). The dose required is in the range of 300 to 600 mg/day. The drug interaction profile is very favorable. No interaction has been found in combining moclobemide with lithium, tricyclics, serotonin reuptake inhibitors, or neuroleptics (Amrein et al., 1992). Moreover, this drug does not require any dieting restrictions regarding tyramine-containing foods. The above feature of the drug increases the possibility of making moclobemide and other reversible MAOIs first-line choices. The drug is expected to be approved by the Food and Drug Adminsitration in 1996.

SLEEP APNEA AND NOCTURNAL MYOCLONUS

In the past two years, I have had the experience of treating more than a dozen cases of patients with DID who have been in long-term psychotherapy and have worked through many of their unresolved issues. However, in the face of various medications, these patients have continued to suffer from insomnia, as well as daytime symptoms of dissociation, amnesia, confusion, flashbacks, repetitive headaches, and depression. A thorough history included information from the patients' spouses and other relatives, revealing nighttime snoring as well as leg-jerking. This resulted in a special referral to the sleep lab for a nighttime polysomnogram, which revealed the diagnosis of obstructive sleep apnea, at times in combination with nocturnal myoclonus. The obstructive sleep apnea is apparently not uncommon in DID and PTSD patients. It interferes with the completion of healthy sleep cycles, including REM sleep, and it reduces oxygen saturation, causing the brain to suffer from brief periods of hypoxia. This results in chronic sleep deprivation, as well as daytime symptoms such as sleepiness and poor concentration. Effective therapy for these cases involved treatment with a continuous pressurized air perfusion machine or bilevel pressurized air perfusion machine. In addition, the patients who were diagnosed with nocturnal myoclonus were successfully treated with small amounts of clonazepam (up to 3 mg at bedtime) or small amounts of sinemet in doses ranging from one tablet of 25/100 mg to 50/200 mg at bedtime. The improvement in the patient's quality of sleep at night resulted in a dramatic improvement in the patient's daytime symptoms, including many of the dissociative symptoms mentioned above, as well as in the patient's level of daytime functioning. Dr. Michael Gainer and myself reported on these findings in the November meeting of the International Society for the Study of Dissociation in Chicago, Illinois, as well as in a recent report in the *ISSD Newsletter* (Gainer & Torem, 1994). Dr. Richard Kluft, who was at our presentation in Chicago, reported that he too has had several cases of DID patients who concommentantly suffered from sleep apnea and whose daytime symptoms were significantly improved following appropriate treatment with the continuous pressurized air perfusion machine. This information suggests that dissociative symptoms in patients with DID, as well as other aggravating symptoms, may be of multiple origins and may require a multimodel approach for successful treatment. It also points out that many DID patients may have comorbidity with other psychiatric disorders, as well as medical disorders.

CONCLUSION

It is important to remember the following points when prescribing medications with patients who suffer from DID:

1. Treat the person, not the illness. I believe that effective therapy of a DID patient involves the whole person and not just DID or any other disease. It is the person as a whole who should be treated, *not* just a disease or symptom.
2. There is no one specific medication or medication combination that cures the core symptoms of patients with dissociative disorders.
3. Medications are used as an aid in reducing the intensity of some symptoms, alleviating other symptoms, and helping the patient to better utilize psychotherapy.

4. In cases where the psychotherapy and the pharmacotherapy are provided by two different clinicians, it is vital for these clinicians to work together as a cooperative team to improve the therapeutic response to prescribed medications.
5. Patients with dissociatve disorders are not immune to other psychiatric diagnoses such as bipolar or unipolar mood disorders, panic disorder, obsessive-compulsive disorder, nocturnal myoclonus, or other conditions which do respond quite well to pharmacotherapy. In cases where comorbidity does exist, pharmacotherapy should be considered and used.
6. Safety should always be of the highest priority. In suicidal patients with histories of overdoses, the administration of new medications should be done cautiously and preferably in an inpatient setting.
7. Taking medication from a caring and empathic physician and making it an experience of mastery for the patient increases the chances for a positive therapeutic outcome.
8. More research is needed in this area of psychopharmacotherapy to determine which combinations of medication adminsitration are the ones that have the best therapeutic outcome in specific patients.
9. Sleep Apnea: In a recent report by Michael Gainer and myself (Gainer & Torem, 1994), we found that in a subgroup of patients who were diagnosed with DID, they also had a comorbidity of sleep apnea. The proper treatment of the sleep apnea significantly reduces the dissociative switching and amnesia during the day.
10. Do *not* be too aggressive with pharmacotherapy. Sometimes the side effects can be worse than the original presenting symptoms. Use a rational benefit risk assessment. When the potential benefits outweigh the potential risks, there is value in prescribing pharmacotherapy or any other therapeutic intervention.

REFERENCES

Amrein, R., Allen, S. R., Guentert, T. W., Hartmann, D., Lorscheid, T., Schoerlin, M. P., & Vranesic, D. (1989). Pharmacology of reversible MAOI. *British Journal of Psychiatry, 144,* 66-71.

Amrein, R., Guntert, T. W., Dingemanse, J., Lorscheid, T., Stabl, M., & Schmid-Burgk, W. (1992). Interactions of moclobemide with concomitantly administered medication: Evidence from pharmacological and clinical studies. *Psychopharmacology, 106,* S24-S31.

Barkin, R., Braun, B. G., & Kluft, R. P. (1986). The dilemma of drug therapy for multiple personality disorder. In B. G. Braun (Ed.), *The treatment of multiple personality disorder* (pp. 107-132). Washington, DC: American Psychiatric Press.

Braun, B. G. (Ed.) (1986). *The treatment of multiple personality disorder.* Washington, DC: American Psychiatric Press.

Braun, B. G. (1990a). Unusual medication regimens in the treatment of dissociative disorder patients: Part I. Noradrenergic agents. *Dissociation, 3,* 144-150.

Braun, B. G. (1990b). The use of naltrexone in the treatment of dissociative disorder patients. In B. G. Braun (Ed.), Seventh International Conference on Multiple Personality and Dissociative States (p. 20). Rush University Department of Psychiatry, Chicago, IL.

Chu, J. (1995). *Successful use if Risperidone (Risperdal) in the treatment of DID patients.* Personal communication.

Coons, P. M. (1986). Treatment progress in 20 patients with multiple personality disorder. *Journal of Nervous and Mental Disorders*, *174*, 715-721.

Evans, F. J. (1985). Expectancy, therapeutic instructions, and the placebo response. In L. White, B. Tursky, and G. E. Schwartz (Eds.), *Placebo: Theory, research and mechanisms* (pp. 215-228). New York: Guilford.

Fesler, F. A. (1991). Valproate in combat-related post-traumatic stress disorder. *Journal of Clinical Psychiatry*, *52*(9), 361-364.

Fichtner, C. G., Kuhlman, D. T., Gruenfeld, M. J., Hughes, J. R. (1990). Decreased episodic violence and increased control of dissociation in a carbamazepine-treated case of multiple personality. *Biological Psychiatry*, *27*, 1045-1052.

Friedman, M. J. (1988). Toward rational pharmacotherapy for posttraumatic stress disorder. *American Journal of Psychiatry*, *145*, 281-285.

Friedman, M. J. (1991). Biological approaches to the diagnosis and treatment of posttraumatic stress disorder. *Journal of Traumatic Stress*, *4*, 67-91.

Friedman, M. J. (1993). Psychobiological and pharmacological approaches to treatment. In J. T. Wilson and B. Raphael (Eds.), *International handbook of traumatic stress syndromes* (pp. 785-794). New York: Plenum.

Friedman, M. J. (1994). Biological and pharmacological aspects of the treatment of PTSD. In M. B. Williams and J. F. Sommor (Eds.), *Handbook of posttraumatic therapy* (pp. 495-509). Westport, CT: Greenwood.

Gainer, M. J. & Torem, M. S. (1994). Clinical corner: Sleep and dissociation—New findings. *ISSD Newsletter*, *12*(4), 8.

Griest, J. H., Jefferson, J. W., Kobak, K. A., Katzelnick, D. J., Serlin, R. C. (1995). Efficacy and tolerability of serotonin transport inhibitors in obsessive-compulsive disorder. *Archives in General Psychiatry*, *52*, 53.

Jacobsen, F. M. (1991). Possible augmentation of antidepressant response by buspirone. *Journal of Clinical Psychiatry*, *52*, 217-220.

Kluft, R. P. (1984). Aspects of the treatment of multiple personality disorder. *Psychiatric Annals*, *14*, 51-55.

Kluft, R. P. (1985). The treatment of multiple personality disorder (MPD). Current concepts. In F. F. Flach (Ed.), *Directions in psychiatry* (pp. 1-10). New York, Hatherleigh.

Kluft, R. P. (1989). Playing for time: Temporizing techniques in the treatment of multiple personality disorder. *American Journal of Clinical Hypnosis*, *32*, 90-97.

Larson, J. K., Gjerris, A., Holm, P., Anderson, J., Bille, A., Christensen, E. M., Hoyer, E., Jensen, H., Mejlhede, A., & Langagergaard, A. (1991). Moclobemide in depression: A randomized, multicentre trial against isocarboxazide and clomipramine emphasizing atypical depression. *Acta Psychiatrica Scandinavica*, *84*(6), 564-570.

Lipper, S., Davidson, J. R. T., Grady, T. A., Edinger, J. D., Hammett, E. B., Mahorney, S. L., & Cavenar, J. O. (1986). Preliminary study of carbamazepine in posttraumatic stress disorder. *Psychosomatics*, *27*, 849-854.

Loewenstein, R. J., Hornstein, N., Barber, B. (1988). Open trial of clonazepam in the treatment of posttraumatic stress symptoms in MPD. *Dissociation*, *1*, 3-12.

Loewenstein, R. J. (1991). Rational Psychopharmacology in the treatment of multiple personality disorder. *The Psychiatric Clinics of North America*, *14*, 721-740.

Montgomery, S. (1993). Venlafaxine: a new dimension in antidepressant pharmacotherapy. *Journal of Clinical Psychiatry*, *54*(3), 119-126.

Orne, M. T. (1959). Hypnosis: Artifact and essence. *Journal of Abnormal Psychology*, *58*, 277-299.

Putnam, F. W. (1986). The treatment of multiple personality: State of the art. In B. G. Braun (Ed.), *Treatment of multiple personality disorder* (pp. 175-198). Washington, DC: American Psychiatric Press.

Putnam, F. W. (1989). *Diagnosis and treatment of multiple personality disorder*. New York: Guilford.

Ross, C. A. (1989). *Multiple personality disorder: Diagnosis, clinical features, and treatment*. New York: Wiley.

Rossel, L. & Moll, E. (1990). Moclobemide versus tranylcypromine in the treatment of depressions. *Acta Psychiatrica Scandinavica, Supplementum*, *360*, 61-62.

Shapiro, A. K. (1960). A contribution to a history of the placebo effect. *Behavioral Science*, *5*, 109-135.

Shapiro, A. K. (1968). Semantics of the placebo. *Psychiatric Quarterly*, *42*, 653-696.

Shapiro, A. K. & Morris, L. A. (1978). The placebo effect in medical and psychological therapies. In S. L. Garfield & A. E. Bergin, (Eds.), *Handbook of psychotherapy and behavior change* (2nd ed., pp. 369-410). New York: Wiley.

Sharpley, A. L., Walsh, A. E., & Cowen, P. J. (1992). Nefazodone—a novel antidepressant—may increase REM sleep. *Biological Psychiatry*, *31*, 1070-1073.

Spiegel, D. (1986). Dissociation, double binds, and posttraumatic stress. In B. G. Braun (Ed.), *The treatment of multiple personality disorder* (pp. 61-77). Washington DC: American Psychiatric Press.

Torem, M. S., & Gainer, M. J. (1993). *Treatment of MPD: A systems approach*. Paper presented at the Eighth Regional Conference on Trauma, Dissociation, and Multiple Personality, April 23-24, Akron, OH.

Torem, M. S., & Gainer, M. J. (1995). The center core: Imagery for experiencing the unifying self. *Hypnos*, *22*, 125-131.

van der Kolk, B. A. (1987). The drug treatment of post-traumatic stress disorder. *Journal of Affective Disorders*, *13*, 203-213.

Versiana, M., Nardi, A. E., Mundim, F. D., Alves, A. B., Liebowitz, M. R., & Amrein, R. (1992). Pharmacotherapy of social phobia: A controlled study with moclobemide and phenelzine. *British Journal of Psychiatry*, *161*, 353-360.

Wolin, R. E. (1994). *Successful use of risperidone (Risperdal) in the treatment of patients with dissociative disorders*. Personal communication.

VII

SPECIAL TOPICS

In this final section of the volume, two areas that have generated heated debate are considered—ritual abuse and forensic interpretation of dissociative disorders. Ritual abuse is discussed by Sakheim in Chapter 27. In this chapter, he begins by defining ritual abuse and discussing modifiers such as "satanism" that have been applied to its description. Calling for more research, he begins by describing reports from a variety of sources related to ritual abuse. He then moves to a metacognition level and examines four of the ways in which people have related to these reports. By utilizing four approaches previously suggested by Greaves, general reactions can be characterized as coming from (1) Nihilists, (2) Apologists, (3) Heuristics, and (4) Methodologists. Unfortunately, Sakheim points out, there are no Methodologists since there are so few hard data at this time. However, the mere description of ritual abuse brings forth many complex and difficult questions for treating such abuse victims. This chapter emphasizes that these occur on both the level of the patient, whose information one must process in therapy, and on the level of the therapist, who must consider his or her own personal reactions to hearing stories of ritual abuse.

Dissociative identity disorder has placed the courts in the strange position of having to consider in what ways a dominant identity is responsible for crimes committed by one of the alters. In Chapter 28, Greaves and Faust give their personal reactions to legal, ethical, and historical development in the field of dissociative disorders. Using a narrative style, they consider, from the perspective of their own experience, the relationship between psychology and the law. This discussion is amplified by presentation of one of the most famous "multiple personality cases"—that of "Billy Milligan." The famous Billy Milligan case is one in which the courts found Mr. Milligan not guilty by reason of insanity after he had committed rapes under the control of one of the alters. For many people, these types of outcomes bring forth the consideration of malingering and further questioning related to the diagnosis of dissociative disorder as well as therapeutic techniques such as hypnosis. In contrast to the current legal interest in dissociative disorders, these authors actually suggest that dissociative disorders will play less of a role in future court cases.

27

Clinical Aspects of Sadistic Ritual Abuse

David K. Sakheim

In recent years, therapists have been confronted with thousands of cases in which both children and adults are alleging horrendous abuse at the hands of satanic cults. These patients have been labeled as "ritually abused" and/or "satanic cult survivors."[1] How to make sense of the memories of atrocities described by such individuals has resulted in tremendous controversy within the field. Unfortunately, both clinicians and researchers tend to take strong emotionally based positions, despite the absence of sufficient empirical data to do so in an educated fashion. This chapter is an attempt to discuss and clarify some of the issues that arise in this area and to give an overview of what is currently known in the field.

TERMINOLOGY

"Ritual abuse" is a new term, yet it has already gone through a number of permutations in meaning. It was originally proposed by Lawrence Pazder and Michelle Smith to describe her cult abuse experiences (Smith & Pazder, 1980). The term was designed to reflect a type of abuse that occurred because of the religious beliefs of the perpetrators. As others began disclosing similar stories, most of

[1]This term will be used to refer to individuals who present for psychotherapy and describe atrocities that were inflicted upon them by secret organized groups of people as part of religious rituals. Female pronouns will be used throughout this chapter when referring to ritual abuse survivors since, at present, the vast majority of survivors in therapy are women.

David K. Sakheim • 1610 Ellington Road, South Windsor, Connecticut 06074.

Handbook of Dissociation: Theoretical, Empirical, and Clinical Perspectives, edited by Larry K. Michelson and William J. Ray. Plenum Press, New York, 1996.

which involved groups practicing satanism, the phrase "satanic ritual abuse" began to be applied in the literature. However, it was immediately noted that virtually any group can as systematically abuse a child as can someone practicing satanism (Lanning, 1989). Kenneth Lanning (1992) also pointed out that it does not make sense to label a crime with the religion of the perpetrator. For example, in speaking about child abuse in the recent Waco Texas cult of David Koresh, people did not describe such abuse as a "Christian crime," and it would not have been useful to do so. Thus, the "satanic" was dropped in most uses.

In a task force summary report, the Los Angeles County Commission for Women defined ritual abuse as follows:

> A brutal form of abuse of children, adolescents, and adults, consisting of physical, sexual, and psychological abuse, and involving the use of rituals. Ritual does not necessarily mean satanic. However, most survivors state that they were ritually abused as part of satanic worship for the purpose of indoctrinating them into satanic beliefs and practices. Ritual abuse rarely consists of a single episode. It usually involves repeated abuse over an extended period of time. (Ritual Abuse Task Force, 1989, p. 1)

Current usage of the term "ritual abuse" has broadened somewhat from the original meaning and usually refers to the extremes of human cruelty in which an individual has experienced the combination of repeated physical, sexual, psychological, and spiritual abuses, usually within a religious context. Jean Goodwin (1993) recently recommended using the term "sadistic ritual abuse" to better capture that the phrase almost always applies to the effects of deliberate and repeated sadism.

Most children who are severely and repetitively abused experience this abuse in nonsatanic situations. In fact, it would appear that most child abuse occurs within the context of the family. Although child abuse in satanic cults is an important area, it would be a major error for the field only to focus on cults and miss the far greater problem of everyday child abuse.

SATANISM

Despite the broadened definition, most ritual abuse survivors who seek psychotherapy describe an involvement with satanism among their tormentors. This has made for some confusion about just who are these groups of perpetrators. As one attends to the details of abuses and the specifics of described practices, it becomes clear that these groups are not the same as any of the currently known satanic worshipers. A definition of "satanism" is not simple because the individuals and groups that get so labeled are actually very heterogeneous. "Satanism" as a religion does not necessitate any illegal or abusive activities. Thus, it is very important to be cautious and specific with how one uses the term (see Table 1).

As can be seen in Table 1, satanism can be a label applied by one group to another or a self-applied designation. It can refer to both known and controversial groups and can imply both legal and illegal practices. Throughout history, when one group was called satanic by another, the label usually was being given to justify

Table 1. Satanism

I. Groups known to exist
  A. Labeled by others
    1. Individuals persecuted due to their beliefs or practices
    2. Groups labeled satanic to justify oppression (typically due to different religious beliefs)
    3. Whole nations labeled satanic to justify their "enemy" status
  B. Self-labeled
    1. Organized legal and open satanic churches
    2. Individual dabblers (often with preexisting psychological problems)
    3. Small, disconnected groups/gangs that dabble in satanic practices
    4. Organized crime groups who practice satanic rituals, often with the belief that this will add to their power

II. Groups that are controversial
  A. Small groups of families or daycare personnel alleged to practice highly illegal and violent rituals
  B. Intergenerational satanic cults alleged to be an interconnected global network and to practice secret murderous/abusive rituals

warfare or oppression. It has usually been a way of saying that the individual or group in question is immoral and evil. For example, Ayatollah Khoemeni recently labeled the United States as "The Great Satan" and informed his followers that their moral duty was to fight this evil enemy.

On the other hand, satanism has been used as a self-definition (see Table 1). There are legal, constitutionally protected religions that practice satanism (e.g., the Church of Satan and the Temple of Set) which do not espouse any illegal activities. It is important to note that these legal and open religious groups are almost never named by ritual abuse survivors as being involved in their abuse.

Individuals and groups that break the law in their practice of "satanism" are heterogeneous as well. There are individuals who become fascinated with satanism or the occult and who may dabble in some homespun version (such as an alienated high school student who dabbles in black magic and drugs). There are groups (such as youth gangs) who get involved in satanism, often as part of their rebellion against authority. There are even organized crime groups that get involved in such practices (such as Adolfo Constanzo's murderous drug ring in Matamoros, Mexico).

It is very important to note that none of the above individuals or groups are the people that satanic cult survivors typically describe in their therapies. What is described is actually quite different from any of the known or documented individuals or groups listed above. Public discussions of satanism typically confuse these various groups. What is controversial is the description provided by ritual abuse survivors in therapy of highly organized intergenerational satanic cults and the extreme atrocities that these groups are alleged to commit. However, the media, for example, in presenting coverage about this controversy, frequently uses examples of the above groups (e.g., the groups in Section I.B of Table 1) to support survivors' reports in therapy or to provide evidence that well-organized intergenerational satanic cults exist. Unfortunately, this only serves to further confuse the issue. There is no question that satanism exists. The only controversial groups in Table 1 are those listed in Section II.

INCIDENCE–PREVALENCE

There have been no well-controlled studies on the incidence or prevalence of satanic ritual abuse reports. However, it is clear that more and more cases are appearing in the mental health system each year. Leon Jaroff (1993) noted that a recent survey found that roughly one third of a national sample of psychologists responded that they had treated at least one case of ritual abuse. He also noted that one referral agency in California alone claimed to receive over 5000 calls each year from survivors. This explosion of cases is not just limited to the United States, but is clearly a worldwide phenomena (Braun, 1989a). The lack of clear research data has not stopped speculation about actual incidence and prevalence figures. However, estimates vary tremendously, with some assuming that this phenomena is non-existent or extremely rare and others suggesting that this is a common occurrence. Dr. Bennett Braun, a noted researcher in the dissociative disorders field, has stated that, based on his experience and research, he would estimate this phenomena to be as frequent as 28% of all patients with multiple personality disorder (Braun & Gray, 1987), or even as high as 50% of all inpatients with multiple personality disorder (Braun, 1989b). Clearly, there is a need for more empirical research to address even such basic questions as how common are these reports in clinical settings.

ALLEGATIONS OF RITUAL ABUSE SURVIVORS

There are primarily two ways in which these extreme types of reports come to light. The first are reports coming from adult women in psychotherapy to deal with child abuse, and the second come from daycare abuse investigations with children. It is important to be clear that survivors are discussing an entirely different type of totalist group experience than any of the known forms of satanism in our culture. It is these descriptions of secret, violent, yet well-organized intergenerational satanic cults that many people find hard to accept and about which there is very little information or evidence.

What is typically described by these groups has nothing to do with those in Section I of Table 1. Instead, there is usually a description of a family or group of families that secretly have been practicing satanism for generations. The reports consistently describe extremely violent paramilitary organizations that indoctrinate their children from birth onward to become part of their belief system. The allegations almost always include the torture and murder of children and adults; sexual, physical, and emotional abuse of children; creation of child and adult pornography; forced impregnations and subsequent abortions of teenagers and adults; drug use and sales; forced participation in deviant sexual activities; forced consumption of bodily wastes; cannibalism; and other extreme forms of deviance and violence. These cults are alleged to be very well organized, to commit extreme abuse and violence, and to go to great lengths to cover up their activities.

The primary factor that has led some clinicians to believe the stories of their patients is that the allegations made by these survivors are quite detailed and consistent and often match those of other survivors who have never met, even in differing parts of the world (Braun, 1989a). The similarities in reports from survivors around the world can be uncanny, even down to the wording of specific prayers, the details and sequences of practices for specific holidays, or the secret coding systems and symbols alleged to be used by these groups. Until recently, such information was not widely available, convincing many clinicians that these individuals had been exposed to the kinds of experiences they claimed.

Reported Beliefs and Practices

Survivors typically describe a similar set of beliefs and practices among their tormentors. Although the reality is often disputed, it is interesting to note the commonalties in specific acts, beliefs, teachings, and motivations.

Katchen and Sakheim (1992) have summarized and catalogued these beliefs and practices. They point out that the belief systems described usually stem from a Gnostic viewpoint, in which the world is believed to be under the influence and control of hostile spirits. Thus, in order to survive in such a world, one must learn to control these spirits by becoming more powerful than they are. Learning "black magick" is believed to be the path to this end. This belief system often includes the notion that a person also can become more powerful by being possessed by one of these powerful evil spirits. "Possession" is seen as a way to obtain the power of such a being. For example, many survivors describe being forced to hold a hot object without reacting. A psychological explanation of such an event would be that the individual had to dissociate from the pain involved and hypnotically shut off his or her feelings. It would also be assumed that the pain was being registered out of conscious awareness. The cult view, on the other hand, is that the person was possessed by a strong demon or spirit who was able to handle such things without reaction. In other words, the psychological view would see this event as traumatic and likely to create later problems, while the cult view would see this as a strengthening experience for the person involved, since it connects him or her with such a powerful spirit. By later reconnecting with this spirit, that individual would be capable of superhuman abilities (e.g., of not feeling pain). Many of the events described by survivors appear designed to create such a "possession" experience, believed to increase the person's power in the world. It is also reported that these experiences are of value to the group because when the evil spirit leaves (the person returns to a normal state), memory of cult activities is usually gone as well (dissociated). This then adds an element of protection for the secret rituals that is also valued by the group.

Rituals

In general, the rituals described by survivors appear to have one of three primary purposes. These are indoctrinating someone into the group, helping someone in the group to attain increased power through possession or other magic, or intimidating a member never to disclose cult-related activities (Hudson, 1990; Katchen & Sakheim, 1992; Young, Sachs, Braun, & Watkins, 1991).

Indoctrination Rituals. There are rituals described at certain ages to convince a child that she is "evil" and therefore a part of the group. For example, most survivors describe death and rebirth rituals in which the child is first tortured and is then placed in a box or coffin, usually along with bugs and dead animals. The child is told that she is being killed and buried. After being left for an extended period of time, she is then dug up (sometimes put inside and then pulled out of an animal carcass) and is told that she is "being reborn unto Satan."

As noted above, there are many other types of tortures described by survivors, usually with the goal of getting the person into an altered state of consciousness so that dissociation (what they regard as possession) can occur. These include such abuses as being raped and/or physically injured, being partially hung, drowned, starved, dehydrated, locked in boxes or closets, given electric shocks and/or drugs, and so on. When the person does dissociate, this is encouraged and the split-off parts of the self are sometimes even given new cult names. The idea is that they can then be called on when a certain strength or ability is needed in the future.

Another way that the cults are reported to attack a survivor's sense of identity is to force her to commit atrocities toward others. This confuses any sense of being a good person, and is reinforced by messages to the contrary, such as telling the person that she is evil and therefore a part of the group.

The descriptions of such rituals make it clear that in order to survive, the person must either become an exquisite liar or must learn to dissociate (or both). For example, patients have described being tortured until they would agree to participate in a ceremony. However, when they finally agree, they are told that this is not good enough because they are only doing so to avoid further pain and not because they "really want" to participate. The torture then continues until the person either convinces the group that she really wants this or until she can split off a part of herself that is able to identify with the group's agenda. This is what the group is hoping to accomplish. If the person can dissociate and create a willing group member, the cult views this as possession by a cooperative spirit and therefore as success.

Many survivors describe elaborate "magic tricks" that are used to convince members of the group's power. For example, a number of patients have described having what is supposed to be holy water (but is actually acid) thrown on them. The high priest secretly makes the switch, and then, when the "holy water" burns the person's flesh, both she and the other group members are convinced that she truly must be evil and therefore have become part of the group. This kind of trick can be especially powerful when members of the group are using hallucinogenic drugs at the same time. Such drug use is a commonly reported part of most ceremonies. Such tricks also add to the later confusion about what is real and what was imagined. For example, child survivors from some of the daycare cases have described impossible events such as seeing other children taken apart and then put back together. Other survivors have reported being able to figure out some of these tricks, but most describe a profound sense of disbelief in their own perceptions that results from such confusing and bizarre experiences.

Acquisition of Power. Many of the descriptions of rituals involve reversals of traditional Christian practices and symbols. Survivors typically report that satanic groups see such desecrations as additional ways to attain the power to do magic. Thus, backward prayers, backward writing (e.g., "nema" instead of "amen"), desecration of church property, inverted symbols (e.g., upside-down crosses), and reversals of most Christian holidays and practices are deliberately embraced. This includes reversals of Christian rites of passage such as baptism. In the cult version, the goal is opposite to the Christian one, and becomes a rite to make the person "impure."

Most survivors also speak about having been forced to participate in rituals involving animal and/or human sacrifices. They claim that the groups view sacrifice as a way of obtaining the life force (power) of the organism being killed. In an attempt to explain the usefulness of sacrifices, Aleister Crowley (1924/1976) wrote:

> It would be unwise to condemn as irrational the practice of those savages who tear the heart and liver from an adversary and devour them while yet warm. In any case it was the theory of the ancient Magicians, that any living being is a storehouse of energy varying in quantity according to the size and health of the animal, and in quality according to its mental and moral character. At the death of the animal this energy is liberated suddenly. (pp. 94–95)

In other words, the younger or more "innocent" and "pure" the victim, the more power is believed to reside there. It is also believed that the more physiological arousal present, the more energy there is to obtain. Thus, survivor descriptions often include not only killing, but the deliberate induction of maximal fear and/or sexual arousal in the victim just prior to its death. Some of the cult practices described in therapy suggest that some groups are far more involved with the elaborate details of these practices, believing that numbers, colors, shapes, symbols, and specific practices all contain important magical significance. Other groups appear far less engrossed in such detail and seem much more involved in the sadism, power, and/or monetary aspects of the various activities.

Prevention of Disclosure. These groups are routinely described as going to great lengths to terrorize the members into complete obedience and silence. Everything from tricks and illusions to blackmail and direct threats are used. Children often report being threatened that any disclosure will result in harm to pets, family members, or to themselves.

Many survivors also describe sophisticated uses of hypnosis ("programming") to insure loyalty to the group. A common report of such programming concerns "magical surgery." This process has been widely described by survivors in therapy (Hudson, 1990; Katchen & Sakheim, 1992; Young et al., 1991). For example, a child is drugged and upon awakening is informed that a bomb was surgically placed inside her that is programmed to explode if she ever tells anyone about the group. She is told that this will kill her as well as the person she tells. This kind of suggestion is very clever since it capitalizes on the person's physiology to enhance its effects. If the child even thinks of telling someone, her nervous increase in heart rate may be misconstrued as the bomb's ticking.

Some clinicians have reported incredibly sophisticated and intricate "programming" involving elaborate attempts at mind control that begin early in a child's life and are reinforced on a regular basis. What makes most of these reports even more controversial is that they often include references to the involvement of CIA and other government intelligence agencies. It is alleged that these groups have been interested in studying mind control in an attempt to develop the perfect assassin, soldier, or messenger, by using deliberately created dissociation. Although US and other intelligence agencies have revealed that they have carried out secret mind control experiments on unsuspecting civilians and have even involved organized crime figures in their research (Marks, 1979; Shefflin, 1993), the present allegations suggest a far more elaborate and organized effort involving long-term experimentation, using a variety of tortures, on hundreds of nonvolunteers, mostly children. If confirmed, it undoubtedly would be the biggest scandal in US history. Clearly, many of these reports sound farfetched. But, once again, what has been convincing to some therapists is that numerous clinicians have validated running into similar detailed descriptions of these mind control strategies and the agencies involved, even down to the same unusual code words and techniques being mentioned and the same individuals being named (Hammond, 1993).

Various types of conspiracy theories abound when it comes to this area, and some writers believe that blaming satanism has become a way to have simple answers for the complex and overwhelming violence and turmoil in our current world as well as disillusionment with current political answers (Hicks, 1991). These authors point to the massive conspiracy theories as examples. For instance, in his book, *The Ultimate Evil*, Maury Terry (1987) postulates interconnections between organized satanic cults, the Process Church, the Manson murders, and the Son of Sam killings.

The Black Mass. The most controversial allegations made by survivors involve reports of forced abortions, infanticide, and cannibalism. These usually have to do with descriptions of a Black Mass. Such depictions are not new, and have emerged in very similar forms throughout recorded history. However, historians are as divided as current researchers as to the significance of such reports (Hill & Goodwin, 1989; Noll, 1989; Raschke, 1990). Some historians believe that these stories are the evidence for an ongoing satanic conspiracy that has been unmasked from time to time. Others see them as fictional accounts designed to titillate (such as the stories from the Marquis de Sade). There are still others who believe that these are primarily the text of tortured confessions produced by inquisitions and are therefore completely unreliable. Finally, there are historians who believe that these reports are genuine criminal acts, but are the actions of isolated groups of mentally unbalanced individuals who happened to hit on similar bizarre behaviors in acting out their perversions. They explain the similarities of reports as being due to the fact that there are a limited number of options available for such extreme sadism and debauchery. Thus, the similarities in reports do not suggest interconnections between groups, but merely similarities among the pathologies of the perpetrators.

Specific descriptions of the Black Mass usually include the reciting of backward prayers, the murder of an infant or the use of an aborted fetus in the ceremony (many survivors report being raped in previous ceremonies so that they will be pregnant and can be aborted in this ritual), the consumption of blood and flesh, the use of alcohol and drugs throughout, and finally, a sexual orgy where children and adults are all involved. The Black Mass allegedly is designed to combine the various rituals that the group believes can enhance their power to do magic.

Summary

Whatever the rationales, it is clear that virtually all of the allegations from survivors are of terrible abuses and tortures by the very people who were supposed to protect them. In fact, virtually every survivor also describes sadistic abuses at home in addition to the traumas that occurred at rituals and cult ceremonies. Whether or not the specific descriptions have all occurred, a picture almost always emerges of a family that is almost exclusively focused on power and control in every sphere of life. The experience that survivors present dramatically portrays having felt completely helpless and alone in a sadistic, controlled, and power-oriented environment. For most clinicians, it is difficult to believe that that experience was not in some way real, even if aspects of the survivor's presentation turn out to be something else.

CREDIBILITY ISSUES

The most common area for discussion about satanic cults in current papers, conferences, and the media is to debate the reality of their existence. The opinions expressed vary from the extreme position assuming 100% accuracy of survivors' recall to the equally extreme alternative position that none of the descriptions of atrocities are real. Clearly, until more investigative work is completed, there can be no definitive answers to this debate. However, it seems likely that there will never be one single answer. Patients will probably range from those who are malingering for secondary gain to those who are delusional or who were tricked and confused. There are likely to be others for whom descriptions of satanism are screen memories, incorporated ideas from readings or support groups, metaphoric communications, or even exaggerated memories. There are likely to be some distortions due to trance phenomena for patients who are highly dissociative, and finally, there are likely to be some individuals who have truly experienced extreme and ritualized forms of abuse.

The situation becomes even more complex when one sees that not only is it probable that patients will differ in these ways, but that even for one individual, different memories may have different meanings. A patient who was actually abused in a cult may have some memories that are distorted due to tricks, confusion, or drug use at the time and other memories that are more clear and unmistakable. Some memories may be more elaborated due to secondary gain, while others may even be able to be corroborated. In other words, each individual will likely experience a variety of influences to memory so that each description has its own complex meanings.

At present, the field is not yet acknowledging this complexity, but is more involved in a debate about whether or not the phenomena are real. Unfortunately our field has a tendency to become polarized in such situations, with some clinicians claiming that every patient's story is true and that the rest of the field is heartless (e.g., "believe the children"), while others claim that every patient's story is delusional, that there is no such thing as dissociation or repression, and that the rest of the field is merely too gullible (e.g., the proponents of a "false memory syndrome"). This argument primarily comes down to how to make sense of two conflicting aspects of these claims. The first is that survivors from all over the world are coming forward with very similar descriptions and reports of abusive practices by satanic cults (Edwards, 1990). The second is that there has not been sufficient forensic evidence found to date that would validate these allegations, especially the more extreme charges of infanticide and adult murders (Hicks, 1991). In an excellent discussion of this dilemma, George Greaves (1992) points out that in the presence of conflicting information and the absence of clear data, therapists, sociologists, historians, anthropologists, police, and other researchers in this area tend to take one of four positions. He calls these the Nihilists, the Apologists, the Heuristics, and the Methodologists.

Ritual Abuse as False Memory

Greaves (1992) refers to the first viewpoint about this area as being "Nihilist." The commonality for this group is that they believe that reports by survivors cannot be true. Some members of this group naively cannot conceive the possibility that human beings could be so violent and cruel to each other. However, the majority of this group's membership are clear-thinking individuals. Some are clinicians who do not work in the trauma field (and are therefore less moved by similarities between these and other trauma survivors), others are police who have become skeptical of survivor reports after failed investigations, and most of the rest are researchers (e.g., historians and anthropologists) who are hypothesizing that false ritual abuse reports are a phenomena that occurs under certain problematic social conditions.

The police in this group point out that in addition to the lack of sufficient physical evidence, ritual abuse reports are usually different from what is currently understood about other types of crime (Van Benschoten, 1990). Ken Lanning of the FBI notes that there are aspects of these crimes that make them hard to accept. For instance, the reports typically describe as many female as male perpetrators, something unseen in the forensic world. The reports also involve multiple-victim, multiple-perpetrator conspiracy crimes in which very dysfunctional individuals are alleged to go for long periods of time maintaining tightly controlled secrets and group loyalties. Lanning points out that these individuals are described as being completely out of control and impulsive at times, yet able to commit massive conspiracy crimes while maintaining total group loyalty and cohesion, as well as being able to cover up all forensic evidence of their crimes. He suggests that this is difficult to accept, especially on such a large scale (Lanning, 1992).

Interestingly, there is a small group made up of therapists and client advocates who take the Nihilist position as well. These individuals are fearful that the more extreme reports of ritual abuse survivors will not be verified in the long run and that this will harm the hard-won credibility of other abuse survivors and of the trauma recovery movement itself.

The Nihilists point out the lack of convincing forensic evidence to date. For example, Hicks (1991) provides an excellent critique of much of the evidence that has been used to support ritual abuse allegations. However, this group has largely been unable to come up with satisfying arguments to explain the allegations themselves of why survivors from around the world are saying such similar things. Some of the explanations generated by this group are shown in Table 2.

George Ganaway (1989) compared the phenomena of patients reporting ritual abuse to those reporting UFO abductions, suggesting that the same psychological mechanisms (the creation of dissociative fantasies and distortions) may be at work for both populations. Of the various writers in this group, he offers the most plausible psychological explanations of why some survivor reports may not be accurate.

The sociologists and anthropologists in the Nihilist group also point out ways that communities can become involved in believing inaccurate reports about satanism. Examples include "urban legends," where interesting but untrue stories get rapidly spread through a population, or rumor panics that effect small rural areas (Victor, 1990). The Nihilists believe that this type of social contagion is not only occurring in the larger society, but is specifically taking shape in the psychotherapeutic community. As satanism is more widely reported, therapists believe they are seeing it and/or patients believe that this must have been their experience (Brunvand, 1986; Hicks, 1991; Mulhern, 1990, 1991; Richardson, Best, & Bromley, 1991; Victor, 1989).

Although it is certainly the case that each of the above hypotheses can account for some cases, therapists working in the field usually do not see them as satisfactory explanations for what they are witnessing clinically. If the Nihilists are correct that this phenomena is completely unreal, there will need to be better psychological explanations for how this can occur. The field simply does not yet have an adequate theory to account for thousands of people making up and believing detailed and consistent stories of horrendous abuse.

Table 2. Nihilist Explanations for Ritual Abuse Allegations

Individual reports
1. Screen memories
2. Incorporation from reading, lectures, or other patients
3. Delusions/hallucinations
4. Therapist influence/suggestion
5. Reinforcement by therapist for severe abuse allegations
6. Errors in hypnotically recovered memories
7. Material from the collective unconscious

Community hysteria about cults
1. Social contagion
2. Urban legends
3. Rumor-panics

George Greaves (1992) calls the second viewpoint about ritual abuse the "Apologists." This group is primarily made up of the clinicians who work with ritual abuse survivors and who insist that patient reports of massive atrocities must be true. These therapists tend to work with incest victims and other trauma survivors, and many have been politically active in pushing the field to understand the psychological impacts of such trauma; they therefore tend to approach abuse reports from an advocacy stance. There is a strong belief that an injustice has been done to trauma survivors in the past because of the field's disbelief in reports of incest and other family abuses (Masson, 1984), and many in this group caution that we not make the same mistakes again. In order to maintain this position, the Apologists must then account for why so few validating data have been available.

Some Apologists argue that in fact there has been forensic evidence to support survivor claims, that numerous cases have even been won in court, but that these data are often unavailable because there is currently no organized police mechanism for collecting such case information (Boyd, 1991; Raschke, 1990; Tamarkin, 1993). However, more typically, in order to explain the paucity of available forensic evidence to support the numerous claims by survivors, Apologists tend to trace the flow of the investigative process, pointing out the problems that occur for ritual abuse survivors at every step of the way.

The Apologists point out that most ritual abuse survivors are too intimidated and afraid to go to the police in the first place, and even if they do go, they often are not taken seriously because of the bizarre nature of the allegations or because the accusations are being made by a child or an adult with a psychiatric history. Even if the police believe the reports, it is noted that they tend to be very hesitant to devote the resources needed to investigate such claims because of limited manpower or because the statute of limitations for prosecution has frequently run out.

When investigations do occur, the Apologists claim that it is not surprising that more information has not been found since the cults use very sophisticated mechanisms to destroy evidence (such as portable crematoriums) and because the police are not trained to investigate these types of groups (just as special units had to be formed to successfully investigate organized crime). The Apologists go on to suggest that when evidence has been found and cases have been pursued, they frequently have been so mismanaged by investigators that they become impossible to pursue to a trial. Most people in the field agree that the cases that have gone to court have been terribly mishandled (such as the McMartin case), making it almost impossible to sort out what really happened. Errors have included leading interviews, contamination between witnesses, premature notification of potential perpetrators, lost evidence, poorly trained therapists and police, to name but a few.

Thus, rather than saying that no confirming evidence has yet been found, Apologists argue that it would be more fair to say that there have not yet been any adequate investigations. Some Apologists even go so far as to suggest that in many of these cases the above problems have been compounded because police or other investigative agencies were infiltrated by cult members who sabotaged attempts to explore cult-related charges.

Many Apologists accurately point out that the cases that reach the court system are frequently "sanitized" so that claims of satanic cult activities are dropped or restated in more traditional legal language. This is done by prosecutors who are afraid that juries will become incredulous at the more extreme charges, so they leave out the controversial aspects of the case and prosecute for "child abuse," "murder," "cruelty to animals," "child pornography," and so on. The result is that if they then obtain convictions, these do not appear to be convictions of "satanic cult cases."

The above explanations account for some cases being inadequately pursued, examined, or followed up. However, these arguments are not sufficiently satisfying to police and others who are trying to understand how it is possible that thousands of survivors (each alleging massive conspiracy crimes that involve multiple murders, abortions, stabbings, kidnappings, etc.) have not resulted in more substantive forensic evidence to date. This criticism becomes more and more problematic as time goes by, especially since some police forces and district attorneys are now willing to pursue these allegations, are providing training to their officers, and are devoting manpower and resources to investigate this area.

Accuracy of Memory as Irrelevant

George Greaves (1992) describes another group of clinicians who claim that it does not matter if this phenomena is real or not. He calls this group the "Heuristics." They point out that these patients seem to get better if they are treated like other trauma survivors and their stories are accepted as truth. In other words, if a clinician acts as if the reports are real and helps the patient to work through her feelings, the patient can recover. It is argued that the clinician is not an investigator and that the veracity of the material is not relevant. Clearly, however, this is not a viable social position because it *does* matter if the reports are real or not. A major problem with this position has come about as more and more of these cases end up in court. One might argue that the truth of such claims can sort itself out in the haven of the consulting office; however, once people's lives and reputations are on the line in court, a different standard becomes essential. In addition, the truth of allegations about children and adults being being raped, killed, cannibalized, or used to make pornography certainly does matter in terms of society's obligation toward protection and prevention.

Positions Based on Research and Data

The last group described by Dr. Greaves (1992) are the "Methodologists." This group is made up of people who base their views on the data. Unfortunately, at the present time this group clearly has no members! There does not yet appear to be sufficient data to come to any solid conclusions about this area. Until there is a more centralized way of disseminating information about investigations of these cases and until such investigations are able to be assessed from beginning to end, it is simply not possible to fairly assess whether adequate efforts have yet been pursued.

In the absence of such clear research data, much of the writing to date is based on clinical experiences, speculations, and preexisting assumptions. However, a careful study of clinical cases would actually suggest that the outcome of this debate may be to endorse a more complex view than any of those described by Dr. Greaves (1992). It may well be that patients presenting as ritual abuse survivors are actually quite a heterogeneous group. Memory is a very complicated, and as yet, little understood process. Some of the known factors affecting recovered memories are shown in Table 3.

There is no question that some patients are lying about having had cult experiences. For example, various kinds of false sexual abuse allegations can occur in some custody battles in order to obtain increased leverage. The truth in such complex legal cases is often impossible to sort out. There are also some patients who appear to be malingering in order to obtain attention, availability of staff, and monetary support or increased psychotherapy time. It is unfortunate but true that current practices in the mental health field sometimes differentially reinforce certain types of problems so that patients can be pushed toward defining themselves in more extreme ways. For example, it is not uncommon for more interest and resources to be expended for a "satanic ritual abuse survivor" than for someone who is "merely" disclosing a history of family violence.

It is also clear that some patients present with delusional disorders, demonstrating primary process thinking. Psychotic patients frequently can include satanism as part of their delusional system. Such a presentation, however, is usually quite different from the degree of specificity, knowledge, and detail described earlier.

Some clinicians have reported seeing instances of incorporation where a patient comes to believe that he or she has experienced ritual abuse (or other trauma) after being exposed to it verbally or after reading about someone else's experiences. The reported instances of this "sponging" of material from another patient usually have been described as occurring for patients who are struggling to make sense of their own vague feelings and symptoms. After reading or hearing a

Table 3. "Memory" as a Complex Process within and across Individuals

1. Conscious lying
2. Malingering for secondary gain
3. Delusional material
4. Screen memories
5. Incorporated memories from others
6. Metaphoric communications
7. Exaggerated memories
8. Misperception based on confusion or trickery
9. Torture or drug-induced distortions
10. Trance phenomena in the creation or retrieval of memories
11. Other, as yet unknown types of distortions (e.g., pseudo-PTSD)
12. Actual experiences

description of another person's experiences, they confuse identification with the feelings with the belief that the same things must have happened to them. It would seem likely, therefore, that even if the descriptive material is not accurate in these instances, it is still important to attend to the feelings behind the descriptions. Thus, it would be a mistake to discount such incorporation as being out of whole cloth. The person is likely struggling to convey something for which they may not have words, but which is about feelings that seemed accurately conveyed when someone else described their experiences. It is certainly possible that some UFO abduction reports and/or past lives descriptions are similar in being attempts to find images to convey something only currently available on a feeling level.

A ritual abuse memory could also turn out to be a screen for more usual family incest experiences. However, this is mostly inadequate as an explanation of these recovered memories because most ritual abuse survivors typically also describe memories of severe abuses within their families. Thus, the idea of a "screen" to protect them from such overwhelming betrayal would not apply (Greaves, 1992).

Some survivors appear to be speaking in the language of metaphor. These individuals do not usually describe details of holidays, coding systems, or the content of prayers. However, their descriptions of rape and other abuses by Satan worshipers may speak to how their nonsatanic childhood abuse experiences actually felt to them. Just like those who incorporate someone else's story, these individuals may be using images and metaphors in an attempt to communicate about experiences and feelings for which they do not currently have the words.

Some trauma survivors defend themselves by minimizing the significance of the abuses they actually experienced. Thus, to convey the horrors of what they felt (and often feel while remembering), there may be some need to exaggerate their story. In other words, the patient is communicating about feelings. For example, they may feel that in order to convey to the listener the degree of horror and taboo experienced as a sexually abused child, they must describe something as extreme as cannibalism or infanticide.

There is also no question that some trauma memories become confused or distorted. People are generally terrible as witnesses, even under ideal circumstances (Orne, 1979). If one is hearing the retrieval of a dissociated memory, 20 years after the fact, that was created under the influence of trickery, fear, torture, pain, terror, and sometimes a variety of drugs, it would be inconceivable to imagine that some distortions do not occur. Thus, it is quite likely that most trauma memories have at least some element of idiosyncratic distortions. This confusion of perception is often one of the most painful aspects for any torture survivor in his or her struggle to sort out what is real.

Hypnosis has been shown to influence memory in a variety of ways. The most significant is that the subject is often able to fill in memory gaps. These can be accurate or inaccurate reconstructions, but the person involved usually increases his or her belief in the material in either case (Bliss, 1986; Orne, 1979). It would make sense that this could occur whether or not the hypnosis was part of a formal induction procedure or happened in the patient's own recovery of a dissociated memory (e.g., in a flashback, dream, body memory, etc.). Many survivors also describe deliberate hypnotic procedures as part of their abuse in which all sorts of distortions of experience were suggested to them. Thus, although this is not well understood, it would appear that some survivor memories may have been influenced by hypnotic distortions or hypnotic artifacts that have occurred from the traumas experienced and other distortions from the memory recovery process itself.

It is clear that some patients describe traumas that external investigations suggest were never experienced. Clinicians have reported examples of this such as a Vietnam veteran who presents with combat-related posttraumatic stress disorder (PTSD), but who, upon external investigation, turns out to never have been in the military, or patients who describe aspects of near-death visions, abuse in a past life, abduction and abuse by space aliens, and so on. It is certainly conceivable that some ritual abuse survivors fall into a similar category. It clearly would provide the field with very useful information to follow such patients in order to see if their symptoms reflect some other type of trauma or are instead more similar to some form of delusional disorder. Following the therapy course for patients with "pseudo-PTSD" would help us understand more about the various categories in Table 3. It would also help us to understand what is helpful in psychotherapy in such cases. For instance, is it necessary for the patient to eventually come to understand their distortions or can therapy be helpful if it never challenges these? Does the psychotherapy for such patients follow a similar or a different course than the therapy for more typical PTSD cases? Some clinicians have reported success in dealing with such material as if it were real; for example, Morse and Perry (1990) and Ring (1984) describe the clinical usefulness of exploring near-death visions, and Feldman (1993) and Ryder (1992) both describe the help to their clients of abreacting "past life" memories as real events. It seems difficult to imagine that treatment could truly be successful without ultimately dealing with whatever is behind such material and the need to disguise it with these metaphors; but this is clearly an empirical question that has not yet been addressed.

Last, for anyone working with this group of patients, it is very convincing that at least some have had the experiences they describe. Many present a clinical picture fitting the profile of a torture survivor, and the course of treatment often supports this view. It seems unlikely that the vast numbers of patients presenting as ritual abuse survivors have all been through such extreme abuses; however, it certainly seems possible that some have. A few patients have even been able to present external evidence to support their claims, with a small minority being able to find some forensic data to support them.

Complexity of Memory

It is very important to appreciate the complexity of this area and it seems likely that even for any particular patient, different memories that surface may fit into different categories in Table 3. In fact, it is probably fair to say that most patients will present with a combination of these factors. The field is only just beginning to acknowledge the complexity of memory (e.g., the American Psychological Association just commissioned a task force to investigate and summarize the data about repressed-recovered memory). Thus, it is very important to recognize that memory has many functions and many forms. If clinicians can keep an open mind about a patient's descriptions, the patient will be far better served than if the clinician comes to his or her work with a preconceived notion about the veracity of recovered information.

A recent example from my practice may help to exemplify this complexity. A woman in her late 20s, who had been in therapy for a few years, had made major positive changes in her life, primarily by working through numerous childhood abuse memories. She and I had been able to validate the accuracy of many of these in discussions with siblings, grandparents, and parents, through medical examinations that documented her internal and external injuries, as well as through obtaining a variety of documents (e.g., school and medical records) and even recovering some of the objects used in the abuse. After a few years in therapy she began to have a memory of being present at the murder of a little boy. This memory was very confusing for her as her perspective was not at all clear. In order to help to clarify her confusion about it, she drew the scene that was in her mind (see Figure 1). Unlike other memories, instead of becoming more and more clear as she worked on it, this one became more and more confused. At times it seemed as though she had been the woman in the drawing, at other times she thought that she had been the little boy, and sometimes she even thought that she had been the priest doing the killing.

The mystery was finally solved when she discovered an almost identical picture in her mother's attic. Upon finding this picture, she remembered that on one of the many times that she was being abused, she had dissociated, left her body, and gone into the nearest picture on the wall (a defense she had used many times

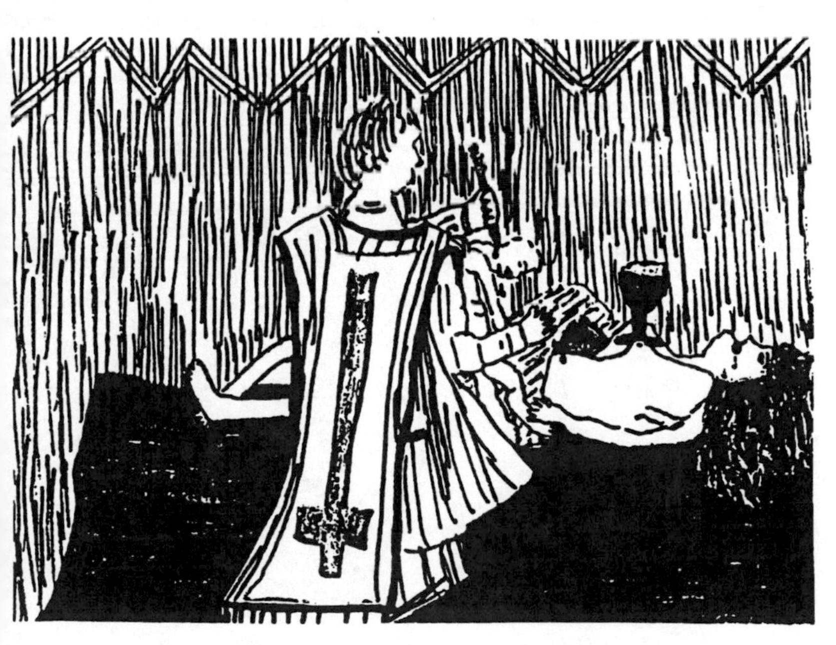

Figure 1. Client's drawing of her "memory."

before). Unfortunately, instead of finding it to be a pleasant scene in which to escape, she found the picture shown in Figure 2. Thus, not only did this leave a dissociated memory of the real abuse, but also left her with the confusing sense that she had experienced what was in this picture.

The above example is not given to suggest that all ritual abuse memories are created in this way. It is given to show the incredible complexity of memory. Even for someone with externally well-validated memories, it is possible to find one that turns out to be something other than directly factual. It is noteworthy that this memory felt different to her, motivating her to continue to pursue its meaning even after she had "recovered" it. However, her case points out the potential danger if a clinician assumes that there is perfect accuracy in recall (especially if the "memory" leads to charges being made against other individuals), as well as the danger of dismissing all recovered memory as fantasy (since many of her other memories had been able to be validated).

The fact that trauma survivors can give very accurate accounts, can speak in metaphor, can lie, can be confused, and so forth should really not be all that surprising to clinicians. Unfortunately, the field's need to see survivors as either being perfectly accurate or as having "false memories" misses this complexity. This can create problems clinically, but especially creates them when survivors enter the legal system. There is no reason to think that the testimony of an abused person cannot have the same kinds of distortions and contaminations as other people's testimony. In addition, it appears that severe abuse can create confusion and a need for distance, which can result in additional distortions. It would be tragic to disallow such testimony, but it would be equally mistaken to assume perfect veracity. Just as we might expect that a crime victim could make errors in identification due to his or her state of emotional arousal at the time of the crime, we must assume that this is possible for severe child abuse survivors. However, we do not

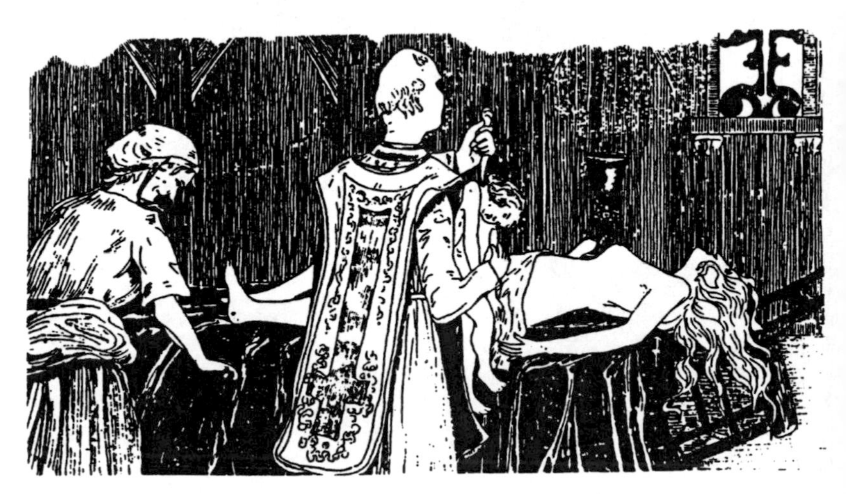

Figure 2. Picture on the attic wall in parents' home.

disallow the testimony of all crime victims just because we know that they can make errors. What is done instead is to insist that there be corroboration via a combination of evidence (including witness testimony) that helps to rule out reasonable doubts about what is being alleged.

It is worrisome that some court systems are beginning to disallow hypnotically refreshed testimony rather than educating themselves about the potential costs and benefits of such a process. The reason this is problematic is that many abuse survivors use their own hypnotic abilities to defend themselves against the abuse. They also use hypnotic processes to recover the memories later on (whether or not this is pursued in conjunction with a therapist). If this defense is then regarded as something that makes them less than credible, we would be denying many victims of violence the possibility of using the courts. Just as fear can create inaccurate recollections for any crime victim, dissociation (use of one's hypnotic abilities to distance from an overwhelming situation) can lead to inaccuracies later on. The answer is not to disallow all testimony contaminated by hypnotic processes any more than it would be to disallow all testimony contaminated by fear. The same principles should apply when it comes to the reports of sadistic abuse survivors as for any other population. Juries should be educated about the kinds of errors and accuracies that can occur with such memories and should then be allowed to assess the whole of the evidence presented.

TREATMENT ISSUES

A discussion of the treatment of ritual abuse survivors is obviously complicated by the fact that, as noted above, ritual abuse survivors are a heterogeneous and complex group of patients. However, it is possible to discuss certain important issues that are likely to emerge in this work. As in any good therapy, the first phase of treatment is assessment. The initial assessment of these patients is not so different from any other evaluations and primarily utilizes a therapist's standard assessment skills and knowledge of posttrauma syndromes. It is important to make a comprehensive evaluation of the patient's presenting problems, as well as to begin to hypothesize about where in Table 3 this patient seems to fit (or which combination of areas apply). Since virtually all of these patients appear to have some kind of trauma history, it is important to examine the areas of functioning known to be affected by such experiences. In reviewing the research and clinical literature on the effects of trauma, Sakheim and Devine (1995) suggest that in addition to the standard psychiatric assessment that would occur for any patient, a comprehensive assessment for trauma survivors should include evaluation of the following areas found in the research and clinical literature to be impacted by trauma and violence: relational disturbances, general distancing defenses, hypnotic distancing defenses, returning memory fragments, physical and physiological consequences, cognitive consequences, aggressive-sociopathic responses, spiritual consequences, aspects of the trauma itself, past and present support, the internal strengths of the patient, and the patient's current external situation.

Unfortunately, many standard psychological assessment techniques are not validated for the impact of severe trauma and can result in a misdiagnosis (Mangen,

1992). However, Mangen (1992) points out ways that psychological testing can be effectively utilized, as well as noting some of the newer, more specific assessment devices that are being developed.

Most clinicians working with severe trauma survivors suggest that in addition to assessment, the early phase of psychotherapy is primarily aimed at establishing a trusting relationship and an environment of safety both inside and outside of the therapy setting (Herman, 1992). This often takes a very long time for people who have been severely abused and betrayed by those who were supposed to protect them.

The stages of therapy with ritual abuse survivors are very similar to those for other trauma survivors with PTSD. Judith Herman's (1992) model of psychotherapy will not be reiterated here, but is a simple and elegant outline for the psychotherapy process that should be must reading for any clinician working in this area. Since virtually all of these patients have experienced severe kinds of abuse, most have utilized dissociative defenses. Thus, in working with this population, it is also important to be familiar with what has been learned in recent years about the dissociative disorders and appropriate treatment interventions (Kluft, 1989; Putnam, 1989; Ross, 1989). In general, the approaches needed with ritual abuse survivors vary only in that these patients often appear to be at the far end of the abuse-torture continuum and therefore require more attention to safety and grounding issues as well as concern about maintaining functioning and stability.

SPECIFIC TREATMENT ISSUES

Much of the treatment of ritual abuse survivors involves an attempt to understand the original adaptive significance of many of the current problematic behaviors of the patient. This search usually reveals that in their original context, these same behaviors were very helpful to the person's survival. Thus, the patient comes to see that she is not "crazy," but rather, has been continuing a defensive strategy that was once adaptive but is no longer necessary or helpful now that she is out of the abusive, controlled context. In such an examination of symptoms, instead of seeing herself as pathological, the patient comes to see herself as having survived a very difficult and threatening time, using creative defenses.

Self-Abuse

One of the symptoms that almost always emerges for such severe abuse survivors is that of self-abuse. This is an area that has been widely misunderstood, but recently has been best discussed by John Briere (1993), who explains such behaviors as "tension reduction" strategies. Briere points out the defensive value of self-abuse in its management of otherwise intolerable affects.

In trying to help someone stop hurting themselves, it is essential to explore what purpose such behavior is serving. Only through an understanding of the costs and benefits of that particular kind of self-abuse, at that particular time, is it possible to really begin to explore realistic alternatives. There are countless reasons why people injure themselves, and Table 4 shows some of the more common patient descriptions of how it can be helpful as a defense.

Table 4. Reasons for Self-Abuse

1. Distraction from painful affect
2. To show others the pain inside, "to make the outside look like the inside feels"
3. To go into a trance
   a. To push away a painful memory/feeling
   b. To bring forward a personality who handled pain by being anesthetized, thereby eliminating current pain
   c. To use a trance state to come back from a flashback
   d. To switch alters to achieve a more tolerable feeling state
   e. To speed up a flashback by jumping to the end via replicating the physically painful part
   f. To self-sooth by leaving the body or otherwise going to an internal safe place
4. To see blood/feel pain
   a. To feel real (instead of some kind of dissociated unreality)
   b. To recreate part of an abuse memory
   c. To ground oneself by becoming aware of one's body and the present instead of being lost in a memory
5. Internal communication
   a. For one alter to punish another
   b. For one alter to try to communicate about a memory (such as by carving a symbol on the body), especially if they are not being heard any other way
6. To express anger
   a. A generalized expression of anger by an alter that doesn't feel pain
   b. If one alter blames another or themselves
   c. To pretend the self-abuse is being done to a perpetrator
7. Physiological
   a. To trick the body into releasing endorphins
   b. To create a feeling that is incompatible with a frightening one (such as creating pain so as not to feel sexual feelings)
8. Confusion of feeling states due to early abuse experiences
   a. Confusion of pain/closeness
   b. Confusion of pain/sexuality
9. Other personal meanings

In order to help someone to find alternatives to self-abuse, one must first understand its idiosyncratic meanings. For example, one woman cut herself vaginally every night before being able to go to sleep. If she did not do this, she was unable to sleep. In exploring this symptom, she remembered that most nights when she was a child, her brother would hide in her room, jump out after she was in bed, and violently rape her. She recalled being unable to fall asleep, knowing this was likely to occur; however, once it was over, she could go to sleep, knowing that she was now "safe" for the rest of the night. Thus, as an adult, she would lie in bed, in a state of hypervigilance, unable to sleep. However, once she cut herself, she could replicate the feelings that she had had that made her feel that the danger was past and that she could let down her guard and sleep. Once this was understood, she was able to find an alternative to the self-abuse. She could remind herself of the safety of her current room and that her brother was no longer in her life. She got a burglar alarm so that she could decrease her need for internal vigilance. She learned and practiced other self-soothing strategies at bedtime, with a special focus on helping the parts of her that had experienced the abuse to be in an internal safe place.

The above example points out the importance of understanding the meaning of any symptom to the person, of learning its original adaptive value, and then of seeing if it is still serving any important functions. One can then work on finding alternatives that achieve similar benefits without the same costs. Alternatives are often relatively easy to find once the symptom is truly understood. For example, if someone is using self-abuse to go into a trance, one can teach them much easier and less harmful way to accomplish this. There are many types of trance induction that are not self-damaging. Slow drawing on the arm with a magic marker may work just as well as slow cutting. In general, self-hypnosis or other relaxation strategies are often just as effective trance induction methods. If the person is trying to show how horrible things are internally, drawing and/or writing may be a good alternative. If an alter is trying to communicate something, encouraging the person to find safe ways to listen to that part of themselves may negate the need for such extreme action. If an alter is expressing anger by cutting, learning that other parts of the person do feel this as well as learning other ways to express such feelings might be helpful. If an alter is blaming themselves or another personality for the abuse, exploration of the incident may help to reframe this misperception. Even if the person is trying to trick the body into releasing endorphins by creating a minor injury [an automatic reaction the body has after any injury (Van der Kolk and Greenberg, 1987)], this same effect can often be accomplished using hypnosis and sometimes by using medications or other self-soothing approaches. If the person is confusing feeling states because of early experiences in which these always occurred together (e.g., pain with sexual feelings), this can be explored in therapy, and ultimately the patient can be encouraged to experiment with experiencing one without the other.

In other words, the solution cannot be prescribed ahead of time, and one person's solutions may not work for someone else. It is critical to explore the personal meanings of the behavior, its original adaptive significance, its current functions, and to explore what might work as a substitute in accomplishing the same goals without the same costs.

Programming

Many patients who describe ritual abuse histories include detailed descriptions of perpetrators using deliberate hypnotic suggestions designed to control their later behaviors. Programming, as described earlier, is an area about which many clinicians disagree. At present, for those clinicians who believe that it does occur, there are primarily three approaches that get suggested to deal with it in treatment. These are attempting to dismantle the program, countering the original programmers with alternative suggestions, and last, treating the program like any other abuse symptom.

The first approach assumes that people are like machines that can be programmed. It is believed that the therapist must understand sophisticated mind control techniques in order to safely deprogram the patient. This approach is similar to defusing a time bomb. It is believed that a wrong move can result in dire consequences. This approach primarily comes from the work of Corrydon Hammond (1993), who describes some patients as having been programmed by the intelligence community, utilizing incredibly sophisticated layers of programs, specialized codes, and protective systems. The second approach views programming as merely hypnotic suggestions that were given to the patient as part of their abuse. Thus, the solution is simply to give countersuggestions. The last approach views programming as hypnotic suggestion, but also sees it as part of an abuse incident that must be abreacted and reframed in order to truly undo its effects. It is viewed here as just another type of abuse.

In the absence of any clinical trials of these approaches, they can only be addressed in terms of personal clinical experiences. Some would argue that the first approach is unnecessary since many clinicians are successfully dealing with this area without being experts on mind control. However, others argue that these clinicians are missing important programs and controls that will cause later symptoms for their patients. The second approach, of trying to outsmart the original programmers, appears to work in many instances, but many clinicians report that this is usually only a short-term solution, and that the patient's belief in the original program will eventually resurface again. In general, most clinicians seem to agree that a long-term solution requires that the patient remember the abuse incident in which such a suggestion was made in order to experience how it was really a trick, and to fully understand how the suggestion affected them. At that point, countersuggestions may not even be needed.

Danger

The issue frequently arises of how much danger exists for both patients and therapists involved in this work. Many clinicians in the field believe that there is great danger from currently active cults. Interestingly, a recent study suggests that there is little direct evidence of harm coming to either patients or therapists who are working on ritual abuse issues (Stanek, 1993). Despite these data, there is often a tremendous degree of fear that is generated in such work, with many patients becoming convinced that they will be killed for disclosing information and many therapists becoming convinced that their own or their family's lives are in danger. It is certainly conceivable that working with this population could pose risks; however, the data noted above would suggest that this has not occurred with any frequency to date. It may well be that both patients and therapists are primarily responding to the intensely projected affects from childhood memories of extreme powerlessness, danger, and fear. This is clearly an important area to investigate further because if the danger is no longer in the present, it would clearly be a disservice to the patient for clinicians to validate such feelings, instead of helping the patient understand them as part of their past experiences.

SUMMARY

Psychotherapy with ritual abuse survivors is very complex and very difficult work. The extremes of human cruelty that are described are bound to affect the therapist in profound ways. Although the work can reaffirm the therapist's faith in human beings and in the ability of love to survive even the most unimaginable horrors (Sakheim, 1993), it can also bring into question many of the therapist's previous beliefs about people and about life in general (McCann & Pearlman, 1990). It is an easy area in which to lose objectivity and to develop countertransference difficulties. The therapist must not be seduced by his or her own needs or by the compelling material and the intensely projected affects to give up a therapeutic role.

The degree to which intergenerational satanic cults exist, conspire, and are organized is not yet clear. However, there is not disagreement about the fact that many of the patients in question have experienced severe forms of abuse and that as therapists we will need to find ways to help them to heal. Clearly, there is a need to investigate the claims of these patients further in order to help ascertain the reality behind the allegations. However, even if we discover that there is no global satanic conspiracy, or that some of the descriptions are metaphors for other types of abuse, we will still need to develop ways to provide treatment for these clients and to investigate and prosecute the criminal acts that have occurred. Too strong a focus on Satan or on any of the other more mystical and sensational aspects of this area can take us away from the sad reality of the extreme sadism and violence that are truly behind the problems that these and many other patients experience.

REFERENCES

Bliss, E. L. (1986). *Multiple personality disorder, allied disorders and hypnosis*. New York: Oxford University Press.

Boyd, A. (1991). *Blasphemous rumors: Is satanic ritual abuse fact or fantasy?* London: Fount.

Braun, B. G. (1989a, April). *Ritualistic abuse and dissociation*. Paper presented at the Second Annual Conference for the California Society for the Study of Multiple Personality and Dissociation, Costa Mesa, CA.

Braun, B. G. (1989b). Letters to the editor. *International Society for the Study of Multiple Personality and Dissociation Newsletter*, p. 11.

Braun, B. G., & Gray, G. (1987). *Report on the 1986 questionnaire: Multiple personality disorder and cult involvement*. Paper presented at the Fourth International Conference on Multiple Personality Disorder/Dissociative States, Chicago, IL.

Briere, J. (1993, June). *Tension reduction behaviors*. Paper presented at the Fifth Regional Conference on Abuse and Multiple Personality, Washington, DC.

Brunvand, J. H. (1986). *The choking doberman and other "new" urban legends*. New York: Norton.

Crowley, A. (1924/1976). *Magick in theory and practice*. New York: Dover. (Reprint 1976)

Edwards, L. M. (1990). Differentiating between ritual assault and sexual abuse. *Journal of Child and Youth Care, Special Issue*, 67-90.

Feldman, G. C. (1993). *Lessons in evil, lessons from the light*. New York: Crown Publications.

Ganaway, G. (1989). Historical truth versus narrative truth: Clarifying the role of exogenous trauma in the etiology of multiple personality and its variants. *Dissociation*, *2*(4), 205-220.

Goodwin, J. (1993). *Sadistic abuse: Pitfalls for victims and therapists*. Paper presented at the Fifth Regional Conference on Abuse and Multiple Personality, June, Washington, DC.

Greaves, G. (1992). Alternative hypotheses regarding claims of satanic cult activity: A critical analysis. In D. K. Sakheim & S. E. Devine (Eds.), *Out of darkness: Exploring satanism and ritual abuse* (pp. 45-72). New York: Lexington Books.

Hammond, C. (1993, June). *Treatment approaches to ritual abuse and mind control*. Paper presented at the Fifth Regional Conference on Abuse and Multiple Personality, Washington, DC.

Herman, J. L. (1992). *Trauma and recovery: The aftermath of violence—From domestic abuse to political terror*. New York: Basic Books.

Hicks, R. (1991). *In pursuit of satan: The police and the occult*. Buffalo, NY: Prometheus Books.

Hill, S., & Goodwin, J. (1989). Satanism: Similarities between patient accounts and pre-inquisition historical sources. *Dissociation*, *2*(1), 39–44.

Hudson, P. S. (1990). Ritual child abuse: A survey of symptoms and allegations. *Journal of Child and Youth Care, Special Issue*, 27–54.

Jaroff, L. (1993, November 29). Lies of the mind. *Time*, 52–59.

Katchen, M. H., & Sakheim, D. K. (1992). Satanic beliefs and practices. In D. K. Sakheim & S. E. Devine (Eds.), *Out of darkness: Exploring satanism and ritual abuse* (pp. 21–43). New York: Lexington Books.

Kluft, R. P. (1989). *Childhood antecedents of multiple personality*. Washington, DC: American Psychiatric Press.

Lanning, K. V. (1989). *Satanic, occult, ritualistic crime: A law enforcement perspective*. Quantico, VA: FBI Academy.

Lanning, K. V. (1992). A law-enforcement perspective on allegations of ritual abuse. In D. K. Sakheim & S. E. Devine (Eds.), *Out of darkness: Exploring satanism and ritual abuse* (pp. 109–146). New York: Lexington Books.

Mangen, R. (1992). Psychological testing and ritual abuse. In D. K. Sakheim & S. E. Devine (Eds.), *Out of darkness: Exploring satanism and ritual abuse* (pp. 147–173). New York: Lexington Books.

Marks, J. (1979). *The search for the "Manchurian Candidate": The CIA and mind control*. New York: Norton.

Masson, J. M. (1984). *The assault on truth: Freud's suppression of the seduction theory*. New York: Harper & Row.

McCann, I. L., & Pearlman, L. (1990). Vicarious traumatization: A contextual model for understanding the effects of trauma on helpers. *Journal of Traumatic Stress*, *3*(1), 131–149.

Morse, M., & Perry, P. (1990). *Closer to the light: Learning from the near death experiences of children*. New York: Ivy Books.

Mulhern, S. (1990, November). *Training courses and seminars on satanic ritual abuse: A critical review*. Paper presented at the Seventh International Conference on the Treatment of Multiple Personality and Dissociative Disorders, Chicago, IL.

Mulhern, S. (1991). *Satanism and psychotherapy: A rumor in search of an inquisition*. In J. T. Richardson, J. Best, & D. G. Bromley (Eds.), *The satanism scare* (pp. 145–172). New York: Aldine De Gruyter.

Noll, R. (1989). Satanism, UFO abductions, historians and clinicians: Those who do not remember the past. *Dissociation*, *2*, 251–253.

Orne, M. T. (1979). The use and misuse of hypnosis in court. *International Journal of Clinical and Experimental Hypnosis*, *27*, 311–341.

Putnam, F. W. (1989). *Diagnositc and treatment of multiple personality disorder*. New York: Guilford Press.

Raschke, C. (1990). *Painted black: Satanic crime in America*. San Francisco: Harper & Row.

Richardson, J. T., Best, J., & Bromley, D. G. (Eds.). (1991). *The satanism scare*. New York: Aldine De Gruyter.

Ring, K. (1984). *Heading toward omega: In search of the meaning of the near-death experience*. New York: Morrow.

Ritual Abuse Task Force. (1989). *Ritual abuse: Definitions, glossary, the use of mind control*. Los Angeles County Commission for Women. September 15.

Ross, C. A. (1989). *Multiple personality disorder: Diagnosis, clinical features, and treatment*. New York: Wiley.

Ryder, D. (1992). *Breaking the circle of satanic ritual abuse*. Minneapolis: CompCare Publishers.

Sakheim, D. K. (1993). Vicarious actualization: Therapist self-development through work with trauma survivors. *Raising Issue*, Winter.

Sakheim, D. K., & Devine, S. E. (1995). Trauma-related syndromes. In C. Ross & A. Pam (Eds.), *Pseudoscience in biological psychiatry: Blaming the body* (pp. 255–272). New York: Wiley.

Shefflin, A. (1993, October). Mind control and hypnosis. Paper presented at Daniel Brown & Associates Annual Seminars & Workshops on Psychotherapy & Hypnotherapy, Cambridge, MA.

Smith, M., & Pazder, L. (1980). *Michelle remembers*. New York: Pocket Books.

Stanek, L. (1993). *Satanic ritual abuse: Therapist's attitudes, beliefs and experiences*. Unpublished masters thesis.

Tamarkin, C. (1993, June). *Investigative issues in ritual abuse cases.* Paper presented at the Fifth Regional Conference on Abuse and Multiple Personality, Washington, DC.

Terry, M. (1987). *The ultimate evil.* New York: Doubleday.

Van Benschoten, S. C. (1990). Multiple personality disorder and satanic ritual abuse: The issue of credibility. *Dissociation, 3,* 22-30.

van der Kolk, B. A. & Greenberg, M. (1987). The psychobiology of the trauma response: Hyperarousal, constriction, and addiction to traumatic reexposure. In B. A. van der Kolk (Ed.), *Psychological Trauma* (pp. 63-87). Washington, DC: American Psychiatric Press.

Victor, J. (1989). A rumor-panic about a dangerous satanic cult in western New York. *New York Folklore, 15,* 22-49.

Victor, J. (1990). The spread of satanic cult rumors. *Skeptical Inquirer, 14,* 287-291.

Young, W. C., Sachs, R. G., Braun, B. G., & Watkins, R. T. (1991). Patients reporting ritual abuse in childhood: A clinical syndrome. Report of 37 cases. *Child Abuse and Neglect, 15,* 181-189.

28

Legal and Ethical Issues in the Treatment of Dissociative Disorders

George B. Greaves and George H. Faust

The whole of the legal matter as regards the status of dissociation and pathological dissociation is that it is more than nine parts lore and less than one part law.

There is abundantly more collective (and contradictory) lore than statutory or judicial law in regard to all aspects of the alleged "special status" that dissociative phenomena—ordinary or pathological in character—purportedly deserve.

As one famous psychiatrist in the field of multiple personality disorder (MPD, now called dissociative identity order, or DID) put it: "We all feel that we need to treat MPD patients in a "special" way, but no one can say exactly why."

Beginning with the publication of *Sybil* (Schreiber, 1973) and continuing with *The Minds of Billy Milligan* (Keyes, 1981), a mystique seemed to grow among many psychiatrists, psychologists, a few judges, some prosecuting attorneys, and a plethora of defense attorneys that individuals undisputedly suffering from dissociative identity and other dissociative disorders deserved special consideration under both the canons of psychiatric standards of care and the civil and criminal and administrative law.

"Special," under this way of looking at things, variously meant differential, preferential, exceptional, and even deferential consideration as to criminal sentencing, or exemplary-punitive rewards as plaintiffs in civil tort actions, or as complainants against therapists in administrative actions against therapists' licenses. It

George B. Greaves • 1175 LaVista Road, Apartment #205, Atlanta, Georgia 30324. **George H. Faust** • 2515 Kemper Place, Shaker Heights, Ohio 44120.

Handbook of Dissociation: Theoretical, Empirical, and Clinical Perspectives, edited by Larry K. Michelson and William J. Ray. Plenum Press, New York, 1996.

became the "uniquely crippled" defense cry in criminal cases and the "uniquely crippled" plaintiff's cry in civil cases.

By about 1985, virtually anybody who proclaimed himself or herself to be an "expert" in dissociative identity disorder could do so, even those who had never published on the subject in a major professional journal, and those who boasted that they had never read the collective scientific literature on the matter, "because it was too dreadfully awful to digest." Whether the "dreadfully awful part" was because of the lurid content of DID patients and their clinical reporters, or because the whole field was regarded as simply bad or trifling science, differed from instance to instance, and continues so to this day. Whatever the case, a prosecutorial mind grew up against the whole notion of dissociative identity as a clinical entity beginning in the mid-seventies and is now, however, grudgingly, relenting to the main clinical facts of MPD/DID (Goettman, Greaves, & Coons, 1994; Greaves, 1993).

The bottom line during the 1970s and 1980s concerning the more severe dissociative disorders was child abuse—not ordinary spanking, but severe child abuse and neglect. We in the forensic area knew the truth. Children locked in closets or bedrooms or chained inside houses for days or years at a time; skeletons of children concealed within walls. There is no reason to be lurid about it. We've been in many trials attempting to defend the child abuser, with no success. The evidence has been overwhelming against our clients. It is recently that criminal physical and negligence charges against children has been strenuously pressed in the courts, and the whole evidentiary matter is usually quick, straightforward, unambiguous, unarguable, and final.

The matter of alleged child sexual abuse is a significantly different matter. We absolutely know, from a forensic standpoint, that actual child sexual abuse of most heinous and unbelievable varieties—even to very young children—actually occurs, though it is beyond the ken of any normal man or woman either to even conceive of it and least of all to carry it out. We know it from the physical evidence, the directly correlated evidence of those confessing to particular details, and from direct and corroborated eyewitness reports other than the child victims themselves.

We also know that children lie outright about many things, distort actual events, confuse dreams and memories and wishes and fantasies, can be rather easily coerced to believe and elaborate on events which never happened, can act as stooges, and can confabulate quite freely about partial events. We utterly refute the ersatz notion that no child, willingly or by default of memory, would lie on the witness stand. We also know that some young children behave in highly sexually explicit ways. To complete the circle, we also know that children of no apparent sexual interests are sexually abused by other children and adults, that even young children may have quite explicit sexual fantasies and desires, and arising out of sexual guilt, may project that guilt onto adults. *The Children's Hour* and *The Sailor who Fell from Grace with the Sea* are exemplary portrayals of the latter phenomenon. Every hypothesis and observation about child sexual abuse is partially true:

1. It actually happens.
2. It is overreported.
3. It is underreported.
4. It is exaggerated in importance.

5. It is diminished in importance.
6. It is lied about.
7. It is covered up.
8. It is denied altogether as ever happening.

What is lacking in the process of the law is the someones who can systematically contrast (1) from (7), and who can convincingly compare and contrast the gradients within the list in matrix fashion.

We get a little closer to the legal tests of truth with child physical abuse because there are forensic indicators in physical as well as psychiatric forms. For all that, the medical and psychiatric politics from about 1960 to 1980, many physicians seemed to eschew the notion of "actual" child abuse. Neglect, maybe, yes, even probably, in some cases. The consensus seemed to be that such reports were vastly overinterpreted and overemphasized by other specialists, including pediatricians, psychiatrists, emergency room physicians, psychologists, clinical social workers, coroners, and others to the extent that it has become an "obsession"—meaning a neurosis—a shared "hysteria" among them. That was to miss the point entirely. It wasn't the reports of abuse that so startled the latter community, it was the direct medical and scientific evidence they were quite involuntarily collecting, publishing about and testifying to (Goodwin, 1985; Greaves, 1989).

Part of the denial of the actually existing, forensically documented cases of child abuse seems to be that psychiatrists and psychologists seem either not to like or not to appreciate scientific, legal, and psychiatric forensics; don't know about it; don't care to know about it; don't want to know anything about it; or don't want to be bothered by knowing anything about it.

But you can bet your last piece of toast on a miserably cold, child-starved day in medieval England, they're all crack experts on the subject once on the witness stand.

Against this backdrop came the American Psychiatric Association's long (both as to time and to size) struggles with producing the third edition of the *Diagnostic and Statistical Manual of Mental Disorders* (DSM-III; American Psychiatric Association, 1980), followed very quickly by a revised edition (DSM-III-R; APA, 1987). While many psychiatrists and clinical psychologists welcomed the new diagnostic work, a large number of well-established practitioners and psychiatry professors loathed it. They felt it was far too radical a departure from the second edition (DSM-II; APA, 1972), which had been the mainstay of psychiatric diagnosis for many years and whose nosology and nomenclature were the natural outcome of psychiatric evolution since the 19th century. They found DSM-III nosologically fractionated and some of its nomenclature and concepts if not actually spurious, certainly debatable. For purposes of this chapter, the grouping of the dissociative disorders was especially ill-received—and the notion of multiple personality disorder being singled out as *ein Ding an sich* as a diagnostic entity rankled many. Many simply dismissed it as an error of the APA nomenclature committees. When subordinate clinicians began to use the diagnosis, their diagnoses were changed. In some instances, the patients were removed from the care of the subordinates and the subordinates were chastised.

The American Psychological Association had, in turn, ventured out on its own grand vision which consumed some ten years of committee work. The purpose was to write the *sine qua non* of psychological ethics as concerned the practice of psychotherapy and related procedures. The new ethical principles and guidelines first appeared in December, 1991, and, like the reception of DSM-III, was anything but universally endorsed by the APA membership. Some vexing ambiguities in past codifications had been gratefully clarified. On the other hand, certain issues which formerly had been relatively clear now became frankly perplexing, especially in the area of dual relationships.

The boy who mows the neighbors' lawns, including the psychologist's, confides in the psychologist that his father is quite depressed after losing his job. If the father were willing, would the psychologist see him? The father follows through and the psychologist accepts him into treatment. Does the psychologist now have to terminate the boy's services in order to avoid a dual relationship with the father? A majority of psychologists in an advanced ethics training seminar soberly answered yes.

Dr. Thatcher is a lifelong Lutheran and attends St. Timothy's in Winslow. She belongs to the pastor's Sunday School class. A new patient moves to Winslow, who is also a Lutheran and also winds up at St. Timothy's and in the pastor's Sunday School class. What are Dr. Thatcher's ethical obligations regarding dual relationships in this situation? More than half the participants stated that Thatcher and her patient should not be in the same Sunday School class, as Dr. Thatcher's expressed religious view in the course of the dialectic of the class may well contaminate therapy. They also felt that they should sit at opposite ends of the church so that Dr. Thatcher's emotional responses to sermons and the liturgy would not show.

The "dual role" matters above are the analogue of an old psychoanalytic problem—quite honestly and seriously debated for years. An analyst sees his last patient of the day and leaves his office. There is a downpour outside as the analyst enters the parking lot. He sees his patient shuddering in the wind. The analyst has a hefty umbrella; the patient has none. Would it be too intimate a thing for the analyst to escort his or her patient to his or her (the patient's) car under the protection of his or her umbrella? Might this be misread as a sexual gesture? Or a gesture to the patient to be overdependent on the analyst? Shouldn't a good analyst just let the patient soak in the downpour, letting him or her know that he or she should take responsibility for him- or herself in the most rudimentary of situations, and to emphasize that the analyst has no real power over anything?

These examples are like straining at a gnat and swallowing the camel to a lawyer's mind. The Council of Nicea actually did a better job of canonizing the many ancient texts known to them which now comprise the Bible.

We have taken on the task and risk of writing this chapter as lawyers, historians, and serious scientific psychologists would look at it: very, very skeptically. The laws of Caesar change slowly.

THE FIRST MAJOR ETHICAL PROBLEM IN MPD: CORNELIA WILBUR AND SYBIL

The most important case recorded in the clinical archives of literature on multiple personality disorder is undoubtedly that of a woman whom Connie Wilbur called Sybil (Greaves, 1993). Frank Putnam, M.D., the National Institute of Mental Health's resident expert on dissociative disorders for many years, calls this case "essential reading" in the field of dissociative disorders (Putnam, 1989).

Flora Rheta Schreiber, the author of *Sybil*, was a professor of English on the faculty of a major school of law in Manhattan. She lived in Gramercy Park until her death some recent years ago. She met Cornelia Wilbur at a women's business group in New York City and the two struck up a spirited friendship, based on a mutual admiration of each other's expertise in their fields.

Wilbur, whose parents were both highly trained scientists, obtained advanced degrees in chemistry, medicine, and psychiatry. She had moved to Manhattan to obtain even more advanced training in psychoanalysis, training which in the 1950s and 1960s, and even today, is available in only a few major cities in the world.

She began to speak to Professor Schreiber of an unusual patient she had been working with for a number of years in Omaha, Nebraska, whom she described as having multiple personalities. Wilbur went on to say that there was no evidence that anyone had ever successfully treated such a condition, but that she felt she could, especially with her new, advanced training and her advanced skills in the knowledge and clinical use of hypnosis.

Wilbur went on to state that the patient had followed her to New York in order to continue treatment.

As Schreiber stated to Greaves in an extensive conversation (personal communication, Schreiber, 1983, paraphrased):

> I was fascinated by her [Dr. Wilbur's] description of Sybil. But when she asked me if I would like to write a book on the subject I replied: "How could I possibly write a book without an ending? She's [Sybil] still in treatment." It was when she persuaded me to meet Sybil that everything changed.

Everything did, indeed, change—in Sybil's life, in Schreiber's life, and in Wilbur's life.

Schreiber was enchanted with Sybil, who came to live with her over quite some course of time. Sybil eventually became well under Wilbur's care, after suffering many years of severe mental illness, and eventually relocated to New England to become art instructor in a small college. Wilbur and Schreiber became enormously famous. Sybil preferred to remain anonymous.

Largely as a result of her work with Sybil, Wilbur was promoted from her advanced New York training and psychoanalytic practice to become Chair of the Department of Psychiatry at the University of Kentucky Medical School in Lexington. She ultimately retired and died there, faithfully admired by a nationwide host of colleagues, most of whom eventually became members of the International Society for the Study of Multiple Personality and Dissociation, an organization founded by Greaves, one of her many followers (Greaves, 1993).

This would seem to add up to a happy ending. Such was not to be the case at all.

The treatment of Sybil occurred over a span of sixteen years. Wilbur went to heroic efforts to treat her. In believing the essential theme of the origins of Sybil's baffling illness—extremely cruel childhood sexual abuse—and her objective checking out of Sybil's accounts, Wilbur gained not only the reputation as a pioneer in the treatment of multiple personality disorder, but a pioneer in the discovery and confirmation of severe child sexual abuse as well.

But Wilbur could not obtain publication of her work with Sybil in mainstream psychiatric journals. Her offerings were repeatedly turned down by editors and reviewers. It was during this period of frustration that she turned to Flora Schreiber for help.

Thus began a series of ironies that persists to this day and continues well into the foreseeable future.

In the book *Sybil*, one reads the most important book about a psychiatrist and patient ever written, a book instructive to tens of thousands of multiple personality patients, their psychotherapists, and the public.

Schreiber's book hit the ground running, selling by now into the millions of copies range, considering its various paperback releases, and was turned into the award-winning four-hour television movie of the same name, starring Sally Field as Sybil and Joanne Woodward as Dr. Wilbur.

Such a book could only have been written by a third party to the proceedings, observing many of the proceedings, and from the unique vantage point of a journalist.

Certain members of the American Psychiatric Association viewed the publication of *Sybil* not with a joyful welcoming of a new day in psychiatry in which a rare and pernicious mental illness known for 150 years had finally been treated successfully by one of their own, but with outrage.

Whether or not Sybil had been cured or not was thrown to the winds. The main issues raised at the time were that:

1. Wilbur should never have allowed to be exposed in the popular press what had not previously been approved and published in scientific journals.
2. Wilbur was seriously "overly involved" with Sybil.

A huge outcry arose within the American Psychiatric Association for the expulsion of Dr. Wilbur from its ranks. Fortunately for science, Dr. Wilbur, and the crucial rediscovery of multiple personality, with all its attending implications in the 1970s and 1980s, the attempted expulsion of Dr. Wilbur was a fiasco.

When put to the vote, the psychiatrists involved in the matter could not agree among themselves what, exactly, "overinvolvement" with a patient would be, or where, exactly, the ethical rule was that one had to publish in a scientific journal before one could release results into the "public" press.

For all the folderol, hype, gossip, rumors, novels, movies, and judicious and injudicious decisions—at all levels of fantasy and the law and professional ethics and personal and journalistic speculation about dissociative disorders—they all owe their contemporary history to the two cases mentioned above: *Sybil* and *Milligan*. All else is footnotes to these guiding cases.

We exclude from our discussion *The Three Faces of Eve* case (Thigpen & Cleckley, 1957), because litigation issues surrounding it arose only much later and were primarily focused on copyright issues (Sizemore & Pittillo, 1977).

Judging Wilbur for ethics violations under present-day APA guidelines:

1. Making living arrangements with Flora Schreiber,
2. Seeing patient outside of office,

3. Traveling with patient to verify abuse,
4. Inadequate training to treat patient,
5. Failure to discharge patient when she was not getting better (16 years is a long treatment),
6. Dual relationships with patient (treating patient while a book was being written about her; becoming a traveling companion with the patient),
7. Numerous "boundary violations," and
8. Probable violations of confidentiality.

But these were the years 1956 to 1972.

Giving an organization a new code of ethics is like giving a child a new BB gun. The very first thing a father teaches a child about a new BB gun, beyond fundamental safety issues, is never to shoot a bird. Shoot a bird and the gun is gone.

Yet the "hallway hangings" of Connie Wilbur we have listened to at professional meetings over many years have been lifted totally out of context, and fraught with a most peculiar vindictiveness. There seems to be a perverse penchant for aiming the sights of the new weapon into the past—like a time traveler.

In these conversations, no distinction was drawn between the present and the past. In the past, Freud loaned or gave money to his patients. In the past Sandor Ferenczi, one of Freud's favorite disciples, either allowed or encouraged patients to sit on his lap and even kissed them, though Freud was disturbed upon learning about this. In the 1960s, hugging patients or students or strangers in "encounter groups" was highly recommended as a therapeutic means of contact, recognition, appreciation, confirmation, and grounding. Earlier in the century, analysts taking the month of August off for vacation were frequently followed or accompanied by an entourage of patients.

That these kinds of relationships with patients sometimes led to immediate or long-term misadventures between therapists and patients gave rise to a constant review of the interpersonal process between them. These systematic observations, in turn, gave rise over the course of many years' evolution to ethical guidelines based on trial and error: what works and doesn't work.

The essence of contemporary ethical guidelines in psychiatry, generically speaking, is that practitioners in a treating or advisory capacity have allegedly been schooled and trained in such a way that they have such vastly superior knowledge, skills, authority, and power, and that they could readily disadvantage a client were they to choose to do so out of malice or cunning, or they could innocently injure their clients out of neglect of the knowledge of the powers or applications of their learning. Ethical principles are therefore proscriptive and restrictive in nature: that is, they do not so much inform a professional practitioner about what to do, but about what not to do as regards a client.

That is as helpful as the beginning of the Hippocratic Oath: *prima non docere*. Very helpful. But no one ever asks how Hippocrates learned that.

THE FIRST MAJOR LEGAL PROBLEM IN MPD: BILLY MILLIGAN

Connie Wilbur ethically malpracticed in her treatment of Sybil? The lore and law of the time said no.

Billy Milligan was a criminal serial rapist? The lore of the time said no. Serial rapist? Undoubtedly yes. *Criminal* rapist? No.

The Milligan case is the most important and least studied of multiple personality cases in the modern lexicon of law. The so-called "Milligan defense" has, in our experience, been tried—both in concept and in court—more often than virtually all other versions of the "amnesia for criminal actions" defense.

First of all, the Milligan felony kidnapping-rape-armed robbery case never went to trial; therefore, it never generated either a jury-verdict opinion or appellate decision.

Second, virtually all courts, appellate courts, and juries trying similar cases have subsequently rejected Milligan-type defenses outright.

For all the dramatic reality of the Billy Milligan case, a popular myth persists in many attorneys' and mental health professionals' minds that Billy Milligan was acquitted for his three major multifelony crimes by a jury of his peers based on "not guilty by reason of insanity," commonly know as the NGBRI (NEEG-bree) plea, in the jargon.

None of these believers in the Milligan form of the NGBRI defense (meaning basically that one person cannot be held criminally liable for the independent and unsanctioned criminal actions of others—in the absence of a criminal collusion between the defendant and others—***even when the "others" happen to inhabit one's own body***), can precis the case correctly.

The history and background of the Milligan case is essentially thus:

During the early autumn of 1977, three young women were abducted from the Ohio State University campus at gunpoint, driven to nearby Delaware County in their own cars, raped, and subsequently robbed. One was an optometry student, the second was a nurse in the huge medical school complex, the third was a twenty-year-old student who has never been identified in the quasi-official public literature on the case beyond the pseudonym of Polly Newton.

Milligan's crime spree, ultimately resulting in numerous felony assaults, lasted perhaps thirteen days, ending with his arrest on or about October, 27, after midnight.

To understand what happened next, one has to understand the culture of Columbus, Ohio. Ohio is a very conservative state and one thing which Columbus, its capital, will not put up with is violence.

It not only had to put up with the Kent state rioting in which four completely unarmed students were needlessly and pathetically killed in May of 1970 by the Ohio National Guard (which was an army, after all, not a police force), but the pride of its enormous public university system—Ohio State—was forced to close during the student rioting following the Kent State tragedy.

It was the apex of civil protest against the Vietnam war, in the capital of the very state which, with Virginia, had produced significantly more than half the elected Presidents of the United States during more than half the nation's formative history. Ohio's version of the tally was: Ohio-8, Virginia-7.

To put the context of the matter somewhat more remotely, historians of the American Civil War would be hard put to find two nobler and greater adversaries than the State of Ohio and the Commonwealth of Virginia. General Lee of Virginia surrendered to General Grant of Ohio after General Sherman of Ohio "broke the back of the Confederacy" in his largely unopposed "march to the sea" from Atlanta to Savannah.

Ohioans never believed that they won the Civil War by themselves or that the Virginians lost it by themselves. But Ohioans believed that they were the phalanx of Union bravery just as Virginia lay at the heart of Confederate bravery.

This would be a gratuitous regression into history except for two things. Ohio came out of the Civil War rich, but sober, and contributed an amazing number of generals, statesmen, presidents, and the first human being to set foot on the moon. Ohio was high-tech to the *N*th degree in agriculture, engineering, education and manufacturing before the Civil War and continued to grow in civil law, social services development and administration, highway development, police science, aviation, communications science, medicine, research, publishing, high technology—you name it—well into the late twentieth century.

But the Kent State massacre virtually undid the state—a festered black eye for all the world to see—chilling Ohio's pride to its core. It had to make up for it in fairness. And Billy Milligan was one of the benefactors of its new moral awareness and campus safety.

By 1977, no one sidled onto the campus of Ohio State University—in whatever imaginable disguise and with whatever alibi—kidnapped young women from the campus between 7 a.m. and 8 a.m., and got very far for very long. The Ohio State University Police force is many times larger than most small town jurisdictions across the country, owing to the population density in the three or four square miles the campus itself encompasses, as well as the adjacent areas. For all that, there were no checkpoints, passports, or passes needed to obtain entry to any part of the campus, except, of course, course registration cards to enter certain training classrooms. It was all high-surveillance.

Given its virtually instant high technology, it took barely two weeks to catch Billy Milligan. Within the first week of his crimes he was labeled as "the campus rapist" around the world. Police artists drew ambiguous sketches of Milligan which appeared on the front pages and magazines everywhere. The closest we can come to in the present time is the vast lore and mystery of the "Unabomber," who has apparently committed his crimes over a period of 17 years.

Once Milligan was firmly established worldwide as the notorious "campus rapist" at Ohio State, all eyes were focused on Columbus to see what would happen next. What did happen was as far from the Kent State debacle as could be imagined, and was born of the strangest conceivable set of ironies.

George Greaves had arrived at the Ohio State campus in the summer of 1970, while the whole of the east side of North High Street across from the main campus was still a shambles—glass and the detritus of mob destruction everywhere, former businesses boarded up. After doing a year of post-doctoral training at the College of Medicine's department of psychiatry, he headed on to gather still more advanced training at the Kitchener-Waterloo Hospital in Ontario, Canada, where he accepted the directorship of the 24-hour psychiatric crisis clinic.

It was there, in January of 1972, that Greaves and his staff encountered their first unmistakable case of multiple personality, an individual they studied and cared for most attentively for a number of months.

In the meantime, Greaves's services were needed back in Columbus. At the invitation of Jim Gibson, executive director of the new Southwest Mental Health Center, Greaves agreed to assume the role of developer and director of the center's several outpatient programs. Included among these was the Southwest Forensic Center, which was contracted with Franklin County in Columbus to provide forensic evaluations for indigent prisoners suspected of suffering from mental disorders. With Greaves's concurrence, Gibson hired Dorothy Turner and Stella Karolin as the first two clinicians in the new program in early 1973.

Once the outpatient programs were up and operational, Greaves received an invitation from the University of California Medical Center in San Francisco as a research psychologist. UCSF was the virtual world's research headquarters for studies in the neurotransmitters, which Greaves saw as the psychiatric wave of the future. Here was yet another opportunity to sharply upgrade his psychiatric knowledge.

Yet half a year later, Ohio called him back: this time to develop and head his own tri-county mental health center, replete with hundreds of thousands of dollars of new facilities construction.

Greaves, who headed the new Gallia-Jackson-Meigs Mental Health Center, quickly made the acquaintance of David Caul, who headed the adjacent Athens-Vinton-Hocking Mental Health Center. They quickly discovered their mutual interest in MPD which, along with a sense of great mutual respect, formed the basis of an abiding friendship which lasted until Caul died in March, 1988, and led them through many adventures and heartaches. Caul was also a protege of Connie Wilbur, who had recently moved into the area, and began drawing Greaves into Wilbur's training seminars in 1975.

To begin to pull some of these peripatetics together as regards the Milligan case, we may begin with the irony that it was the Southwest Forensic Program that first recognized Billy Milligan as having multiple personality disorder, possibly the result of Greaves' sojourn in Canada and subsequent oral accounts of the condition.

The next remarkable event that happened in the Milligan case was that Judge Jay C. Flowers, the Common Pleas Court assigned to the case, sought his own special expert for advice on the case, once it appeared that Billy Milligan was likely a multiple. It was both the most conservative and wisest decision possible for a judge in terms of what was quickly shaping up as a unique legal case.

His selection for an advisor was neither a crony, nor *pro forma*. Instead he enlisted the consultation of a physician who was undisputedly the most respected psychiatrist in the state: George Harding, Jr. Harding came from a transgenerational family of psychiatrists, much like the Menningers in Kansas, and, as director of the Harding Hospital on Columbus' north side, he was in a position to be philanthropic in the service of justice. He undertook the diagnosis and treatment of Milligan, creating a special treatment team, and sought consultation with Drs. Caul and Wilbur.

Dr. Harding wrote an eloquent report detailing the reality of Milligan's clinical condition. This was backed up by depositional testimony by Drs. Wilbur, Caul, and Kaolin and by Ms. Turner. Mr. Yavitz, the Franklin County prosecutor, declined any attempt at prosecution in the face of such evidence. Judge Flowers ruled Mr. Milligan not guilty by reason of insanity (under *M'Naghten*) and the inability to refrain from his acts (under *Durham*).

The only thing now that remained was the disposition of the detainee.

David Caul was willing to treat Billy Milligan as an inpatient at the Athens Mental Health Center, with the concurrence of his state superiors.

Milligan prospered under the care of Drs. Harding and Caul and soon became so well that he was moved into what was called "transitional care." He was moved out of the hospital to live on his own recognizance nearby, with daily check-ins at the hospital. He rented a nearby farm with the extraordinary money he had been making from his extraordinary oil paintings. He contacted Daniel Keyes to write his side of the story of what had gone wrong, but Keyes would have nothing to do with anything of the sort. He was not a "ghost writer" or a "subwriter." Keyes was an honest-to-goodness "real writer." As such, he called the shots. And Milligan, who would otherwise have composed a completely self-serving work, was all the better for Keyes' objectively written work.

Then, suddenly, the bottom fell out.

David Caul was removed from the Milligan case abruptly, almost as soon as he had brought about an amelioration of Milligan's MPD disorder, though he was following Ohio State and Joint Commission for Accreditation of Hospitals treatment policy. The crucial policy was that as patients improved in their conditions, they should be transferred to the least restrictive environment consistent with their care.

Milligan is not what one would call your average good mental patient. He went AWOL on occasions. It is claimed that he was found drunk in a neighboring town and was in a fight past curfew hours and had no reason to be there anyway.

Months later, as Caul put the whole incident and many others to Greaves, described his whole treatment of Milligan, and pointed out on the Athens Mental Health Center campus exactly when and where Milligan got drunk on a pass or fled up this hill or that as a prank, he became gravely despondent. His eyes were red and he sniffed in the cold hilly air. He never quite bounced back from the Milligan case.

His heart was not so much sorrowed by Billy Milligan's ongoing teenage, sociopathic betrayals—Caul knew very well Milligan was a sociopath and was far too wise to commingle his heartstrings with those of his capricious patient—but by what he felt were the betrayals by his own kind. Psychiatrists and psychologists up to this time had been standing shoulder to shoulder with Caul, along with many defense attorneys and state attorneys and judges.

Now, given Milligan's deliberately annoying escapades, Caul began to be second-guessed. He was treating Billy too "special." He was overindulging him. He was "allowing him" to act out. Caul was perfectly willing and able to pull the reins in on Billy (and Milligan freely agrees with this), but he was never given the chance. Milligan was a political hot potato. He came to be regarded as a treatment failure under Caul and was removed from the Athens Mental Health Center altogether to the Dayton Forensic Center. From there he was transferred to the Lima State Hospital for the Criminally Insane. Finally, he was transferred to the new Timothy B. Moritz Correctional Center, a barbed wire compound on the grounds of Central State Hospital in Columbus.

The Cases Come In

While Milligan was being shifted from pillar to post, appellate decisions of the Milligan-type began to appear.

In *State v. Darnell* (1980, Oregon), in a flagrant case of male multiple personality, the jury found Darnell "responsible and guilty" of the murder of his father.

Kirkland v. State (1983, Georgia) became the classic case which still prevails. It was uncontested that the bank robber was psychiatrically ill from MPD. But under *M'Naghten*, whatever part of the consciousness of the person who committed the crime knew that he or she was committing a crime by way of objective evidence (e.g., elaborate plans for escape and evasion of capture).

In *State v. Rodrigues* (1984, Hawaii), the lower court judge ruled for acquittal in an MPD case. The state appealed and the higher court reversed the judge, stating "a defense of multiple personality syndrome (MPS) does not per se require a finding of acquittal."

In *State v. Brooks* (1986, Ohio), Ohio itself had a second look at the Milligan-type defense. The defendant was convicted on three counts of aggravated murder, but defense appealed on the basis that he suffered from amnesia. Despite that, and given that the defendant was mentally ill at the time, descriptions of his behavior at the times of the crimes made it perfectly clear to everyone that the murders were conscionably premeditated. *State v. Dillard* concurred (1986, Idaho) with *Rodrigues* the same year.

During 1988, *United States v. Davis*, 11 Cir., a federal appellate court cited Greaves in its findings that he would never attribute second-hand facts to his decisions about whether or not an individual person might or might not be suffering from multiple personality; and if that was even his clinical diagnosis, upon direct examination—that a certain person suffered from MPD—that did not, in itself, preclude a person from knowing what he or she was doing was criminally wrong (under *M'Naghten*).

Numerous other appellate cases have evolved regarding MPD/DID and the other dissociative disorders. The best annotated list is found in *Multiple Personality and Dissociation, 1791-1992: A Complete Bibliography* (Goettman, Greaves, Coons, 1994). Virtually all the criminal topics can be subsumed under two rubrics: 1) whatever personality or personalities commit a crime shall be subject to examination and adjudication, in full, on the M'Naghten rule; and 2) the existence of multiple personality disorder in an individual may be used as a mitigating diminished-capacity defense to avoid a sentence of death.

What Ever Happened to Billy Milligan?

In December of 1977, the director of the Franklin County Mental Health and Mental Retardation Board in Columbus called George Greaves at his office in Atlanta.

"We have certain problems with the Billy Milligan case," the director began forthright. "You come widely recommended as a person to serve as a consultant on this case and to conduct an evaluation of Mr. Milligan."

He went on to explain that they had had Milligan in the system for a decade now, but were not sure he belonged there or how to get him out. Ironically, Billy had served more time in mental health incarceration than he likely would have served doing straight time (a la *One Flew Over the Cuckoo's Nest*) and, well, there was another problem. Billy had become the prison "attorney." Making use of the prison library, he was filing lawsuits, motions, and briefs which were resulting in increasing mayhem in the Franklin County State and Common Pleas Courts.

After negotiating fees, parameters, expectations, and the like, Greaves agreed to evaluate Milligan during the first part of February, 1988, and to furnish a report.

In addition to his familiarity with Milligan through press reports, Keyes' book, and David Caul, Greaves spent four hours at the Moritz center poring through a large stack of hospital reports, the so-called official records. For the next four hours, he took Milligan through a far-ranging interview, specially designed to uncover remnants of dissociated personality elements. There were none. Milligan himself was a bright, engaging, likeable sort, with a keen sense of humor. Obviously, he was on his best behavior—but even good-natured people can grow testy after four hours of questions, some quite personal, out of the blue. But Milligan didn't flinch. The only time he became bitter was when he related how the state had seized the $350,000, which was his half of the profits from *The Minds of Billy Milligan*, to apply to his "treatment costs." It had taken a special act of the Ohio Legislature to do this. "One should not be able to capitalize from a crime" was the principle. Greaves knew that what he was telling him was true, because he had followed the whole matter through the national news. As he sat with Milligan, he couldn't help but wonder about the Watergate bunch.

Greaves phoned the director once he had returned to Atlanta and told him what he had found.

"Mr. Milligan does not have MPD which is the disorder which sparked his legal troubles, and I take it that he has not had it for some time. The records and my interview do not reflect that he has any present mental disorder, nor is he being treated for any; yet you have him incarcerated in a high-security mental facility. In my opinion he is being held unlawfully."

"You'll send me that in writing with a discharge plan, a transitional care plan, and a treatment/follow up plan?"

"Before the week is out."

"It's done then. Thank you. Send me your bill."

Within the month Milligan was a free man, with a new identity and a new job.

IT WAS NEVER ABOUT MULTIPLE PERSONALITY ANYWAY

When Faust and Greaves began their collaboration in 1984, both were fully aware that multiple personality was a faux appellation.

What concerned them from a forensic standpoint was they were by no means sure that psychiatrists, psychologists, social workers, and attorneys generally understood this. In fact, they heard dozens of persons speaking both in the parlors and from the podium as if different persons actually shared the same body. "Bad facts make bad law," we both said over and over, and for years we lived in rue of the day that some civil court would accept this impossible premise as a given and some appellate court would uphold it. Fortunately this never happened and now likely never will, thanks to DSM-IV nomenclature. But there was a run of some twenty years when some metaphysically handicapped practitioners were willing to put God's forswearance to the point.

Greaves was thoroughly trained in British analytic philosophy, as well as personality theory, and was fully aware of the absurdity of the notion of multiple personality. It was one of those unfortunately inherited psychiatric terms from the past, as misleading as hysterical conditions said to arise out of the involuntary wanderings of the uterus within a woman's pelvis, giving her the most frightening jitters and phantasms. No one really believed this nowadays—quite—though the fact remained that hysteria was still overwhelmingly a female family of psychiatric illnesses.

Of the score or so of civil and criminal MPD cases Greaves took on in the 1980s and early 1990s, as expert consultant, he was cautious with attorneys in helping them to understand that they were not dealing with different people in these clients, but with different aspects of a single person. For all that, he found attorneys separately deposing different "personalities," becoming frustrated when one or another personality refused to cooperate, or feeling at their wit's end when a particular personality refused to sign a release for legal documents.

Given the needless perplexities the terms "multiple personality" and "multiple personality disorder" were generating in all sorts of arenas, Greaves set out in 1990 to reconceive of and attempt to rename the related clinical disorders. He completed this project by 1993 and published his revisions in an American Psychiatric Press text, edited by Richard Kluft and Catherine Fine.

Greaves proffered two novel modifications to the clinical concept of MPD. First, instead of conceiving of MPD as a neurosis, as was the historical lore, Greaves conceived of MPD as an organized series of "recurrent episode psychoses." Secondly, he held that the hallmark of MPD was not that of multiple personality, but that of multiple identity process. He suggested the disorder be renamed *multiple identity disorder*.

A year later, when DSM-IV appeared, MPD had been changed to *dissociative identity disorder*. Whether this happenstance was a matter of parallel evolution, synchronicity, or the fact that Greaves's editor was a member of the Dissociative Disorders Committee for DSM-IV is of minor importance. The major importance is that for the first time in nearly 200 years a major, elusive mental illness was finely given a name descriptive of it.

It was actually Richard Kluft who said it best, quoting an unnamed colleague at Harvard:

> The problem with MPD is not that the person has too many personalities, but that they don't even have one functional one.

THE PARTICULAR HAZARDS IN TREATING DID PATIENTS

Numerous clinical authors have written about and catalogued the hazards of working with certain DID patients. On the one hand, the issue of physical violence has been stressed (e.g., Watkins & Watkins, 1984, 1988; Young, 1986). On the other hand the emotional viciousness of the DID patient toward the therapist has been stressed. The classical paper in this genre is that of Chris Comstock and Diane Vickery (1992), entitled "Therapist as Victim."

The active hatred of some patients toward their putatively neutral or nurturing therapist is by no means a new topic in psychotherapy. Freud was familiar with the transference phenomenon in which the therapist was projected to be *the bad object*.

But in the early days of treating multiple personality, as far back as Eve (Thigpen & Cleckley, 1967) and through most of the early 1980s, little was reported about the physically and emotionally violent proclivities of MPD patients. If anything, they were regarded as rather exemplary patients to work with from a relational standpoint.

Then Richard Horevitz and Bennett Braun (1984) began taking notice of the borderline personality features of many MPD patients, followed by George Ganaway (1989). Even Frank Putnam, in his 1989 classic, talks about frank sexual attacks by MPD patients (p. 192) and the proclivities for some patients to "bad mouth" their present and former therapists (p. 194). Putnam's counsel is to take all such reports with a grain of salt.

But by 1994, based both on survey and personal experience, the cat was out of the bag. We let them speak for themselves:

> Direct attacks, apart from verbal and physical assaultiveness to the therapist, have included unusual behavior such as leaving dead animals on the therapist's porch, poisoning and/or releasing of therapist's dogs, attacks on the therapist's possessions and/or person, and shooting guns in the therapist's office or home. More usual types of attacks have taken the form of filing frivolous or malicious lawsuits and reports to supervisors or Ethics Boards, harassing telephone calls, violating the therapist's space by refusing to leave, refusing to pay, and bringing guns or knives to the therapist's office.

We could supplement with our own direct knowledge a list of aggressions and transgressions: death threats to the therapist and family; threatened kidnapping of children; broken windows; slashed tires; egging and scratching of cars' surfaces; breaking, entering, and theft; telling other patients wildly-fabricated stories about therapy sessions; phoning therapists' parents with sordid details of sexual abominations in the therapist's office; actual stabbings and other unanticipated sudden injuries of therapists; numerous false and concocted late night crises (e.g., massive drug overdoses which never occurred); wholesale blackmail (e.g., "If you ever let on to a soul what I did last night, I'll march right down to the police station and holler rape at the top of my voice.").

How each and every of these types of crises is worked through therapeutically is of the gravest importance, and there is not the slightest doubt that to fail to recognize these gambits for what they are and to fully resolve each example can lead not only to an escalation of such crises, but to the most painful misadventures possible on everyone's part (Chu, 1988; Greaves, 1988).

But there is a glitch in all this, a glitch we will elaborate on at length below.

When a DID patient makes a *de nouveau* attack upon a therapist, there arises a general suspicion among fellow practitioners that the therapist has somehow made a therapeutic mistake or invited or provoked the attack. And the worse the attack, of course, the more grievous must have been the therapeutic error that caused it. Now, while it is all quite true that the failure to come to a complete understanding and resolution of the attack is a therapeutic error, it does not follow that the attack itself was provoked by therapeutic error. When a therapist is seeing a number of DID patients, a number of *de nouveau* attacks are possible, inflamed by contagion effects. Where there is smoke there must be fire. Now there is a therapist out of control.

The answer to this small riddle is quite simple. Therapists schooled in the nature and psychotherapeutic treatment of the neuroses simply do not believe in vicious, *de nouveau*, aggression. Neurotics simply do not behave that way unless some gross therapeutic error or series of errors has occurred, in which case such outbursts would be reactive in nature and not *de nouveau* at all.

Almost no one but psychoanalysts and a few psychiatrists are thoroughly schooled in the psychodynamics of pre-oedipal psychopathology, including its object inconstancy, splitting phenomena, narcissistic omnipotence, and ego-syntonic rage. Greaves had drawn these conclusions about MPD character structure as early as his 1980 "Mary Reynolds" paper, but it had either not been understood for what it implied or had not been taken seriously.

The point to be made is that in dealing with pre-oedipal character pathology, unprovoked rage is the norm in the therapy situation, not the exception. Unsuspecting therapists working with DID patients were completely taken aback by this—and sometimes emotionally quite injured—while their equally unsuspecting colleagues began to suspect they were working with Job.

It is considered to be the therapist's responsibility to set and maintain the therapeutic boundaries in therapy. Yet as has correctly been observed, the internal boundary chaos of DID patients, due to their nearly boundaryless upbringing, have poor external boundary control because of their impoverished internal boundaries. Boundary establishment on the part of the therapist is thus felt to be an important corrective element of the treatment in and of itself.

But some DID patients, i.e., those with severe underlying pre-oedipal character disorders, will agree to any boundary, and adhere to none. When such acting out against boundaries is limited to noncompliance with therapy, termination of therapy may well be warranted, though some therapists, wisely or unwisely, are willing to tolerate quite wide degrees, or "exceptions," to noncompliance. But when the acting out takes the form of criminal behavior, there may be no remedy short of arrest and criminal action. One therapist we have followed was so severely put upon by his patient in such an obsessive and aggressive way, that he was able to obtain a permanent Superior Court injunction barring the patient from any further contact by any means whatever, direct or indirect.

Except for examples as extreme as the last, it is not commonly said that the patient trashed boundaries, or refused to honor boundaries, or violated boundaries, or repeatedly crossed boundaries, or the many other permutations of the concept. What is most commonly said is that the therapist did not hold or enforce boundaries. By way of example, one of Greaves' patients eloped from her day care program by driving her car to another state and by remaining secluded in the mountains at a motel for several days.

The question put to Greaves was not why this errant event had taken place, but why he had let her do it.

A therapist's purely conceptional and fictional omnipotence in maintaining the therapeutic framework is no match whatever for a patient's real rageful, infantile omnipotence. People tend to forget that outpatients, in particular, are free to exercise the full range of their civil rights.

The Worst Nightmare of All

In this last section on the law and ethics as pertaining to the dissociative disorders, we are going to take the reader through some totally unfamiliar territory—through a chamber of horrors as it were. Yet it exists. We've followed these cases firsthand from our vantage point as members of the Legal and Ethics Committee for the International Society for the Study of Dissociation for several years (Faust was cochair), until the Committee was disbanded. In the meantime we verified Comstock and Vickery's suspicions quite thoroughly. During one sixteen-month period we became aware of 86 lawsuits, licensing board actions, and other administrative actions lodged against those treating DID patients.

Paul Dell was not the first to notice, but was the first to systematically study the other side of the equation: not the patients' hostilities toward their therapists, but colleagues' hostilities toward MPD therapists (Dell, 1988, 1988a). The papers were both riveting and sad commentaries on the sociological aspects of scientific discovery toward the end of the century.

As in the cases of *Sybil* and *Milligan*, however, a couple of paradigm cases and a couple of spinoff cases are wholly adequate to make our point.

Over the years, quite out of idle curiosity, we have asked a wide variety of people upon what, historically, the American legal system is based. Nearly always we receive the answer: the English Common Law.

This is quite a remarkable notion given that until very recently virtually every county and state court house, and every state capitol, and most all civic buildings and post offices were built in Romanesque architecture. Virtually all technical legal terms are in Latin. The American legal heritage, like the English legal heritage is Roman through and through. It is based on statutory and judicial law, much of it unchanged for more than 2,000 years.

Physicians, psychiatrists, psychologists, social workers, and others seem to quake at the day they may be called to court to answer a lawsuit.

In point of fact, to be sued in Caesar's court is the finest place on earth to be sued. The reason is quite simple. First of all, if one is a practitioner, one has insurance to cover lawyers' fees for the litigation. Secondly, there are strict rules of procedure which assure that the adversarial game is played fairly, with all the cards on the table. The orderly process of the discovery of relevant evidence, and its sharing with both sides, mitigates against ambush. Rules of evidence mitigate against gossip, hearsay, innuendo, and past reputation being considered in the present dispute. Since the entire case is laid out in advance of the trial, there normally is no trial. The judge and attorneys can read the matrix which is often quite clear on one side or the other. Agreements are made, and assuming the judge concurs, the matter is settled and put permanently to rest.

Try this matter by contrast:

Dr. Jones is visited, by appointment, by the State Board of Licensing Examiners whereupon it is revealed that a complaint against him has been lodged on behalf of Ms. J. Smith. He is informed that the identity of the complainant or group of complainants is confidential. He is also told that he will not be permitted to read any portion of the complaint, nor any paraphrasing of the complaint, nor will he be furnished with any bill of particulars until the time of any hearing which may come about. He is asked a few perfunctory questions and told that he may proffer an affidavit in the matter. This he does, on advice of counsel, though the affidavit is, by necessity, general in nature.

Six months later, the same thing happens. This time it is in regard to a Ms. Thomas. Another six months goes by with no word or action. Friends call the board to see if Jones is under investigation. One friend calls the President of the Board, and is told that Jones has not been and is not being investigated.

Nearly a year later, Jones is summoned to meet with the Board to answer charges of sexual misconduct and "such other concerns as the Board may wish to address."

Attorneys are employed. They are told that they have 10 days in which to conduct discovery, though the board has been conducting discovery in secret for two years. A prosecution list of 21 witnesses is presented, about a third without any identifying information, addresses, or phone numbers. Only one witness has waived her confidentiality privilege, but she refuses to testify at the hearing if Jones is present. The hearing officer allows full television presence throughout the hearings, subject to several provisions: (1) the witnesses would have their faces blocked out; (2) their hands would not be photographed; (3) they would all be given aliases; (4) Jones could be photographed in full at any time; and (5) the television station would be given full editorial discretion over whatever it chose to broadcast. The defense team puts forth 21 motions pertaining to due process in the hearings, and all were denied. The prosecution's chief expert witness states that the keystone case should not be included in the hearings for *ex post facto* reasons. The witness who has declined to face Jones on the witness stand has her current therapist testify in her behalf—a complete hearsay testimony over the strenuous objections of the defense. A second expert witness for the state admits that while Jones has done nothing technically wrong regarding the main charge, that he nevertheless feels that Jones has behaved unethically, because the Ethical Code is too liberal in that regard. When confronted by the defense that his views are in a small minority and do not reflect the will or tenor of the American Psychological Association, he freely recognizes that fact, but still feels he is right and the majority is wrong.

Jones was being vilified by both these "make up the rules as you go" procedures and by the local TV channel in "investigative" news the week before the hearings. Jones and his attorneys had no choice but to pull the plug, as the stress was beginning to take a toll on Jones' physical health as well. Jones' professional liability insurance had no provision for attorneys' fees in administrative actions, and with procedures varying so extremely from normal civil procedures, his legal fees were mounting rapidly. False, collusory charges; no viable defense.

Jones and his attorneys entered into a consent agreement to revoke his license with no finding of guilt or innocence. Jones lost his means of livelihood, his home, his solvency, and his retirement, and was forced into bankruptcy.

There is a interesting aftermath to the story, however. Every subsequent lawsuit arising from this fiasco fizzled in Caesar's court. And it did not cost Dr. Jones a dime to be tried in a *civil* court. One very short story more and we will have proved our point.

Dr. Jane did not trust Ms. Betsy's father because of his reputation as a tyrant. She decided that it would be safest if she tape-recorded every therapy session between them to which Ms. Betsy agreed. About a year later, Ms. Betsy's father got it in his head that Dr. Jane and his daughter were conspiring against him and that he was going to teach Dr. Jane a lesson. Given the vagaries of the situation, he knew that the law could not help him, but he was advised that the State Board of Psychology could get to the bottom of things and it wouldn't cost him a dime.

Dr. Jane hired Greaves as a consultant. The Board had ordered her to turn over all her therapy records in written form. Her taping had thus backfired, as it cost her nearly $5,000 to have the transcripts made within the time frame allowed her by the Board.

Greaves was able to obtain, in this case, a copy of the letter of complaint, as in that state jurisdiction, complainees were furnished with those details.

Quite innocently, believing the Board to be the psychologist's friend, Dr. Jane had been corresponding freely with the Board with no idea of the implications of doing so. It cost another $5,000 in attorney's fees just to get negotiations on track. She had no clue that Ms. Betsy's father was out to kill her license and career.

Then came the matter of Greaves's piecing together a multi-page rambling complaint against several hundred pages of transcript. As it turned out, Greaves was able find copious examples within the transcripts which were diametrically opposite to the father's contentions, but it required dozens of tedious hours and thousands of more dollars by the time Greaves finished his lengthy report to the State Board. The point is not in the least subtle, though it is grim. Hundreds of people with both honorable and evil intentions are learning to use the free services of the State Boards of Licensure for both corrective and nefarious purposes.

RECOMMENDATIONS

We have come full circle in this chapter, from how law and ethics affect DD patients to how they affect DD practitioners.

The past ten years make no bones of the fact that concentrating in the treatment of DID patients is a high-risk enterprise, no matter how earnest, able, trained, or honest a practitioner may be.

It is in the nature of kangaroo courts that by their very nature they are meant to be expeditious, not fair. They are meant to make a quick end to some real or perceived trouble forthwith and are based on power plays, not equanimity. Yet this is precisely where practitioners are at highest risk. Lose a lawsuit, you lose money, perhaps some degree of reputation. Lose your license and it is catastrophic to all of a purely material nature one has built, as well as having to shelve years of finely honed skills.

1. The first change we would make in the status quo is to include in professional liability policies provisions for legal coverage for administrative hearings, at minimum State Licensing Board proceedings. Given the antipsychotherapy and

hate groups we have seen organized within the past decade, it is no longer possible to believe that licensed professionals and professional boards are not being systematically abused.

2. Secondly, we would add an entire new section to the APA Code of Ethics having to do with psychologists serving in adjudicative roles. Among issues addressed should be the following:

a. No psychologist will serve in an adjudicative capacity in any forum in which a colleague is denied right of counsel.

b. No psychologist will serve in an adjudicative capacity in which there is unequal due process in terms of evidentiary discovery and sharing.

c. No psychologist will serve in an adjudicative capacity in which a full bill of particulars is not amply served upon a colleague.

d. No psychologist will serve in an adjudicative capacity in areas esoteric to his or her field of training in the absence of an acknowledged expert defense witness.

e. No psychologist will serve in an adjudicative capacity who holds "nullification views" towards relevant portions of the Code of Ethics under which his colleague is being tried.

f. Every psychologist serving in an adjudicatory role will remain cognizant at all times of time frames of alleged unethical behavior, and will in no case apply superseding standards in an *ex post facto* manner.

3. Thirdly, we maintain that all actions against professional licenses be mandated to conform to the rules of the uniform civil code for the state; preferably that actions against professional licenses be handled as matters of personal chattel and assigned to the jurisdiction of Superior or Common Pleas Courts.

REFERENCES

American Psychiatric Association (1972). *Diagnostic and statistical manual of mental disorders* (2nd ed.). Washington, DC: Author.

American Psychiatric Association (1980). *Diagnostic and statistical manual of mental disorders* (3rd ed.). Washington, DC: Author.

American Psychiatric Association (1987). *Diagnostic and statistical manual of mental disorders* (3rd ed., rev.). Washington, DC: Author.

American Psychiatric Association (1994). *Diagnostic and statistical manual of mental disorders* (4th ed.). Washington, DC: Author.

Chu, J. A. (1988). Ten traps for therapists in the treatment of trauma survivors. *Dissociation, 1*, 24-32.

Comstock, C., & Vickery, D. (1992). The therapist as victim: A preliminary discussion. *Dissociation, 5*, 155-158.

Dell, P. F. (1988a). Professional skepticism about multiple personality. *Journal of Nervous and Mental Disease, 176*, 528-531.

Dell, P. F. (1988b). Not reasonable skepticism, but extreme skepticism: A reply. *Journal of Nervous and Mental Disease, 176*, 537-538.

Ganaway, G. K. (1989). Establishing safety and stability within an inpatient milieu. *Trauma and Recovery, 2*, 2-5.

Goettman, C., Greaves, G., & Coons, P. (1994). *Multiple personality and dissociation, 1791-1992: A complete bibliography* (2nd ed.). Lutherville, MD: Sidran Press.

Goodwin, J. (1985). Credibility problems in multiple personality and abused children. In R. Kluft (Ed.), *Childhood antecedents of multiple personality* (pp. 1-19). Washington, DC: American Psychiatric Press.

Greaves, G. (1980). Multiple personality: 165 years after Mary Reynolds. *Journal of Nervous and Mental Disease*, *168*, 577-596.

Greaves, G. (1988). Common errors in the treatment of multiple personality. *Dissociation*, *1*, 61-66.

Greaves, G. (1989). Observations on the claim of iatrogenesis in the promulgation of MPD: A discussion. *Dissociation*, *2*, 99-104.

Greaves, G. (1993). A history of multiple personality disorder. n R. P. Kluft & C. G. Fine (Eds.), *Clinical perspectives on multiple personality disorder* (pp. 355-380). Washington, DC: American Psychiatric Press.

Horevitz, R. P., & Braun, B. G. (1984). Are multiple personalities borderline? An analysis of 33 cases. *Psychiatric Clinics of North America*, 7, 69-88.

Keyes, D. (1981). *The minds of Billy Milligan*. New York: Random House.

Kirkland v. State, 304 S.E.2d 561 (Ga. App. 1983).

Putnam, F. (1989). *Diagnosis and treatment of multiple personality disorder*. New York: Guilford.

Schreiber, F. R. (1973). *Sybil*. Chicago: Henry Regnery Company.

Schreiber, F. R. (1983). Personal communication.

Sizemore, C., & Pittillo, E. (1977). *I'm Eve*. Garden City, NY: Doubleday & Company.

State v. Brooks, 495 N.E.2d 407 (Ohio 1986).

State v. Darnell, 614 P.2d 120 (Oregon App. 1980).

State v. Dillard, 718 P.2d 1272 (Idaho App. 1986).

State v. Rodrigues, 679 P.2d 615 (Hawaii 1984).

Thigpen, C. H., & Cleckley, H. (1957). *The three faces of Eve*. New York: McGraw-Hill.

United States v. Davis, 835 F.2d 274 (11th Cir. 1988).

Watkins, J. G., & Watkins, H. H. (1984). Hazards to the therapist in the treatment of multiple personalities. *Psychiatric Clinics of North America*, 7, 111-119.

Watkins, J. G., & Watkins, H. H. (1988). The management of malevolent ego states in multiple personality disorder. *Dissociation*, *1*, 67-72.

Young, W. C. (1986). Restraints in the treatment of a patient with multiple personality disorder. *American Journal of Psychotherapy*, *50*, 601-606.

Index

Printed in the United Kingdom
by Lightning Source UK Ltd.
120527UK00005B/9